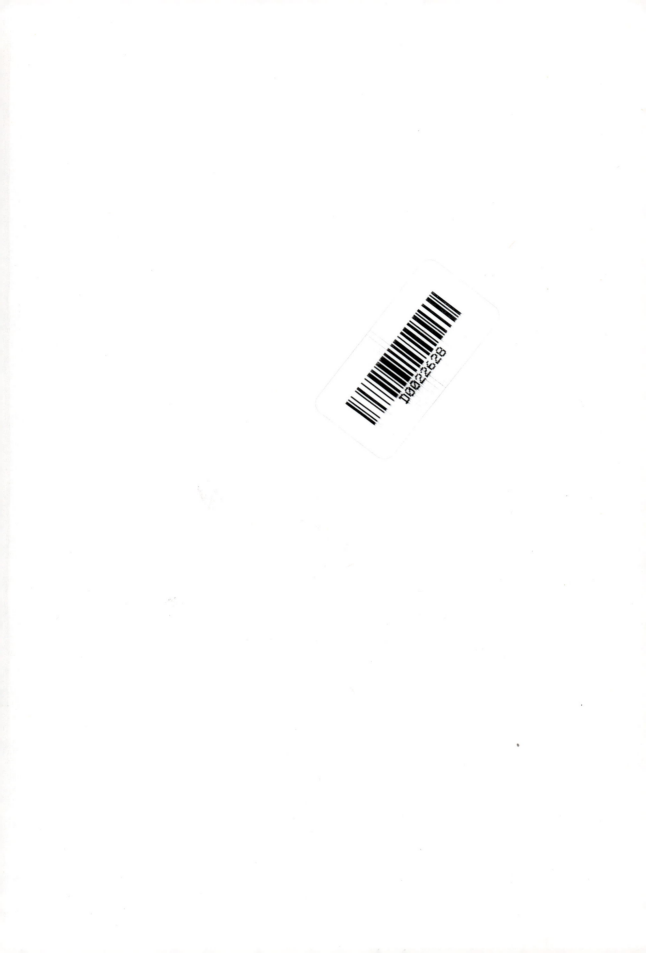

REHABILITATION OF THE ADULT AND CHILD WITH TRAUMATIC BRAIN INJURY

Second Edition

REHABILITATION OF THE ADULT AND CHILD WITH TRAUMATIC BRAIN INJURY

Second Edition

Mitchell Rosenthal, Ph.D.
Director of Psychological Medicine
Marianjoy Rehabilitation Center
Wheaton, Illinois
Associate Professor of Psychology and
    Physical Medicine and Rehabilitation
Rush Medical College
Chicago, Illinois

Ernest R. Griffith, M.D.
Co-ordinating Editor
Professor and Head
Department of Physical Medicine and
    Rehabilitation
University of Illinois at Chicago College of
    Medicine
Chicago, Illinois

**Michael R. Bond, M.D., Ph.D., FRCS,
    MRC Psych., MRCP, DPM**
Professor and Chairman
Department of Psychological Medicine
University of Glasgow
Scotland, United Kingdom

**J. Douglas Miller, M.D., Ph.D.,
    FRCSE, FRCPSG, FACS, FRCPE**
Professor of Surgical Neurology
Chairman, Department of Clinical
    Neurosciences
University of Edinburgh
Consultant Neurosurgeon
Western General Hospital
Astley Ainslie Hospital
Royal Infirmary of Edinburgh
Scotland, United Kingdom

Foreword by Bryan Jennett

 F. A. DAVIS COMPANY • Philadelphia

Printed in the United States of America

Last digit indicates print number: 10 9 8 7 6 5 4 3 2

Library of Congress Cataloging-in-Publication Data

Rehabilitation of the adult and child with traumatic brain injury / [edited by] Mitchell
    Rosenthal ... [et al.].—Ed. 2.
        p.   cm.
    Rev. ed. of: Rehabilitation of the head injured adult. c1983.
    Includes bibliographies and index.
    ISBN 0-8036-7626-3
    1. Brain—Wounds and injuries—Patients—Rehabilitation. 2. Brain—dam-
aged children—Rehabilitation. I. Rosenthal, Mitchell, 1949–
II. Rehabilitation of the head injured adult.
    [DNLM: 1. Brain Injuries—rehabilitation. 2. Head Injuries—rehabilita-
tion.   WE 706 R3445]
    RD594.R44   1989
    617.5′1044—dc20
    DNLM/DLC
    for Library of Congress   89-7929
                                                                         CIP

For our patients with brain injury and their families. They have taught and inspired us more than they can know.

FOREWORD

Although head injuries are ten times more frequent than spinal injuries, there is much less chance that the victim of head injury will be fortunate enough to find a coherent and expertly conceived rehabilitation program. The problems of paraplegia are fairly stereotyped and well understood, with well-tried schemes of management available for most of them. The disabilities caused by head injury are more complex and varied, but this is seldom fully recognized. Even when the disabilities are well analyzed and adequately diagnosed, their management is often difficult. The main reason for this is that mental deficits dominate, and these deficits interfere both with the patient's ability to cope and with his capacity for cooperation with those trying to help him. No wonder the therapists who are not sensitive to the subtleties of brain damage often tend to reject head-injured patients; even families and friends can find them a trial. The aggressive muscular approach that so often pays off with paraplegic or orthopedic patients is doomed to failure with most head injuries. Yet many patients make a good recovery, whereas others can be taught to cope with their altered selves and to make a new life by capitalizing on their remaining assets. Head-injured patients therefore present a challenge, responding to which can prove most rewarding for those therapists who are prepared to make the effort.

There is a welcome awakening in the therapeutic community on both sides of the Atlantic to the needs of the head-injured patient. Courses on this topic have been consistently over-subscribed, and by a broad spectrum of disciplines—physicians, nurses, neuropsychologists, and social workers, as well as those more conventionally associated with rehabilitation.

This book is for all of the health-care professionals interested in rehabilitating head-injured patients. It endeavors to explain the many facets of head injury in the acute and late stages, with a view to improving understanding of how to plan both rehabilitation and studies in rehabilitation. The latter are needed not only so that new techniques can be devised and tested, but also so that methods already in use can be re-examined with a view to discarding those found to be ineffective. In the call for more rehabilitation, however, there is a need to resist the temptation to indulge in action for its own sake, or to accept as self-evident that more rehabilitation must always mean more benefit for patients. Rehabilitation depends on the intensive use of that scarcest of all resources—skilled personnel. We should therefore seek to deploy such skills in an appropriate manner, that is, in circumstances in which they are both necessary and effective. Only in that way will patients and society benefit most from our efforts.

Bryan Jennett, M.D., FRCS
University of Glasgow,
Glasgow, Scotland, United Kingdom

PREFACE TO THE SECOND EDITION

Why publish a second edition of our textbook on rehabilitation of the head-injured adult? And why expand the scope of the book to include pediatric aspects? Dr. Rosenthal's preface to the first edition merits rereading as an introduction to the answers to these questions. Our first book was a response to a long-identified need for a current state-of-the-art text on the subject. The awakening of a professional and public consciousness to the presence of a "silent epidemic" has become a dramatic reality in the 6 years since our first publication. That former silent epidemic is now an audible, visible, and palpable epidemic. A number of textbooks relating to rehabilitation of the head-injured patient have appeared, with notable emphasis on psychosocial aspects. Two books on pediatric head trauma have been published. However, no single work encompassing the spectrum of disabilities resulting from brain injury in adults and children has been assembled—until now.

Meanwhile a worldwide quest continues for enhanced knowledge and skills of rehabilitation and related professionals in this discipline. The genesis of an international head trauma society, the appearance of two scientific journals devoted exclusively to brain injury, continuing productivity of educational seminars throughout the United States and in other countries attest the mounting attention that is accorded the topic. Specialization of brain injury rehabilitation is expanding with the development of national systems of care, and increasing numbers of head trauma units within hospitals, rehabilitation centers, and other facilities. Other forms of rehabilitation programs proliferate, ranging from those within intensive care units to community-based educational, vocational, behavioral, residential, and respite programs. Training fellowships for physicians and other rehabilitation professionals are increasingly available.

The National Head Injury Foundation (NHIF) has become a potent and articulate voice in patient and family advocacy, dissemination of information, and reformation of legislative and public policy[1]. The National Institute of Disability and Rehabilitation Research (formerly NIHR) has designated head injury as a priority area of research. A federal interagency agreement has been concluded in order to promote coordinated research and training. Standards of care for rehabilitation of traumatic brain-injured patients have been adopted by the Commission on the Accreditation of Rehabilitation Facilities (CARF). A Special Education Task Force has produced a manual for educators. In addition, NHIF has promulgated the development of revised disability criteria by the Social

Security Disability Insurance Administration, thereby allowing more equitable assessment of brain injury clients. The Foundation has provided evidence to third-party payers of the urgency of funding post-acute rehabilitation services.

The Head Injury Task Force has assumed an influential and productive role as a national organization of concerned educational, research, and care provider professionals. The standards of care for head injury adopted by CARF were generated by this body. It has developed close liaisons with NHIF, the American Congress of Rehabilitation Medicine, and other organizations concerned with head injury. The Task Force has focused on such subjects as innovations in service delivery, coordination of educational and research activities, and dissemination of information and resources among professionals. The Head Injury Special Interest Group of the American Academy of Physical Medicine and Rehabilitation is an organization of concerned physiatrists. This body has produced major academic courses at the Academy annual scientific meetings. It is currently addressing academic issues including standards of training and education in head injury for residents and fellows, and research priorities.

Here, then, are some instances of the accelerating interest and activity engendered by this provocative field. The spirit of inquiry, of exchange of information, of advancing expertise proceeds unabatedly; what has been more art is evolving into an applied science, with many questions yet to be answered.

How will this book compare and contrast with its predecessor? In response to constructive criticisms of the first edition, we have attempted to rectify omissions, upgrade information, and delete material that seemed unessential. Hence, several chapters have been omitted, a number added, surviving chapters extensively rewritten, and a section on pediatric head injury appended. Our authors include many who contributed to the first edition and a host of new contributors, experienced and knowledgeable in the discipline. We have sought to retain the essence of the first book: a resource of practical information to aid clinicians and students who work with the brain injured in all of the health care and related professions.

The original editorial team remains intact. My colleagues, Drs. Rosenthal, Bond, and Miller have adhered to the core of our mission: to provide a book of quality and practicality that will compare favorably with the original. The expansive presence of the Atlantic Ocean notwithstanding, we have communicated closely and harmoniously throughout the preparation. I salute each of these scholars and friends for his estimable work as author and editor. My grateful appreciation extends to each of the contributing authors for his or her thoughtful, enthusiastic participation. Once again, we have enjoyed a fully supportive relationship with F.A. Davis Company, particularly with Jean-François Vilain, Senior Editor. To Brenda Thomas, my secretary: profound thanks for your devoted efforts. To my wife, Anna and children, Ann, Jean Ellen, Drew, and Wesley: Bless you for your steadfast love and support. And to you, the reader, our ultimate gratitude: for the study and application of the contents of this book for the benefit of your patients and their families.

Ernest R. Griffith

Reference

1. Rosenthal, M, and Berrol, S: From the editors. J Head Trauma Rehabil 2(1):viii, 1987.

PREFACE TO THE FIRST EDITION

For the victim, family member, and health-care professional, head injury has always been something of a "puzzle." The event creating the injury occurs suddenly without warning. From that instant, the course of medical and rehabilitative management proceeds, but ultimately may not resolve the nagging questions posed by family members: "Will he ever be the same person again?" "What kind of life can he have now that he is brain-damaged?" Head injury often strikes persons within the prime of their lives—aged 16 to 35 years. Often, these victims are, at the time of injury, in the midst of carving out social, vocational, and economic patterns that typically last a lifetime. Yet, in the case of severe head injury, all of this has changed—often permanently. Within the past few decades, the advances in neurosurgical diagnostic and management techniques have enabled many persons to survive the immediate consequences of the injury. However, this newly head-injured person and the family are then faced with the difficulties inherent in continued survival and the challenge of regaining a measure of productivity and happiness.

Those professionals concerned with rehabilitation have only recently truly awakened to the plight of head-injured persons. That is not to say that head-injured persons have not received rehabilitative services for the past 30 years. Instead, I would suggest that the impression of "irreversibility of damage to brain tissue" has led many to behave as if rehabilitation efforts were rarely successful in restoring the person to a meaningful, productive existence. The public has also been frightened by head injury, perhaps because of its close association with the concept of brain damage, which has often incorrectly been equated with "mentally retarded," "emotionally disturbed," "physically crippled," and the like. Though the process of neural reconstitution and recovery from head injury is still not fully understood, those practicing within the medical and allied health community appear to be more hopeful about the future prospects of head-injured patients.

The "puzzle" of head injury is partly attributable to the extraordinary array of physical and mental sequelae of the injury, and the lack of adequate, scientifically based methods of treating these deficits in a systematic, effective manner. The fact that no two head injuries result in the exact same sequelae precludes broad generalizations for rehabilitation management and necessitates individualized treatment programs. In the not-so-distant past, many well-meaning practitioners equated head injury with stroke and dealt with these t-

populations in a similar manner. However, the research and clinical experiences gained in the past decade have highlighted the important differences in the initial neurologic insult and eventual residual deficits. One such finding—namely, that head injury usually results in diffuse brain damage, while stroke often is focal and unilateral in its locus—has helped to explain the greater variety of physical and mental deficits following head injury. For example, a stroke patient with a right brain insult may experience motor paralysis on the left side, spatial disorientation, dysarthria, and emotional lability. In contrast, a closed head injury impacting on the right hemisphere may cause a "contre-coup" effect, which may result in diffuse damage. The manifestations of this injury could include bilateral motor weakness, subtle language deficits, post-traumatic amnesia, motor slowing, impaired perception, emotional blunting, altered sensation, and so forth. In addition, the head-injured victim often sustains associated injuries, which may include leg fractures, spinal cord injury, and facial lacerations.

The sum total of head injury may often be the temporary or permanent displacement of the victim and family. The victim may struggle for many years to accept and understand what has really happened. Life can become a series of frustrations and obstacles that often lead to exasperating failures. Head-injured persons return to the community to find that previous friendships and rewarding activities have been greatly restricted. After the euphoria accompanying discharge from the hospital subsides, relationships with spouse, family members, and significant others become strained. Economic hardship becomes a new reality. Some head-injured persons describe their houses as "feeling like a prison." A fight for emotional, social, and economic independence is likely to be a long, painful one.

The initial impetus for the writing of this text comes from our collective involvement in the Annual Post-Graduate Course on the Rehabilitation of the Brain Injured Adult, sponsored by the Medical College of Virginia. When initiated in 1977, no other annual course on head injury was ongoing in the United States. The first program was planned with the hope that 50 to 100 rehabilitation professionals would attend. More than 250 applications were received for that course. By 1981, at least 10 major hospitals had initiated annual courses in head injury, involving more than 2000 health-care professionals per year. Clearly, the compelling nature of the topic has been established. No fewer than 30 hospitals and rehabilitation centers have opened specialized head-injury units within the past 5 years.

A second motivating force for producing this book has been the dearth of previous texts or articles directed toward educating the rehabilitation professional about head injury. The last book of this type was published in 1969. Drs. Walker and Caveness edited a book entitled *The Late Effects of Head Injury,* which was a compilation of papers from a symposium. At each meeting about head injury, rehabilitation professionals posed the question, "Why doesn't someone publish a book about rehabilitation and head injury?" Finally, we decided to answer this question by compiling the current volume.

Since this book is the first text on head-injury rehabilitation in many years, we have attempted to be as comprehensive as possible. The attempt to adequately cover such a broad topic is fraught with perils. By presenting a comprehensive overview of the subject, we have not been able to provide as much depth on some topics as we would like. Thus, the physician may be disappointed at the relatively few chapters devoted exclusively to medical assessment and management. Yet other texts may fulfill this need, such as the recently published book by Bryan Jennett and Graham Teasdale, *Management of Head Injuries* (F. A. Davis, 1981). Certain rehabilitation professionals may feel that their specialty area, such as nursing or physical therapy, has not been given adequate space. Regrettably, the field of head injury encompasses so many disciplines that the volume would have exceeded 1000 pages if material was presented for every group of professionals involved with brain injury— for example, nutrition, law, recreational therapy, education, psychiatry, and orthopedic surgery. Nonetheless, we are of the opinion that the content of the book will be valuable for all those concerned with head injury, regardless of their specific area.

Another difficulty in writing this book was to strike a balance between an academic and a clinical point of view. Predictably, the point of view varies depending on each chapter's author. We have designed the book not only to highlight important research advances of the past decade but to allow clinicians to find it useful as a guide to clinical practice. It is our sincere hope that each reader will find something of value that will generalize to his or her clinical practice.

This book owes its existence to a great many people. First and foremost, we are indebted to our contributors, whose long and hard labors have resulted in this text. I am personally grateful to the indefatigable efforts of my co-editors, Drs. Griffith, Bond, and Miller. Without their assistance, the book would likely still be in the planning stages. The support and editorial assistance provided by Mr. Bob Martone has been exceedingly valuable. I would like to express my deep appreciation to my colleagues who had a major role in planning and running the series of head-injury courses that led to the volume, especially Richard and Christi Eisenberg, Linda Diehl, Rita Riani, Robin McNeny, Jean Cerny, and others at the Medical College of Virginia. I also appreciate the support and encouragement provided by my colleagues at the Department of Rehabilitation Medicine, Tufts-New England Medical Center—especially my chairman, Dr. Bruce Gans. My thanks are also extended to Dr. Roberta Trieschmann, Dr. Cynthia Dember, and Dr. Paul Karoly, all of whom were important influences in my early career as a graduate student. The assistance of Mrs. Sarah McGillowey in typing the final manuscript is gratefully acknowledged. Finally, I express my heartfelt appreciation to my wife Peggy, daughter Michelle, and parents Morris and Edythe for their love, support, and encouragement.

Mitchell Rosenthal

CONTRIBUTORS

Brenda B. Adamovich, Ph.D.
Director, Regional Rehabilitation Center
Mercy Hospital
Springfield, Massachusetts

Yehuda Ben-Yishay, Ph.D.
Associate Professor, Clinical
    Rehabilitation Medicine
Assistant Chief Behavioral Sciences
Director, Head Trauma Program
New York University Medical
    Center, Rusk Institute
New York, New York

James P. Berger, M.A., C.T.R.S.
Director, Therapeutic Recreation Services
Rehabilitation Institute
Detroit, Michigan

Sheldon Berrol, M.D.
Associate Clinical Professor
University of California
San Francisco
Chief, Rehabilitation Medicine
San Francisco General Hospital
San Francisco, California

Michael R. Bond, M.D., Ph.D.
Professor and Chairman
Department of Psychological Medicine
University of Glasgow
Glasgow, Scotland, United Kingdom

Catherine F. Bontke, M.D.
Director, Head Injury Program
The Institute for Rehabilitation and Research
Assistant Professor of Rehabilitation
Baylor College of Medicine
Houston, Texas

Joyce D. Brink, M.D.
Associate Professor, Clinical Pediatrics
University of Southern California
    School of Medicine
Medical Director, Rehabilitation Center
Children's Hospital
Los Angeles, California

Professor D. Neil Brooks, Ph.D.
Director, Wellcome Neuroscience Group
University of Glasgow
Glasgow, Scotland, United Kingdom

Derek A. Bruce, M.B.Ch.B.
Director, Pediatric Neurosurgical Institute
Humana Advanced Surgical Institutes
Humana Medical City
Dallas, Texas

Larry E. Cervelli, B.S., O.T.R.
Chief Operating Officer
AMS-Rehab, Inc.
Northampton, Massachusetts

Anna J.L. Chorazy, M.D., FAAP
Clinical Assistant Professor, Pediatrics
University of Pittsburgh School of Medicine
Medical Director, The Rehabilitation
    Institute of Pittsburgh
Children's Hospital of Pittsburgh
Pittsburgh, Pennsylvania

Sally B. Cohen, M.Ed.
Cognitive Rehabilitation
Clinical Facilitator
The Rehabilitation Institute of Pittsburgh
Pittsburgh, Pennsylvania

Sandra Cole, A.A.S.E.C.T., C.S.E., C.S.C.
Professor and Director
The Sexuality Training Center of the
    University Hospital
Department of Physical Medicine and
    Rehabilitation
University of Michigan
Ann Arbor, Michigan

Theodore M. Cole, M.D.
Professor and Chairman,
Department of Physical Medicine and
    Rehabilitation
University of Michigan
Ann Arbor, Michigan

Joy V. Cook, M.A.
Acquired Brain Injury Specialist
Glendale Community College
Glendale, California

D. Nathan Cope, M.D.
Vice President for Medical Affairs
NeuroCare, Inc.
Concord, California

Linda N. Diehl, R.N., M.S., CNAA
Director of Program Development
Sinai Rehabilitation Center
Faculty Associate of Maryland
School of Nursing
Baltimore, Maryland

Jean C. Dise, M.S., O.T.R.
Supervisor, Rehabilitation Division
Occupational Therapy Department
Medical College of Virginia Hospitals
Richmond, Virginia

Pamela Duncan, M.A., P.T.
Department of Physical Therapy
Duke University Medical Center
Durham, North Carolina

Peter Eames, M.D., MRCP, MRC Psych
Consultant Neuropsychiatrist
Burden Neurological Hospital
Bristol, England, United Kingdom

Bruce M. Gans, M.D.
Professor and Chairman
Department of Physical Medicine and
    Rehabilitation
Wayne State University School of Medicine
President and Chief Executive Officer
Rehabilitation Institute, Inc.
Detroit Medical Center
Detroit, Michigan

Douglas E. Garland, M.D.
Chief, Central Nervous System Division,
Department of Surgery, Rancho Los Amigos
    Medical Center
Clinical Professor Orthopedics
University of Southern California
Downey, California

Ziya L. Gokaslan, M.D.
Research Fellow
Department of Neurosurgery
Baylor College of Medicine
Houston, Texas

Ernest R. Griffith, M.D.
Professor and Head
Department of Physical Medicine and
    Rehabilitation
University of Illinois at Chicago College of
    Medicine
Chicago, Illinois

Michael E. Groher, Ph.D.
Assistant Chief, Audiology/Speech Pathology
Veteran's Administration Medical Center
New York, New York
Professional Associate, The Department of
    Rehabilitation Medicine
The New York Hospital
New York, New York
Adjunct Faculty
Adelphi University
Garden City, New York

William J. Haffey, Ph.D.
Executive Director
Rehabilitation Services
Sharp Healthcare
7901 Frost Street
San Diego, California

Douglas E. Harrington, Ph.D.
Consulting Neuropsychologist
Traumatic Head Injury Program
Coastline Community College
Fountain Valley, California
Director, Mental Health/Rehabilitation
(MH/R) Associates
Irvine, California

Ross M. Hays, M.D.
Assistant Professor, Rehabilitation Medicine
Adjunct Assistant Professor, Pediatrics
University of Washington School of
    Medicine
Associate Director, Department of
    Rehabilitation Medicine
Children's Hospital and Medical Center
Seattle, Washington

Lawrence J. Horn, M.D.
Medical Director, Brain Injury Rehabilitation
    Program
Magee Rehabilitation Hospital
Clinical Assistant Professor
Department of Rehabilitation Medicine
Thomas Jefferson University
Medical Director
Remed Recovery Care Center
Philadelphia, Pennsylvania

Kenneth M. Jaffe, M.D.
Associate Professor, Rehabilitation Medicine
Adjunct Associate Professor, Pediatrics and
    Neurological Surgery
University of Washington School of
    Medicine
Director, Department of Rehabilitation
    Medicine
Children's Hospital and Medical Center
Seattle, Washington

John A. Jane, M.D., Ph.D.
Alumni Professor and Chairman
Department of Neurosurgery
University of Virginia
Health Sciences Center
Box 212
Charlottesville, Virginia

Bryan Jennett, M.D., FRCS
Professor of Neurosurgery
Institute of Neurological Sciences
University of Glasgow
Glasgow, Scotland, United Kingdom

Patricia A. Jones, Dip. Phys., M.Sc.
Research Associate
Department of Clinical Neurosciences
University of Edinburgh
Edinburgh, Scotland, United Kingdom

Kenneth I. Kolpan, J.D., P.C.
Attorney at Law
One Winthrop Square
Boston, Massachusetts

**Martin G. Livingston, M.D., MRC
    Psych**
Senior Lecturer in Psychological Medicine
University of Glasgow
Consultant Psychiatrist
Gartnabel Hospitals
Glasgow, Scotland, United Kingdom

William J. Lynch, Ph.D.
Program Chief, Brain Injury
    Rehabilitation Unit
Veterans Administration Medical Center
Palo Alto, California

Nancy R. Mann, M.D.
Assistant Professor and Acting Chairman
Department of Rehabilitation Medicine
Tufts University School of Medicine
Boston, Massachusetts

Joyce P. Mastrilli, O.T.R./L.
Occupational Therapist
The Rehabilitation Institute of Pittsburgh
Pittsburgh, Pennsylvania

Nathaniel H. Mayer, M.D.
Director, Drucker Brain Injury Center
Moss Rehabilitation Hospital
Professor, Department of Physical Medicine
    and Rehabilitation
Temple University School of Health Sciences
Philadelphia, Pennsylvania

Robin McNeny, O.T.R.
Occupational Therapist-Head Trauma Unit
The Medical College of Virginia Hospitals
Richmond, Virginia

**J. Douglas Miller, M.D., Ph.D.,
    FRCSE, FRCPSG, FACS, FRCPE**
Professor of Surgical Neurology
Chairman, Department of Clinical
    Neurosciences
University of Edinburgh
Consultant Neurosurgeon, Western General
    Hospital
Astley Ainslie Hospital and Royal Infirmary
    of Edinburgh
Edinburgh, Scotland, United Kingdom

Cindy Black Molitor, P.T., MS
Physical Therapist, Private Practice
Greensburgh, Pennsylvania

Craig A. Muir, Ph.D.
Assistant Research Professor
UCLA Center for the Health Sciences,
    Neuropsychiatric Institute
Los Angeles, California

Raj K. Narayan, M.D.
Chief of Neurosurgery
Ben Taub General Hospital
Assistant Professor of Neurosurgery
Baylor College of Medicine
Houston, Texas

James T. Nelson, Ph.D.
Neuropsychologist
The Rehabilitation Institute of Pittsburgh
Pittsburgh, Pennsylvania

**Brian Pentland, B.Sc.(Hons),
    M.B.Ch.B., FRCPE**
Consultant Neurologist
Department of Rehabilitation Medicine
Astley Ainslie Hospital
Department of Clinical Neurosciences
University of Edinburgh
Edinburgh, Scotland, United Kingdom

George P. Prigatano, Ph.D.
Chairman, Neuropsychology and Clinical
    Director, Neuropsychological
    Rehabilitation
Barrow Neuropsychological Institute
St. Joseph's Hospital and Medical Center
Phoenix, Arizona

Anne E. Regalski, C.T.R.S.
Recreational Therapist
Macomb Hospital Center
Warren, Michigan

Rebecca W. Rimel, R.N., N.P.
Pew Charitable Trusts
Philadelphia, Pennsylvania

Mary Anne Rinehart, M.S., P.T.
Director, Physical Therapy
Santa Clara Valley Medical Center
San Jose, California

Mitchell Rosenthal, Ph.D.
Director of Psychological Medicine
Marianjoy Rehabilitation Center
Wheaton, Illinois
Associate Professor of Psychology and
    Physical Medicine and Rehabilitation
Rush Medical College
Chicago, Illinois

Shirley F. Szekeres, Ph.D., CCC-SLP
Director, Speech-Language Therapy
    Department
The Rehabilitation Institute of Pittsburgh
Pittsburgh, Pennsylvania

Anne S. Valko, M.D., FAAP
Physiatrist
Director of Outpatient Rehabilitation
   Medicine
The Rehabilitation Institute of Pittsburgh
Clinical Assistant Professor of Pediatrics and
   Orthopedics
University of Pittsburgh School of Medicine
Pittsburgh, Pennsylvania

John Whyte, M.D., Ph.D.
Staff Physiatrist and Assistant Professor of
   Rehabilitation Medicine
New England Medical Center Hospitals and
   Tufts University School of Medicine
Director of Research and Associate Director
   of Rehabilitation Medicine
The Greenery Rehabilitation and Skilled
   Nursing Center
Boston, Massachusetts

Mark Ylvisaker, Ph.D.
Program Director
New Medico Rehabilitation and Skilled
   Nursing Center of the Capital District
Schenectady, New York

Barbara Zoltan, M.A., O.T.R.
Consultant in Private Practice
Saratoga, California

CONTENTS

Chapter 32   **EDUCATIONAL STRATEGIES** **476**
Douglas E. Harrington, Ph.D.

Chapter 33   **RETURNING TO WORK AFTER TRAUMATIC HEAD INJURY** **493**
Joy V. Cook, M.A.

NATURE OF THE PROBLEM

Michael R. Bond, M.D., Ph.D., Editor

Chapter 1

Scale and Scope of the Problem

BRYAN JENNETT, M.D.

Head injuries are very common. Just how common they are is difficult to discover because many are not serious enough to warrant admission to the hospital, and statistics about emergency room attenders are unreliable and incomplete. Deaths, however, are readily documented, providing a guide to the relative frequency of injuries in different geographic regions. In different parts of the United States, there are 22 to 25 fatal head injuries per 100,000, more than twice as many as in Britain, Sweden, or Japan.[1] About 7 million head injuries are estimated to occur annually in the United States,[2] with about 500,000 persons admitted to the hospital.

Many patients admitted to the hospital are only mildly injured and stay for only a few days; in Britain more than two thirds are discharged in 2 days or less. Yet each of these numerous patients, passing rapidly through the hospital emergency room and wards, may suffer for several weeks from symptoms and impaired function; a few will develop an accident neurosis that can last for months or even years. At the other end of the scale are patients who remain in coma for several days, even weeks. During that period they require assiduous assistance from physiotherapists if they are not to develop pulmonary complications that may be fatal or limb contractures that may cause lasting disability. Most of these seriously injured patients will have major disabilities for some months, and many of them will never be the same people again; some will have a major disability, mental or physical, for the rest of their lives. Since their average age is under 30 years this means many

years of disability. This remains a problem long after patients lose contact with the original hospital system that treated them in the acute stage.

Although the number of these severe injuries that occur in any one district or community hospital is relatively small, the population of disabled survivors of head injury in the community is much greater than the statistics on the annual occurrence of new cases might suggest. Exactly how many patients this amounts to at any one time (the prevalence of disability due to head injury) is difficult to calculate. One estimate in Britain arrived at a figure of 150 markedly disabled persons per 100,000 population. As head injuries are much less common in the United Kingdom than in many parts of the world, the number of disabled survivors will be higher than this elsewhere (for the United States approximately 400 per 100,000).

A word of warning is needed regarding the epidemiology of head injury—about counting the numbers of head injuries that occur, the nature of the victims, and the causes of the accidents that led to injury. The basis of the calculation should be the community, rather than a hospital or a specialist service. This is because a variety of selection processes operate to determine where patients go after injury. Many of these processes are unrecognized, and some are difficult to determine even if they are looked for. The distribution of causes, for example, is quite different in the emergency room than in the intensive care unit or the autopsy room; this is because the cause is related to the severity of the injury. Thus,

3

traffic accidents are the major cause of serious head injuries, whereas minor head injuries are mostly due to falls and fights.

SEVERITY OF INJURY

The problems of management, both in the acute stage and for later rehabilitation, are so different for injuries of different severity that it is vital to understand how to assess severity. It is obviously brain damage that matters, not scalp lacerations or skull fractures. The brain damage may be primary, sustained at the moment of impact; or it may be secondary, the result of subsequent pathologic processes. These processes include brain swelling, intracranial hematoma, and the effects on the brain of extracranial events such as blood loss, arterial hypotension, and pulmonary complications. The most common combined effect of these various secondary processes is to produce widespread ischemic brain damage. This can occur within hours after injury, perhaps even in the first few minutes. In some cases, it is obvious that secondary brain damage is dominant, in that the patient was clearly not severely affected soon after injury; for example, the patient may have talked before lapsing into coma. In other cases it is a matter of conjecture how much of the brain damage has resulted from primary as distinct from secondary factors. In either event, the therapist has to deal with the net effect of these two kinds of damage.

Of most importance for rehabilitation are the nature and location of the brain damage. Not only is secondary ischemic damage widespread throughout the brain but in most cases the impact damage also affects many parts of the brain. Wherever the blow on the head or the location of the skull fracture, there are usually contusions of the cortex in both frontal and temporal lobes; and there is commonly widespread disruption or stretching of nerve fibers in the white matter of the cerebral hemispheres and the brainstem.[3, 4] Even when there is a clear focal lesion, such as an intracranial hematoma causing hemiplegia, this is seldom the only site of brain damage. This is one reason for the difference in the disability produced by head injury as compared with that produced by cerebrovascular accident. The latter is usually a strictly focal lesion, and the main rehabilitation issue is the focal neurophysical deficit. By contrast, the widespread nature of the brain damage after head injury is probably responsible for the dysfunction that affects so many aspects of mental activity.

The most consistent effect of diffuse brain damage, even when it is mild, is impairment of consciousness. The best guide to the severity of this damage is the degree and duration of altered consciousness. In the emergency room, it is useful to classify patients into those who are already talking when they arrive and those who are not. The talkers can be divided into those who have a period of amnesia following their injury and those who can remember everything clearly. In those who are unconscious on arrival, the depth and duration of coma provide the best guide to the severity of the diffuse damage, and this is readily recorded in terms of the Glasgow Coma Scale (see Chapter 5 for further discussion). It should be noted that a severe compound depressed fracture with brain issuing from the wound can occur without there having been any loss of consciousness or any amnesia whatever. This is because the brain damage was focal.

After the patient has recovered, the best guide to the severity of the diffuse damage is the duration of the post-traumatic amnesia (PTA). An advantage of this indicator is that it can be assessed in conversation with the patient months after injury and without reference to records relating to the early management of the patient. This makes it of particular value to the rehabilitation team that inherits the patient some time after injury, often from another institution. Patients are asked how long it was before they "came to," in that they themselves became aware of their surroundings. Doctors must confirm that patients are not reporting what their relatives have told them about this. Relatives usually equate awareness with when patients first began to talk, and that is usually long before the beginning of continuous memory for day-to-day events. There is no need to seek a very accurate figure for PTA; what matters is whether it lasted minutes, hours, days, or weeks (Table 1–1). There is now abundant evidence that the duration of PTA correlates well with late outcome as well as with the interval before patients return to work; it also influences

Table 1–1. DURATION OF POST-TRAUMATIC AMNESIA (PTA) AND SEVERITY OF INJURY

PTA Duration	Severity
Less than 5 min	Very mild
5 to 60 min	Mild
1 to 24 hr	Moderate
1 to 7 days	Severe
1 to 4 weeks	Very severe
More than 4 weeks	Extremely severe

the occurrence of late traumatic epilepsy (see Chapter 7).

NATURE OF THE DISABILITY

After both mild and severe injuries it is useful to distinguish between the mental and physical components of disability, while acknowledging that what matters is the net effect of these on the overall social functioning of the individual. It is also important to distinguish between persisting complaints or deficits that reflect incomplete recovery and those that develop anew. The latter include traumatic epilepsy, as well as secondary psychosocial problems resulting from reactions of the patient and family to the accident and its consequences. Although there is a certain amount of overlap between the disabilities suffered after mild and severe injuries, the differences are more striking than the similarities.

The symptoms that predominate after mild injury (often dubbed the postconcussional syndrome) are seldom suffered after severe injury. Indeed such patients usually deny ever having had headaches, dizziness, or even anxiety. That is not to imply that the symptoms complained of after mild injury are either imaginary or psychologically induced, as was once believed. Indeed there is now ample evidence that these symptoms are based on physiologic disorders, albeit short-lived. This knowledge comes from better means of testing the ability of these patients to process information, and of measuring mild vestibular abnormalities and other physiologic functions. There is also pathologic evidence that even mild concussion causes visible structural damage in the brain; evidence of stretching and rupture of nerve fibers can be found in the white matter of the brains of patients who die from other causes after having recovered from mild head injury. If the symptoms of these mildly injured patients are ignored or are unsympathetically dealt with, there is a real risk of secondary anxiety and depression that can lead to long-lasting neurosis.

After severe injury the disability is frequently characterized by a combination of mental and physical deficits. This often leads to a greater degree of social disability than would be expected from the separate deficits. In most cases the mental dysfunction predominates in contributing to the social handicap. This also impedes the rehabilitation of the physical deficits because motivation is reduced and some patients even reject the efforts of those trying to help them. The physical deficits comprise those related to cerebral hemisphere function (sensorimotor hemiplegia, dysphasia, and epilepsy) and those caused by damage to the brainstem and cranial nerves. Mental deficits include memory disorder on a day-to-day or even hour-to-hour basis, cognitive impairments that can be measured by psychometric tests, and personality disorders. The latter are both the most common and often the most disabling; they frequently occur in patients who have little or no physical deficit and whose performance on formal psychologic tests is not greatly impaired.[5] Yet personality change may not be immediately evident, unless care is taken to invite family and friends to compare the patient's present overall behavior with that before injury. Personality change is also the disability that is least influenced by therapeutic intervention.

A further factor that contributes to the overall disability of the head injured patient in many cases is the patient's pretraumatic psychosocial status. The victims of head injury are not a random sample of their age group; they include an undue proportion of people with some kind of social deviancy. Some are risk-takers in cars and on motorcycles, and some are drinkers or declared alcoholics. And although the young brain may have more potential for recovery than an older one, youth is less helpful in the social sense. Some of the younger patients are still facing the turmoil of adolescence and greatly resent the enforced dependence on their parents that is often the result of brain damage. Others are on the threshold of their careers and cannot expect special arrangements to be made by employers, who might be sympathetic to persons with years of good service to the firm behind them. Those who are married have seldom been so for long, and these marriages frequently break down under the stress of brain damage. By contrast, for example, the older man with a stroke, married for many years and perhaps already expected to retire soon, may be more readily accepted by his wife when he is left with hemiplegia; he may also be more ready himself to adopt a dependent role.

RECOVERY AFTER HEAD INJURY

Little is understood about the process of recovery after head injury. By any standards this is a remarkable phenomenon. A patient who is lying unconscious, temporarily apneic and pulseless immediately after injury, may get up and walk away only minutes later. Other patients may be in a coma for several days, and it may be weeks before full consciousness is restored. While some such patients make a full recovery, many never do get back to their own selves, or anything like them. Rehabilitation aims to influence this process favorably, either to hasten the restoration of function or to ensure that recovery is eventually more complete than it would have been without therapy. This treatment can be rationally based only if it is founded on some hypothesis of the process of recovery.

It seems probable that different biologic activities operate at different stages of the injury. Recovery of consciousness after a stunning blow takes only minutes, whereas there are severely injured patients who report continuing improvement in some neurologic functions a year or more after the injury. Changes in the first minutes after injury presumably indicate the resolution of transitory dysfunction that may not have any structural component. Recovery after several days is more likely to be due to the resolution of temporary structural abnormalities such as edema and vascular permeability. The mechanism that underlies recovery over months or years is much less

easily explained. The extent to which alternative, perhaps normally redundant, pathways are brought into action as a substitute for structures that have been rendered permanently functionless is uncertain. Whether recovery is due to restoration of activity in structures that are recovering or to diversion to other pathways, it seems likely that some of the restoration of function is essentially a learning process. The poorer prospects for recovery in older patients may have several explanations: a reduced capacity to learn, a less resilient vascular system, and a more limited neuronal reserve by way of available alternative pathways.

Just as there are different biologic processes taking place at different times after injury, so do the objectives and techniques of rehabilitation differ as the time since injury increases. In the first month after severe injury the aim is to prevent complications—those in the chest that may threaten life and that can cause additional brain damage in survivors, and those in the limbs that may cause permanent crippling.

It is in the next 3 to 6 months that therapeutic rehabilitation interventions seem likely to have their greatest impact. As the recovery process slows down and it becomes evident that severe permanent disability is likely (even though some further improvement is expected) the time comes to decide to abandon efforts to restore old skills to damaged parts in favor of teaching how to substitute new skills using unaffected parts. The success of rehabilitation for permanent paraplegics may derive in part from the certainty that walking will never be possible, so that no time is lost before turning attention to what can be done without walking. It may be that after brain damage therapists should be readier to recognize when such a point has been reached with specific deficits such as hemiplegia or dysphasia, and to seek substitution rather than flogging a functionally dead horse. This is certainly the theme of rehabilitation after 6 months or more, when the need is to analyze not only the patient's disability but also his or her remaining capability. Only then is it clear how to encourage patients to adapt physically and mentally to their changed physical and mental status, so that patients and their families may adjust socially in an appropriate way. This is no easy matter when it is the mental and emotional sphere that is most drastically changed; but unless that effort to adjust is made there may be little to look forward to.

The importance of family and friends can hardly be overestimated. It is therefore an additional but vital responsibility of therapists to influence the attitudes of the family, to prepare them for the difficult months ahead, to support and counsel them during these months, and to help them to understand their brain-damaged family member. If this is accepted as a part of rehabilitation from the outset it should be possible to anticipate the most harmful of secondary psychologic reactions (and interactions) of the patient and family. These reactions can be a serious impediment to optimal recovery, and efforts to minimize them are well worth making. An important element in this counseling is the setting of realistic goals that are based on properly calculated predictions rather than on false hopes. To hold out promises of substantial further functional recovery once the likelihood of this has passed is not only unkind but can be a positive hindrance to a sensible attitude both to rehabilitation and to life in the future.

An aspect of rehabilitation that is too often neglected is research—into how effective present methods are, as well as into new approaches. The obvious emotional need of the family and of the caring professionals to respond to disability by action can lead to unquestioning acceptance of the belief that more therapy means better recovery. This is a costly assumption, considering that rehabilitation is a labor-intensive activity that depends on skilled personnel, a resource that even money cannot always buy. The effectiveness of therapy, whether an organized system or a single technique, can be judged only if there are reliable means of describing the state of recovery at given (fixed) times after injury, and so of comparing the rate of recovery with and without specific methods of rehabilitation in different patients (see Section IV).

There is need also to be able to quantify the treatment given—its type, its dose, and its timing—and to distinguish between skill-specific therapy and the general benefits of enthusiastic amateurs, whether these be other health professionals or members of the family. Only if all these factors are recognized is it possible to plan a rehabilitation program that is realistic and economic, rather than pretentious and expensive.

If rehabilitation is to be taken seriously by health care providers, like a potent drug or an effective surgical procedure, then it deserves to be assessed by the same standards. That entails seeking answers to the same kinds of questions. What is the best method, and what is the most effective dose? When should treatment start, and when should it finish? Are there adverse effects of some forms of rehabilitation, and can some patients become addicted?

One of the most important goals is to provide continuity of care for a program that is likely to be intensive for a few months but that may require some continuing input for the rest of the patient's life. Family members are the only persons able to provide this. They should be recruited as members of the therapeutic team as soon as possible after the patient emerges from coma. They should be taught what to do and encouraged to do it; as time passes, they should be told what they may now need to do differently. This is not just economically sensible but the only way to ensure that the patient can adapt within the family and to the community in general rather than relating primarily to some therapeutic or supportive group.

REFERENCES

1. Jennett, B and MacMillan, R: Epidemiology of head injury. Br Med J 282:101, 1981.
2. Frankowski, RF: Descriptive epidemiological studies of head injury in the United States 1974–84. Adv Psychosom Med 16:153, 1986.
3. Jennett, B and Teasdale, G: Management of Head Injuries. Contemporary Neurology Series, Vol 20. FA Davis, Philadelphia, 1981.
4. Adams, JH et al: Brain damage in fatal non-missile head injury. J Clin Pathol 33:1132, 1980.
5. Jennett, B et al: Disability after severe head injury: Observations on the use of the Glasgow Outcome Scale. J Neurol Neurosurg Psychiatry 44:285, 1981.

Chapter 2

Characteristics of the Head Injured Patient

REBECCA W. RIMEL, R.N., N.P.
JOHN A. JANE, M.D., Ph.D.
MICHAEL R. BOND, M.D., Ph.D.

Over the years there has been a steady increase in the number of individuals sustaining head injuries. More die on American highways each year in automobile accidents than were lost in the entire Vietnam conflict, and central nervous system (CNS) trauma is the single most common cause of death in these accidents. The head is injured in more than two thirds of all automobile accidents, and head injury is the cause of death in about 70 percent of fatal cases.[1] Trauma is currently the third most common cause of death in the United States and is the primary cause of death in persons under age 38.[2] Because of its potentially devastating physical, psychologic, and social consequences, head injury is one of the most critical problems facing the health care system.

The medical problems of patients who survive head injury are enormous, and the socioeconomic impact on our society is staggering. Even though head injury is recognized as a major international health problem, the epidemiology is not well described because of problems in patient identification and definition of the severity of injury. Over the past decade, the epidemiology of head injury has received greater attention, and as a result, a wide range of incidence figures has been obtained.[3–12] Studies that are confined to small geographic localities are felt to be the most reliable because there tend to be fewer methodologic problems. Such studies, however, may not be entirely representative of other or larger populations. It is difficult, therefore, to give valid general incidence rates for CNS

trauma. The variation in estimates of head injuries in the United States and other countries is demonstrated in Table 2–1. There is value in comparing the statistics for head injuries across countries and this has been done in various ways—for example, between the United States and Britain. Jennett and MacMillan[5] showed that head injury deaths per 100,000 are twice as numerous in San Diego and central Virginia as in Britain (22 and 25 per 100,000 versus 9 per 100,000). These figures cannot be accounted for by known variations in the age structure of the population. Further differences emerged in this study on consideration of hospital admission rates which are lower in San Diego (245 per 100,000) and Charlottesville (216 per 100,000) than in Scotland, the explanation being that fewer patients with mild injuries were admitted in the American centers. A survey conducted by the National Institute of Neurological and Communicative Disorders and Stroke, the largest survey of its kind in the United States, provided data on the occurrence of new cases of head injury, type and cause of injury, admission and duration of hospital stay, and frequence of existing cases of injury.[6] Comparisons of these and other findings, and data collected at the University of Virginia,[13–15] are discussed in this chapter, which provides an overview of the characteristics of head injured patients. Each person, whether practicing in an acute care or rehabilitation setting will be involved not only with patients sustaining head trauma but also with families. Therefore, a better

Table 2–1. INCIDENCE OF HEAD INJURY

Source	Description	Incidence/100,000	Total USA
National Surveys and Estimates:			
National Center for Health Statistics[6]	All injuries except death	3900	8,111,000
Caveness[7]	Excluding lacerations of scalp and face	915	1,900,000
Health Interview Survey[22]	Household interview survey	600	1,275,000
Research Triangle for NINCDS[12]	Hospitalized patients	185	422,000
Hospital Discharge Survey[23]	Hospitalized patients	170	353,000
Annegers, Grabow, and Kurland[8]	Traumatic unconsciousness or post-traumatic amnesia or skull fracture	↑ 300 est.	
England and Wales[3]	Hospitalized patients	430	
San Diego County[9]	Death or hospitalization	295	

knowledge of the characteristics of the patients, the mechanism of injury, outcome in the short and long term, and implications for management is useful for providing improved patient care as well as education and counseling directed at the patient, the family, and the public.

In September 1977, the Department of Neurosurgery at the University of Virginia began to develop a prospective data bank of patients with CNS injuries in central Virginia.[13-15] The major emphasis of the project was the identification and study of all patients who sustained injury in a well-defined geographic area. The University, located in central Virginia, offers the only neurologic coverage for 13 counties in which all head injuries requiring neurosurgical care are treated at one center, thus providing an opportunity for population-based studies where the bias of selection factors is minimized. During the 20-month period from October 1, 1977, to May 30, 1979, a prospective study resulted in a data bank of 1248 patients from which the data presented here are derived.

PATIENT CHARACTERISTICS

Age and Sex

All studies have reported that head trauma is two or three times more common in males than in females. In the Virginia series, occurrence of CNS trauma in males was approximately twice that in females for most age categories and, even though male predominance exists in most categories, the differences between the sexes are greatest between ages 15 and 24.

For the age distribution of CNS injuries, three age groups were found to exceed the overall incidence of 24 percent per 10,000 population in the Virginia study. This was demonstrated first in age groups 15 through 29 years, with the highest risk group, aged 15 through 19 years, showing an incidence of 42 per 10,000. Another high-risk group was age 75 and over, in which the incidence was 30 per 10,000 population. Lowest incidence of injury occurred in the 5 through 9 age group. These figures are very comparable with those reported by Jennett and MacMillan[5] and Field[3] for Britain. The overall age distribution for head injuries on the Virginia study can be seen in Figure 2–1. In this series and others, there was no significant difference in the occurrence of head injuries between the white and nonwhite population based on local census data.

The reason for assessing demographic and epidemiologic data is that certain important characteristics will become evident that will help identify a population at risk. Such is the case when looking at age distribution, but examination of the frequency of the age dis-

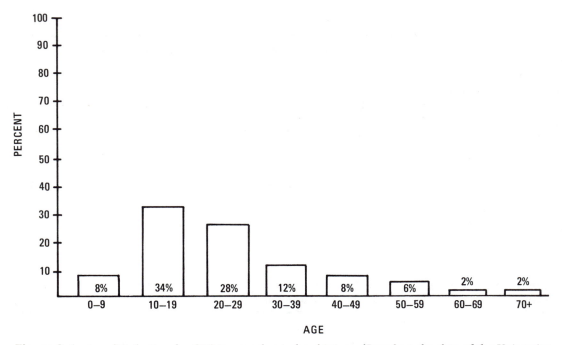

Figure 2–1. Age distribution for CNS trauma due to head injury. (Based on the data of the University of Virginia study.[13, 14])

tribution can be quite deceptive. As expected, the greatest number of patients is between ages 10 and 19 (34 percent). The elderly population comprises a very small percentage, with fewer than 4 percent of the patients over age 65. However, calculation of the incidence figures based on the population for the central Virginia catchment area shows that two age groups are at risk for head injury. They are the 10 to 30-year-olds, as anticipated, and the elderly population.

Socioeconomic Status

Other significant descriptive characteristics were evaluated, including marital status, type of employment, and overall socioeconomic status. Of those injured, 59 percent were single, which is 20 percent higher than the population base as a whole. Twenty-nine percent of the patients were married, and the remainder were either widowed or divorced. In this series, the majority of patients (75 percent) earned less than $10,000 a year. Differences in salaries within specific geographic areas must be considered, however; therefore, the em-

ployment status provides a more objective overview of the group's socioeconomic status. The largest category is that of "student," which comprises 24 percent of the population (the existence of a large university in Charlottesville results in a greater proportion of students in the population). The "unemployed" patients are particularly noteworthy, as their incidence of CNS trauma is almost three times that of their proportion in the total population.

Data on education revealed that approximately 25 percent of patients had fewer than 8 years of education, 50 percent had 8 to 12 years, and 25 percent had 12 years or more of education. In the Virginia study, the patients who sustained head trauma were predominantly from a lower socioeconomic class. Selecki and coworkers[16] found that among neurosurgical admissions in New South Wales, Australia, laborers and craftsmen were disproportionately represented, and similar observations have been made in Britain.[5] Persons in the lower socioeconomic classes in both countries had considerably more head injuries caused by assaults and household accidents. Traffic accidents were not related to socioeconomic class and in Britain socioeconomic status appears to have little, if any, effect among those over 65 years of age.

Medical History

In the Charlottesville series, 31 percent of all patients studied were previously hospitalized for a head injury. The question that presents itself is whether people who have already had a head injury are at high risk for a second injury. The literature seems to vary on this question. Partington[1] found no increased risk for a second head injury in children who had previous insult. However, in a study conducted in Minnesota,[8] the incidence of a subsequent head injury in adults was about three times that of a first head injury in a general population. Among those who had sustained more than one head injury, the incidence of a subsequent head injury was eight times that of the general population. Therefore, based on these data and on the Virginia experience, it seems that adult patients who sustain a single head injury are at high risk of another insult.

In evaluating other aspects of the medical history, 25 percent of the Virginia patients interviewed stated that they had received some type of professional treatment for alcohol abuse. A significant number (20 percent) had also been treated for heart disease or high blood pressure or both. These and other disorders requiring treatment, such as psychiatric illness (11 percent), seizures (4 percent), and drug abuse (4 percent), are all characteristics suggesting a possible increase in the risk for head trauma among those afflicted. With such information available, preventive educational programs could be directed at those physical illnesses in the hope of decreasing the rate of readmission for successive injuries.

CAUSE OF INJURY

High-risk groups for head trauma may be identified by the analysis of the causes and mechanisms of injury. A review of the literature shows that the major causes of serious injury are similar in Australia, Britain, Canada, and the United States. In the majority of series, more than half the patients are involved in traffic accidents, with falls being the next major cause of injury.[3, 17] Some interesting data are available demonstrating how the cause of injury differs with the age of the patient. In the Charlottesville series, when age-specific incidence rates were evaluated based on the cause of injury, there was an overwhelming predominance of motor vehicle accidents, and most cases of head injury occurred in the age group between 15 and 24 years. Most cases of head injury from falls in the National Institutes of Health (NIH) series[6] were seen in the group under age 15. In the Charlottesville study, falls were the second most frequent cause of injury, with a definite rise in incidence in those age 70 and over. Contrast this with information from Scotland,[5] which reveals the importance of taking local cultural factors into account when discussing the causes of injury. Thus, among Scottish men aged 15 to 24 treated in accident departments, assaults were twice as common as traffic accidents. Also, road victims accounted for only a minority of attendances at accident and emergency departments but they were responsible for more than half the serious injuries and deaths.

Causality data are valuable in proposing programs designed to reduce traffic accidents and minimize their consequences. One strategy should be to encourage the use of safety measures such as seat belts and protective helmets. Of patients admitted to the Charlottesville medical center, fewer than 14 percent reported that they were wearing seat belts at the time of injury. Of those involved in motorcycle accidents, only 58 percent were wearing helmets, even though Virginia has a requirement for such equipment. In Britain, with a compliance rate of well over 90 percent for several years, the wearing of front seat belts is compulsory as is the wearing of a motorcycle helmet. The consequence of legislation enforcing these safety measures has been a significant decline in the number of head and facial injuries in car drivers and passengers and also in head injuries among motorcyclists. One might argue that those who care for the head injured patient in the United States must become actively involved in designing preventive programs and supporting legislation for mandatory and improved safety measures nationally. In Virginia automotive accidents, it was the driver (71 percent) who most frequently sustained a head injury, and this injury was often the result of a single-car accident (58 percent). More than half the patients who were injured reported that the vehicle was traveling in excess of the 55 mile per hour speed limit. Most frequently, the victim was riding in the front seat (87 percent) of a full-sized (calculated from the wheel-base size) car (75 percent). Only 12 percent of Charlottesville patients were injured as a result of interpersonal violence; which is quite a marked difference from the Scottish figures. Approximately 80 percent of all assaults, including gunshot wounds, beatings, and knife wounds, were either self-inflicted or a result of domestic strife. This picture differs significantly from that in larger urban areas in the United States where assaults are more often the result of violent crimes.

Alcohol use is the most significant contributing factor to all accidents in Western countries. In the Charlottesville study blood alcohol levels were obtained on 86 percent of all patients studied, with 72 percent having a blood alcohol level of 0.10 percent or higher. However, a Scottish study[18] revealed that disorientation does not occur, at least in Glasgow patients, until the blood level of alcohol is at least 200 mg/100 ml, and this may well reflect the high level of heavy drinking and alcoholism in the population of that city.

LOCATION OF INJURY

As expected from the large number of accidents, more than half (58 percent) of the head injuries in Virginia occurred on the highway. Most took place on small two-lane roads and secondary highways, and only 5 percent on the major interstate highways or freeways. In part, this is because there are fewer major highways in the localities studied and also because safety conditions on secondary roads are often poor. Twenty-six percent of the injuries occurred at home or school, and an additional 8 percent took place at work. These injuries, in some cases, could have been prevented with educational safety programs directed at hazards found in the home and at industrial sites. Therefore, health care professionals should take an active role in community-oriented programs directed toward preventive measures for the population at risk for head in-

jury. These include legislative changes and an increase in public awareness of the risks of driving while intoxicated.

TIME OF INJURY

Most studies show an increase in head trauma during the summer. For example, in the Minnesota study,[8] the occurrence of head trauma was highest in the summer and fall. Bicycle and motorcycle accidents were highest in the summer, whereas falls were slightly more common in the winter than in other seasons. In the Virginia series, the incidence of head injury was highest in September, partly because of the large number of students returning to school, followed closely by the three summer months. December, January, and February were found to have the lowest occurrence of injury.

As might be expected, nearly half all CNS injuries occurred during the weekend. Peak periods were Saturday (25 percent) and Sunday (20 percent). Similar data on time of occurrence can be very useful for health care planning and staffing for emergency departments and trauma wards. The daily occurrence of CNS injury shows a definite pattern, with the low point being between 5 and 6 AM and the peak occurring between 3 and 7 PM (26 percent). After 7 PM the occurrence rate progressively declines from midnight until 5 AM. Separating injured children from injured adults reveals that the former are injured most often after school hours, with a more extended time scale from 5 PM to midnight in the case of adults.[3]

SEVERITY OF INJURY

As mentioned previously, the University of Virginia is in a rural locality with a large geographic catchment area. Four community hospitals strategically located throughout this area refer all head injuries to the medical center. There is an area of approximately a 100-mile radius surrounding the University which is devoid of hospitals or emergency medical care. Because of the referral patterns, long periods of time occur between injury and treatment by either rescue squad personnel or community hospitals. Thus, 65 percent of the patients waited

30 minutes or longer for treatment and 20 percent did not receive emergency care for 3 hours or longer. More than 30 percent traveled distances greater than 30 miles to the hospital from the site of injury. It should be remembered that often events occurring during the first hour after injury decide the eventual outcome for the patient. Therefore, rapid transfer of the head injured patient to the hospital is important, and a long period in which the patient is susceptible to additional insults to the nervous system should be avoided. At the University of Virginia, the local hospital is assisted in arranging transfer by direct collaboration with the neurosurgical service. Through implementation of programs with early prehospital intervention, the morbidity and mortality of head injured patients can be greatly reduced, as shown many years ago in Britain. If further advances in this direction are to be made, individuals skilled in the management of head trauma must take an active role in training programs, seminars, and clinical practice sessions for personnel working in the prehospital and acute care areas and in rehabilitation.

In contrast to the situation in the larger metropolitan areas, all emergency vehicles and ambulances in central Virginia are staffed totally by volunteers and contain only equipment bought with contributions from community sources. The training of volunteer personnel in the care of the head injured patient at the site of injury is undertaken by the Department of Neurosurgery. The long transport times to the medical center mean that often the emergency medical technician (EMT) is responsible for the care of patients during the most critical time. Therefore, the major emphasis in training programs is placed on maintenance of the airway, ventilation, and adequate circulation with attention to the history, physical assessment, and various transport techniques. The importance of aggressive early management of the head injured patient cannot be overemphasized. Less than an hour's attention to the principles of basic life and brain support at an early stage may reduce the cost of later hospital care and rehabilitation by hundreds of days, thousands of man-hours, and tens of thousands of dollars. More importantly, appropriate critical care at the right time can conserve valuable human faculties that would otherwise be lost forever to the victim, the family, and the community. (See Chapter 3 for further discussion of acute management.)

GLASGOW COMA SCALE

At one time the study of the epidemiology, treatment, and outcome of head injuries was impaired because of difficulty in defining the type and severity of injury. It was only after the development of a method of grading the severity of injury that accurate figures on the incidence and outcome from head trauma could be obtained. In order to accomplish this goal and compare data among centers, the use of an injury severity scale has been implemented. Changes in the level of consciousness constitute the earliest sign of neurologic deterioration after head injury, and in order to measure this and thereby define the severity of head injury and predict its outcome, Teasdale and Jennett,[18] developed the Glasgow Coma Scale. It relates "consciousness" to motor response, verbal response, and eye opening (see Table 3–4, Chapter 3, and Chapter 5 for further discussion of the scale).

Of patients studied at the University of Virginia, 25 percent were in a coma at admission, with a Glasgow Coma Scale (GCS) of 8 or less according to the Teasdale and Jennett criteria, meaning that they had a severe brain injury.[18] The remaining patients had altered levels of consciousness, with 49 percent sustaining "minor head injuries" indicated by a GCS score of 12 or better. Those with scores of 9, 10, or 11 had moderate injuries. Much investigation has been directed toward severe head injuries (a Glasgow Coma Scale score of 8 or less). The Charlottesville study demonstrated that even patients sustaining minor head trauma were left with significant morbidity 3 months after discharge, but this observation has not been confirmed by others.[19]

In addition to the GCS scores, data were collected on loss of consciousness at the time of injury. Of all patients studied, 93 percent were unconscious following their injury; but only 42 percent of them were still unconscious upon arrival at the hospital. The majority of patients (54 percent) remained unconscious for 30 minutes or less. However, such data tend to be unreliable unless collected from a family member or close friend who witnessed the event. The duration of unconsciousness in many cases was also influenced by the prior alcohol intake of the patients.

CLINICAL COURSE

It is often the case that in a busy emergency department, head injured patients remain in diagnostic or holding units for long periods of time. In the Virginia study, 40 percent of the head injured patients remained in the emergency department for 4 hours or longer. The reasons for long delays in the emergency department are varied. Usually, however, the head injured patient presents a difficult diagnostic and management problem. The majority of patients studied received a skull roentgenogram (94 percent) while in the emergency department, and 34 percent underwent computed tomography (CT) scanning.

Two percent of those included in the study died in the emergency department before hospital admission, and of those admitted to the hospital, 22 percent required observation in an intensive care unit. During hospitalization, 39 percent underwent additional surgical procedures and 52 percent were assessed by a clinical service other than the hospital's neurosurgery department. Most frequently orthopedic surgery was involved because of the high incidence of fractures and concomitant spinal injuries. Many patients require a multidisciplinary approach to varied problems; this often involves designing a program to maximize the patient's abilities and at the same time developing plans that are feasible for the staff resources. Of the patients studied, 31 percent required physical therapy during their hospitalization, 17 percent needed occupational therapy, and 8 percent required speech therapy. Ideally such programs should be initiated during the acute management of the head injured patient to ensure that the patient has the maximum opportunity to recover. Through anticipation of the needs of the head injured patient, a comprehensive plan of care can be instituted resulting in a decrease in secondary physical and psychologic problems which

may require prolonged hospitalization and rehabilitation.

LENGTH OF HOSPITAL STAY

The majority of the Charlottesville patients (51 percent) were in the hospital for 7 days or less; however, 17 percent of those studied were hospitalized for more than 15 days. In the National Head and Spinal Cord Injury Survey,[6] patients under age 15 had the shortest stay, and those in the 15- to 24-year age group were in hospital for the longest periods. In the older population, medical complications often result in prolonged hospitalization. In the University of Virginia study, as well as that reported by the NIH, men remained in hospital longer than women. These findings suggest that not only are men more frequently the victim of head injuries than women, but also their injuries tend to be more severe.

OUTCOME

In the majority of outcome studies, mortality is based on patients sustaining nonpenetrating injuries to the head, which excludes gunshot wounds. At the University of Virginia, mortality among patients admitted with a Glasgow Coma Scale score of 8 or less was 70 percent overall; however, when gunshot wounds were excluded from the analysis, the mortality in the same group was reduced to 48 percent. In a further analysis of patients with nonpenetrating injuries, the mortality dropped dramatically with increasing Glasgow Coma Scale scores. Thus, in patients admitted with a score of 9, 10, or 11, mortality was 6 percent; in patients with scores of 12 and 13, mortality was 1 percent; and no patient with a score of 14 or 15 died. These data and those presented by others demonstrate the value of the Glasgow Coma Scale as a prognostic indicator of mortality after head injury.

The most important goal in the care of the surviving head injured patient is to maximize the chance for a good recovery, and every therapeutic intervention should be directed to this end. This demands a detailed knowledge of patterns of morbidity changes with time. In the past 10 to 15 years research studies of the natural history of the outcome from severe and minor brain injuries have shed a great deal of light on the process of recovery in terms of patients' short- and long-term physical, mental, behavioral, and social strengths and weaknesses. However, in contrast, there are relatively few hard scientific data on the way in which various methods of rehabilitation affect "natural recovery"; that is, recovery with minimal intervention.

Outcome at Discharge

Attempts have been made in many centers to categorize late outcome after head trauma, and the Glasgow Outcome Scale (GOS), developed by Jennett and Bond,[20] is widely used for this purpose (see Chapter 5). The scale served as a baseline method for assessing the degree of recovery achieved by the head injured patients in the Charlottesville study, and the survivors were placed in one of four categories depending on the degree of function and independence they attained. However, the scale is intended to provide only broad categories of morbidity and does not evaluate the often subtle cognitive impairment of the patient for which other measures are required. The results of the Glasgow Outcome Scale assessments at discharge for the patients in the study are summarized in Table 2–2.

Seventy-two percent of the patients returned home after discharge from acute care centers and 7 percent required additional hospital care at another facility. During this time, 14 percent of the entire head injured patient population were not considered self-sufficient in activities of daily living. Of these patients, 50 percent required institutional care and 50 percent were cared for by a family member. These figures demonstrate clearly that many patients with significant problems in their daily lives were in fact sent home without the benefit of rehabilitation. This was due in part to a shortage of appropriate facilities for the large number of injured seen each year.

The time taken for outcome to become stable has yet to be fully established. Studies using the GOS reveal that patients' overall levels of disability and dependence become stabilized within a year of injury.[21] However, caution is required when interpreting such an observation because, given the wide range of functions (physical, intellectual, and behavioral) times to stabilization vary considerably, being shortest for neurologic disabilities and longest for behavioral problems.

Outcome at 3 Months

In order to improve assessment of the impact of head trauma on the patient and family and to gain some knowledge about the recovery over time, all patients were seen in a follow-up University of Virginia clinic 3 months postinjury. At the clinic, the patient's physical and psychologic status was assessed. Data were collected from 79 percent of the injured on various outcome measures including the Glasgow Outcome Scale, employment status, and physical complaints expressed by the patients. The GOS was used as a baseline assessment of recovery at 3 months from time of injury, and the results are given in Table 2–3, from which it can be seen that 88 percent were only moderately disabled or had made a good recovery at this point.

Other factors noted in the assessment of

Table 2–2. GLASGOW OUTCOME SCALE (AT DISCHARGE), UNIVERSITY OF VIRGINIA STUDY

Dead	7%
Vegetative	4%
Severely disabled	8%
Moderately disabled	12%
Good recovery	69%

Table 2–3. GLASGOW OUTCOME SCALE (3 MONTHS POSTINJURY), UNIVERSITY OF VIRGINIA STUDY

Vegetative	4%
Severely disabled	8%
Moderately disabled	22%
Good recovery	66%

outcome were changes in employment and financial status caused by the injury. Thirty-three percent of the patients interviewed 3 months after discharge were unemployed because of their injury, and an additional 4 percent had changed their employment. Sixty-two percent of the total patients contacted at follow-up had some change in their financial status owing to their injury. In patients with multiple injuries, it was difficult to determine the extent to which the associated injuries affected the length of unemployment.

SUMMARY

The reason for evaluating epidemiologic data is that certain characteristics may thereby become evident which can be used in the identification of populations at risk for head trauma. Such information can be of value to individuals involved in the prevention of accidents leading to injury; in the stimulation of increasing awareness of the potential problems after hospital discharge for the patient, family, and community at large; and in rehabilitation.

REFERENCES

1. Partington, MW: The importance of accident-proneness in the aetiology of head injuries in children. Arch Dis Child 35:215, 1960.
2. It's an emergency. Newsweek, Nov. 21:105, 1977.
3. Field, JH: Epidemiology of head injuries in England and Wales. Her Majesty's Stationery Office, London, 1976.
4. Jaggar, J et al: Epidemiology of central nervous system trauma: Preliminary findings presented at 107th APHA Meeting, November 1979.
5. Jennett, B and MacMillan, R: Epidemiology of head injury. Br Med J 282:101, 1981.
6. Kalsbeek, WD et al: The National Head and Spinal Cord Injury Survey: Major findings. J Neurosurg 53:519, 1980.
7. Caveness, WF: Incidence of craniocerebral trauma in the United States in 1976 with trends from 1970 to 1975. Adv Neurol 22:1, 1979.
8. Annegers, JF et al: The incidence, causes, and secular trends of head trauma in Olmstead County, Minnesota, 1935–1974. Neurology 30:912, 1980.
9. Klauber, MR et al: The epidemiology of head injury: A prospective study of an entire community—San Diego County, California, 1978. Am J Epidemiol 113:500, 1981.
10. Krause, JF et al: The incidence of acute brain injury and serious impairment in a defined population. Am J Epidemiol 119 (2):186, 1984.
11. Whitman, S, Conley-Hoganson, R, and Desai, BT: Comparative head trauma experience in two socioeconomically different Chicago communities: A population study. Am J Epidemiol 119(4):570, 1984.
12. Frankowski, RF, Annegers, JF, and Whitman, S: The descriptive epidemiology of head injury in the United States. In Becker, DP and Povlichock, JT (eds): Central Nervous System Research Status Report, 1985, p 33.
13. Rimel, RW et al: Disability caused by minor head injury. Neurosurgery 9:221, 1981.
14. Rimel, RW et al: Completing the clinical spectrum of brain trauma. Neurosurgery 11:344, 1982.
15. Rimel, RW: Understanding the complete spectrum of head trauma. Presented at meeting of American Association of Neurological Surgeons, Washington, DC, April, 1983.
16. Selecki, BR et al: A retrospective study of neurotraumatic admission to a teaching hospital: Part 1. General aspects. Med J Aust 2:113, 1967.
17. Galbraith, S et al: The relationship between alcohol and head injury and its effect on conscious level. Br J Surg 63:138, 1976.
18. Teasdale, G and Jennett, B: Assessment of coma and impaired consciousness: A practical scale. Lancet 2:81, 1974.
19. Gentillini, M et al: Neuropsychological evaluation of mild head injury. J Neurol Neurosurg Psychiatry 48:137, 1985.
20. Jennett, B and Bond, MR: Assessment of outcome after severe brain damage. Lancet 1:489, 1975.
21. Bond, MR and Brooks, DN: Understanding the process of recovery as a basis for the investigation of rehabilitation for the brain injured. Scand J Rehab Med 8:127, 1976.
22. National Center for Health Statistics: Acute Conditions. Incidence and Associated Disability, United States, July 1974–June 1975. Vital Health Statistics, Series 10, No. 99, DHEW Publ. No. (HRA) 75-1526. Washington, DC, US Government Printing Office, 1977.
23. National Center for Health Statistics: Utilization of Short-Stay Hospitals. Annual Summary for the United States, 1975 Vital and Health Statistics, Series 13, No. 31, DHEW Publ. No. (HRA) 77-1783. Washington, DC, US Government Printing Office, 1977.

Section I Conclusion

MICHAEL R. BOND, M.D., Ph.D.

THE NATURE OF THE PROBLEM

The information contained in the two chapters in this section, describing the scale and scope of the problem of head injury and the characteristics of the injured, reveal quite clearly that the majority of those who are severely traumatically brain injured are adolescents and young adult males in the lower social and economic groups in society, irrespective of their country of origin. Also, they represent a relatively small proportion of the total number of those who suffer head injuries. However, the way in which their injuries occur and the problems of the severely injured and their families do vary with their country of origin, as the contrast between patients from the United States and those from Scotland reveals. Despite these differences, however, commonly accepted measurements of the severity of injury and outcome used in several countries show that in terms of the severity of injury, outcome in physical and cognitive terms does not differ appreciably, whatever the cause of the injury and the origins of the person impaired. In other words, effects and injury on the brain produce features common to all and, presumably, reflect structural brain damage. The initial consequences of injury are greater among those in the older age groups, but sex differences do not appear to occur. It will be revealed in later chapters that for longer-term outcome, the behavioral and emotional consequences of injury and the degree of adaptation to deficits are more prominent than are physical problems. The former vary to a great extent among individuals and are related to the personal, family, and professional resources available to them. Looked at in a different way, the recovery of physical function takes place over a relatively short period, and the greater part of it is completed within the year of injury. In contrast, emotional and behavioral changes vary much more in terms of the times at which they appear. In fact, some of the emotional and behavioral changes that appear soon after injury lessen with time, whereas others worsen, and new ones develop as the process of recovery takes place. The extent to which the physical, emotional, behavioral, and social problems can be ameliorated depends upon the amount and nature of rehabilitation available. Rehabilitation is a matter not only of quantity but also of quality, and this raises a final question—namely, does rehabilitation profit the brain injured patient and if so, in what ways and by what mechanisms?—a question that is considered later in detail in this book.

EARLY METHODS OF ASSESSMENT AND EVALUATION

J. Douglas Miller, M.D., Ph.D., Editor

Chapter 3

Early Evaluation and Management

J. DOUGLAS MILLER, M.D., Ph.D.
BRIAN PENTLAND, B.Sc.(Hons), M.B.Ch.B.
SHELDON BERROL, M.D.

The final outcome in any patient who suffers head injury is governed by three groups of factors: the preinjury status of the brain, the total amount of immediate damage done to the brain by the impact of the head injury (primary brain damage), and the cumulative effect of secondary pathological damage to the already injured brain, produced by systemic and intracranial mechanisms that come into play at various times after the accident that caused the head injury.[1] The outcome from such a complex of brain injury can be considered in terms of mortality and of morbidity in surviving patients. The rate and extent of recovery in survivors is also influenced by rehabilitation measures, the form that they take, and the timing of their application. Ideal management of head injured patients is aimed at minimizing the primary impact damage to the brain and preventing or treating secondary insults so as to provide the best possible milieu for recovery consistent with the premorbid status of the brain, then beginning the process of neurobehavioral assessment and rehabilitation as soon as feasible.

This chapter describes the pathophysiology of head injury—the ways in which primary and secondary brain damage are produced. A system of assessment and diagnosis is presented that provides for rapid triage of cases so as to provide urgent treatment to those patients who most require it. The principles and practice of managing head injured patients are described, starting at the scene of the accident and following the patient in transit, through the emergency room to the intensive care unit and the ward. Indications for surgical treatment are defined and surgical procedures described briefly. Prognosis of head injury is considered, particularly factors that forecast disability in survivors. The principles of early assessment for rehabilitation are described together with the earliest measures. The criteria for transfer of recovering head injured patients to the neurorehabilitation unit are also considered.

PATHOPHYSIOLOGY OF HEAD INJURY

Premorbid Status of the Brain

Although head injuries occur most commonly in young men, they can and do affect all sectors of the community, including persons who may have already sustained some form of brain damage. In virtually all forms of head injury—mild, moderate, and severe—variable numbers of cerebral neurons and axons are irreversibly injured. When a head injury occurs to a person who has already lost a sizeable number of neurons because of previous brain disease or injury, but has made a good recovery from that prior insult, the result of the second head injury is usually much worse.

A 54-year-old man slipped while cleaning a chicken coop, striking his head on a concrete floor. The patient was unconscious for 15 minutes but thereafter recovered consciousness fully. He was admitted to the hospital for observation because he had been unconscious and because skull x-ray films revealed a linear skull fracture. When a full history was obtained, it transpired that 1 year previously the same patient had been involved in an automobile accident and had sustained a closed head injury that had rendered him unconscious for 5 days. The patient had made a good recovery from this injury and had returned after 2 months to his occupation of farming, functioning apparently as well as he did prior to injury. Following this second, evidently less severe injury, however, the patient never fully recovered. His personality changed completely; he was unable to manage any of his own affairs, never ventured out of the house unless accompanied by someone else, was incapable of making even the simplest decisions, lost interest in all social and sexual activities, and was described by his wife as having become a completely different person.

For similar reasons, in patients who have already suffered stroke, hydrocephalus, or meningoencephalitis, a relatively minor head injury can be crippling. In addition, the older the patient who sustains a head injury, the less satisfactory recovery is likely to be. A particular problem is head injury in elderly patients who are already on the verge of senile dementia. (This problem is discussed at greater length in Chapter 17, Minor Head Injury.)

Thus, when assessing the potential for recovery of any head injured patient, it is important to establish the preinjury status of that patient. This can be derived from school or college tests, previous medical examinations, results of job interviews, or interviews with members of the family. This status defines the upper limit for recovery for that particular patient, and in a number of head injured patients, that limit may fall far short of "normal."

Primary Impact Damage to the Brain

Depending on the nature, direction, and magnitude of the forces applied to the skull, brain, and body at impact, primary damage to the brain may be of any or all of the following three types.[2]

LOCAL BRAIN DAMAGE

Local damage refers to a brain injury that is localized to the site of impact on the skull. The damage may take the form of contusion or laceration, or both. It may be superficial or it may extend deeply into the brain from the surface. It may be mild, consisting of slight subpial hemorrhage, or severe, with extensive brain necrosis, pulping, hematoma, and a surrounding area of perifocal brain edema. Because of such edema, the damaged area may swell and act as an intracranial space occupying lesion. When the local injury has been of sufficient severity to interrupt the pial surface so as to cause laceration of the brain, then secondary bleeding may produce subdural or intracerebral hematoma, or both. In the early stages the propensity of such local lesions to be associated with telltale neurologic signs depends entirely upon the location of the injury. When, for example, the local injury is over the motor cortex, contralateral weakness of the face and arm may be expected. On the other hand, when the lesion is frontal, there may be little or no evident neurologic dysfunction, unless the process involves both frontal lobes, in which case there is likely to be considerable behavioral disturbance.

When perifocal brain swelling progresses to the point at which brain shift and herniation occur, then a new set of neurologic signs may emerge, the so-called false localizing signs. These include oculomotor or abducent nerve palsies and unilateral weakness of the arm and leg, which may be ipsilateral to the swollen hemisphere.

POLAR BRAIN DAMAGE

When the head is subjected to acceleration or deceleration, the brain can move within the skull and dural envelope to a limited extent. When this motion is suddenly arrested, the frontal and temporal lobes impact against the walls of the anterior and middle cranial fossae, and damage is done to the tips and undersurface of the temporal and frontal lobes. This damage is also in the form of contusion and/or laceration to the brain. Damage to the occipital pole can also occur but is much less common. Just as with local brain injury, these polar lesions can swell, be subject to hemorrhage and form sizeable intracranial mass lesions. Because of their frequent anterior and unilateral location, such lesions are often not associated with abnormal neurologic signs until the mass effect produces brain distortion and shift. This process may take 2 or 3 days. These polar lesions are one reason for delayed deterioration after head injury. Hemorrhage within a polar lesion may also explain a lucid interval, in which a patient who has been briefly comatose recovers consciousness but then deteriorates into coma once more.

A 45-year-old man fell in the street after a drinking bout, was briefly unconscious, and was admitted to the hospital in a lethargic state, able to speak but confused and disoriented. No focal neurologic signs were detected. There was a linear skull fracture in the right temporal bone. On the second day after injury, the patient was recognized to have expressive dysphasia, right homonymous hemianopia, and mild weakness of the right face and arm. Angiography revealed a large right temporal mass that proved at operation to be a combination of contused brain and subdural and intracerebral hematoma.

DIFFUSE BRAIN INJURY (FIG. 3–1)

As a further consequence of the movement that the brain may make inside the cranial cavity during head injury, widely

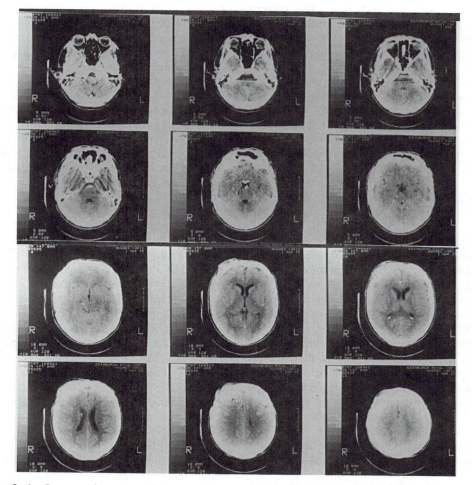

Figure 3–1. Computed tomography series in a patient with diffuse brain damage. The patient was rendered immediately and deeply comatose (E1, M2, V1) by high-speed traffic accident. There are small hemorrhages scattered widely in the brain but the ventricular system shows no compression or shift, indicating that intracranial pressure is not increased at this time.

scattered shearing of axons within their myelin sheaths may occur.[3] This damage to the subcortical white matter is not intense in any single location. The cumulative effect of diffuse axonal injury is, nevertheless, dramatic. In patients who have suffered this form of brain injury in relative isolation from focal and polar damage, the neurologic picture is fairly typical. The patient is deeply comatose from the time of injury, with abnormal motor function consisting most frequently of extensor posturing of both the upper and lower limbs, occurring spontaneously or in response to painful stimulation.[4] The coma results from impairment of function of the reticular activating system in the brainstem. The patient remains in this state for many weeks, during which time spontaneous eye opening returns. This patient does not, however, give any evidence of an organized response to the environment, and recovery is limited to a severely disabled or vegetative state. If death occurs, usually because of an intercurrent infection or other medical problem associated with prolonged coma, autopsy reveals a brain that looks externally normal, but in which there is a moderate degree of ventricular enlargement. Microscopic examination of such a brain reveals scattered axon retraction balls in the white matter and microglial stars with demyelination in those areas where the scattered axons converge into tracts, for example, the cerebral peduncles.[5] Common accompanying injuries are tearing of the corpus callosum, gliding contusions of the medial side of the cerebral hemisphere and dorsolateral contusion of the mid-brain, all produced when the mobile brain impacts or moves against relatively rigid dural structures.[3]

When this type of diffuse brain injury is particularly severe, the areas of damage may be larger, forming distinct petechial hemorrhages in the white matter. With increasing severity of injury such lesions extend inward from the subcortical white matter to the mid-brain and brainstem. In some cases there is a deeply placed area of hemorrhage or contusion located in the basal ganglia.

A 24-year-old competition motorcyclist fell from his machine while racing at a speed of over 100 mph. He was found in an opisthotonic posture with spontaneous extension of all four limbs and arching of his back. His crash helmet was intact and the skull was not fractured. Urgent CT showed no intracranial hematoma, and intracranial pressure was only moderately increased. Three weeks later he was opening his eyes, but both arms were held in an abnormal flexed posture while his legs remained rigidly in extension. Three months later, CT showed moderate ventricular dilatation and he had neither spoken nor obeyed any command.

Primary Impact Damage to the Scalp, Skull, Dura, and Other Structures

In head injury, the brain is seldom, if ever, injured in isolation. Injuries to the structures that surround the brain are significant for two reasons. They may provide a clue as to the site and nature of the impact, and they may in themselves be responsible for complications that can play a major role in affecting the outcome from injury. Examples would be epidural hemorrhage complicating linear skull fracture to produce severe brain compression, or meningitis complicating a basal skull fracture.

Fractures of the skull may be linear (Fig. 3–2) or depressed (Fig. 3–3). The significance of a fracture of the skull is often a hotly debated medicolegal issue. To the layperson, the presence of a skull fracture signifies that a great deal of force has been exerted against the skull; hence, there must also be a considerable degree of brain damage and thus a severe head injury. While this is true in a number of cases, there are important exceptions to the rule. When no motion is imparted to the head but the skull has been crushed, extensive linear fractures can result with little or no associated brain damage. More importantly, however, absence of a skull fracture cannot be taken as proof that no significant brain damage has taken place. In children, the capacity of the skull to bend in relation to a distorting force can permit considerable brain injury to occur in the absence of skull fracture. When the accelerating or decelerating force is widely applied to the whole head, considerable brain damage in the form of diffuse axonal injury may occur in the absence of any identifiable skull fracture. Conversely, when damage to the skull is extremely localized, as that produced, for example, from a blow from a hammer or axe, there is local damage

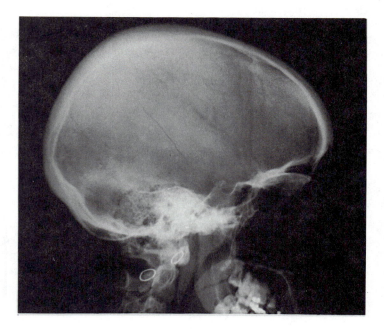

Figure 3–2. Lateral skull x-ray film showing a linear fracture in temporoparietal area. The clear, straight line of the fracture contrasts with the softer, wavy outline of the normal skull vascular marking.

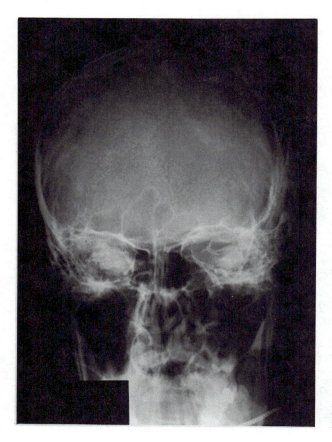

Figure 3–3. Anteroposterior skull x-ray film showing depressed fracture.

to the skull in the form of a depressed fracture with in-driven bone fragments. There may be severe focal damage in the underlying brain, yet brain function elsewhere may be undisturbed (Fig. 3–4). Thus, 50 percent of patients who sustain depressed skull fractures have either never been unconscious, or have been unconscious for only a few moments.[6] This is because the localized injury does not disturb the reticular formation of the brainstem. Four fifths of the 67 cases of depressed fracture of the skull seen at the University of Edinburgh in a 2-year period have been in patients classified as having a minor head injury with only a brief or no loss of consciousness.[7]

The principal significance of damage to the skull is that it may be associated with bleeding that, if inside the cranial cavity, soon becomes an urgent problem in its own right because of the limited space available for expansion of the hematoma.[8] There is a strong association between the presence of a skull fracture and the presence of an intracranial hematoma (Table 3–1). Of particular importance is the combination of skull fracture with any depression of the level of consciousness, with focal neurologic signs, or the presence of a seizure. In all of these instances, the risk that the fracture is associated with an intracranial hematoma is high

and CT scanning should be a matter of urgency.[9]

If a compound skull fracture is associated with dural tearing, introduction of infection

Table 3–1. ASSOCIATION BETWEEN SKULL FRACTURE AND PRESENCE OF INTRACRANIAL HEMATOMA

	Hematoma	None	Total
Severe			
Skull fracture	47 (43%)	63	110
None	32 (33%)	64	96
Total	79 (38%)	127	206
$\chi^2 = 1.91$; n.s.			
Moderate			
Skull fracture	31 (23%)	105	136
None	19 (7%)	247	266
Total	50 (12%)	352	402
$\chi^2 = 20.24$; p <0.001			
Minor			
Skull fracture	19 (7%)	253	272
None	12 (0.6%)	1955	1967
Total	31 (1.4%)	2208	2239
$\chi^2 = 71.13$; p <0.001			

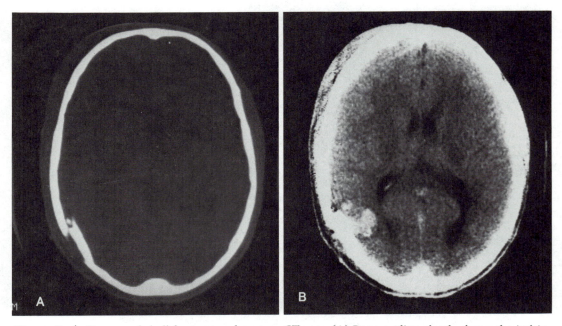

Figure 3–4. Depressed skull fracture as shown on CT scan. (A) Bone outline clearly shows the indriving of the skull. (B) Brain tissue images show an underlying hemorrhagic contusion.

into the intracranial cavity is facilitated.[6] The integrity of the dural envelope is of considerable importance. If the dura remains intact, intracranial infection as a complication of head injury is extremely rare: if the dura is torn, infection is an ever-present possibility.

> A 4-year-old boy was admitted from an infectious diseases hospital to the neurosurgical unit with meningitis and a small puncture wound in the forehead that oozed watery fluid. Five days previously, he had fallen in the home and impaled himself on the axle of a toy truck. This had been pulled out by the mother. When the child became ill 3 days later with headache, vomiting, and fever, the injury was not mentioned to the family doctor, and the patient was referred to the infectious disease hospital as a case of meningitis. The puncture wound in the forehead extended through the skull and dura mater into the frontal lobe. The meningitis was clearly related to this injury.

Secondary Insults to the Injured Brain

The energy requirements of the brain are extremely high. The blood flow to the brain accounts for one fifth of resting cardiac output and its oxygen consumption is one sixth of that consumed by the whole body, despite the fact that the brain represents only one fiftieth of total body weight. There is no capacity for storage of energy-rich substrates so that the supply of oxygen and glucose to the brain must be not only plentiful but continuous. Interruption of the supply is followed within 15 seconds by neurologic dysfunction and within a few minutes by neuronal damage that soon becomes irreversible if the substrate supply is not restored. It is unfortunate that following severe head injury, several conditions occur frequently, all of which conspire in one way or another to decrease the energy supply to the injured brain.[10] These insults may be of systemic or of intracranial origin (Table 3–2).

Secondary brain insults of systemic origin are frequently related to the presence of concomitant injuries elsewhere in the body. In patients with head injuries, multiple injuries are extremely common. In 1986 in the Head and Spinal Injury Unit in Edinburgh, 60 percent of 113 cases of severe head in-

Table 3–2. SECONDARY SYSTEMIC AND INTRACRANIAL INSULTS IN THE INJURED BRAIN

Systemic	Intracranial
Arterial hypoxemia	Hematoma—extradural, subdural, intracerebral
Arterial hypotension	
Hypercapnia	Raised pressure—brain swelling, brain edema, acute hydrocephalus
Anemia	
Pyrexia	
Hyponatremia	Infection—meningitis, abscess/empyema
Hypoglycemia	
	Epilepsy
	Vasospasm

jury and 40 percent of 193 cases of moderate head injury had one or more additional systemic injuries. These figures are typical for case series reported from North America, Europe, and Asia.

Arterial Hypoxemia

The most common of the systemic brain insults is arterial hypoxemia. This is present in more than one third of severely head injured patients when they arrive at a major hospital from the scene of the accident.[11] Its prevalence after arrival in the hospital, during transit between the emergency room and other departments, and in the neurosurgical intensive care unit, is as yet unknown. Until recently, establishment of the presence of hypoxemia depended upon withdrawal of an arterial blood sample and measurement of arterial Po_2 With the recent advent of continuous transcutaneous pulse oximetry, more comprehensive data on the prevalence of hypoxemia after head injury can be obtained. When arterial Po_2 falls below 7 kPa (approximately 55 mmHg) desaturation of arterial blood begins to occur, with a consequent fall in the volume of oxygen carried per unit volume of blood. Under normal circumstances, this fall in oxygen content would be compensated for by a brisk cerebral vasodilatation. In the damaged brain, however, a compensatory boost in blood flow does not occur or occurs to a lesser extent, with the net result that there is a reduction in carriage of oxygen to the most severely injured parts of the brain.[12]

Causes of arterial hypoxemia range from obstruction of the airway by blood or foreign bodies to poor positioning of the patient so that the tongue falls back to obstruct the airway; inhalation or aspiration of regurgitated gastric contents is an ever-present risk in the head injured patient, and injury to the chest may result in pneumothorax, hemothorax, or pulmonary contusion. Brain injury is associated with impairment of the rhythm and depth of respiration and is also associated with abnormalities in the relationship between ventilation and perfusion of the lung. The majority of head injured patients have normal lung function prior to injury so that it is somewhat of a surprise to find that nearly all severely head injured (comatose) patients have some degree of impairment of oxygenation in the lung. In the majority of cases this can be compensated for by increasing the fraction of inspired oxygen, but in severe cases the hypoxemia is progressive and leads to pulmonary edema or adult respiratory distress syndrome, or both. The combination of abnormalities in the rate and rhythm of respiration and in oxygenation in the pulmonary vascular bed is a strong argument in favor of artificial ventilation of the severely head injured. Thus, hypoxemia can be regarded as a complication either of head injury alone or of multiple injuries that include the upper abdomen and thorax.

Arterial Hypotension

In the normal person in whom arterial blood pressure is progressively reduced, compensatory cerebrovascular dilatation preserves cerebral blood flow in the normal range despite the fall in perfusion pressure. Under these normal conditions, cerebral blood flow does not fall until systolic arterial pressure is less than 80 mmHg and mean arterial pressure less than 60 mmHg. In the injured brain this capacity for maintenance of normal cerebral blood flow, autoregulation, is impaired or abolished, either on a focal basis or globally if the injury is of sufficient severity.[13] The severely head injured patient is, therefore, extremely vulnerable to the effects of a reduction of blood pressure below the normal range, because any fall in blood pressure can lead to a reduction in cerebral blood flow. It is likely that in the head injured patient systolic blood pressure levels of less than 100 mmHg and mean arterial pressure levels of less than 80 mmHg will be associated with reduced cerebral blood flow.

Arterial hypotension is seldom produced by head injury alone. In virtually all cases, arterial hypotension results from another injury concomitant with the head injury.[14] The most frequent sources of arterial hypotension are intra-abdominal visceral injuries and fractures of the pelvis associated with large volume blood loss.[15] Because of the high frequency of multiple injuries in head injured patients arterial hypotension occurs in approximately 1 in 6 severely head injured patients. Systolic pressure levels less than 90 mmHg occurred in 16 percent of 225 severely head injured patients presenting to the Medical College of Virginia hospitals and in 15 percent of 206 severely head injured patients presenting to the Head and Spinal Injury Unit in Edinburgh. In all hypotensive cases, the patients had suffered significant additional major systemic injuries that included fractures of the pelvis, injuries to the abdominal and thoracic viscera, and major long bone fractures. When systolic arterial pressure is less than 100 mmHg in an adult head injured patient, an assiduous search should be made for a source of blood loss and in most cases this should include peritoneal lavage or minilaparotomy to detect occult intra-abdominal bleeding. In a series of 60 consecutive severely head injured patients in whom peritoneal lavage was carried out, intra-abdominal blood was detected in 10 cases. Subsequent intra-abdominal exploration confirmed a major source of hemorrhage in all 10 patients.[15]

Under special circumstances, low arterial pressure may be the result of head injury alone. In young children, blood loss from a scalp laceration or intracranial hematoma may attain a sufficient fraction of the total blood volume to cause arterial hypotension. In patients who sustain a high cervical spinal cord transection in addition to the head injury, spinal shock may be associated with arterial hypotension. Rarely, traumatic section of the pituitary stalk may produce late arterial hypotension. Finally, in patients who have severe and unrelieved brain compression, the onset of brain death can be associated with terminal arterial hypotension due to impending failure of the vasopressor centers in the brainstem.

Anemia

While traditional teaching is that traumatic hemorrhage is followed only sometime later by significant hemodilution and lowering of the hematocrit, a reduced hematocrit is not uncommon as a finding in head injured patients on admission to the hospital. Hematocrit levels of less than 30 percent were present in 10 percent of a series of 225 severely head injured patients seen in the Medical College of Virginia. The presence of a low hematocrit in a person who was not considered to be anemic prior to injury should prompt a search for blood loss that may also include peritoneal lavage.

Hyponatremia

Following severe head injury the blood electrolytes must be carefully monitored. Of particular significance is the serum sodium level, which must not be allowed to fall below 120 mEq/1. The danger of hyponatremia lies in the accompanying reduction of serum osmolality and the tendency of damaged brain to imbibe water osmotically from the bloodstream. This can result in severe brain swelling. Causes of hyponatremia include the retention of body water because of stress-induced natriuresis followed by secretion of antidiuretic hormone, or inappropriate secretion of antidiuretic hormone, a complication of certain types of brain damage. Another cause is dilutional hyponatremia, due to replacement of mixed electrolyte and water body fluid losses by overinfusion with dextrose solutions.

Intracranial Hematoma Following Trauma

An important concept in head injury management is the definition of "avoidable" factors that may lead to death or disability. This concept is most graphically illustrated in the case of patients who "talk and die."[16] These are patients who are observed to be talking after the injury but who later lapse into coma and die. In such cases the primary brain injury is not great, as the patients are able to talk but the secondary insult is gravely disabling or fatal.

Late diagnosis of intracranial hematoma stands out as the most important avoidable factor in all reports.[17-19] Whatever the severity of the injury, ranging from the mildest bump with no loss of consciousness to the most severe injury associated with instant and prolonged loss of consciousness, there is always some risk that intracranial bleeding may complicate the injury, producing coma and threatening life. Such hemorrhage most commonly begins at the time of injury: by the time of hospital admission, on average 3 hours later, a 40 percent incidence of intracranial hematoma was recorded in two series of 160 and 225 comatose head injured patients.[11, 20]

The classic clinical picture of intracranial hematoma after head injury is of a short period of unconsciousness immediately after impact, followed by partial or full restoration of consciousness then a secondary loss of consciousness, now due to compression of the brain by the expanding hematoma. A "lucid interval" occurs in only a portion of head injured patients. Many more patients with intracranial hematomas are in coma from the outset. If the hematoma remains undetected and untreated, such patients will show progressive deterioration of neurologic function, then of respiratory and cardiovascular function, leading to death.

Intracranial hematomas may be subdivided into those that are extradural and those that are intradural; or, alternatively, into those that are intracerebral and those that are extracerebral. In practice the simplest subdivision is into extradural (or epidural) hematoma, subdural hematoma, and intracerebral hematoma classifications.

The epidural hematoma is formed of solid clotted blood and in adults is virtually always associated with a fracture of the skull (Fig. 3–5). Bleeding occurs when the fracture line traverses the middle meningeal vessels or other vascular channels. As the hematoma expands, the dura mater is stripped from the inner surface of the skull. The most common location for an epidural hematoma is in the temporal region (70 percent), but they are also found in the frontal and occipital regions, at the vertex, or in the posterior cranial fossa.

Also formed of solid clotted blood, the acute subdural hematoma develops between the inner surface of the dura and brain (Fig. 3–6). Subdural hemorrhage may originate from veins linking the brain surface with the dura. They are torn by the motion of the

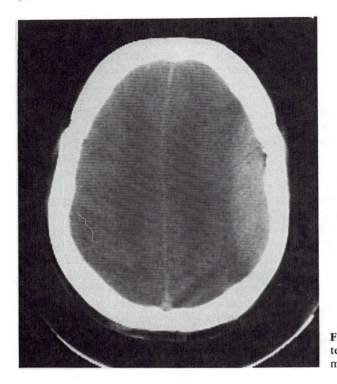

Figure 3–5. CT scan showing the characteristic biconvex density of an epidural hematoma.

Figure 3–6. CT scan showing an extensive acute subdural hematoma, concave-convex in shape, and of mainly increased radiodensity, confirming its composition of solid clotted blood. The contralateral ventricle is shifted and dilated, indicating that intracranial pressure will be high.

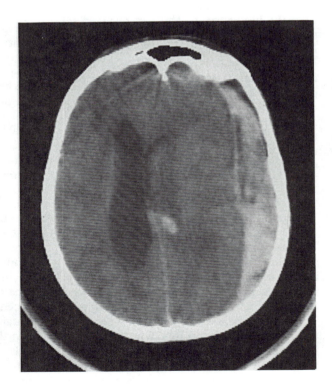

brain relative to the inside of the skull that occurs with sudden acceleration or deceleration. The lesion is more likely to occur when the brain is atrophic, as seen in the elderly or in persons who are suffering from alcohol-induced brain atrophy (Fig. 3–7). Another source of acute subdural hemorrhage is bleeding from a small sclerotic artery on the surface of the brain. The most common source of acute subdural hemorrhage, however, is bleeding from the edges of a cerebral laceration. In such cases there is usually a combination of subdural and intracerebral blood clot. This event occurs not infrequently at the frontal or temporal pole when it is characterized by the term "burst temporal lobe."

Intracerebral hematomas may form as described in conjunction with acute subdural hematoma or in isolation deeper within the brain. Patients who are receiving anticoagulant therapy are at particular risk of developing intracerebral bleeding related to contusions (Fig. 3–8).

Brain Swelling and Edema

In acute head injury, an increase in brain bulk is commonly identified on CT scans carried out within the first 24 hours. Such swelling can be identified by collapse of the ventricular system with loss of the image of the third ventricle and loss of the cerebrospinal fluid (CSF) cisterns around the midbrain. This appearance on CT carries a strong association with the development of raised intracranial pressure.[21] The appearance is often loosely referred to as posttraumatic brain edema. In fact, this is a misnomer. The true definition of brain edema is an increase in brain volume because of an increase in brain tissue water content, but there is no evidence that in this early form of brain swelling the brain tissue water content is increased. The evidence suggests rather that the increase in brain bulk is congestive brain swelling due to an increase in the cerebral blood volume. This is not to state that true brain edema never occurs following trauma. It does so later and may take one of several different forms.[22]

Vasogenic brain edema is due to outpouring of protein-rich fluid through damaged vessels related to cerebral contusions. The process is most pronounced at the periphery of the contusion and results in the appearance of a "halo" of perifocal edema.

Cytotoxic edema is found in relation to hypoxic and ischemic brain damage and is

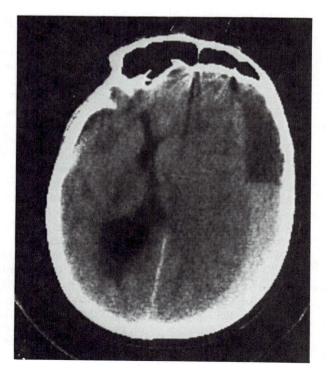

Figure 3–7. CT scan showing a chronic subdural hematoma, distinguished from the acute hematoma by its radiolucency, indicating that the contents are liquid. In this case there is layering of the contents, with thicker blood settling to the lower part of the hematoma cavity.

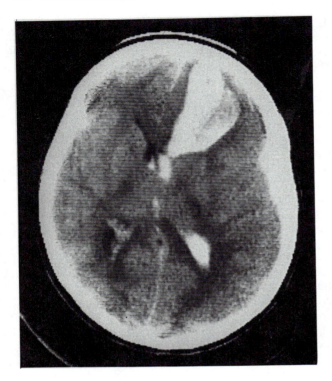

Figure 3–8. CT scan showing an extensive traumatic intracerebral hematoma in the subfrontal region. There is also intraventricular hemorrhage. This patient had impairment of the blood clotting mechanisms.

produced when the energy supply to the cells fails, resulting in malfunction of the cell wall pumping systems and imbibition of water by the dying cells. Cytotoxic edema is therefore intracellular in location, in contradistinction to vasogenic edema which is extracellular and tends to be located mainly in white matter, where it is easier for the extracellular fluid to percolate among the white matter tracts.

Hydrostatic edema is produced when previously compressed brain is subjected to surgical decompression, followed by a rapid increase in cerebral perfusion pressure due to a surge of arterial hypertension or to sudden reduction of intracranial pressure. Cerebral perfusion pressure is equivalent to the difference between these pressures and can therefore be equally affected by changes in arterial or intracranial pressure. In this form of edema the cerebral resistance vessels are usually impaired functionally, with impaired autoregulation, and the increased head of intravascular pressure is transmitted into the capillary bed with a net outpouring of water. The fluid in this form of edema is protein poor, however, and thus distinct from vasogenic edema.

Hypo-osmotic edema may occur when hyponatremia becomes severe. This is a diffuse process.

Raised Intracranial Pressure

Because intracranial hemorrhage and brain swelling occur in what is virtually a rigidly enclosed space, it is not surprising that intracranial pressure (ICP) should frequently be elevated in patients with head injury. In two consecutive series of severely head injured patients in whom ICP was monitored, abnormal elevations of ICP were recorded at some time in more than 50 percent of patients.[11, 23] Based on this experience, indications for monitoring ICP in head injured patients are shown in Table 3–3.

In the normal adult, pressure in the subarachnoid or intraventricular CSF spaces should remain in the range of 0 to 10 mmHg in the recumbent position. Pressures over 20 mmHg are definitely abnormal, and when ICP reaches 40 mmHg there is neurologic dysfunction and impairment of brain electrical activity in head injured patients. This is because, at pressures over 40 mmHg,

Table 3–3. INDICATIONS FOR ARTIFICIAL VENTILATION AND FOR CONTINUOUS RECORDING OF INTRACRANIAL PRESSURE

1. After evacuation of intracranial hematoma if patient in coma (GCS ≤8) beforehand
2. No hematoma but patient in deep coma (GCS ≤6)
3. Patient in coma (GCS ≤8) and CT shows signs of raised ICP (absence of third ventricle and of perimesencephalic CSF cisterns)
4. Combination of moderate/severe head injury (GCS ≤12) and severe chest or facial injuries

ICP becomes a limiting factor in the regulation of cerebral blood flow. A minimum cerebral perfusion pressure of 50 mmHg is necessary in the normal subject. In the head injured patient, the minimum required perfusion pressure may be much higher. While severe elevations of ICP, over 60 mmHg, almost always result in death, even the milder elevations of ICP from 20 to 40 mmHg are associated with increased morbidity in survivors.[23, 24]

Intracranial Infection

Intracranial infection as a complication of a head injury is always a tragedy.[25] Such an occurrence should be preventable; moreover, meningitis, suppurative encephalitis, or brain abscess all add rapidly and insidiously to morbidity and mortality. The development of meningitis in a comatose head injured patient is extremely hard to detect. Nuchal rigidity and mild elevation of body temperature (to 38.5°C [101.3°F]) are common sequelae of traumatic subarachnoid hemorrhage. The only feature that indicates that these signs are due to meningitis and not to subarachnoid blood is unexplained deterioration in the neurologic status of the patient. If the patient is already deeply comatose, this deterioration may take the patient to the point of death before the meningitis is detected.

Intracranial infection can arise because of compound injuries of the skull via a scalp puncture or laceration; basal skull fractures may be compound if the fracture extends into one of the paranasal air sinuses or the middle ear. Postoperative intracranial infection may occur because of inadequate debridement of a contaminated wound, or as a complication of surgery. Introduction of intraventricular or subdural catheters for measurement of intracranial pressure is another potential source of intracranial infection. The dura mater is an extremely effective barrier to the development of intracranial infection. When it is breached either traumatically or surgically, the possibility of meningitis or abscess formation must always be considered.

Cerebral Arterial Vasospasm

Narrowing of cerebral arteries, associated with focal or general reduction in cerebral blood flow and impairment of neurologic status, is a well-recognized sequel of spontaneous subarachnoid hemorrhage. Despite the fact that trauma is the most common cause of blood in the subarachnoid space, the possibility of post-traumatic cerebral vasospasm is less well recognized. It has, however, been well described, but replacement of cerebral arteriography by CT as the most common radiologic investigation of the head injured patient has meant that information as to the prevalence of cerebral vasospasm in severe injuries is no longer obtained. Nevertheless, the clinician should be aware of this possibility.[26]

Hydrocephalus

The normal pathways by which CSF passes from the ventricular system over the surface of the brain to be absorbed into the cerebral venous sinus system can be obstructed as a result of copious subarachnoid hemorrhage following head injury, or during the resolution of basal meningitis. When the CSF pathways have been obstructed in this way, the ventricular system expands at the expense of the cerebral white matter. The process of recovery in the head injured patient ceases and is followed by further slow deterioration in mentation, gait, and urinary control. This is a relatively rare occurrence after severe head injury but it is important to detect because a rather simple CSF shunting operation can reverse the neurologic deterioration and allow further recovery.[27]

Unfortunately, by far the most common cause of an increase in the size of the ventricular system in the head injured patient is the so-called *hydrocephalus ex vacuo* in which the ventricles enlarge secondary to post-traumatic loss of white matter. In this circumstance the enlarged ventricles are merely the consequence of loss of brain substance. Not surprisingly, this form of ventricular enlargement is strongly correlated with the presence of severe neuropsychologic disability in head injury survivors. CSF shunting procedures have no influence whatsoever on the outcome of such cases.[28]

Post-traumatic Epilepsy

Epileptic seizures always pose a threat to the brain—particularly the injured brain. At a time when increased neuronal activity associated with the seizure discharge is making demands for more blood, oxygen, and glucose, the patient is likely to become hypoxemic because of respiratory difficulties associated with the seizure. Even when satisfactory oxygenation is maintained by artificial ventilation, the affected neurons can still become hypoxemic because their excessive metabolic demand outstrips the supply of blood. The ensuing hypoxic brain damage may destroy any chance for a useful recovery from a severe head injury.

Epileptic seizures can occur any time after head injury, from a few minutes after impact to several years after the original injury. Early epileptic seizures are particularly common in young children. Seizures that develop later than 1 week from the time of injury are defined in the United Kingdom as late onset epilepsy. Such later developing seizures are more likely to recur and to persist. More detailed information on the causes, significance, and management of post-traumatic epilepsy may be found in Chapter 7.

SECONDARY DAMAGE TO THE INJURED BRAIN

Brain Distortion, Shift, and Herniation

When an intracranial mass lesion such as a hematoma develops, brain in the immediate vicinity exhibits viscoelastic properties, becomes distorted, and tends to flow away from the deforming mass. The cerebral cortex under an epidural hematoma will show concave indentation, which remains for several minutes or even hours after the hematoma has been evacuated. Neurologic dysfunction appropriate to the indented area is probably due to vascular compression on the surface of the brain. Thus, a temporoparietal epidural hematoma situated over the motor strip is commonly associated with weakness of the contralateral side of the face and arm.

In the initial compensatory phase during expansion of an intracranial mass lesion, the brain tends to fill spaces normally occupied by CSF; the subarachnoid space becomes obliterated and the lateral ventricles become smaller, particularly on the side of the mass lesion. As the process continues, the brain herniates from one intracranial compartment and protrudes into others.[24] The cingulate gyrus on the side of the mass lesion herniates under the free edge of the falx. This subfalcine hernia may even occlude one or both anterior cerebral arteries.

The medial portion of the temporal lobe ipsilateral to the mass lesion herniates through the gap between the mid-brain and the free edge of the tentorium cerebelli. This process compresses and distorts the cerebral peduncle causing progressive motor dysfunction of the opposite limbs. First there is hemiparesis; then, because of the interruption to the rostral modulating influences, abnormal motor activity emerges as abnormal flexor or extensor responses. Impairment of the rostral inflow to the reticular activating system of the brainstem also produces loss of consciousness. As herniation progresses, the oculomotor nerve, located in the immediate path of the herniating brain, becomes compressed between the posterior cerebral and superior cerebellar arteries, causing a third nerve palsy ipsilateral to the mass lesion. This is manifested by dilatation of the pupil with loss of that pupil's response to light shone into either eye. Ptosis and lateral deviation of the eye may also become evident, the latter owing to unopposed action of the abducens nerve and lateral rectus muscle.

There is also downward axial displacement of the brainstem toward the foramen magnum. Movement and compression of the brainstem interfere with its blood supply from the basilar artery. This ischemic process is associated with impaired respiration, leading ultimately to apnea, and elevation of the blood pressure, which can rise to enormously high levels; the heart rate usually slows. Medullary impairment is intensified by development of tonsillar herniation, when the cerebellar tonsils prolapse through the foramen magnum and directly compress the medulla oblongata.

Secondary brainstem damage can be identified in fatal cases of brain compression in the form of hemorrhages located centrally in the mid-brain, pons, and medulla. These secondary hemorrhagic lesions are thought to result from downward traction on the central perforating branches of the basilar artery, producing either direct rupture of the vessels or bleeding into areas of ischemic necrosis.

Hypoxic and Ischemic Brain Damage

In addition to the brain damage that is a direct result of trauma or is secondary to the compressing effects of an intracranial mass lesion, a third form of post-traumatic brain damage has received much attention. This damage results from severe hypoxic or ischemic insults to the brain. It is exceedingly common in head injury. Graham and his colleagues[29] recorded ischemic brain damage in 91 percent of 151 patients who had died from severe head injuries. Ischemic brain damage is widespread, occurring most commonly in the hippocampus (81 percent of cases), basal ganglia (79 percent), and in scattered sites of the cerebral cortex, both in the arterial distribution zones and in the watershed areas between them. Ischemic brain damage also affects the cerebellum.

The nature and distribution of these pathologic changes suggest multiple etiologies. These include arterial hypotension and

hypoxemia, both of which are common in patients with severe head injury, particularly when complicated by multiple injuries. Other contributory causes are raised intracranial pressure, cerebral vasospasm, brain edema, and the combination of these physiologic insults with disordered cerebrovascular regulation. Dysregulation of cerebral blood flow is a frequent accompaniment of cerebral trauma. When this is combined with any reduction in cerebral perfusion pressure, caused by either a fall in arterial pressure or a rise in intracranial pressure, there is no longer sufficient compensatory vasodilatation and cerebral blood flow may fall to ischemic levels. The cerebral vasodilator response to hypoxemia is also impaired by trauma. The head injured patient is therefore in the particularly dangerous situation of suffering frequently from hypoxemia and low perfusion pressure while often lacking the necessary defense mechanisms that protect the brain against such insults.

DIAGNOSIS IN HEAD INJURY

Determinants of Head Injury

The diagnosis of acute head injury is not usually in doubt. Nevertheless, occasions arise in which a patient is found comatose at home or in the street and it is uncertain whether or not a significant head injury has been sustained. Doubt is often increased when alcohol or drugs are invoked as possible causes of the patient's coma. In such circumstances, the correct procedure is to treat the patient as if he or she had sustained a serious head injury. This management protocol will be appropriate for the patient who is suffering from drug-induced coma, but the converse does not hold true. Galbraith and his colleagues found that the majority of male patients with head injury seen at a major city hospital had some degree of alcohol intoxication. Extremely high blood alcohol levels were encountered in a number of patients who were not in coma. Several patients with high blood alcohol levels in whom this had been thought responsible for coma were subsequently found to be harboring large intracranial hematomas. The assumption that coma in any patient in whom head injury is suspected is due to alcohol rather than brain injury is more often wrong than right.[64]

Epilepsy is another common source of confusion in patients who have sustained a head injury. The sudden onset of coma due to the rapid enlargement of an intracranial hematoma may be wrongly attributed to epilepsy in which the clonic phase of the seizure is assumed to have occurred unobserved. Valuable time may be wasted awaiting return of consciousness in a head injured patient who is in fact continuing to deteriorate rapidly because of progressive brain compression. Unilateral pupillary dilatation is not caused by epilepsy, but bilateral dilatation often is.

In summary, the correct way to manage lethargic or comatose patients in whom no clear history of head injury has been elicited but in whom injury is suspected, is to proceed as if the patient had sustained a head injury and to apply without delay the appropriate diagnostic measures. The urgency with which this process is carried out depends upon the level of consciousness of the patient when first seen at the hospital and during subsequent evaluation. What is required is a practical method of diagnostic triage of patients who are known or suspected to have suffered a head injury. This process is best achieved by assessment of the level of consciousness using the Glasgow Coma Scale.

Evaluation of the Head Injured Patient

It is impossible to make a valid assessment of neurologic function in a patient who is hypoxemic or in shock. The very first step, therefore, is to ensure that the patient has an adequate airway, is well oxygenated, and has satisfactory arterial blood pressure and peripheral circulation.

The neurologic evaluation of the comatose patient must be brief and objective.[30] The first determination is the level of consciousness.[31] The Glasgow Coma Scale (GCS) consists of three elements of response: eye opening, motor responses, and verbal responses to standard stimuli (Table 3−4). The initial stimulus is always verbal. If there is no response, the preferred pain

Table 3−4. ASSESSMENT OF CONSCIOUS LEVEL (GLASGOW COMA SCALE)*

	Examiner's Test	Patient's Response	Assigned Score
Eye Opening	Spontaneous	Opens eyes on own	E4
	Speech	Opens eyes when asked to in a loud voice	3
	Pain	Opens eyes upon pressure	2
	Pain	Does not open eyes	1
Best motor response	Commands	Follows simple commands	M6
	Pain	Pulls examiner's hand away upon pressure	5
	Pain	Pulls a part of body away upon pressure	4
	Pain	Flexes body inappropriately to pain (decorticate posturing)	3
	Pain	Body becomes rigid in an extended position upon pressure (decerebrate posturing)	2
	Pain	Has no motor response to pressure	1
Verbal response (talking)	Speech	Carries on a conversation correctly and tells examiner where he/she is, who he/she is, and the month and year	V5
	Speech	Seems confused or disoriented	4
	Speech	Talks so examiner can understand victim but makes no sense	3
	Speech	Makes sounds that examiner cannot understand	2
	Speech	Makes no noise	1

*Coma Score $(E + M + V) = 3$ to 15.

stimulus consists of application of heavy pressure on the nailbed of the little finger. To compare the motor response on both sides, it may also be necessary to apply pain to the sternal area. In addition, it is important to include a painful stimulus in the supraorbital area to identify the patient who is quadriplegic from concomitant neck injury: unresponsive to painful stimuli applied to the limbs, yet conscious and responsive to pain applied above the neck. Coma is defined as a state in which there is no eye opening even to pain, failure to obey commands, and inability to utter recognizable words.[32]

The Glasgow Coma Scale has been extensively tested for inter-rater variability and shows a high level of agreement, an issue of obvious importance when multiple observers may be sequentially observing the same patient.[33] Based on the Glasgow Coma Scale, patients may be rapidly assigned to the categories of severe, moderate, and minor head injury. Patients with severe head injury are in coma. These patients score E1 M5 V2 (or lower) on the Glasgow Coma Scale. If the score is summated for the three responses this means that severely head injured patients score 8 or less on the GCS. However, eye opening must be absent; if a patient scores 8 but has eye opening to painful stimuli the predicted mortality is only one fourth of that of the patient who has no eye opening.[7, 33] Moderately head injured patients score from 9 to 12, whereas patients with minor head injury score from 13 to the maximum of 15 points on the Glasgow Coma Scale. Thus, patients with minor head injury either may be fully alert with spontaneous eye opening, obeying commands and fully oriented in time and place, or may be disoriented with eye opening only to command. This system of classification of head injuries can be made rapidly and, as will be seen, has profound implications for the urgency with which investigations take place.

In the initial neurologic examination the other important elements are the pupillary responses to light and the eye movement reflexes. These are tested to give an indication of cranial nerve and/or brainstem dysfunction. These will be discussed in more detail in the following chapter.

The patient must be examined from head to toe for other injuries since a high proportion of head injured patients, particularly those who have sustained their injuries in falls from a height or in automobile accidents, will have other major injuries. Signs of head injury include swelling of the scalp, which may indicate an underlying fracture, and bleeding from the nose or ear, particularly if this is mixed with CSF. Cerebrospinal fluid may be suspected if the blood-stained fluid, allowed to drip onto filter paper or a piece of gauze shows that the drop is surrounded by a pale halo. Presence of CSF otorrhea or rhinorrhea, or both, is proof not only that the patient has sustained a basal skull fracture but also that the dura and arachnoid surrounding the brain are torn. Tell-tale bruising in the periorbital areas and behind the ears appears only after several hours and is not usually present on this first assessment in the emergency room. When these signs are present, however, they provide indication of fracture of the anterior cranial fossa, in the case of "raccoon-eyes" bruising, or of the middle cranial fossa in the case of bruising behind the ear (Battle's sign). In examining the rest of the body particular care must be taken to detect spinal injury and soft tissue injuries around the major joints, looking for evidence of instability. The possibility of occult intra-abdominal hemorrhage must always be remembered. This is the case even in patients whose blood pressure is still normal.

This initial assessment of the head injury patient is completed in the emergency room. Plain x-ray films should be taken of the skull, cervical spine, and any other part of the body in which bony or ligamentous injury is suspected. The importance of detecting skull fracture is twofold. The presence of a skull fracture considerably increases the risk that a patient is harboring an intracranial hematoma, particularly if there is also depression of consciousness, abnormal neurologic signs, or early epilepsy. If the skull fracture is compound through the vault of the base of the skull, the risk of intracranial infection must always be kept in mind. Skull radiography is useful to detect not only fractures but also intracranial foreign bodies or intracranial air. The latter is always an abnormal finding and indicates the presence of dural tearing and communication between the outside and subarachnoid space commonly via fractured paranasal air sinuses. The x-ray films of the cervical spine should be scrutinized not only for fractures or dislocations of the spine but also for swelling of the prevertebral soft tissues. This may be the only clue that the patient has a previously dislocated and unstable cervical spine that happens to be aligned in the normal position while the patient is recumbent.

When these examinations have been concluded, and provided that the patient is in stable condition—with a good airway, adequate oxygenation, and normal blood pressure—it is safe to transfer the patient from the emergency room for further diagnostic or therapeutic measures. By far the most important further diagnostic measure is computerized tomography (CT).

This noninvasive method of investigation has represented a major advance in head injury care, making it possible to detect intracranial hematomas, those lying outside the brain in the epidural or subdural spaces and intracerebral hematomas, that lie entirely within the substance of the brain.[34] Occasionally, the hematoma may be difficult to distinguish from brain substance on CT. Nevertheless, the mass effect of the hematoma is detectable by the distortion of the ventricular system and the shift of identifiable structures such as the choroid plexus and pineal gland. CT also enables identification of hemorrhagic or lucent areas in the brain suggestive of contusion, infarction, edema, intracranial foreign bodies, intracranial air, and fractures of the skull. Finally, CT permits identification, with a high degree of reliability, of those patients in whom raised ICP will be a problem. In such cases the third ventricle and the CSF cisterns around the mid-brain can no longer be seen.

The urgency with which CT is obtained depends upon the grade of severity of the head injury. In severely head injured patients (GCS 8 or less) the incidence of intracranial hematoma detected on CT is at least 40 percent. In all severely head injured patients, therefore, CT should be carried out as soon as the patient is judged safe to be moved from the emergency room. In cases of moderate injury (GCS 9 through 12) CT should be carried out soon after admission and immediately if the patient also has a skull fracture, has focal neurologic deficits, or has had seizures. In cases of minor head injury (GCS 13 through 15), CT should also be carried out early if the patient has a skull fracture, has focal neurological deficit, or

has had seizures. Even if these factors are absent, CT should be carried out if the patient does not regain the full score of 15 points on the Glasgow Coma Scale within 24 hours of admission to the hospital.

In a small number of patients an epidural hematoma develops only after the individual has been admitted to the hospital and after the first CT scan has been negative. In any patient who suffers neurologic deterioration or unexplained intracranial hypertension in the ward, repeat CT scan should be carried out.

MANAGEMENT OF SEVERE HEAD INJURY

Early Measures at the Scene of the Accident and in Transit

The most important single objective at this early stage is the establishment and maintenance of a clear airway. The mouth and throat must be cleared of blood, secretions, dentures, and any other foreign bodies. All patients with head injury should be considered as potentially having concomitant injuries to the cervical spine. The patient must be moved into the ambulance with extreme care to avoid unrestrained motion of the head and neck. If circumstances dictate that the patient should be transported lying supine, then an adequate artificial airway must be in position to prevent the tongue and lower jaw from falling back and occluding the airway. An oral or esophageal occlusive airway is adequate for this purpose. If the patient does not have to be transported lying supine, then the preferred position is three-quarters prone because in this position the tongue does not fall back, the airway is kept clear, and should vomiting occur during transit the risk of aspiration of vomitus or blood into the airway is much less. In the three-quarters prone position the patient is put on his or her side, then turned more face down with the uppermost leg drawn up so as to prevent the patient rolling entirely on to the face. The head is turned slightly to one side, and the tongue and lower jaw will tend naturally to fall forward.

If oxygen is available, it should be administered during transport to the hospital. Suction should be available in the ambulance to clear the oral and nasopharynx of blood, vomitus, or secretions. Arterial blood pressure and heart rate should be checked; if arterial blood pressure is low, intravenous crystalloid fluids should be given. Bleeding from the scalp can be arrested by firm pressure. The patient's level of consciousness should be checked using the Glasgow Coma Scale. If possible, this information should be relayed to the receiving hospital in advance of the arrival of the ambulance.

Management in the Emergency Room

At this stage the goals of management are to provide normal levels of arterial oxygen tension and arterial blood pressure with an adequate peripheral circulation, while assessment of neurologic status and extent of injuries proceeds. In the comatose patient, an endotracheal tube should be inserted as soon as possible and the cuff inflated. This provides the best possible security for the airway. During insertion of the endotracheal tube, it must be remembered that the cervical spine may be unstable owing to injury, and excessive extension of the neck should be avoided. It may be necessary to perform nasotracheal intubation, a task that should be handled by an expert. Intravenous lines must be established (if not already in place), and the bladder catheterized.

The emergency room physician must be in a position to declare whether the patient is safe to move for further diagnostic or therapeutic measures. The patient must not leave the emergency room until a secure and stable respiratory and circulatory status has been attained. If the patient is to be artificially ventilated, sedative and muscle relaxant drugs will be given but should be administered only after an adequate examination of neurologic status and level of consciousness has been carried out. The administration of these drugs precludes any further evaluation of neurologic status other than assessment of the pupillary light response.

The location, extent, and severity of all injuries should be carefully documented, preferably using a chart with outlines of the body. The results of the neurologic examination and the levels of arterial pressure, heart rate, and any early laboratory data should all be noted on a chart. The neurologic examination should be repeated every 15 or 30 minutes if the patient remains for any length of time in the emergency room, so that any trend toward deterioration or improvement in status can be detected.

If a decision has been made to provide prophylactic anticonvulsant therapy (indications are detailed in Chapter 7) it should be started early, the loading dose being given while the patient is in the emergency room, with the aim of achieving a prophylactic anticonvulsant blood and tissue level as quickly as possible. If phenytoin is administered intravenously the infusion should be given slowly, with continuous monitoring of the ECG to guard against the occurrence of cardiac arrhythmias. In the United Kingdom, steroid therapy is no longer used in cases of head injury because of lack of published evidence of its efficacy.[35] Intravenous mannitol solution should not be given until there is more information, from CT, about the intracranial pathology. In cases when severely head injured patients are secondarily referred to a head injury and trauma center from a primary hospital, intravenous mannitol may well have been given at the first hospital. This can cause a temporary improvement in the neurologic status of the patient and lull the emergency room staff in the secondary hospital into the false belief that the head injury was not as severe as originally described over the telephone. If mannitol is given, its use should be recorded in writing.

If CT shows an intracranial hematoma that will require surgical decompression because of the extent of brain shift, a large dose of mannitol should then be given as a rapid intravenous infusion of 1 g/kg body weight. This allows the beneficial effect of the mannitol to cover the patient through the relatively hazardous phase of transport from the radiology department to the operating room, induction of anesthesia, and positioning on the operating table. Exceptions to this rule are made in patients who show rapid deterioration after admission either to the primary or secondary hospital, developing signs of tentorial herniation, deteriorating level of consciousness, and unilateral pupillary dilatation. In such cases it is recommended that the patient receive a full dose of mannitol immediately to cover the time required for CT diagnosis of the location of the lesion.

Operative Management of Head Injury

There are three main indications for surgical treatment in patients with head injury. The first is to provide relief from brain compression due to an intracranial hematoma or a swollen contused and hemorrhagic lobe. This is virtually always an emergency, and decompressive surgery must be performed as soon as possible. The operation entails a full craniotomy with exposure of the frontal lobe, temporal lobe, and part of the parietal lobe.[35] All large extracerebral hematomas should be evacuated and, if necessary, necrotic swollen brain tissue amputated. Intracerebral hematomas are treated with more circumspection.

The second broad indication for surgery is the prevention of infection by debridement and lavage of compound wounds. These procedures include excision and repair of penetrating wounds to the scalp and dura, repair of depressed skull fractures and persistent dural fistulas communicating with fractures at the base of the skull, and the surgical management of penetrating missile wounds of the head. Although it is important that surgical measures for the prevention of infection from compound wounds be carried out relatively urgently, these need not be emergency procedures. It may be preferable to wait a few hours to permit the patient to be adequately ventilated and for measures to be taken to reduce brain swelling and increased ICP prior to the surgical procedure. Such measures minimize the amount of brain tissue lost at the time of the surgical cleansing. If surgery is delayed for much more than 24 hours, however, the risk of intracranial infection is increased.

There is no evidence that surgical treatment of depressed skull fractures or penetrating injuries of the brain affects the incidence of epilepsy at a later date. Prevention of post-traumatic epilepsy is not, therefore, an indication for surgical treatment.

The third surgical indication is to insert a device for monitoring the intracranial pressure. All methods, including an implanted transducer, or a subdural or intraventricular catheter connected to an external transducer, require insertion via a burr hole, usually in the right frontal bone. The indications for insertion of a monitoring device are shown in Table 3–3.

Management in the Intensive Care Unit

In the comatose patient, the underlying principle of care is prevention of further neurologic deterioration due to secondary brain insults. Because the potential causes of such deterioration include hypoxemia, arterial hypotension, intracranial hypertension, fluid and electrolyte imbalance, infection, and elevations of body temperature, indicators of these complications must be monitored carefully and continuously in the intensive care unit and any adverse trends corrected as rapidly as possible.[36]

VENTILATION

Assisted respiration should be provided for all patients who exhibit any evidence of abnormal respiration.[37] Hypoxia and hypercapnea must be avoided. During the initial stages of management mechanical ventilation is generally required to maintain a Pao$_2$ greater than 70 mmHg, and controlled hyperventilation to provide a Paco$_2$ of 25 to 30 mmHg.[38]

Common nursing interventions such as suctioning may increase intracranial pressure. If the ICP exceeds 30 mmHg, suctioning should be discontinued for brief periods of time. Small amounts of sedation, or mild manual hyperventilation, may be necessary prior to reinstituting the procedure.

In some centers artificial ventilation via an endotracheal tube is used in all comatose patients for periods of 3 days to 3 weeks after injury. In the Head and Spinal Injury Unit in Edinburgh, artificial ventilation is used in patients who have been comatose (GCS 8 or less) prior to the evacuation of an intracranial hematoma, in patients without hematomas who score GCS 6 or less, and in comatose patients in whom CT is indicative of raised ICP. In addition, patients with less severe head injuries that occur in combination with significant injuries to the face, chest, and/or abdomen are artificially ventilated. For all patients in whom artificial ventilation is used, arterial pressure must be monitored continuously from an indwelling arterial catheter and intracranial pressure should be monitored continuously from a subdural or intraventricular catheter or a subdurally implanted pressure transducer.

The intra-arterial line is used for intermittent withdrawal of blood samples for measurement of arterial blood gases, and transcutaneous pulse oximetry is used to provide a continuous measure of tissue oxygenation. In patients in whom artificial ventilation is likely to be required for more than 2 weeks, or if extensive faciomaxillary surgery is required, tracheostomy is performed.

When instituted, artificial ventilation is maintained for a minimum of 3 days before temporary discontinuation of the sedative and relaxant drugs in order to obtain an updated assessment of neurologic status. If this reveals persistent abnormal motor activity, spontaneous hyperventilation, or vegetative disturbance, then artificial ventilation is reinstituted for another 3 to 4 days before the neurologic status is reassessed. During the intervening period, the pupillary light reflexes are assessed hourly, and whenever possible a record is obtained of brain electrical activity using some form of condensed EEG recording such as the cerebral function analyzing monitor.

Weaning from the respirator may proceed when there is evidence of a decreasing intermittent mandatory ventilation (IMV), improved tolerance for altering IMV and a longer duration of lower IMV, improvement in mean expiratory force, an improved vital capacity and a decreasing fraction of inspired air (FIO_2) or decreasing positive endexpiratory pressure (PEEP).

In some patients the passive respiration induced by the breathing apparatus may be habit-forming. The level of O_2 and the number of breaths per minute provided by the respirator may have to be gradually reduced to allow adequate adaptation to independent breathing. Some patients may experience "air hunger," which exacerbates oxygen demand and thus prolongs the weaning process.[37]

In moderately or severely head injured patients who do not require artificial ventilation, the key factor in management control is frequent reassessment of clinical neurologic status. The factors recorded are the three elements of the Glasgow Coma Scale (eye opening, motor response, and verbal response), pupil reaction to light, eye movement reflexes (oculocephalic or oculovestibular), and comparison of limb power of the four extremities. These items should all be recorded half-hourly, then hourly in comatose patients, increasing the interval between examinations as the patient's conscious level improves. The results are noted on a neurologic watch sheet along with the blood pressure, heart rate, body temperature, and ICP (if this is being recorded) (Fig. 3–9). In this way, trends of improvement or deterioration can be detected.

TREATMENT OF RAISED INTRACRANIAL PRESSURE

When ICP becomes elevated over 25 mmHg mean, or when any elevation of ICP appears to be accompanied by neurologic deterioration, measures should be taken to reduce the pressure.[39] Hyperventilation is used first to bring arterial PCO_2 down from 4 to 3 kPa (30 to 22.5 mmHg). If this is unsuccessful in reducing ICP, a choice must be made between the administration of osmotic therapy or of sedative therapy (Table 3–5).[40]

Osmotic therapy consists of the intravenous administration of mannitol, usually in a starting dose of 0.5 g/kg body weight. This infusion is followed by administration of a diuretic such as furosemide and then stable plasma protein solution. Sedative or hypnotic drug therapy consists of administration of barbiturates or other similar drugs (in France and in the United Kingdom, gammahydroxybutyrate may be used) that reduce cerebral blood flow and cerebral blood volume and thereby reduce ICP.

Hypnotic drug therapy must be undertaken with extreme care because most agents tend to lower arterial blood pressure.[41] This effect is extremely dangerous in the head injured patient, as brain ischemia is likely to ensue.[42] It may be necessary to monitor not only central venous pressure but also pulmonary artery and pulmonary capillary wedge pressure to ensure that there is no degree of hypovolemia present prior to the administration of sedative drugs, since it is under this circumstance that arterial hypotension is most likely to complicate sedative drug therapy.

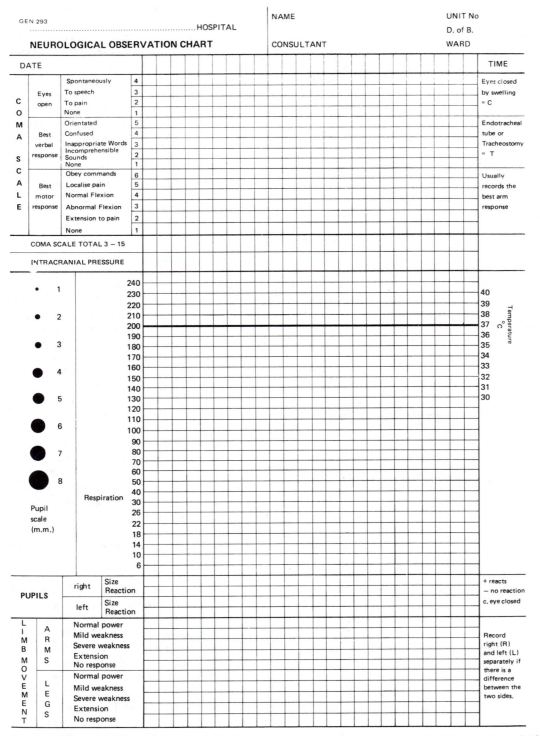

Figure 3–9. A typical neurologic watch sheet, incorporating observations on the Glasgow Coma Scale, for use in sequential monitoring of head injury patients in the intensive care unit or in the ward setting.

Table 3–5. MANAGEMENT OF RAISED INTRACRANIAL PRESSURE

General Measures	Specific Measures
Check—head position airway blood gases temperature	**Osmotherapy**—best for edema Mannitol Furosemide Plasma protein solution **Vasoreductive therapy**—best for swelling Hyperventilation Thiopentone Gammahydroxybutyrate

FACE AND NECK INJURIES

A contusion of the neck in the region of the larynx and cervical emphysema secondary to a tear of the upper airway are signs of a laryngeal injury. Voice pitch will be affected once vocalization has been established. If the larynx is fractured, endotracheal intubation is usually contraindicated and immediate tracheostomy is preferred for securing the airway. Open reduction or placement of a stent will adequately treat these fractures.

The nasal bone is the most frequently fractured facial bone. Such an injury has the potential to cause disruption of the orbital floor resulting in a blow-out injury and damage to the eye. Thus these patients should have thorough and repeated ophthalmologic assessment until such injury has been satisfactorily ruled out.

Next in vulnerability to fracture is the mandible. Because of its U shape, multiple fractures are the rule, and contrecoup fractures are common. If one fracture is noted, careful radiologic studies are required for additional fractures. The patient who later complains of malalignment of the teeth may well have sustained a mandibular fracture. Ecchymosis in the floor of the mouth is almost pathognomonic of mandibular fracture.

Flattening of one cheek warrants suspicion of zygomatic complex fracture, and may be accompanied by unilateral nose bleed. Dysconjugate gaze with periorbital ecchymosis and subconjunctival hemorrhage may also be present. In addition to appropriate maxillofacial management, routine ophthalmologic follow-up is essential.

Mid-face fractures can be quite complex. With severe disruption, CSF rhinorrhea is common. Prophylactic antibiotic therapy, while controversial in CSF rhinorrhea without mid-face fractures, is indicated. Early reduction and stabilization of the fractures rapidly heals the CSF leak.[43]

General and Metabolic Care of the Head Injured Patient

An indwelling urinary catheter is important so that the exact volume of urinary output on an hour-to-hour basis can be measured. Serum electrolyte levels should be checked daily, and any tendency toward hyponatremia speedily corrected.

For the first days after severe head injury the nasogastric tube is used to keep the stomach empty so as to minimize the risk of aspiration of gastric contents into the lungs. Once bowel sounds return, usually after 72 hours, nasogastric tube feeding begins, with half-strength milk at first, gradually working up to the full daily calorific requirement. In head injured patients the required caloric intake is surprisingly high, averaging 3000 kilocalories per day for an adult. Spontaneous abnormal motor activity will increase this requirement.

The regular nursing care of patients with severe head injury includes frequent changes of position, with attention to skin care and aspiration of secretions from the airway. Vigorous physiotherapy will ensure that the lung fields remain clear and atelectasis does not occur, and that all moveable limbs can be put through a full range of passive movement.

Respiratory therapy should include vibration, percussion, and postural drainage (as ICP levels permit). Stretching and massage should be directed to the accessory muscles of respiration. There may at times be a need to increase the intermittent mandatory ventilation during therapy. The use of a rocking or rotating bed has been suggested as a prophylactic measure to mechanically increase pulmonary drainage, as well as for its potential to reduce the incidence of thrombophlebitis, and reduce prolonged pressure on skin. Changes in bed position do not differentially affect ICP. Rotation of the bed from right to left through its natural arc does not appear to alter ICP.[44]

OTHER EARLY MEDICAL PROBLEMS

Pulmonary

Neurogenic pulmonary edema has been reported to occur in severe head injury, in subarachnoid hemorrhage (SAH), and in the presence of elevated ICP. It is a well-documented complication of fatal SAH.[45] The question of centrally mediated pulmonary edema has been a point of controversy in the literature. Theodore and Robin felt that increased ICP may be closely related to acute lung congestion.[46] Elevations of extravascular lung water are associated with pulmonary embolism in 50 percent of patients with severe head injury. Levels appear to peak after 48 hours but the clinical course is prolonged. Increased pulmonary microvascular permeability may be the underlying pathogenic factor. Mackersie and coworkers believed that the role of ICP is probably quite limited.[47]

Fat embolism may be an early complication of long bone fractures in 10 to 25 percent of multiple trauma victims. Eighty to 100 percent of patients who die of various causes after fractures of long bones have had fat emboli in their lungs. It may be, therefore, that fat embolism occurs more commonly after trauma than has been previously thought.[37]

Severe hypophosphatemia as the result of respiratory acidosis is an unusual complication of mechanical ventilation. Hyperphosphatemia causes a wide variety of musculoskeletal and CNS disturbances that can complicate neurosurgical management and obscure the accurate assessment of the neurologic status. This electrolyte disturbance can be resolved with correction of the hyperventilation that induced acid-base abnormalities.[48]

Hyperthermia

Fever may be the only sign of meningeal irritation in patients in deep coma.[49] Fever may also occur with intracranial abscess, subdural empyema, pulmonary or genitourinary infection, and retained bone fragments in cerebral tissue, among other conditions. The most common extracranial source of infection is the respiratory tract, followed by the urinary tract. Early removal of the indwelling catheter and institution of an intermittent catheterization program should be the treatment of choice to avoid urinary tract infections. Adequate bladder filling should be allowed between catheterization to maintain normal filling tonus, but overdistention should be assiduously avoided. Iatrogenic causes of fever include inadequate hydration and a variety of medications. Hypothalamic injuries may be responsible for temperature elevations in some cases. An adequate evaluation for other causes of fever should include consideration of the aforementioned entities as well as thrombophlebitis, pulmonary embolism, heterotopic ossification, and wound infections. Thus the diagnosis of temperature dyscontrol secondary to cerebral injury is often one of exclusion. If fever is associated with hypertension and tachycardia as a component of generalized autonomic dyscontrol, propranolol may be effective in controlling the fever as well as the other aspects.

Corporal temperature control appears to be centered in the mid-brain. In the presence of impending tentorial herniation, fever of central origin may arise as an irritative phenomenon. One must also be aware that fever associated with a hypermetabolic state may occur as a result of generalized spasticity. Severe elevations in tonus should be controlled in the presence of febrile episodes.

Control of body temperature to a normal or moderately subnormal range (33 to 36°C [91 to 97°F]) may help lower intracranial pressure by decreasing cerebral metabolism. However, generalized shivering that may ensue can sometimes elevate ICP owing to generalized increase of muscular contractions and elevation of systemic and central venous pressures.

Hyperthermia increases the metabolic demands of the brain. Temperatures in excess of 38°C (100°F) must be avoided because this may create further brain damage. Nutritional requirements should be carefully modulated since caloric needs increase in the presence of hyperthermia. It is essential to treat the fever immediately and then search for cause. Treatment approaches include adequate hydration, antipyretic agents (frequently by suppository), alcohol sponging and cooling blankets, and cessation of suspected drugs.

Hypothermia (32°C [89.6°F]) is associated with cardiac arrythmias and an increased incidence of hypoxia in unconscious patients. Therefore, the use of cooling blankets should be carefully monitored if used in the management of hyperthermia. Other causes of hypothermia include sedative overdose or coexisting hypothyroidism. Because of its depressant action on cerebral circulation and metabolism, hypothermia may exert a protective effect on the brain in some circumstances.[50]

Hypertension

Hypertension is second only to elevated cardiac output as a cardiovascular response to head trauma. The blood pressure elevation is often transient or a result of spasticity.[51] Thus noxious stimuli frequently result in the production of systemic hypertension. An endotracheal tube, pressure sores, constricting bed clothes, poorly fitting splints, and other seemingly innocuous factors may be responsible.

Loss of autoregulation of cerebral blood flow produces an increase in the blood-brain volume, which is the prime cause of increased brain bulk resulting in intracranial hypertension.[52] Systemic arterial hypertension can result in blood-brain barrier disruption followed by extravasation of proteins and transudation of water, causing or augmenting brain edema.

All significant elevations of blood pressure must be treated. Frequently sedation may be all that is required. Sodium nitroprusside, commonly used to control systemic hypertension, may have a negative effect on cerebral perfusion pressure because of the cerebrovascular dilatation that results. If the drug is used ICP must be monitored closely. (Hypertension is further discussed in Chapter 9.)

Tachycardia

Tachycardia in head trauma may be a response to acute blood loss, fever, or anemia, or to the development of pulmonary embolism. Pre-existing causes such as hyperthyroidism should be ruled out. Commonly after head injury, the normal cyclic changes in heart rate are decreased. There appears to be a direct correlation with an increase in ICP.[53]

Various regions of the CNS from the diencephalon to the myelencephalon are involved in control of the heart rate. Cardioregulatory centers have been localized in the medullary tegmentum in the region of the fourth ventricle. Information from the mechanoreceptors supply feedback.

Considerations involved in cardiac rate include respiration rate and pattern, temperature, level of arousal, medications that suppress the CNS or block vagal activity—any factor that may inhibit variability. The more severely involved patients demonstrate periodicity of instantaneous heart rate.

Cardiac monitors determine heart rate by the number of beats per unit of time. There is normally a continual change in the beat-by-beat rate (R-R interval) that is lost in severe head injury.[53]

THE PROCESS OF RECOVERY FROM HEAD INJURY

In the comatose patient who is being managed in the intensive care unit by artificial ventilation and continuous monitoring of arterial and intracranial pressure, orderly progress in the transition from dependence on life support systems to independence from them is crucial if optimal recovery is to be attained. When ICP has been consistently below 20 mmHg for more than 24 hours (including at least one overnight recording) this monitoring system can be discontinued. The process of discontinuation of artificial ventilation and restoration of spontaneous respiration is potentially hazardous and needs to be carefully supervised. In a number of patients there may be a period during which the endotracheal tube remains in situ but the patient breathes spontaneously. At this stage addition of dead space will increase the end tidal volume and arterial Pco_2 and encourage a larger minute volume. To facilitate adequate oxygenation, continuous positive airway pressure (CPAP) may be helpful. Thereafter, provided that minute volume and arterial blood gas tensions are satisfactory, the endotracheal tube may be removed. Before it is finally removed, however, the anesthetist will wish to ensure that the patient has an adequate cough and gag reflex. On occasion, a head injury is complicated by lower cranial nerve palsies; such patients are in grave danger of regurgitating and aspirating gastric contents into the airway. Tracheostomy may be required to provide lasting protection to the airway until adequate cranial nerve function returns.

The eye opening response may recover through the stages of the Glasgow Coma Scale, but in any case, spontaneous eye opening usually begins after about 2 weeks even in otherwise unresponsive patients.[54] Roving eye movements are common and may be wrongly interpreted by members of the family as following movements. Patients who remain in the permanent vegetative state usually have spontaneous eye opening with regular sleep-wake cycles and roving eye movements. However, such patients do not speak any recognizable word, nor do they obey commands.

The best early indication of recovery of consciousness is the motor response, which in adult patients ascends through the stages listed in the Glasgow Coma Scale. In some patients who have had pronounced abnormal flexor or extensor posturing, the early phase of recovery may be accompanied by the emergence of abnormal spontaneous movements of a dystonic, athetoid, or choreiform nature. Rhythmic tremors may also emerge at this time, but these abnormal movements virtually always subside spontaneously after a period of days or weeks.

As with the motor response, the verbal response usually returns through the stages noted on the Glasgow Coma Scale. The patient may go through a stage of shouting and uttering expletives, then through a stage of confusion and disorientation during which there may even be florid delusions. At this stage relatives may remark that the patient's voice sounds different from the way it sounded preinjury. Subsequent testing indicates that while in this confusional state, which may last for days or weeks, the patient remains amnesic and will have no subsequent memory of conversation or events that occurred during this period (post-traumatic amnesia, or PTA).

Emergence from coma is generally marked by the return of speech or an equivalent signal from the patient and by the capacity to obey spoken commands. The return of continuous memory and the end of PTA do not occur until much later. Duration of PTA is commonly three or four times that of the period of observed unconsciousness. Until the patient has emerged from the period of PTA, he or she is not accessible for psychometric evaluation. The Galveston Orientation and Amnesia Test (GOAT) has been developed to provide guidance for the clinical psychologist during this period.[55] Until the patient can score 75 out of a possible 100 points on this scale, detailed attempts at psychometric evaluation are not worthwhile. Other aspects of the rehabilitation process can, however, begin at a much earlier stage.

SELECTION OF PATIENTS AND TIMING OF TRANSFER TO THE NEUROREHABILITATION UNIT

There are no generally accepted criteria for the selection of patients or for determining the optimal timing of transfer from the acute surgical ward to the neurorehabilitation unit. One reason for this is the varied nature of available rehabilitation facilities; the resources allocated to this aspect of care differ considerably among countries, and even within one nation there are often dissimilar institutions addressing differing aspects of the complex spectrum of problems that may follow brain injury. Even if one restricts the discussion to physical medicine establishments, important variables remain. Some units are sited in the same hospital as the acute service while others are freestanding institutions. Early transfer may be easier in the former where surgical and radiologic expertise are on hand, whereas in the latter a greater certainty of medical stability may be required before the patient is moved. The number and training of staff in different rehabilitation departments will also determine some aspects of operational policy such as the ability to accept patients requiring ventilation, tube feeding, and other skilled nursing input.

The process of restoring to patients their maximal capabilities begins in the trauma unit, and rehabilitation is a continuum ranging from this acute stage to reintegration into the community. In the acute setting a program of care is instituted that takes account of environmental influences on the brain injured patient, adopting and evaluating neurostimulation techniques when appropriate. Some would argue that individuals at this early stage should be taken to a specific rehabilitation unit for this purpose. More commonly selection and timing of transfer is determined by two principal considerations: medical stability, and ability to respond to a rehabilitation program.

The individual who is in need of neurosurgical procedures or who has other major injuries requiring surgical or radiologic attention is often best served by remaining in the surgical ward while things are being "done to" him or her. Once the approach changes to one of "doing things with" him or her to increase the patient's independence, this is often the optimal time for transfer. This strategy is also beneficial to the patient's family, who can now feel that the life-threatening phase is over and their loved one has graduated to a better level. If the patient has to be returned to the acute unit for further surgical or diagnostic procedures this can add to the relatives' distress and confusion.

Determining who will and who will not respond to a rehabilitation program is not easy and certainly does not imply that only cooperative patients should be admitted to a neurorehabilitation unit. Even the most severely impaired patients should be assessed to decide whether or not they are responsive at that time. The comprehensive interprofessional assessment of the individual's disabilities and abilities is an integral part of rehabilitation. Even if leading to the conclusion that the patient is so damaged as to require total nursing care, this process is of value for planning future management and counseling the family. Such a decision should never be regarded as irrevocable within the first 3 months after injury, and provision should be made for readmission for future reappraisal.

Rehabilitation, when properly done, is a labor-intensive and hence an expensive service. It should therefore involve a continuous critical evaluation of what is being

achieved. The aims are to prevent or minimize chronic secondary disabilities, both physical and psychosocial, while restoring the individual to the optimal level of function. There is no rigid time limit that can be set to achieve these aims in all cases. Some individuals may benefit significantly from the maintenance of an intensive approach over some months, but the majority of patients probably require less time as an inpatient in the rehabilitation unit. The sooner the patient can spend some time at home in a familiar nonmedical environment, the better from the point of view of morale and orientation. Initial home visits are usually on weekends, and the final return home can be preceded by a full appraisal of the rehabilitation aids required in the home. Ideally, the inpatient rehabilitation ward is backed up by an outpatient facility providing a coordinated goal-directed service following discharge.

In the context of selection and timing of transfer it is appropriate to describe briefly the experience of the rehabilitation unit of the neuroscience service in Edinburgh.[56] Reference has already been made to the constraints resulting from staff levels and structural resources. These are considerable in that head injured patients at the Astley Ainslie Rehabilitation Hospital are accommodated in an open ward with a wide range of other neurologically disabled individuals; numbers of nursing, remedial therapy, and clinical psychology staff are low and patients are admitted from throughout Scotland as well as directly from our own neurotrauma unit. In the four calendar years 1983 to 1986, 183 new cases of head injury were admitted to the unit. These comprised 81 percent male and 19 percent female patients with a median age of 29 years (range 15 to 89 years). All patients had significant physical disability and of the 145 patients with an acute Glasgow Coma Scale Score recorded, 70 percent had scores of 8 or less. The median time from injury to admission on the neurorehabilitation ward was 47 days. This figure is significantly influenced by a number of patients coming from remote parts of the country.

Patients returned home in 81 percent of cases, and about half of the patients stayed in the unit for less than 1 month (Table 3–6).

There is much truth to the suggestion

Table 3–6. REHABILITATION AFTER SEVERE HEAD INJURY (LENGTH OF STAY IN EDINBURGH UNIT)

Length of Stay in Unit	Patients From Edinburgh Area	Patients From Other Parts of Scotland	Total
<1 month	62	33	95
1–2 months	24	19	43
2–3 months	10	5	15
3–6 months	7	14	21
6–10 months	2	7	9
Total number	105	78	183

that the real problems following head injury start once the patient leaves the hospital. There is, no doubt, however, that the needs of the individual change over the year or so following injury. From neurophysiologic studies as well as from clinical experience, there is evidence to justify intensive, aggressive health care involvement in the first few months that is expensive in human and monetary terms. With the passage of time, however, the needs of the head injury survivor become more predominantly psychologic and social with attention directed more toward adjusting to long-term disability and addressing vocational and social needs.

EARLY PREDICTION OF OUTCOME FROM SEVERE HEAD INJURY

Several carefully performed studies, comparing the early clinical status of large numbers of head injured patients with the outcome at 6 months or later, have shown general agreement concerning the significance for outcome of a number of clinical factors (Table 3–7).[57–60] One of the most important is the age of the patient. The younger the patient, the more likely he or she is to survive following head injury; the older the patient, the more likely he or she is to die. This increase of mortality with age is related largely to the chances of dying from a medical complication of prolonged coma. In addition, older patients are more likely to have intracranial hematomas,

which carry a higher mortality. The age of the patient does not appear to be a powerful predictor of severe disability or prolonged vegetative state in survivors of severe head injury. This is probably because older patients who might have suffered injuries severe enough to render them severely disabled or vegetative are more likely to die from pneumonia or other intercurrent problems. The level of consciousness as determined on the Glasgow Coma Scale is also a powerful predictor of outcome. Of the three elements in the scale, the most powerful in predicting a poor outcome (death, vegetative state, or severe disability) is the motor response.[58, 61] There is a very large increase in mortality and in morbidity among patients who have abnormal flexor, extensor, or absent motor responses to painful stimulation as compared with those who are able to obey commands, localize, or even withdraw the limbs in a normal fashion from a painful stimulus. The presence of brainstem dysfunction as shown by bilateral absence of the pupillary light response or abnormal eye movement reflexes is also associated with a much worse outcome from injury. In the case of brainstem dysfunction, however, the prognostic significance is that an increase in mortality rather than an increase in the incidence of severe disability is forecast.

The CT scan is not only of value to indicate the presence of intracranial pathology in the acute stage but also has predictive value.[62] Of most adverse significance is the presence on CT of lesions of increased density in the brain parenchyma particularly when these occur in both hemispheres. Patients with such lesions show an increase in severe disability and mortality. CT at a later

Table 3–7. FACTORS IMPORTANT FOR OUTCOME FROM SEVERE HEAD INJURY

Age
Motor response
GCS
Pupils
Eye movements
Presence of hematoma
Secondary insult
Intracranial pressure
Cerebral blood flow/metabolism
Brain electrical activity
Enzyme/chemical markers

stage, more than 2 weeks after injury, may show enlargement of the ventricular system; this appearance is associated with a poor outcome. Most instances of ventricular enlargement represent compensatory ventricular dilatation consequent on loss of white matter. This is related to extensive diffuse white matter brain damage. Focal lucent areas on CT may represent cerebral infarcts and correlate with focal neurologic abnormalities. Enlargement of the fourth ventricle is associated with cerebellar atrophy and persisting ataxia in survivors, while dilatation of the temporal horns of the lateral ventricles is associated with severe memory problems after injury.

Intracranial hypertension is common after injury, particularly in those patients who have already required surgical decompression because of an intradural hematoma. In one quarter of these patients and in about 15 percent of all comatose head injured patients this intracranial hypertension is progressive, cannot be controlled by management measures, and progresses until intracranial pressure attains the level of arterial pressure. At this point cerebral perfusion pressure is zero and the cerebral circulation is arrested, resulting in brain death. Half of all head injury deaths in the hospital are by this mechanism. Milder degrees of intra-

cranial hypertension, between 20 and 40 mmHg, are also of adverse prognostic significance even when this moderate intracranial hypertension is controlled by treatment. Patients who suffer this moderate degree of raised intracranial pressure show a higher proportion of severe disability among the survivors than do patients with normal ICP.

Based on the known outcome of many hundreds of patients with severe head injury, the combined influence of these clinical variables can be assessed using Bayesian or other statistical models.[58, 63] For any individual patient about whom the various factors are known, it is now possible to predict with considerable accuracy the probability of death, severe disability, or better-quality survival in that particular patient. It remains to be seen whether control or reversal of those adverse factors will significantly improve on the predicted outcome. It is already possible, within a day or two after injury, to identify those patients who are likely to require prolonged and intensive rehabilitative measures and to start these measures as early as possible. Continuing and critical assessment of the influence of the rehabilitation measures upon outcome is now one of the most important tasks in head injury research.

REFERENCES

1. Miller, JD: Physiology of trauma. Clin Neurosurg 29:103, 1982.
2. Adams, JH: Head injury. In Adams, JH, Corsellis, JAN, and Duchen, LW (eds): Greenfield's Neuropathology, ed 4. Edward Arnold, London, 1984, p 85.
3. Adams, JH et al: Diffuse brain damage of immediate impact type. Brain 100:489, 1977.
4. Strich, SJ: Diffuse degeneration of the cerebral white matter in severe dementia following head injury. J Neurol Neurosurg Psychiatry 19:163, 1956.
5. Oppenheimer, DR: Microscopic lesions in the brain following head injury. J Neurol Neurosurg Psychiatry 31:299, 1968.
6. Miller, JD and Jennett, B: Complications of depressed skull fractures. Lancet 2:991, 1968.
7. Miller, JD and Jones, PA. The work of a regional head injury service. Lancet 1:1141, 1985.
8. Mendelow, AD et al: Risks of intracranial haematoma in head injured adults. Br Med J 287:1173, 1983.
9. Miller, JD: Minor, moderate and severe head injury. Neurosurg Rev 9:135, 1986.
10. Miller, JD, et al: Early insults to the injured brain. JAMA 240:439, 1978.
11. Miller, JD et al: Further experience in the management of severe head injury. J Neurosurg 54:289, 1981.
12. Lewelt, W, Jenkins, LW and Miller, JD: Effects of experimental fluid percussion injury of the brain on cerebrovascular reactivity to hypoxia and hypercapnia. J Neurosurg 56:332, 1982.
13. Lewelt, W, Jenkins, LW and Miller, JD: Autoregulation of cerebral blood flow after experimental fluid percussion injury of the brain. J Neurosurg 53:500, 1980.
14. Kohi, YM, Mendelow, AD and Teasdale, GM: Extracranial insults and outcome in patients with acute head injury in relationship to the Glasgow Coma Scale. Injury 16:25, 1984.
15. Butterworth, JF et al: Detection of occult abdominal trauma in patients with severe head injuries. Lancet 2:759, 1980.
16. Reilly, PL et al: Patients with head injury who talk and die. Lancet 2:375, 1975.
17. Rose, J, Valtonen, S and Jennett, B: Avoidable fac-

tors contributing to death after head injury. Br Med J 2:615, 1977.

18. Jeffreys, RV and Jones, JJ: Avoidable factors contributing to the death of head injury patients in general hospitals in Mersey region. Lancet 2:459, 1981.

19. Marshall, L, Toole, B and Bowers, S: The National Traumatic Coma Data Bank: Part 2. Patients who talk and deteriorate: Implications for treatment. J Neurosurg 59:285, 1983.

20. Becker, DP et al: The outcome from severe head injury with early diagnosis and intensive management. J Neurosurg 77:491, 1977.

21. Teasdale, E et al: CT scan in severe diffuse head injury: Physiological and clinical correlations. J Neurol Neurosurg Psychiatry 47:600, 1984.

22. Miller, JD: Clinical management of cerebral oedema. Br J Hosp Med 20:152, 1979.

23. Miller, JD et al: Significance of intracranial hypertension in severe head injury. J Neurosurg 47:503, 1977.

24. Miller, JD and Adams, JH: The pathophysiology of raised intracranial pressure. In Adams, JH, Corsellis, JAN, and Duchen, LW (eds): Greenfield's Neuropathology, ed 4. Edward Arnold, London, 1984, p 53.

25. Miller, JD: Infection in head injury. In Vinken, PJ and Bruyn, CW (eds): Handbook of Neurology. Vol. 24. Injuries of the Brain and Skull, Part II, edited by R Braakman. North Holland, Amsterdam, 1976, p 215.

26. Macpherson, P and Graham DI: Correlation between angiographic findings and the ischaemia of head injury. J Neurol Neurosurg Psychiatry 41:122, 1978.

27. Girevendulis, AK et al: Serial CT as an indication of prognosis in patients with severe head injury. Neuroradiology 15:242, 1978.

28. Levin, HS et al: Ventricular enlargement after closed head injury. Arch Neurol 38:623, 1981.

29. Graham, DI, Adams, JH and Doyle, D: Ischaemic brain damage in fatal non-missile head injuries. J Neurol Sci 39:213, 1978.

30. Fisher, CM: The neurological examination of the comatose patient. Acta Neurol Scand 45:5, 1969.

31. Teasdale, G and Jennett, B: Assessment of coma and impaired consciousness. Lancet 2:81, 1974.

32. Jennett, B and Teasdale, G: Aspects of coma after severe head injury. Lancet 1:878, 1977.

33. Teasdale, G, Knill-Jones, R and Vander Sande, JP: Observer variability in assessing impaired consciousness and coma. J Neurol Neurosurg Psychiatry 41:603, 1978.

34. Roberson, FC et al: The value of serial computerised tomography in the management of severe head injury. Surg Neurol 12:161, 1979.

35. Dearden, NM et al: Effect of high dose dexamethasone on outcome from severe head injury. J Neurosurg 64:81, 1986.

36. Becker, DP et al: Diagnosis and treatment of head injury. In Youmans, JR (ed): Neurological Surgery, ed 2. Volume 4. WB Saunders, Philadelphia, 1982, 1938.

37. Gildenberg, PL, and Frost, EAM: Respiratory care in head trauma. In: Becker, DP and Povlishock, JT (eds): Central Nervous System Trauma: Status Report. NINCDS, NIH, Washington, 1985, p 161.

38. Bowers, SA and Marshall, LF: Severe head injury:

39. Miller, JD: ICP monitoring: Present position and future directions. Acta Neurochir 85:80, 1987.

40. Miller, JD: Therapy for raised intracranial pressure in patients with severe head injury. Neurotraumatology 10:247, 1987.

41. Ward, JD et al: Failure of prophylactic barbiturate coma in the treatment of severe head injury. J Neurosurg 62:383, 1985.

42. Miller, JD: Head injury and brain ischaemia—implication for therapy. Br J Anaesth 57:120, 1985.

43. Bertz, JE: Maxillofacial injuries. CIBA Clin Symp 33:1, 1981.

44. Gonzalez-Arias, SM et al: Analysis of the effect of kinetic therapy on intracranial pressure in comatose neurosurgical patients. Neurosurgery 13:654, 1983.

45. Wilkins, RH: The possible role of the hypothalamus in the development of intra-cranial arterial spasm. In Wilkens, RH (ed): Cerebral Arterial Spasm. William and Wilkins, Baltimore, 1980, p 266.

46. Theodore, J and Robin, ED: Speculation on neurogenic pulmonary edema. Am Rev Respir Dis 113:405, 1976.

47. Mackersie, RC et al: Pulmonary extravascular fluid accumulation following intra-cranial injury. J Trauma 23:968, 1983.

48. Gadisseux, P et al: Severe hypophosphatemia after head injury. Neurosurgery 17:35, 1985.

49. Caronna, JJ: The Neurologic Evaluation. In Rosenthal, M et al (eds): Rehabilitation of the Head Injured Adult. FA Davis, Philadelphia, 1983, p 65.

50. Pearn, JH, Bart, RD and Yamaoka, R: Neurologic sequela after childhood near drowning. Pediatrics 64:187, 1979.

51. Clifton, GL, Robertson, CS and Grossman, RG: Management of the cardiovascular and metabolic responses to severe head injury. In Becker, DP and Povlishock, JT (eds): Central Nervous System Trauma: Status Report. NINCDS, NIH, Washington, 1985, p 139.

52. Langfitt, TW, Weinstein, JD and Kassell, NF: Vascular factors in head injury: Contribution to brain swelling and intracranial hypertension. In Caveness, EF and Walker, AE (eds): Head Injury. JB Lippincott, Philadelphia, 1966, p 172.

53. Lowensohn, RI, Weiss, M and Hon, EH: Heart rate variability in brain damaged patients. Lancet 1:626, 1977.

54. Minderhoud, et al: The pattern of recovery after severe head injury. Clin Neurol Neurosurg 84:15, 1982.

55. Levin, HS, O'Donnell, VM and Grossman, RG: The Galveston Orientation and Amnesia Test: A practical scale to assess cognition after head injury. J Nerv Ment Dis 167:675, 1979.

56. Pentland, B and Miller, JD: Head injury rehabilitation in Edinburgh. Health Bull 44/2:105, 1986.

57. Jennett, B and Bond M: Assessment of outcome after severe brain damage. A practical scale. Lancet 1:480, 1975.

58. Jennett, B et al: Prognosis of patients with severe head injury. Neurosurgery 4:283, 1979.

59. Braakman, R et al: Systematic selection of prognostic features in patients with severe head injury. Neurosurgery 68:362, 1980.

60. Born, JD et al: The relative prognostic value of best

motor response and brain stem reflexes in patients with severe head injury. Neurosurgery 16:595, 1985.

61. Miller, JD: Prediction of outcome after injury—a critical review. In Vigouroux, R (ed): Advances in Neurotraumatology. Vol 1. Springer-Verlag, Berlin, p 229, 1986.

62. Rao, N et al: Computerised tomography head scans as predictors of rehabilitation outcome. Arch Phys Med Rehab 65:18, 1984.

63. Stablein, DM et al: Statistical methods for determining prognosis in severe head injury. Neurosurgery 6:243, 1980.

64. Galbraith, S et al: The relationship between alcohol and head injury and its effect on the conscious level. Br J Surg 63:128, 1976.

Chapter 4

The Neurologic Evaluation

J. DOUGLAS MILLER, M.D., Ph.D.
BRIAN PENTLAND, B.Sc.(Hons), M.B.Ch.B.

In the acute phase it may be difficult to evaluate head injured patients neurologically as they are often critically ill, unconscious, or confused and uncooperative at examination. The awareness that the comatose individual's brain may be in a state of failure, with death or permanent neurologic disability as imminent possibilities, adds stress and urgency to the situation. The essentials of the early multidisciplinary management of the acutely head injured patient are outlined in the previous chapter. This early management involves interaction between a number of medical and nonmedical personnel with varying levels of training and experience. The neurologic evaluation of the head injured patient stands at the center of all of the patient care activities in the early stage, and the need for clear unequivo-cal descriptive terminology is crucial. The extent of the neurologic evaluation that is possible depends at any stage upon the degree of accessibility of the patient to verbal, painful, or other stimuli (Table 4–1). This in turn depends not only on the depth of coma or impairment of consciousness produced by the injury but also on any sedative and muscle relaxant drugs that may be in use to facilitate artificial ventilation. At all stages, however, information about the patient's neurologic status must be transmitted between members of staff directly in person, by telephone, or by written report and it is vital that the terminology used be objective and exact. In modern parlance this means that the repeatability and the interrater reliability of the neurologic findings must be tested and found satisfactory. This

Table 4–1. NEUROLOGIC ASSESSMENT AFTER SEVERE
HEAD INJURY

Early Phase	Later Phase

1. Level of consciousness
   a. Eye opening
   b. Verbal response
   c. Best motor response
2. Worst motor response
3. Motor power and tone
4. Orbicularis oculi reflex
5. Pupil size and light response
6. Resting eye position
7. Reflex eye movement
   a. Oculocephalic reflex
   b. Oculovestibular reflex
8. Oculocardiac reflex
	1. Sense of smell and taste
	2. Visual acuity and fields
	3. Eye movements
	4. Facial sensation and motor function
	5. Hearing
	6. Phonation and swallowing
	7. Limb coordination, power, and dexterity
	8. Gait and balance

approach to the evaluation of neurologic examination has only relatively recently come into use but it has amply proved the worth of the most widely used scale for determining the level of responsiveness of the recently head injured patient, the Glasgow Coma Scale.

THE GLASGOW COMA SCALE

This three-part scale was developed by Teasdale and Jennett in response to a growing dissatisfaction with the several unidimensional scales that were at that time used to describe level of consciousness.[1] Whereas some numerical scales gave higher scores for higher levels of consciousness, others awarded higher numerical value to increasing depths of coma; thus, the potential for misunderstanding was great. The Glasgow Coma Scale is based on the concept that consciousness represents a state of arousal and awareness of the external environment linked to the capacity to react to changes in that environment. It is dependent upon interaction between the ascending reticular activating system, with the cortex, thalamus, and hypothalamus above and the cerebellum, medulla, and spinal cord below. The state of arousal is assessed in terms of the eye-opening response, and the capacity to respond to changes in the environment is tested by assessing the motor response and the verbal response. The observed responses are expressed in categorical and objective terms. The coma scale completely avoids the use of terms such as "comatose," "stuporous," "semipurposeful," as these are all largely subjective and when tested for inter-rater reliability have been shown to perform poorly in statistical terms. Scoring on the Glasgow Coma Scale, in contrast, shows a high degree of repeatability and inter-rater reliability, as further elaborated upon in Chapter 5. In empirical terms the scale is a highly effective descriptor of the severity of head injury. Head injured patients who score between 3 and 8 on the Glasgow Coma Scale have a 40 percent mortality, between 9 and 12 a 4 percent mortality, and between 13 and 15 a 0.4 percent mortality. The Glasgow Coma Scale is therefore a powerful prognostic instrument.

Determination of the Glasgow Coma Scale score is, however, only part of the neuro-logic assessment of the head injured patient. To this information must be added any asymmetry in response indicating hemiparesis or monoparesis and evaluation of a number of aspects of brainstem function. For the purpose of recording the level of consciousness the best responses to stimulation on the coma scale are used, but valuable information about focal neurologic deficits can be obtained from noting the worst responses. During the examination the observer must remain aware that any conclusions from neurologic assessment are of doubtful value unless hypoxemia or arterial hypotension associated with the injury are first corrected. The influence of drugs on the neurologic findings must also be accounted for, particularly sedative and muscle relaxant drugs; and the neurologic observer must always bear in mind the possibilities of blindness, deafness, and complete spinal cord lesions affecting the determination of neurologic status.

The Eye Opening Response

It is a prerequisite to the definition of the state of coma and the classification of a severe head injury that there be no eye opening, even in response to painful stimuli. Eye opening to pain or on command indicates that arousal is possible and, therefore, that the patient is not comatose. Jennett and Teasdale emphasize the importance of loss of the eye opening response in the definition of severe head injury.[2] This has been supported by Miller and Jones, who showed that in patients with severe head injury, defined as a total coma score of 8 or less, the mortality was 45 percent in those with no eye opening but only 10 percent in patients whose eyes opened to pain (but who had a slightly worse motor response).[3] Eye opening cannot be assessed when the eyes are swollen shut owing to anterior cranial fossa or local injury, and when such is the case this part of the coma scale assessment is left blank. This does emphasize, however, the importance of early assessment on the Glasgow Coma Scale, which may be possible when the patient is first seen in the emergency room before the periorbital swelling closes the eyes. The value of the eye opening response as an index of the severity of the head injury is limited to the first 10 to

14 days after injury. After this time spontaneous eye opening returns even in patients who fail to make any other significant improvement and who remain permanently in the vegetative state.

The Best Motor Response

The motor response to command or to painful stimulation of the trunk, face, or limbs is the single most important part of the neurologic evaluation of the comatose patient. The response to pain should be elicited in all four limbs and by stimulating the supraorbital ridge. The latter stimulus must be included because absence of response to painful stimulation in the limbs may be the result of spinal cord damage. The most important cutoff point on the motor scale is the differentiation between normal flexion and abnormal flexion. The characteristics of the abnormal flexor response include pronation of the wrist, flexion of the wrist, and frequently tucking of the thumb across the palm of the hand. If there is doubt about the nature of the response then several forms of painful stimuli should be applied at multiple sites. These will include heavy pressure on the nailbed of the little finger, using a pencil or other hard object, pinching of the skin of the upper arm in the axilla, heavy pressure with the knuckle of the examiner's fist rolled over the sternum, and thumbnail pressure on the supraorbital ridges. Extensor responses of the arm and leg imply extension at the elbow and knee, respectively. These may not always be the same as the classic decerebrate response, in which there is elbow extension, pronation of the arm, and flexion at the wrist. On occasion, extension of the arm may be accompanied by supination.

Even in patients with no voluntary motor response, it is possible to assess motor power by comparing the strength of motor response in the facial and limb muscles between the right and the left side. A unilateral motor weakness is an important sign of focal neurologic dysfunction.

Although most adult patients ascend and descend the six points on the motor scale in order, the position may be different in very young children. In babies, the state of coma may be accompanied by flaccidity of the upper limbs, and during recovery the limb motor response may improve without interruption from flaccidity to a flexor response.

Motor function cannot be adequately tested in limbs immobilized by splints or plaster casts, nor when the patient is receiving muscle relaxant drugs during artificial ventilation. For some hours after withdrawal of these drugs there may be difficulty in deciding when it is valid to begin testing the motor response. This is best determined by the use of an electrical peripheral nerve stimulator to see whether satisfactory muscle contractions can be obtained by electrical stimulation. Within the definition of coma a wide range of responses is possible on the motor scale, ranging from localization of pain down to no response whatever. Ability to obey commands is, however, incompatible with a definition of coma.

The Verbal Response

By definition, patients in coma do not utter recognizable words. Either no noise is elicited, even to painful stimulation, or there may be unintelligible sounds. As patients recover, ascending the verbal scale, they reach the stage of confused speech. It is important to recognize that such patients are almost certainly within the period of post-traumatic amnesia and will not subsequently remember the events of the time. Nor will such patients be amenable to detailed neuropsychologic evaluation. The Galveston Orientation and Amnesia Test can be used to indicate emergence from post-traumatic amnesia at the end of the confusional period.

The examiner must be aware of the possibility that expressive or receptive dysphasia may totally alter the interpretation of the verbal response scale. It is also clear that when the patient has an endotracheal tube in situ a verbal response is unobtainable. However, when spontaneous eye opening has returned it may be possible to test the patient's capacity to accept and analyze information by using eye blinking, hand gestures, or writing instead of speech. At an earlier stage the data on verbal response are simply recorded as missing.

The verbal response scale is concerned with the content of the verbal response rather than the nature of articulate speech. After a severe head injury, a number of patients suffer from dysarthria or dysphonia. While such abnormalities in combination with truncal ataxia are important indicators of brainstem or cerebellar dysfunction, these alterations of speech are not considered in the assessment of the verbal response as part of the coma scale.

In children younger than 2 years old who have not yet reached the stage of producing formed speech, the verbal response scale cannot be fully evaluated. It is considered by some that crying may be the infantile equivalent of words on the adult coma scale.

TESTS OF BRAINSTEM FUNCTION

In cases of blunt acceleration/deceleration injury of the head, it has been proposed that with increasing force applied to the head the brain injury is centripetal; i.e., the greater the injuring force, the more deeply do the diffuse white matter injuries extend toward the brainstem.[4] Therefore, the presence of brainstem dysfunction in a comatose patient is evidence of a considerable force of injury and carries a correspondingly worse prognosis. Even in the unconscious patient it is possible to test a number of brainstem reflexes, of which the most important are the pupil responses to light and the eye movement reflexes. In the belief that there is an anatomic and pathophysiologic hierarchy of brainstem reflexes indicating the caudal extent of the traumatic dysfunction in the brainstem, Born and his colleagues proposed the addition of a fourth element—brainstem reflex scale—to the three elements of the Glasgow Coma Scale.[5] This Glasgow-Liege Scale has been subjected to rigorous tests of repeatability, inter-rater reliability, and prognostic power. It has been shown to amplify the information provided by the standard Glasgow Coma Scale, particularly in comatose, severely head injured patients.

The fourth scale is based on the observation that with deepening levels of coma there is an orderly and progressive loss of certain brainstem reflexes. In descending order these are the orbicularis oculi reflex elicited by the glabellar tap; the vertical oculovestibular reflex induced by simultaneous bilateral irrigation of the ears with

cold water; the pupillary light reflex; the horizontal oculovestibular reflex stimulated by unilateral caloric testing; and, finally, the oculocardiac reflex consisting, in the normal subject, of production of bradycardia with orbital pressure.

THE PUPILLARY LIGHT RESPONSE

The examiner will be concerned both with the size and equality of the pupils at rest and with the response of the pupils to light shone first into one eye and then into the other. As the examination is usually done in bright surroundings it is important to use shading and a good light source.

To test the pupillary responses a bright light is shone into each eye individually, observing the direct response in the ipsilateral eye and the consensual reflex in the opposite eye. If there is an afferent lesion involving the optic nerve, light shone into the affected eye fails to produce a response in either eye. This contrasts with an efferent defect involving the third nerve, in which light shone into either eye fails to produce a response in the affected eye while light shone into the affected eye produces constriction of the opposite pupil.

After testing each eye separately the light is moved rapidly from one pupil to the other. This so-called swinging flashlight test is done to detect a partial lesion of the optic nerve. It depends on eliciting the Marcus-Gunn sign in which there is dilatation of the pupil of the abnormal eye when the light is shone briefly into it after oscillating between the two eyes for about a second at a time. Under normal conditions there should be constriction in the illuminated eye even with a brief exposure to light.

Bilateral small or pinpoint pupils in a comatose patient are usually an indication of a destructive lesion in the pons but it is important to remember that opiates can produce the same appearance. Elderly people often have bilateral senile miosis but their small pupils do react to light. Widely dilated pupils which are unreactive to light occur in end-stage cerebral hypoxia or ischemia. Nonreactive, mid-position pupils bilaterally are indicative of mid-brain damage. Bilateral pupil dilatation can, of course, be the result of mydriatics such as atropine and scopolamine, which paralyze the pupillary response.

Wide pupillary dilatation on one side only is usually the result of a third nerve palsy, particularly if it is accompanied by ptosis and lateral deviation of the eye owing to the unopposed action of the abducens nerve. Apart from an isolated third nerve palsy or local damage to the eye or optic nerve, other causes of unequal pupils should be considered, including the installation of pharmacologic agents into one eye or the presence of a tonic pupil. One form of tonic pupil occurs in Adie's syndrome, in which there is a unilateral dilated pupil that reacts only very slowly to light stimulation and is often accompanied by a decrease in the tendon reflexes. Other, less common causes of tonic pupil are infection of the ciliary apparatus and diabetes mellitus. Inequality of the pupils may, of course, be the result of unilateral miosis. This may be found in Horner's syndrome, resulting from damage to sympathetic pathways as may occur in neck trauma cases. The small pupil in patients with Horner's syndrome does, however, constrict in reaction to bright light. It is also well to remember that a slight difference in the size of pupils occurs in about 15 to 30 percent of normal individuals, so-called physiologic anisocoria. Such pupils should both react normally to light.

RESTING EYE POSITION

Conjugate deviation of the eyes is seen with posterior frontal cortical contusions when the eyes deviate to the affected side. Brainstem lesions can also produce conjugate deviation, but in these circumstances the eyes deviate to the opposite side. Skew or dysconjugate deviation of the eyes indicates a lesion in the brainstem involving the medial longitudinal fasciculus. Minor degrees of movement of the orbital axes can be detected by shining a light from a distance of 1 meter directly between the eyes. The position of the reflected point of light within each pupil should be compared. The point of light should be in the same position for both pupils.

EYE MOVEMENTS

A considerable amount of neurologic information is available from studies of eye movements. In the conscious patient the action of each extraocular muscle can be individually assessed simply by asking the patient to look in the appropriate directions. The saccadic and pursuit systems can be tested by eliciting optokinetic nystagmus. This test is done by moving a series of identical dark objects on a tape or drum in front of the eyes in one direction. Under normal circumstances the eyes will pursue the moving object then quickly flick back in the opposite direction to pick up the next moving object. This normal response is indicative of an intact oculomotor pathway coupled with intact visual apparatus. If optokinetic nystagmus is not elicited the defect may be in the visual or the oculomotor apparatus.

When it is not possible for the patient to obey commands and thus to cooperate in these tests of eye movement, some form of testing reflex eye movements becomes necessary. The most widely used are the oculocephalic and oculovestibular responses. The oculocephalic, or doll's eye, maneuver is carried out by moving the patient's head rapidly from side to side to elicit lateral eye movements. With the patient supine the normal position of the eyes is looking directly upward and when the head is moved quickly to one side the eyes swing back to regain this normal orientation. Thus, if the head is turned to the left side, the eyes should move in a conjugate manner back toward the right side to resume the vertical orientation. A similar phenomenon occurs when the examiner moves the patient's head up and down, provoking compensatory vertical movement of the eyes. These responses result from stimulation of the vestibular system, so that this system, as well as the central and peripheral oculomotor apparatus, must be intact to get a normal response. Absence of response or a dysconjugate response indicates defects in either or both of these systems. Oculocephalic reflex testing cannot be done when there is suspicion of damage to the cervical spine or any other factor that impedes mobility of the head and neck.

The oculovestibular reflexes depend on stimulating the vestibular system by applying either cold or warm water to the tympanic membrane on either side. In comatose patients it is usual to apply ice cold water by syringe in the external auditory meatus. Under these circumstances the normal response would be conjugate deviation of the eyes toward the irrigated ear. Simultaneous irrigation of both ears should produce a vertical movement of both eyes. Absence of response or a dysconjugate response indicates a lesion of the vestibular and/or oculomotor apparatus, which may be peripheral or central in the brainstem.

Caloric testing in a conscious patient should be done with much less strong stimuli. Irrigation with warm water (44°C [101°F]) produces nystagmus with the quick phase to the irrigated side and the slow phase away from the irrigated ear. Irrigation with cool water (30°C [86°F]) results in quick movements to the opposite side and the slow phase toward the irrigated ear. As nystagmus is traditionally named after its quick phase, irrigation of the right ear with warm water produces nystagmus to the right, and with cold water, nystagmus to the left (Cold Opposite, Warm Same—COWS). Caloric testing cannot be done in the usual way if the tympanic membranes are not intact or if blood or cerebrospinal fluid (CSF) is coming from the ear. If there is any suspicion that the tympanic membrane is not intact, it is still possible to stimulate the ear by inserting a blind-ended needleholder into the ear and irrigating cold saline into that.

LESIONS OF THE FACIAL AND AUDITORY NERVES IN HEAD INJURY

In patients with fractures involving the petrous temporal bone nerve deafness occurs frequently. When the fracture is transversely across the petrous bone the deafness is most likely to be permanent and may be accompanied by a lower motor neuron type of facial palsy. In some cases the facial palsy appears only after a delay of 2 or 3 days from the time of the injury and is considered to represent the effects of swelling of the nerve within the facial canal. In such cases there is usually a recovery of facial nerve function after some months. At the time when the patient is still unconscious it will not be possible to detect deafness in the usual way but its presence may be indicated by unsuccessful attempts to elicit an auditory evoked potential from the affected ear.

Lesser degrees of damage to the auditory

and vestibular system may be the basis of complaints of dizziness and vertigo experienced by a number of patients recovering from head injury.

LESIONS OF THE LOWER CRANIAL NERVES

Injury to the last four cranial nerves— glossopharyngeal, vagal, accessory, and hypoglossal—as a result of trauma is rare. When present, such injuries are usually associated with fractures of the basisphenoid and basiocciput. When there are persisting disorders of phonation and swallowing, these are of considerable importance in the intensive care unit because of the danger of regurgitation and aspiration of gastric contents, with consequent lung complications. These abnormalities are commonly associated with marked truncal ataxia and probably then represent brainstem damage rather than a specific lesion of the cranial nerves themselves.

AUTONOMIC DISTURBANCES

As well as altering consciousness level, lesions of the upper brainstem and hypothalamus may result in disruption of the central control of various autonomic functions leading to vasomotor disturbances, disorders of body temperature, and altered respiratory patterns. Pulse, blood pressure, temperature, and respiratory recordings must be monitored carefully, and adequate ventilation and support of the circulation are clear priorities in the management of head injured patients. The various disturbances of autonomic control from brainstem damage are important but of limited diagnostic value in localizing the site of the lesion.

COORDINATION OF MOVEMENT, BALANCE, AND GAIT

As severely head injured patients recover in the early stages a variety of abnormal motor postures and movements may be observed. In some cases these can include emergence of frankly abnormal motor movements of a choreoathetoid or ballistic nature. There is difficulty with performing rapid or precise movements and at rest the limb may be held in abnormal positions. Hand-eye coordination is impaired, and the impairment of motor control can be emphasized when the patient's eyes are closed.

In patients who have markedly abnormal limb motor responses, the gait is frequently abnormal with considerable difficulties for the patient in achieving standing balance, coordinated walking, and control of the body when changing direction. These types of abnormality all appear to correlate with the presence of brainstem damage.

NEUROLOGIC EVALUATION DURING RECOVERY

Detailed neurologic assessment may not be possible in the earliest stages after head injury but it is essential that, as the patient recovers consciousness and orientation, full neurologic evaluation be made. Smell and taste should be tested and accurate measurement of visual fields, visual acuity, and hearing are necessary. There is also the need for frequent re-examination, as the recovery from one disability may unmask another of important diagnostic or prognostic significance. The complex constellation of possible neurologic deficits that can follow head injury is such that accurate assessment and documentation throughout the recovery period is vital in planning the rehabilitation goals of the individual at different stages and necessary for the early detection of neurologic complications such as intracranial infection, hydrocephalus, and chronic subdural hematoma.

REFERENCES

1. Teasdale, G and Jennett, B: Assessment of coma and impaired consciousness: A practical scale. Lancet 2:81, 1974.
2. Jennett, B and Teasdale, G: Aspects of coma after severe head injury. Lancet 1:878, 1977.
3. Miller, JD and Jones, PA: The work of a regional head injury service. Lancet 1:1141, 1985.
4. Ommaya, AK and Gennarelli, TA: Cerebral concussion and traumatic unconsciousness: correlation of experimental and clinical observations on blunt head injuries. Brain 97:633, 1974.
5. Born, JD et al: Relative prognostic value of best motor response and brain stem reflexes in patients with severe head injury. Neurosurgery 16:595, 1985.

BIBLIOGRAPHY

Bickerstaff, ER: Neurological Examination in Clinical Practice, ed 4. Blackwell-Scientific, Oxford, 1980.
De Jong, RN: The Neurologic Examination, ed 4. Harper and Row, Hagerstown, MD, 1979.
Harrison, MJG: Neurological Skills. Butterworths, London, 1987.
Kunze, K, Zangemeister, WH and Arlt, A: Clinical Problems of Brain Stem Disorders. Georg Thieme, Stuttgart, 1986.
Plum, F and Posner, JB: Diagnosis of Stupor and Coma, ed 3. FA Davis, Philadelphia, 1980.

Chapter 5

Standardized Methods of Assessing and Predicting Outcome

MICHAEL R. BOND, M.D., Ph.D.

WHY MEASURE OUTCOME?

Prior to 1965, little was known about the complex physical, emotional, and social changes that contribute to the process of recovery from severe closed head injury. Nevertheless, there had been several approaches to devising methods of assessing the outcome of severe closed injuries, but they were based mainly on measures of physical handicaps and ability to return to work. In contrast, the problems posed by patients' mental difficulties for themselves and their families were neglected. Finally, assessments of outcome were often made only once, usually many months or even years after the injuries occurred. By this time, much of the recovery process had taken place and been missed, and the opportunity to develop indices of prognosis had been lost. Therefore, it is not surprising that there was uncertainty about the nature of recovery from injury in the minds of caring professionals and the families of the injured. For example, relatives were often told that they could expect the injured person to continue to recover for 2 years or more but were not given detailed information about the nature of the recovery they might expect. Vague statements of this kind, especially when made in the first few weeks after injury, are upsetting to relatives who later discover that many of the patient's deficits are established within a few months after in-

jury and do not disappear later as they had hoped.

The primary focus of head injury research in the past 15 to 20 years has been to provide information for the prediction of the length and extent of the recovery process.

THE PROCESS OF MEASUREMENT

Because many persons are unclear about how to measure disability, it is worth considering the possibilities and the scientific restraints placed upon the one who measures. Measurements in head injury research usually take one of two forms. Patients may be grouped in a general way according to a predetermined characteristic—for example, their level of "general dependency," a factor that forms the basis of the widely used Glasgow Outcome Scale (Table 5–1).[1] This is a global scale and as such has strength insofar as it gives a straightforward and readily understood picture of any group of patients studied; however, it reveals little about the subtle balance between physical incapacity and disturbances of behavior or of mental life.

The grades of the original scale are wide, and although not too precisely defined, the results gained are very useful for painting the broad canvas. An increase or decrease in sensitivity may be needed, and the means of

59

Table 5–1. THE GLASGOW OUTCOME SCALE IN ITS ORIGINAL FORM AND IN EXTENDED AND CONTRACTED FORMS

Extended Scale	Original Scale	Contracted Scales			
Dead	Dead	Dead	Dead or vegetative	Dead or vegetative	Dead
Vegetative	Vegetative	Dependent	Severely disabled		Survivors
Degree of disability: 5	Severely disabled				
4					
3	Moderately disabled	Independent	Independent	Conscious	
2					
1	Good recovery				
0					
Total categories 8	5	3			2

From Jennett et al,[9] with permission.

achieving this are shown in Table 5–1. Detailed information is obtained differently by means of scales built on carefully defined items or questions that, for example, may assess individual components of behavior or attitudes and that, as a result, offer greater precision in rating deficits and the effects of treatments on them.[2] Further, psychological tests used to assess these functions have items within their structure that may be identified according to their purpose as instrumental (i.e., measuring aspects of behavior), as affective (i.e., measuring emotional characteristics), or as cognitive (i.e., measuring aspects of intelligence).

When selecting tests, the experimenter must choose ones that will answer questions or hypotheses defined beforehand. Therefore, the tests selected must be valid. This means that they should measure what the experimenter wishes to measure or, in other words, actually predict the criterion of whatever is intended to be measured. Tests selected should also be reliable, which means that the observations made should be dependable, self-consistent, and stable. A test should yield results that are consistent, even when measured by more than one observer, and should be pertinent to the specific purpose the experimenter has in mind. As many of the physical and mental functions measured are part of a spectrum or range of functions, which in some cases are in continuity with normality, it is important to have information about the performance of normal individuals of comparable age, education, and, perhaps, sex. This enables the measurer to determine whether or not a group of head injured individuals differs significantly from normal and, if so, to what extent. It is a general rule, therefore, that tests of this type must have been standardized in a normal population. Finally, each test should be within the capacity of the testee at the start of testing, thereafter increasing in difficulty to the point where limits of ability are reached. In the case of head injured persons, tests should not be too lengthy, because fatigue and impaired concentration interfere with performance and may invalidate results. It is commonly a fault among inexperienced researchers to design the "full and perfect" battery of tests, only to find that patients cannot and/or will not complete it. Selection of appropriate tests, especially of mental functions, may be very difficult simply because of the large number of tests available for a single function such as memory (Table 5–2).

In general terms, the selection of tests depends on the kind of information required. Tests, or instruments (as they are often called), may be structured, semistructured, or unstructured. Structured instruments define exactly what is to be asked or read; semistructured instruments provide leading questions but rely on the interviewer to gain the needed information; and unstructured interviews may define only the area to be examined and allow complete personal judgment by the interviewer. The former are easy to score and provide standard, comparable information. The latter permit the interviewer to follow leads and explore a new area. Unstructured instruments also are used to gain new ideas, whereas the structured instruments are used to test definitive theories. Finally, the instruments may be administered by a professional or trained interviewer, may be self-administered by the patient, or may be given to a close relative or friend, someone who

Table 5–2. TWENTY-TWO TESTS OF LEARNING AND MEMORY

Wechsler Memory Scale
Auditory-Verbal Learning Task (Rey)
Selective Reminding (Buschke)
Paired Associates Test (Inglis)
Babcock Story
Recurring Figures Test (Kimura)
Visual Retention Test (Benton)
Memory for Designs Test (Binet)
Memory for Designs Test (Graham-Kindall)
Rey-Osterrieth Complex Figure Test
Digit Symbol Test (WAIS)
Symbol Digit Modalities Test (Smith)
Facial Recognition Test (Milner)
Posner Task Test
Knox Cube Imitation Test
Block-Tapping Test (Corsi)
Recency-Primary Test (Corsi)
Boston Retrograde Amnesia Test
Tactile Performance Test
Tactile Nonsense Figure Test (Milner)
Memory Battery (Squires)
University of Wisconsin Memory Battery

knows the patient well and plays a significant part in the patient's life.

AIMS OF MEASUREMENT

The purposes of applying measurements to various aspects of the physical, emotional/behavioral, and social consequences of severe head injury are as follows:

1. Assessment of the severity of injury at the time of admission to hospital
2. Assessment of the physical, mental, and social deficits during the process of recovery
3. Assessment of global outcome and its relation to specific deficits mentioned in Newcombe and Fortuny.[2]
4. Assessment of the effects of the injury on family members
5. All measures (1 through 4) may be incorporated into programs designed to evaluate rehabilitation techniques

MEASURES OF OUTCOME

It is impossible to describe here all the instruments available for the assessment of head injured patients; therefore, a small number have been selected because they are often used and fulfill most of the criteria of suitability described earlier, and because they illustrate recent discoveries about the process of recovery and means of predicting outcome. The measures have been selected from clinical neurologic, psychologic, and social schedules in common use.

Assessment of Severity of Injury

Severity of injury is an important guide to short- and long-term outcome, although in the latter case it will be shown that so far our methods permit any given patient's prognosis to be drawn only in broad terms—especially with reference to the patient's ultimate possession and use of the higher social skills needed in everyday life; for example, to maintain a home, to maintain good relations with others, or to hold down a job.

Assessment of Post-traumatic Amnesia

In 1932, the late Professor Ritchie Russell[3] of the University of Oxford proposed that the time taken to recover full consciousness is a measure of the quantity of brain tissue destroyed by a head injury. He based his observation on the fact that return of memory for day-to-day events on a continuous basis is the last stage in the restoration of full consciousness. The time between injury and recovery of continuous memory is the period known as post-traumatic anmesia (PTA). Retrograde amnesia refers to the period of memory loss prior to injury and seems to be of less value as a measure of severity. When estimating PTA, which is a retrospective measure that can be used months or years after injury, it is important to establish when full memory for day-to-day events was restored. Prior to this, patients may have isolated memories—for example, a visit from a relative or friend—but this is only an "island" in a "sea of forgetfulness." In many cases, the full return of memory is related to an important event in the patient's life, presumably reflecting a period of increased arousal; for example, transfer from one ward or hospital to another, or going home. In this context, full consciousness may be restored more quickly in children in whom it is prolonged, by sending them home to a familiar environment. It has been suggested that in patients without dysphasia the duration of PTA is approximately four times the period taken to speak after injury. Relatives are able to date its end to the time the patient becomes lucid and clearly remembers recent conversations and events. The ability to recall recent events and the presence of correct orientation for

Table 5–3. THE GALVESTON ORIENTATION AND AMNESIA TEST

Name _____   Date of Test ⊔⊔⊔ mo day yr

Age _____ Sex M   F   Day of the week s m t w t f s

Date of birth ⊔⊔⊔ mo day yr   Time   AM   PM

Diagnosis _____   Date of injury ⊔⊔⊔ mo day yr

GALVESTON ORIENTATION & AMNESIA TEST (GOAT)   Error Points

1. What is your name? (2) _____ When were you born? (4) _____   ⊔⊔
   Where do you live? (4) _____
2. Where are you now? (5) city _____ (5) hospital _____   ⊔⊔
   (unncessary to state name of hospital)
3. On what date were you admitted to this hospital? (5) _____   ⊔⊔
   How did you get here? (5) _____
4. What is the first event you can remember <u>after</u> the injury? (5) _____   ⊔⊔
   Can you describe in detail (e.g., date, time, companions) the first event you can recall
   after injury? (5) _____
5. Can you describe the last event you recall <u>before</u> the accident? (5) _____   ⊔⊔
   _____ Can you describe in detail (e.g., date, time, companions) the
   first event you can recall <u>before</u> the injury? (5) _____
6. What time is it now _____ (−1 for each ½ hour removed from correct time to max-   ⊔⊔
   imum of −5)
7. What day of the week is it? _____ (−1 for each day removed from correct one)   ⊔⊔
8. What day of the month is it?_____ (−1 for each day removed from correct date to   ⊔⊔
   maximum of −5)
9. What is the month? _____ (−5 for each month removed from correct   ⊔⊔
   one to maximum of − 15)
10. What is the year _____ (− 10 for each year removed from correct one to maximum   ⊔⊔
    of − 30)

                                              Total Error Points ⊔⊔⊔
                        Total Goat Score (100-total error points) ⊔⊔⊔

From Levin et al,[5] with permission.

time and place form the basis of tests recently designed to determine the end of PTA, in other words, tests that take us from retrospective to prospective assessment.[4] The Galveston Orientation and Amnesia Test, developed by Levin et al,[5] has been used widely in the United States in recent years to measure PTA (Table 5–3).

In his original paper, Russell related the duration of PTA to the severity of injury in the following way:

PTA <1 hr   = mild injury
PTA 1–24 hr = moderate injury
PTA 1–7 days = severe injury
PTA >7 days = very severe injury

In a study of 1000 severe head injuries in Glasgow, it was shown that all patients had a PTA lasting more than 2 days, 94 percent more than 1 week, 80 percent more than 2 weeks, and 60 percent more than 4 weeks.[6]

There is often concern about the accuracy of this method because it involves a retrospective assessment; however, all severe injuries have a PTA exceeding 1 day. The longer the period of amnesia, the less need there is for a precise estimation of its end. In fact, it is usually impossible to estimate PTA without accepting that the figure is within days or, in the case of the severest injuries, a month or two of its end. With regard to milder injuries, more precise estimations of PTA are possible, and Fortuny and others[4] have presented an expanded scale for minor injuries that may be used in association with their test for its duration. The gradings are as follows:

PTA <10 min   = very mild injury
PTA 10–60 min = mild injury
PTA 1–24 hr   = moderate injury

Their study concerns patients who were admitted to a British hospital over a period of 6 months; the proportions in each of the three categories given were 46.7 percent, 17.3 percent, and 20.8 percent, respectively. Only 6.6 percent of patients had a PTA greater than 24 hours.

Measurement of Coma Duration

It should be remembered that an interest in measures of severity is related to a desire for one measurement that will predict immediate and late outcome with the highest possible accuracy from the time of the injury onward, and that the use of coma duration has been perhaps the most popular universal measure of the severity of head injury. However, until 1974, a satisfactory and universally acceptable means of defining coma was lacking, chiefly because there was no agreement regarding the hierarchy of physical signs indicating the depth of coma and reflecting the severity of brain injury. Unconsciousness and wakefulness are not two mutually exclusive states. As the patient recovers, one state gradually shades into the other. Therefore, the process of return to awareness is continuous; during its course, a number of signs of specific neurologic dysfunctions may be detected, and each has significance in terms of the severity of brain damage.

Using the principle of the different significance for life or death of a number of the signs that may occur and for the degree of overall disability they predict later in recovery, Teasdale and Jennett[7] made the most significant contribution so far to our understanding of the assessment of disordered consciousness in the immediate postinjury period. They also developed, to a high level of accuracy, means of predicting the early outcome of injury, and both achievements were made through the construction of the Glasgow Coma Scale (see Table 3–4, Chapter 3). The attraction of the scale lies in the fact that those who use it—whether nurses, general surgeons, neurosurgeons, or physicians—obtain consistent results. The instrument is relatively impervious to the effects of language and, therefore, has a high level of inter-rater and cross-cultural reliability. It enables us to define coma in descriptive terms without reference to supposed anatomic sites of dysfunction or to levels that depend on the concurrence of certain degrees of responsiveness with other features such as pupil reactions or respiration abnormalities. After considerable research involving all disorders of neurologic function that can be measured during unconsciousness and from which a hierarchy of responses can be obtained, three items proved to be the most sensitive measures of severity and predictors of outcome. They are eye opening, motor response, and verbal performance; each is graded independently. Coma is defined as (1) not opening the eyes, (2) not obeying commands, and (3) not uttering understandable words. The responses to the tests are scored separately, giving a total derived from $E + M + V$ with a range of 3 to 15 points. Of the three subscales, the assessment of motor function has proved to be the most powerful predictor of short-term outcome. This is a useful fact because occasionally it is impossible to obtain accurate measures or any measure at all on the eye opening or verbal scales because of the nature of the patient's injuries. Conscious patients get the highest scores; 90 percent of those with scores of 8 or less are in coma, and none of those with scores of 9 or more are in coma. This critical point in the scale is an important watershed because patients with scores of 8 or less are regarded as having had a severe injury, if the low score is maintained for at least 6 hours from impact or is reached at the end of a period of post-injury lucidity during which the patient talked. Approximately 50 percent of these patients will die. Patients with scores higher than 12 are regarded as having had minor injuries, although a significant number of them have residual deficits up to 3 months after injury (see Chapter 2). By exclusion, patients with scores from 9 through 11 have injuries of moderate severity. The critical reader will have realized that despite the effectiveness of the scale in giving a continuous measure of the features of coma, there is no absolute measure of what constitutes a severe injury. However, the definition given is widely accepted on the basis of the relationship between the score of 8 or less and the certainty of the presence of unconsciousness and the significance of scores below this level in terms of the chances of survival or death (Table 5–4).[8] The power of

Table 5–4. OUTCOME ASSOCIATED WITH BEST LEVEL OF RESPONSIVENESS IN FIRST 24 HOURS AFTER COMA

Coma Response Sum	n	Dead or Vegetative (%)	Moderate Disability or Good Recovery (%)
11	57	12	87
8/9/10	190	27	68
5/6/7	525	53	34
3/4	176	87	7

From Jennett et al,[8] with permission.

the coma scale is increased by use of scores of individual responses in the E, M, and V components. (For further information, the reader should consult Chapter 14 of Jennett and Teasdale.[9])

Neurologic Assessment of Outcome

Until recent times, neurologic assessment was virtually the sole measure of the early and late outcome of brain injuries. As a result, there are many scales of widely varying complexity for the assessment of all aspects of neurologic functions encompassed by the broad areas of motor and sensory function, extrapyramidal activity, and higher-level mental activities, although in the last group interest has been confined chiefly to disorders of speech and consciousness. If the nature of the tests is examined in general terms, they appear to form three basic categories.

First, there are tests based on a "points system" in which numerical values are assigned in a graded system to each physical parameter to be assessed. The total number of points gained either for an individual function—for example, the extent of motor dysfunction in a limb—or for all disabilities is used to represent the patient's neurologic status at any given time. Assessment of this type may be used to describe recovery, to predict the speed and eventual extent of recovery, or to evaluate the effects of treatment.

A second approach was described by Roberts.[10] His large-scale retrospective survey of war veterans with head injuries depends upon very careful and detailed neurologic assessments. Analysis of his results leads to the formulation of patterns of disability, which in turn leads to the construction of central neural disability profiles. For example, Roberts identified the hemiparetic, brainstem cerebellar, and athetoid pseudobulbar patterns, as well as a fourth pattern that incorporates mental handicap, decerebrate dementia. This is a familiar and traditional neurologic "grouping" process, but the validity of Roberts' "patterns of disability" awaits confirmation and acceptance by others.

Finally, there are several methods of assessing neurologic function by mechanical, electrical, or photographic techniques. For example, the first two of these are often used to assess muscle tone and power, and the latter—currently improved by the use of videotape equipment and computer analysis—to examine patterns of movements such as gait.

The question of which instrument to use depends on the objectives or aims of the assessor, but for everyday clinical use, relatively short scales that are reliable and easily performed by professionals with varying levels of experience are most acceptable. An example of a simple scale is given in Table 5–5,[11] in which only the degree of deficit is rated and there is no presumption about the central lesion responsible because "localization" is not of much value in studies of severe closed head injuries that cause widespread damage. However, the scale does make a number of judgments about the significance of each deficit for return to activities of daily life. The information gathered

with this type of instrument has proved very useful in studies of the process of recovery from head injury. For example, scores of neurologic disability may be related to a measure of the severity of injury (PTA) (Fig. 5–1) and to overall levels of social disability (Fig. 5–2).[11]

Assessment of Mental Outcome

COGNITIVE AND PERCEPTUAL FUNCTIONS

Psychologic measures of outcome are attractive because of their high degree of specificity, validity, and reliability. However, it is their very specificity that reduces their potency as predictors of the ways in which individuals will use their residual skills and adapt to changes in their personal lives. The

Table 5–5. A NEUROPHYSICAL SCALE

Deficit	Score
Motor	
Monoparesis	1
Monoplegia	2
Hemiparesis	3
Hemiplegia	4
Sensory	
One arm/leg, partial	1
One arm/leg, full	2
One arm/leg and part trunk	3
Arm/leg and trunk	4
Speech	
Partial aphasia	2
Complete aphasia	4
Ataxia	
Each limb Mild/Moderate	1
Severe	2
Dysarthria Mild/Moderate	1
Severe	2
Dysphagia Mild/Moderate	1
Severe	2
Cranial Nerves except	1 for each involved
Vision	2 for each eye
Hearing	2 for each ear
Physical Dificits	
Mild/Moderate	1
Severe	2

From Bond,[11] with permission.

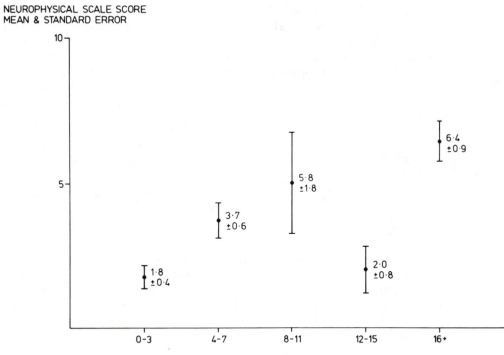

Figure 5–1. Relationship between physical disability following severe head injury duration of post-traumatic amnesia (PTA). (From Bond,[11] with permission.)

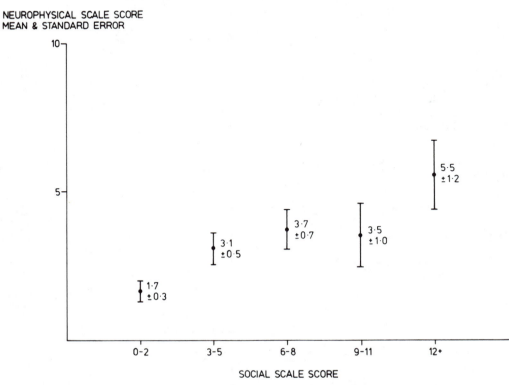

Figure 5–2. Relationship between physical disability after severe head injury and social outcome. (From Bond,[11] with permission.)

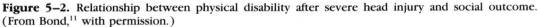

best known of all instruments are those that measure cognitive functions. However, recent studies of tests of intelligence, perhaps the most widely used of all, reveal that residual intelligence levels relate only broadly to an individual's ultimate capacity to cope with work, except perhaps among those who earn their living chiefly by using their intellectual skills. It seems clear that memory and learning tasks are more sensitive measures of cognitive change, at least after closed head injuries, than are conventional intelligence tests. In fact, performance on memory and learning tasks tends to correlate significantly with the severity of head injury. It is important to remember that measurements of intelligence are affected by the subject's educational level and age and that often tests must be completed within a given time. This means that patients may make lower scores than if given unlimited time to complete tests because mental slowness is one of the most common and persistent intellectual deficits of severe

head injury. Other factors, including a poor ability to sustain attention and the tendency to develop mental fatigue, influence performance on tests of all kinds; they also affect activities of daily living, perhaps accounting for the hesitancy and lack of confidence shown by many head injured individuals. For this reason, increasing attention is being given to measuring these difficulties, and it has been found that levels of fatigue are often high in the early months of recovery but lessen with time.

Despite the problems mentioned and the discrepancies between performance in the laboratory and activities in everyday life, neuropsychologic tests of cognitive function have provided an immense amount of information about the way basic mental functions recover after injury. For example, these tests have been used to explore the concept of recovery curves, as shown in Figure 5–3.[12] These reveal the way in which verbal and nonverbal forms of intelligence, as measured by the Mill Hill Vocabulary

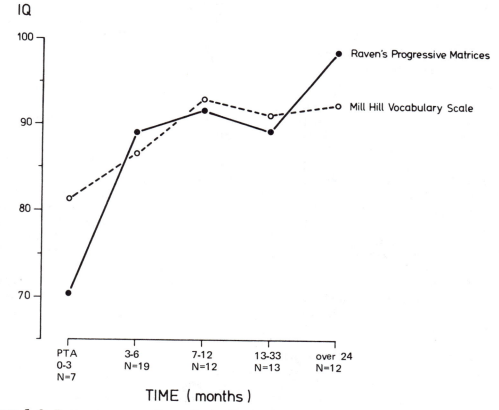

Figure 5–3. Recovery curves: changes in intellectual function after severe head injury. (From Bond and Brooks,[12] with permission.)

Scale and Raven's Progressive Matrices tests, respectively, improve during the first year after injury. Although such measures are valuable in studying groups, it is clear that the results are applicable only in a general way and may not fit the progress of a given individual. This fact emphasizes the need for caution when attempting to extend general rules to individual cases and the desirability of constructing a recovery profile from the results of a carefully chosen battery of tests.

In addition to tests of cognitive function, assessments of perception are needed because it is known that perceptual deficits (for example, of visual-spatial orientation) often subtle in nature, may interfere quite substantially with practical activities of everyday life.[2] When severe, these deficits are very noticeable, leading to such difficulties as inability to dress or to locate one's body in space, thereby making even sitting or lying a task of great difficulty. However, these deficits are almost certainly neglected in most "routine" follow-up examinations in surgical clinics. The full contribution of perceptual deficits to patients' difficulties has yet to be determined.

Assessment of Personality and Behavior

Of all the possible mental consequences of severe head injury, changes in personality and behavior are the most damaging in terms of their effects on family life and reintegration into society. The fact that changes in personality are a more serious barrier to effective rehabilitation and functional recovery than cognitive or intellectual changes was reported 45 years ago by Goldstein[13] and was investigated again 24 years ago by Luria,[14] the famous Russian neuropsychologist. The latter described a lack of self-monitoring after frontal lobe damage, and clearly, changes of this type pose great challenges to rehabilitation. Therefore, means of accurately assessing alterations in personality and abnormal behavior represent a central issue in rehabilitation research. So far, almost all published work on this subject has been based on a descriptive approach to the assessment of personality change; at this level, there is general agreement about the nature of the changes that may occur, and

an account of these changes is given in Chapter 13.

Apart from the descriptive method, there are few scales for assessment of personality after head injury, although there are many for use among normal people and psychiatric patients. However, as these rely on an individual having insight into his or her own characteristics, they cannot be used where this facility is absent or distorted, as is often the case with head injured patients. Moreover, the problem is compounded by the fact that there are many theories of personality but none that is universally accepted. Finally, several of the traits produced by brain injury are not constituents of normal personality (for example, the presence of apathy or persistent euphoria and loss of social restraint). In view of the difficulties described, it has become common practice to examine changes in personality by means of checklists devised with the possible complications of head injury in mind. These are completed by close relatives who provide information about the patient's current mental state and past character. Similar results may be achieved by means of analogue scales (Fig. 5–4); these instruments may also be used to measure the extent to which a given characteristic is present or how much that characteristic has changed as a direct result of injury.

Self-administered tests also have been used, with the Minnesota Multiphasic Personality Inventory (MMPI) being particularly popular. Administered some time after injury when emotional disturbances have stabilized considerably, the test provides results that reveal a positive relationship between psychopathology and cognitive deficits, and some of the residual emotional changes.[15–17] Clearly, the use of this measure is not ideal. Also, certain psychiatric scales have been used with populations of brain injured patients. For example, Levin and others[18] used selected scales from the Brief Psychiatric Rating Scale (BPRS) devised by Overall and Gorham[19] to assess behavioral disturbances in brain damaged patients 1 year after injury. They found that chronic disability was related to the scales for thinking disturbance, emotional withdrawal and depression, and motor retardation, but the levels of anxiety and depression detected bore no relationship to the severity of the injury or overall quality of outcome.

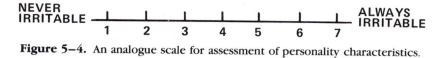

Figure 5-4. An analogue scale for assessment of personality characteristics.

Behavior-rating scales are more practical instruments and are being developed in many rehabilitation centers. In brief, they are used to define broad areas of behavioral change and, within the, sub-behavioral units which become the foci or targets for behavior modification therapies or shaping procedures. For example, one area might be "psychosocial behavior change"; within this the identifiable sub-behaviors include an individual's poor insight into his or her own abilities, a poor reaction to criticism, inability to tolerate frustration, demands for excessive attention, feelings of persecution, self-abuse, and sudden changes of mood. Another area, "aggressive behavior," might be assessed in terms of violent or threatening behavior, offensive language, damage to property, impulsiveness, and premeditated attacks on others. By means of empirically defined grades of severity, usually involving a short numerical scale, behavioral profiles may be constructed to form a basis for assessing the effects of therapy. Alternatively, they may be used for an entirely different issue—namely, to examine the natural history of a particular behavior, as a step toward accurately predicting future events or forming a prognosis.

The advantage of these techniques lies in their great flexibility of design and the fact that they can be assembled or packaged to suit individul patients in therapy and at the same time be made sufficiently reliable (eventually) to form the basis of a universally accepted range of instruments. As an example, the shortcomings and the benefits of certain parts of the BPRS mentioned earlier led Levin and his coworkers[18] to develop a new instrument, a neurobehavioral rating scale (NRS), with which to evaluate behavioral changes caused by brain injury. The NRS retains certain subscales from the BPRS, and its validity and reliability have been established.[18]

The development of techniques like the NRS brings us much closer to the type of instrument required for the assessment of post-traumatic behaviors. For example, factor analysis of their results by Levin and coworkers[18] revealed four major behavioral components detected by the scale (Table 5–6). The scale may be used to monitor the process of recovery and change. To date, its use has not been reported outside the Galveston group. The potential value of the scale as a means of providing a qualitative profile of behaviors is clear (Fig. 5–5). Those wishing to use it are reminded that as a studied interview is required, preliminary

Table 5-6. PRINCIPAL COMPONENTS ANALYSIS OF RESULTS GAINED WITH THE NEUROBEHAVIORAL RATING SCALE (NRS) USED WITH BRAIN INJURED PATIENTS

Factor I   "Cognition/Energy"

Consists of items evaluating the coherence of cognition, efficiency of memory, behavioral slowness or motor retardation and emotional withdrawal

Factor II   "Metacognition" (knowledge of one's cognitive processes)

Reflects inaccurate self-appraisal, unrealistic planning, and disinhibition

Factor III   "Somatic Concern/Anxiety"

Concerns physical complaints, anxiety, depression, and irritability

Factor IV   "Language"

Consists of scales for rating expressive and receptive language deficits

From Levin et al,[18] with permission.

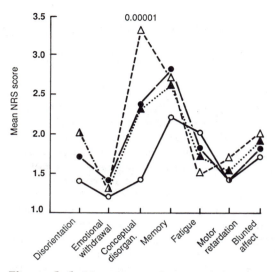

Figure 5–5. Mean scores for neurobehavioral rating scale variables for 101 patients on factor I. This factor evaluates the coherence of cognition and efficiency of memory, together with emotional retardation and emotional withdrawal. (From Levin et al,[18] with permission.)

Assessment of Overall Outcome

The final overall social outcome of severe head injuries has been defined in several ways. Terms such as good, fair, poor, acceptable, practical, worthwhile, and tolerable have been used by various writers. Others have taken a rather different view and expressed outcome in terms of ability to return to work, a matter that depends on many factors other than the residual mental or physical deficits of the patient, availability of work and family attitudes to the injured person being only two that may have a marked effect. Because many of the verbal scales tended to emphasize the more severe effects of injuries, uneven grading was often used (Table 5–7). To overcome this, Jennett and Bond[1] removed value judgments as expressed in terms like "worthwhile" and avoided the pitfalls of outcome based upon return to work, when they constructed the Glasgow Outcome Scale (GOS) (see Table 5–1). In addition to avoiding the objections

training in its administration is needed to ensure accurate assessment and interpretation of results.

to earlier scales, this scale was also devised to facilitate multicenter studies on outcome and to predict outcome accurately. It is now widely used in Europe and North America. The scale is valid and has a high degree of inter-rater reliability; in a recent study, there was a 95 percnt level of agreement between two observers rating 150 severely head injured patients.[6] As Table 5–1 shows, the scale is flexible, which means that its three best categories may be expanded to six without loss of reliability if more closely defined groups are needed. It has proved to be valuable in studies of the natural history of recovery. Large-scale surveys have revealed that the greater part of recovery is achieved between 3 and 6 months after injury and that of those who by 12 months have made a good recovery or who are moderately disabled, almost two thirds have already reached this level within 3 months after injury and 90 percent have done so by 6 months. Only 10 percent of patients who are severely or moderately disabled at 6 months will be in a better category 1 year after injury.[12] These observations correspond with the pattern of recovery of many aspects of cognitive and physical function described earlier, thus adding to the accumulating evidence that the greater part of the recovery of those functions directly attributable to activity of the brain takes place within 6 months after injury.

The overall picture of outcome after head injuries of all degrees of severity is shown in Table 5–8 from data obtained in Charlottesville, Virginia, 3 months from injury (see Chapter 2). Later improvements do occur but to a lesser extent.

On the other hand, considerable and increasing use of coping strategies of every kind, both mental and social, and the resultant interactions with others play an important role in late outcome. For this reason, measures of initial severity of injury, such as coma duration or the length of posttraumatic amnesia, weaken as predictors of psychosocial outcome if used later than 6 months after injury. However, this does not mean that PTA cannot be used to predict late outcome as measured by the GOS.

The relationship between these measures in patients, as reviewed by Jennett and Teasdale[9] at least 1 year after injury, is given in Table 5–9, from which it is clear that severe disability does not result unless PTA lasts

Table 5–7. CLASSIFICATION OF DISABILITY DUE TO BRAIN DAMAGE (CONSCIOUS SURVIVORS)

Acute Brain Damage (Traumatic or Not)	Head Injury			Stroke	
Glasgow Scale Jennett and Bond (1975) (1980) 3-point 6-point	*Najenson (1974)*	*Stover and Zeiger (1976)*	*Roberts (1979)*	*Rankin (1957)*	*Adams (1963)*
Severe disability 5 4	2	2 3 4 5	4 3.5 3	4 3	3 2
Moderate disability 3 2	3 4	6	2.5 2 1.5	2	1
Good recovery 1 0	5	7 8	1 0.5	1	

From Jennett et al,[6] with permission.

longer than 14 days. Moreover, no more than 17 percent of patients with PTA shorter than this will be moderately disabled; the remaining 83 percent will have made a good recovery despite the fact that they were all patients with severe injuries according to the criteria used at the time of admission.

Thus, it seems we have reached a position where measures of early severity primarily foretell the probability of life or death in the first days after injury (especially in the case of the Glasgow Coma Scale) or indicate the likelihood of damage to certain psychologic

Table 5–8. OUTCOME AMONG SURVIVORS 3 MONTHS AFTER HEAD INJURY

Outcome Grade (GOS)	% Total Population (n = 1248)
Vegetative	4
Severe disability	8
Moderate disability	22
Good recovery	66

and neurologic functions that arise directly from activity in the brain. However, they do not forecast late outcome in other than broad terms.

Assessment of the patient's ability to cope with the necessities of everyday life—or their "quality of life"—requires a more detailed approach. "Quality of life" has several interpretations, which indicates that the problem of how to define this concept has not yet been solved.

One approach that is commonly used centers on assessment of the efficiency with which an injured person can perform essential activities of daily life (i.e., cope with feeding, dressing, and toileting) using an activity of daily living (ADL) scale. As there are many instruments of this kind, the difficulty for the assessor lies in the selection of a valid and reliable scale.[21, 22]

This matter was reviewed by Sheikh and others,[23] who produced an instrument with these qualities, also providing scores in the hospital and at home that correlate significantly. As mentioned, the Glasgow Outcome Scale provides a global rating of a patient's dependency level. Livingston and Livingston,[24] members of the Glasgow group, have

Table 5-9. PTA AND OUTCOME AT 6 MONTHS

PTA	n	Severely Disabled (%)	Moderately Disabled (%)	Good Recovery (%)
<14 days	101	0	17	83
15-28 days	96	3	31	66
>28 days	289	30	43·	27

From Jennett and Teasdale,[9] with permission.

devised a second scale combining assessment of physical symptoms and signs, personality/behavioral change, cognitive status, activities of daily living, and occupational status. The Glasgow Assessment Schedule (GAS) was designed to provide a problem-orientated evaluation rather than being focused on the cause of particular forms of impairment. For example, walking ability is rated in preference to determining whether ataxia is the result of brain damage or a psychologic/motivational consequence of injury. The instrument has been subjected successfully to tests of rating reliability, and it has face validity (i.e., it measures what it is intended to measure). The designers of the schedule feel that it could be developed further by incorporating in it a simple psychiatric rating scale for use with patients who have organic impairment.

As stated earlier, the GOS is a coarse measure and, for that reason, other means of assessing outcome may be needed when more detail is required. Therefore, at this point it is important to bring yet another assessment scale to the reader's notice because its use spans the full period of recovery "from coma to community"[25] and because it covers a wide range of functional areas. The Disability Rating Scale (DRS) was devised by Rappaport and others.[25] It is in widespread use throughout brain injury rehabilitation units in the United States. The DRS is a 30-point scale, covering the following eight dimensions: eye opening; verbalization; motor responsiveness; cognitive skills needed for feeding, toileting and grooming; overall level of dependence; and employability. The scores may be classified into one of ten categories of disability ranging from death to no disability. A study by Hall and coworkers[26] showed that among a population of 70 head injured patients, there was a significant correlation between DRS and GOS scores at hospital admission and discharge. As expected, the DRS was noted to be the more

sensitive measure of recovery, with 71 percent of patients showing improvement on the DRS and only 33 percent showing improvement on the GOS. The DRS may be regarded as showing validity, and it has also been demonstrated to have a high level of inter-rater reliability.

As life consists of many elements, it could be argued quite reasonably that an ADL scale is inadequate because it gives information only about practical skills and that the GAS or even the DRS is not broad enough (although the addition of a psychiatric subscale to the GAS, as suggested, would increase its practical value further). Perhaps what is needed is further information on the injured persons' state of well-being as judged by a close relative or friend and an evaluation of changes in his or her various roles in life (e.g., spouse, employed person) by using a social adjustment inventory. The use and value of the latter remains to be discussed, but there is evidence already that the social impact of head injured persons in families is measurable by using such an inventory. For example, detailed studies of social disruption and change among the wives and mothers of head injured men have been reported by Livingston and others.[27]

Assessment of Social Adjustment

In response to the therapeutic movements in psychiatry during the past two decades away from care in large institutions to an expanding concept of community care, a number of scales for the assessment of social adjustment have been developed. At first, they were used with schizophrenic patients and their families, and for the evaluation of psychotherapy among outpatients. In 1973, a joint Food and Drug Administration–American College of Neuropsychopharmacology (FDA-ACNP) group was formed to develop guidelines to evaluate psychotropic drugs, which entailed examining social adjustment scales. The first review of the latter was produced by Weissman[28] in 1975, who described the reliability, validity, and use of 15 social adjustment scales. Since that time, many more have appeared, but only a small number might be of value in assessing head injured patients and their families.

Social adjustment has been defined by Weissman and Sholomskas[29] in broad terms as "the interplay between the individual and the social environment." These authors point out that an individual's major roles are the product of several interacting factors including age, marital status, family constellation, and mental constitution. For example, a normal adult tends to fill an occupational, marital, and community role at different times. When a person is ill (mentally or physically) or disabled, symptoms often alter roles, but in some cases the individual functions relatively normally despite their presence; this may happen in those who make a good recovery where evidence of residual symptoms exists following a severe brain injury. On the other hand, it is well known that those who have had trivial head injuries often may function poorly. Thus, social adjustment is based on an individual's interactions with others and one's satisfaction and performance in roles that are molded by personality, family, and cultural expectations.

The instruments used to assess social adjustment may be of the self-report type. They depend on an interview or may be completed in the form of a postal or telephone assessment. A number of tests are only for patients, but others may be completed by a relative or close friend. Although it is not the function of this chapter to review tests in detail, it is worth mentioning two in order to demonstrate the nature and purpose of instruments that may be of value in head injury rehabilitation research and yet may be unfamiliar to readers.

The Katz Adjustment Scale–Relatives Form (KAS-R)[30] is a 205-item scale used to assess behavior and the life-situation adjustment of patients. Each item is rated on a 4-point scale. In more detail, there are five sections that cover (1) performance at socially expected tasks, (2) relatives' expectations for performance of the tasks, (3) free activities, (4) relatives' rating of performance, and (5) rating of symptoms and social behavior. The main weakness of the scale is its lack of coverage of marital, parental, and extended-family relationships. Therefore, as a supplement, the Social Adjustment Scale–Self Report (SAS-SR) might be used. It measures instrumental and affective performance and the performance of various roles, which include social and leisure activities, relationships with the extended family, marital role, parental role, and family unit and economic independence. This is a stable, valid, and reliable test that has been used extensively in psychiatric and social research, where it has been shown that there is a significant correlation between self-reports and reports by others. This factor makes the test attractive for head injury assessments.

CONCLUSION

Considerable progress has been made in recent years in defining ways of measuring the outcome of severe head injuries for the victims and their relatives. In the process, much has been learned about recovery from injury and the consequences for families of having an injured person among them. Although much has been achieved, there is a need for further research into the nuances of the emotional and social consequences of injury during the later states of recovery, and the matter of designing and critically assessing methods of rehabilitation using valid and reliable tests has only just begun.

REFERENCES

1. Jennett, B and Bond, MR: Assessment of outcome after severe brain damage. Lancet 1:480, 1975.
2. Newcombe, F and Fortuny, LAI: Problems and perspectives in the evaluation of psychological deficits after cerebral lesions. Int J Rehabil Med 1:182, 1979.
3. Russell, WR: Cerebral involvement in head injury. Brain 55:549, 1932.
4. Fortuny, LAI et al: Measuring the duration of post-traumatic amnesia. J Neurol Neurosurg Psychiatry 43:377, 1980.
5. Levin, HS, O'Donnell, VM and Grossman, RG: The

Galveston orientation and amnesia test: A practical scale to assess cognition after head injury. J Nerv Ment Dis 167:675, 1975.

6. Jennett, B et al: Disability after severe head injury: Observations on the use of the Glasgow Outcome Scale. J Neurol Neurosurg Psychiatry 44:285, 1981.

7. Teasdale, G and Jennett, B: Assessment of coma and impaired consciousness. Lancet 2:81, 1974.

8. Jennett, B, Teasdale, G and Braakman, R: Prognosis in a series of patients with severe head injury. Neurosurgery 4:283, 1979.

9. Jennett, B and Teasdale, G: Management of Head Injuries. FA Davis, Philadelphia, 1981, p 317.

10. Roberts, AH: Severe Accidental Head Injury: An Assessment of Long-Term Prognosis. Macmillan, New York, 1979.

11. Bond, MR: Assessment of the psychosocial outcome after severe head injury. In Porter, R and Fitzsimons, DW (eds): Outcome of Severe Damage to the Central Nervous System. Ciba Foundation Symposium 34 (New Series). Elsevier–Excerpta Medica–North Holland, Amsterdam, 1975.

12. Bond, MR and Brooks, DN: Understanding the process of recovery as a basis for the investigation of rehabilitation for the brain-injured. Scand J Rehabil Med 8:127, 1976.

13. Goldstein, K: The two ways of adjustment of the organism to cerebral defects. J M Sinai Hosp 9:504, 1942.

14. Luria, AR: Restoration of Function after Brain Injury. Pergamon Press, Oxford, 1963.

15. Fordyce, DJ, Roueche, JR and Prigitano, GP: Enhanced emotional reactions in chronic head trauma patients. J Neurol Neurosurg Psychiatry 46:620, 1983.

16. Dikmen, S and Reitan, RM: Emotional sequelae of head injury. Ann Neurol 2:492, 1977.

17. Dikmen, S and Reitan, RM: MMPI Correlates of adaptive ability deficits in patients with brain lesions. J Nerv Ment Dis 165:247, 1977.

18. Levin, HS et al: The neurobehavioural rating scale: assessment of the behavioural sequelae of head injury by the clinician. J Neurol Neurosurg Psychiatry 50:183, 1987.

19. Overall, JE and Gorham, DR: The brief psychiatric rating scale. Psychol Rep 10:799, 1962.

20. Levin, HS et al: Long term neuropsychological outcome of closed head injury. J Neurosurg 50:412, 1979.

21. Garraway, WM et al: Observer variation in the clinical assessment of stroke. Age Ageing 5:233, 1976.

22. Smith, ME et al: Measuring the outcome of stroke rehabilitation. Occup Ther 46(3):51, 1977.

23. Sheikh, K et al: Methods and problems of a stroke rehabilitation trial. Br Med J 41:262, 1978.

24. Livingston, MG and Livingston, HM: The Glasgow Assessment Schedule: Clinical and research assessment of head injury outcome. Int Rehabil Med 7:145, 1985.

25. Rappaport, et al: Disability Rating Scale for severe head trauma: Coma to community. Arch Phys Med Rehabil 63:118, 1982.

26. Hall, K, Cope, DN and Rappaport, M: Glasgow Outcome Scale and Disability Rating Scale: Comparative usefulness in following recovery in traumatic head injury. Arch Phys Med Rehabil 66:35, 1985.

27. Livingston, MG, Brooks, DN and Bond, MR: Patient outcome in the year following severe head injury and relatives' psychiatric and social functioning. J Neurol Neurosurg Psychiatry 48:876, 1985.

28. Weissman, MM: The assessment of social adjustment. Arch Gen Psychiatry 32:357, 1975.

29. Weissman, MM and Sholomskas, D: The assessment of social adjustment by the clinician, the patient and the family. In Burdock, EI, Sudilovsky, A and Gershon, S (eds): The Behaviour of Psychiatric Patients. Marcel Dekker, New York, 1982, p 177.

30. Katz, MM and Lyerly, SB: Methods of measuring adjustment and social behaviour in the community: 1. Rationale, description, discriminative validity and scale development. Psychol Rep 13:503, 1963.

Section II Conclusion

J. DOUGLAS MILLER, M.D., Ph.D.

The processes of resuscitation, assessment, management, rehabilitation, and evaluation of outcome from severe head injury should form a continuum of care in which the component parts overlap in time. The goals of early management must be to provide, as soon after injury as possible, the optimal milieu for neuronal recovery and for the least amount of permanent brain damage. The process of rehabilitation assessment and treatment should begin early, while acute management measures are still in progress. The members of the multidisciplinary rehabilitation team are much better able to assess and treat the patient and to advise the family if they are armed with a full understanding of the nature of the head injury, the initial neurologic status of the patient, the diagnostic and management measures that were employed, and details of any complications marring early progress. A sense of continuity of care and the idea that there is a single extended team involved in the care of the head injured patient are reassuring and comforting concepts for the family.

This section of the book has focused on the nature of traumatic brain damage, how secondary brain insults can add to this damage, how clinical examination and modern imaging techniques are combined to delineate the full extent of functional and structural brain disorder, and the principles of surgical and intensive medical management of severely head injured patients. Objective, accurate, and reliable measures are required to describe the neurologic status of the patient, and are essential if they are to be used as a basis for early management decisions, for evaluation of progress, and for early determination of the prognosis of the head injury in the individual patient. Triage of patients into cases of severe, moderate, and minor head injury is based on the score on the Glasgow Coma Scale; this widely used scale is at the heart of almost all systems of sequential neurologic observation of head injury patients as used by medical, nursing, and allied health personnel. Because of the inability of many head injured patients to cooperate actively in the examination process, the emphasis in the neurologic evaluation of head injury is upon standardized stimulus and measured response to test arousal, motor, verbal, and reflex functions.

Additional methods of assessment include CT, MRI, intracranial pressure monitoring, and measurements of brain blood flow, energy metabolism, and electrical activity. These techniques amplify considerably the information on brain function yielded from the neurologic examination, or in some cases substitute for it, to show evidence of both structural (CT and MRI) and functional brain disorder.

The issues of validity, objectivity, and reliability apply with equal force to the assessment of outcome from head injury. A compromise often has to be struck between descriptions of outcome status that are adequate to delineate the difficulties of thinking, remembering, feeling, balancing, and doing things quickly, and the use of a number of outcome categories that is sufficiently limited to enable any individual recovering patient to be consigned to a single category with confidence.

The importance of clear, unequivocal, and standardized descriptions of severity and of the outcome from head injury cannot be overemphasized. These underpin the development of algorithms for determining the prognosis of severe head injury. The identification of pathologic factors important in the determination of a poor outcome from injury guides in the development of newer strategies of treatment of head injury patients, and may identify at an early stage groups of patient in whom particular rehabilitation measures are appropriate. These principles are also of fundamental importance if groups of head injured patients are to be compared. Like must be compared with like regarding the distribution within the groups of features associated with a good or a poor outcome, such as age, prevalence of reflex dysfunction, and the level of motor response. Evaluation of the adverse effects of brain insults or the beneficial effects of therapy upon outcome is possible only when the head injury populations have been adequately defined in terms of neurologic status and outcome category. The same principles apply to evaluation of the benefits of the many facets of rehabilitation therapy, whether by group analysis or in single case study design.

The development among the members of the health care team of a sound understanding of the factors governing the prognosis of severe head injury should result in the provision of more accurate forecasts of the outcome expected in individual patients. This can be of considerable help to the family of the head injured patient by avoiding overly pessimistic and depressing statements on the one hand and on the other, unrealistically optimistic statements that only raise false expectations and lead to later bitterness. Finally, the provision of realistic, objective, and accurate information instills in the family a reassuring sense of the competence, experience, and professionalism of the health care team. That reassurance is immensely comforting and creates a feeling of collaboration and understanding support that will be crucial for the later stages of the rehabilitation process, after the head injury survivor returns home.

SPECIFIC PROBLEMS RELATED TO HEAD INJURY

Michael R. Bond, M.D., Ph.D., Editor

Chapter 6

Mechanisms of Recovery of Function Following CNS Damage

JOHN WHYTE, M.D., Ph.D.*

Without the potential for recovery, the process of rehabilitation would be meaningless. Yet recovery is rarely complete, and perceptible recovery may fail to occur at all. Webster's dictionary defines recovery as the "process of bringing back to a normal condition." The relative contributions of learned adaptations and biologic healing in this recovery are a matter of continued debate.

The concept of "function" is also problematic. If the function under consideration is independent mobility, then effective use of a prosthesis or wheelchair may be seen as recovered function in that it meets that end. One interested in means will point out that the function of spontaneous ambulation with normal motor control has not recovered at all. This example is an obvious one, but the literature is rife with more subtle forms of this debate.

Earlier theories of strict localization of function, such as phrenology, held that *tasks* were localized in discrete regions of brain (e.g., reading in one area, reasoning in another). Those theories had great difficulty accounting for recovery from damage to one such region. Subsequent attempts to understand the brain in terms of mass action

(i.e., abilities are distributed throughout the brain in an unspecialized manner) better accounted for recovery, but accounted poorly for specific persisting deficits. Modern theories of localization of function still struggle to describe *what* is localized in particular regions, and secondarily, how the brain can adapt to loss of that region.

For many years it was believed that the CNS had virtually no ability to undergo biologic modifications in response to injury. Thus, all recovery of function had to be understood in psychologic terms, as learning. The clinical corollary was that recovery of function occurred entirely in the first few months after injury and was accounted for by recovery of reversible factors affecting tissue that was sick but not dead. Any later changes were viewed as "merely" psychologic. For those working in rehabilitation and particularly in head injury, however, it is clear that meaningful recovery continues for much longer than was previously thought. Thus, new mechanisms must be sought to explain such long-term changes.

In this chapter, mechanisms that have been proposed to account for recovery of function will be considered individually along with evidence that supports and refutes them. The roles that each of these mechanisms may play in human recovery after head injury will also be considered. Next, the many theoretical problems that challenge our ability to account definitively

*The author gratefully acknowledges the critical reading and suggestions of James A. Whitlock, Jr., M.D., and Robert L. Mapou, Ph.D., in the preparation of this manuscript.

79

for the observed recovery will be discussed. Finally, areas of research will be identified that suggest clinical implications.

PROPOSED MECHANISMS OF RECOVERY OF FUNCTION

Any proposed theory of recovery must meet certain conditions to be plausible as a mechanism of recovery. First, it must be shown that a specific type of CNS lesion results in a clear behavioral deficit. Next, it must be shown that recovery of the behavioral deficit is accompanied by a biologic or psychologic change that plausibly accounts for the behavioral recovery. Finally, the role of the mechanism must be confirmed by showing that factors that prevent the mechanism also prevent the behavioral recovery. As shall be seen, the amount of human research that can meet these strict criteria is small. Therefore, this chapter, unlike others in this book, concentrates largely on animal research to support firm conclusions. Human data will be cited as supporting or confirming evidence.

Resolution of Temporary Factors

Following CNS injury a variety of factors may impair the functioning of brain structures that have not been irreversibly damaged. In the case of head trauma, edema, focal hematomas, increased intracranial pressure, and hypoxia may all contribute to reversible impairments of function. Furthermore, there is animal evidence for depression of metabolic enzyme activity lasting about a week in regions remote from a cortical lesion, which may relate to acute reversible functional changes.[1] Thus, some early recovery may be due to the renewed activity of temporarily dysfunctional tissue.

Modifications of Neural Connections

The ability of the mature CNS to undergo modification of its axonal/dendritic connections is of increasing research interest. Such changes have been documented in a variety of species and brain systems, but their gen-

erality and particularly their role in behavioral recovery remain unclear. There are two types of neuroanatomic modifications in the CNS that are analogous to their more familiar counterparts in the peripheral nervous system. *Regeneration* implies that fiber processes that have been disrupted grow back from their cell bodies of origin and reestablish preinjury or modified synaptic connections. In contrast, *collateral sprouting* implies that neurons that are intact produce axonal branches that come to occupy synaptic sites left vacant by dying neurons.

Axonal regeneration has been noted in various species.[2] Although there is evidence in some situations that axons "search for" appropriate locations for synapsing, other experiments suggest relatively random regenerative efforts. Furthermore, regenerating axons may become misrouted through chemical attraction to blood vessels, glial cells, and other irrelevant tissues.[2] Regeneration may have the greatest functional role in infancy, but evidence exists that regenerated connections may at times be dysfunctional. For example, infant hamsters with anomalously regenerated visual pathways may orient *away* from food rewards.[3] In addition, attempts at regeneration must overcome the physical barriers of glial scarring or collagen deposition.[4] In recent years there has been an attempt to promote regeneration through the transplantation of fetal brain tissue into lesioned areas. Several experiments show behavioral recovery attributable to such transplants, and show neural processes from the transplants growing into host brain tissue.[5] However, it remains unclear whether such transplants operate via specific neural connections or through generalized release of neurotransmitters into surrounding tissue.

The role of collateral sprouting in behavioral recovery has been more clearly demonstrated. Focal lesions that denervate a target zone may result in expansion of the synaptic territory of neighboring neural systems. Such collateral sprouting is highly specific. Collateral sprouts may not cross certain anatomic boundaries[6] and there appear to be orders of priority in terms of which surviving system will sprout to occupy the available space.[7]

Goldberger and Murray[8] have shown that deafferentation of a cat's hind limb results in a flaccid paralysis, which recovers in association with collateral sprouting of descending neural pathways.[8] But if one afferent root is left intact, it will be this root, not the descending pathways, that expands its synaptic territory. In either case, it is noteworthy that the new collaterals represent expansion of connections in regions normally innervated, not growth into novel CNS domains. Research on recovery from Brown-Sequard spinal cord injury has some striking parallels to the aforementioned research, suggesting that collateral sprouting may play a role in human movement recovery.[9]

Other experiments suggest that collaterals may at times make *novel* connections that promote recovery. For example, hippocampal destruction in the rat results in behavioral deficits that are ameliorated by ingrowth of noradrenergic fibers from the superior cervical ganglion.[10] Sectioning of these fibers reinstitutes the deficit. It is possible that the noradrenergic fibers promote recovery in a nonspecific modulatory fashion rather than by substituting for the specific lost function.

Collateral sprouting cannot account for the broad array of recovery in various neural systems. For example, destruction of portions of the retina in an adult cat leads to a visual scotoma, followed by recovery. However, this recovery is *not* accompanied by expansion of the remaining retinal fiber synapses in the partially denervated lateral geniculate nucleus.[11] Much remains to be learned about the role of axonal regeneration and collateral sprouting in different species and neural systems.

Modifications of Synaptic Function

Von Monakow observed in 1914 that undamaged portions of the CNS may suffer reversible depression following a focal insult.[12] This form of neural shock has been termed "diaschisis." The mechanism of shock was not specified by von Monakow. In modern times, diaschisis is explained by the fact that intact regions that normally receive inputs from the damaged tissue decrease their activity when those inputs are lost or altered.[13] Evidence exists for such widespread reversible depression in humans and other mammals.[1, 14, 15]

In order to account for recovery from neural shock, mechanisms must be found by which the neural depression can be reversed. Potential mechanisms include increased neurotransmitter synthesis by remaining neural inputs, decreased metabolic inactivation of the transmitters that are released, and increased synthesis of neurotransmitter receptors.[12] Of these, changes in receptor production have received the most attention. Temporary overstimulation of adrenergic receptors leads to an abnormal decrease in their numbers. When the stimulation ends, augmented receptor production ensues.[16] Similarly, rats with unilateral lesions to a dopaminergic pathway appear to recover by increased receptor production.[17]

Increased receptor density as a recovery mechanism requires some remaining source of neurotransmitter. Thus it would seem that this mechanism is primarily relevant in cases of *partial* damage of an input. It may also account for generalized effects of transmitter analogue drugs, or transmitter-releasing transplants. Indeed pharmacologic treatment with neurotransmitter agonists has been shown to promote recovery in some animal and human studies,[18, 19] though not in others.[20]

As with the previously discussed mechanisms, modification of synaptic activity cannot account for all instances of behavioral recovery. Rats given a lesion to the primary cholinergic input to the cortex show profound learning deficits, which recover over time. Yet cholinergic activity remains depressed after recovery, and cholinergic receptors do not undergo compensatory increases.[21] Similarly, lesions to dopaminergic sensorimotor pathways in the rat produce behavioral impairments. Recovery is associated with increased production of dopamine receptors. Lithium prevents this behavioral recovery without preventing the receptor production.[22]

Redundancy

Neurophysiologic redundancy implies that latent neural connections capable of subserving a particular function may exist. These connections may be at a different hierarchical level of the CNS, or they may be a reflection of the diffuseness of organization of the particular function throughout the CNS.[12] Redundancy has been most rigorously studied as a mechanism of acute adaptation to CNS insult. This is because if recovery occurs over a longer time course it is difficult to prove that the responsible connections were present in latent form prior to injury rather than occurring through regeneration or sprouting.

Perhaps the most dramatic example of redundancy comes from an experiment in which the spinal cords of cats were reversibly anesthetized. Before anesthesia, neurons in the dorsal column were identified which responded only to stimulation of the cat's foot. Immediately after anesthesia, the same neurons responded to stimulation of the cat's abdomen. When the anesthesia wore off, stimulation of the abdomen could no longer cause firing of the dorsal column cells.[2] Clearly the responsible neural connections must have been present throughout the experiment in latent form.

Specifying the role of redundancy in recovery of function would require a thorough knowledge of complex and overlapping neural circuitry. This is challenging enough in experimental animals but is virtually impossible through the types of experimentation available in humans. Thus, at present, the role of redundancy in human recovery remains obscure.

Vicarious Functioning

Vicarious functioning means that neural tissues *not normally involved* in the performance of a particular task *alter their properties* to subserve that function. This differs from collateral sprouting or redundancy in that the tissue promoting the recovery was not previously structured for the task.

On the surface there is a great deal of evidence for vicarious functioning from two-stage lesion studies. Such studies, using a variety of species and tasks, involve the lesioning of a specific brain area to create a behavioral deficit. After behavioral recovery ensues, lesioning of an adjacent or systematically related region can often recreate the deficit, despite the fact that, if lesioned alone, this second region would not have caused the deficit. This suggests that the newly lesioned region had assumed the recovered function. Although such experiments demonstrate that a new brain region is involved in task performance, they do not

show that the properties of that region have been altered. Indeed, as shall be seen later, it is possible that the properties of the task have been altered to fit the brain region rather than the reverse.

Spear and Baumann[23] have shown that recovery of visual pattern discrimination following occipital cortex lesions in cats can be attributed to "take over" of that function by the lateral suprasylvian (LS) visual area. Single-unit recording from cells in the LS area shows that they retain their native physiologic properties, and do not adopt the receptive field properties characteristic of neurons in the primary visual cortex. A similar experiment in motor function also suggests that neighboring tissue that subserves recovery does so through normal, unaltered mechanisms.[24]

There is considerable evidence that the adult brain lacks the capability to alter its organization even when such alterations would be highly adaptive. In the monkey, the sensory cortex contains a spatial map of the surface of the palm such that adjacent points on the cortex respond to stimulation of adjacent points on the palm. When the monkey's median nerve is cut and allowed to regenerate, this organized mapping is disrupted, presumably because the regenerating nerve fibers become "scrambled" as they reinnervate the skin surface. There is no evidence of cortical reorganization to restore the spatial map of the palm despite the fact that the disorganization prevents tactile localization, stereognosis, and so forth.[25] Similarly, adult monkeys with reversal of their biceps and triceps tendons do not appear to reorganize the corresponding neural regions to compensate function. The best they can do is inhibit elbow flexion *and* extension.[26]

Even in humans, there is considerable evidence that much recovery results from increased functioning of residual tissue in the damaged area, or of related tissue already involved in the process, rather than adoption of the function by unrelated brain structures.[27–29] This conclusion will be examined further in the next section.

Functional Substitution

Functional substitution refers to the overt or covert adoption of a different strategy to achieve a desired goal. This will result in recovery of ends, not recovery of means. Altered strategies as means to an end may be grossly obvious (as when a paraplegic "climbs" stairs on his or her buttocks) or very subtle (as when a person with a visual field defect resorts to increased eye movements to circumvent visual disability).[30] Functional substitution differs from vicarious functioning in that the tissue subserving recovery does not alter its properties to do so. Rather, it simply uses its intrinsic properties to achieve the goal in a different way.

Animal evidence for functional substitution is extensive, but a few examples will be illustrative. Goldberger and Murray[8] showed that cats with various forms of deafferentation and spinal cord injury recover their mobility as measured by ability to walk across a narrow wooden beam. Reflexes lost in the surgery, however, do not return; rather, the cats rely increasingly on reflexes surviving the surgery to guide movement. Monkeys who suffer from hemispatial neglect after unilateral frontal eye field lesions recover their ability to detect stimuli in the neglected field. This recovery is associated with new patterns of visual scanning and with head movements.[31] Finally, rats who receive lesions to their lateral hypothalamus do not eat or drink and will die unless maintained with enteral feedings. However, rats who have very limited access to water *preoperatively* (20 min/day) are quicker to drink spontaneously postoperatively. This is not the case in rats who experience complete water deprivation preoperatively. The rats who have limited access, unlike those with complete deprivation, learn to be very attentive to the water bottle, and are conditioned to become behaviorally active when it appears.[32] Thus, it would seem that recovered drinking is mediated by a set of behaviors and habits different from those that guided it before the lesion.

Evidence of functional substitution exists in humans as well. Bach-y-Rita[33] describes evidence for this in congenitally blind, non–brain injured individuals learning to use the Tactile Vision Substitution System (TVSS). This is a device which transforms visual information from a video camera into a pattern of vibrating points on the skin. Subjects not only learn a variety of visual perceptual concepts (such as perspective), but also report the subjective sense that what they "see" is out in the world rather than on their skin. Thus it appears that they have learned to use a different sensory modality (tactile) as a substitute for the information normally acquired through sight.

Humans with visuospatial neglect resulting from a right cerebrovascular accident (CVA) showed recovery of function over time as measured by an increased ability to copy drawings symmetrically. However, other indices of visuospatial function failed to improve, and the patients still showed a strong right sided position preference in responding to the tasks.[34] Once again, it appears that recovery *of a task* occurred without recovery of the underlying mechanism, suggesting that the task was now accomplished through the use of novel strategies.

LeVere and LeVere[35] suggest quite a different perspective on functional substitution. Some of the behavioral deficit observed after brain injury may result precisely from the attempt to solve a task by an alternate but inferior means. Thus, a visually impaired rat may try to solve a maze through nonvisual cues despite the fact that remaining visual information might better guide performance. Recovery in such instances may be accompanied by return to the impaired but still useful strategy.

The sharp contrast made here between vicarious functioning and functional substitution may be to some extent a semantic one. It has been argued that the major difference between the two mechanisms is that vicarious functioning involves the reorganization of neural tissue to adapt to new task demands, whereas functional substitution involves the modification of the task to fit the organization of the remaining neural tissue. Yet clearly any learning must involve some change in neural organization at the electrophysiologic, chemical, or anatomic level. Thus, functional substitution must involve *some* modification in the brain structures newly subserving the task. Perhaps at this point, the difference is best thought of in terms of the magnitude of the change required. Thus, change of the type found in general learning would suggest functional substitution as a mechanism, whereas change of a more fundamental type would suggest vicarious functioning. Further clarification of these mechanisms must await a more thorough understanding of the precise neural changes found during normal learning.

Summary

After considering the broad array of proposed mechanisms of recovery of function, it is difficult to create a coherent picture of how recovery proceeds. It appears likely that all of these mechanisms may play a role in recovery in some species, with some types of CNS lesions, performing some tasks, at some times, under some conditions. It should not be surprising that simple rules of recovery have not been forthcoming. Before attempting a synthesis of these various mechanisms, therefore, it is advisable to consider the limitations of the research on which our conclusions are based.

THEORETICAL OBSTACLES TO AN UNDERSTANDING OF RECOVERY OF FUNCTION

Localization of Function

Theories of localization of brain function have profound influences on theories of recovery. At one extreme, if all functions are distributed equally throughout the CNS, then explaining recovery is straightforward: the greater the damage, the more widespread the impairment *in all tasks* and the slower and more imperfect the recovery. At the other extreme, if specific *tasks* (e.g., reading) are localized to specific brain regions, then recovery might be predicted to be limited to regeneration of that specific region. Although these two extremes are obviously false, they indicate that the conceptualization of localization of function will affect the types of recovery models generated.

Modern views of localization hold that particular capacities (e.g., "serial processing," "spatial attention," and so on) are localized, and that many such capacities participate in any given task. In clinical work the effects of CNS injury or recovery are rarely defined with reference to just one task. Rather the effects of injury and recovery are considered with reference to an array of tasks that depend to various degrees on the impaired capacity(ies). Yet much animal literature defines injury with respect to impairment on one task and complete recovery as success on that one task. The use of multiple tasks in testing animal recovery may help clarify the localization of the ca-

pacities of interest and the strategies being used during recovery.

Heterogeneity of Brain Systems

Brain structure and function have changed throughout evolution. Therefore, it is not a safe assumption that recovery mechanisms that operate in one species apply to another. Furthermore, the human brain was not "designed" as an integrated system de novo. It evolved through the addition of new systems to pre-existing structures. Thus, it is not safe to assume that all parts of the human brain share the same mechanisms of recovery. In fact, it has been suggested that most regeneration in the adult mammal is found in phylogenetically old, unmyelinated brain systems.[2] Therefore, generalizations about recovery mechanisms from one species to another or one human brain system to another must be made with caution.

Age Differences

There is a wealth of research assessing age-dependent variables in CNS recovery of animals and humans. The bulk of this research suggests that young organisms recover more completely than older ones. There are a number of possible explanations for this. First, it appears that normal CNS maturation involves the production of excess numbers of neuronal connections which are then lost as functional connections take precedence.[2] This might allow for the maintenance of alternate connections in the event of early brain damage. Second, there is evidence that some of the changes in neurotransmitter receptor density in response to CNS injury occur to a greater extent in younger organisms.[16] The most dramatic example of CNS plasticity in humans comes from research on patients with hemispherectomies (removal of an entire cerebral hemisphere). This surgery, while profoundly disabling in adulthood, is compatible with relatively normal cognitive function in children.[36]

Several caveats regarding the greater recovery in youth are in order. First, there are instances in which lesioned infants "grow into" their deficits, indicating that a deficit was not apparent until the developmental point was reached at which the damaged region would have assumed a role in the behavior of interest.[37] There are also cases in which lesions in aged animals have *less* effect because the lesioned area has already ceased to mediate the behavior of interest. Finally, age effects do not adequately distinguish between biologic and behavioral plasticity in youth. Just as the synapses of the young may be more subject to change, so are the young in a natural process of exploring strategies for accomplishing their goals. They also may be more amenable to altering those strategies in response to injury.[38]

Task Differences

As discussed previously, the choice of tasks to study can profoundly influence views of recovery of function. Tasks that are very simple will make it appear that full recovery occurs quickly, though more complex tasks might reveal persisting deficits. Tasks that are very complex will make it appear that no recovery occurs, though a simpler task might show some improvement. It has been shown that verbal abilities recover more quickly following head injury than nonverbal ones, as measured by standardized intelligence tests.[39] Although there are several possible explanations for this, one explanation is simply that the verbal measures rely more heavily on overlearned information and depend less heavily on speed than the nonverbal measures (i.e., they are "easier").

Both animal and human studies of recovery must ensure that the tasks under investigation are of the appropriate level of difficulty to identify deficits when present, yet identify improvement when it occurs. Furthermore, animal researchers should consider the approach of clinical neuropsychologists who seek to clarify the nature and extent of impairment and recovery through appropriately selected *combinations* of tasks. In this way, strategy changes during recovery can be systematically addressed.

Environmental Effects

It has been shown that an enriched and stimulating environment has positive effects both on performance of various learning tasks and on brain anatomy and chemistry in animals.[20] Whether these effects require the active involvement of the animal or the mere presence of stimulation is unclear. Nutrition also has effects on brain function and recovery.[40] Once again, however, it is not clear *how* these environmental factors affect recovery. Stimulation, for example, may aid recovery *because of* its biologic effects on the brain, and/or because an enriched environment offers an animal more ways to find alternate strategies, and/or because it encourages an animal to use its impaired functions.

In summary, a variety of factors represent obstacles to the creation of a simple model of recovery from CNS injury. Although some progress may be made in the development of comprehensive models, it appears likely that more complex theories that incorporate the manifold individual variables will need to be developed. The response to the question, "How does reeovery of function occur?" may need to be another question: "Recovery of what function in whom after what type of injury over what time period?"

CLINICAL IMPLICATIONS

The extent to which we can apply the results of research on recovery of function directly to clinical treatment is very limited at present. This limitation will continue until research designs are developed for humans that can provide the types of information available from more invasive animal research designs. There are, however, some reasonably sound conjectures that can be made now.

It is reasonable to assume that different recovery mechanisms have different time frames of operation. Thus, resolution of temporary factors and presence of redundant systems may be relevant in the first days postinjury. Changes in synaptic function would be expected to operate at an intermediate time frame, and regeneration, or vicarious functioning, over the longest time frames. Functional substitution would be expected to occur more in relation to specific eliciting experiences than to any fixed time scale.

Second, the nature and severity of the injury would be expected to influence the predominant mechanisms of recovery. For example, if a particular white matter fiber tract is *partially* injured, it is likely that modifications in synaptic function can play an important role in recovery because some of the neurons producing the neurotransmitter remain intact as do those receiving it. Thus simple changes in sensitivity can restore activity. On the other hand, if a fiber tract is *completely* disrupted or if grey matter injury predominates, it is less clear that alterations in synaptic function can play a major role.

There appears to be little evidence for vicarious functioning in its strictest definition as an important mechanism of recovery. Rather, it appears that most of what passes for vicarious functioning is a combination of recovery of incompletely damaged tissue and functional substitution involving alterations in how the task is performed. Thus it would appear prudent to tailor rehabilitation not toward "reorganizing" brain regions, but toward characterizing how they *are* organized, and using this information to help reorganize tasks in compatible ways.

Implications for the Future

Current research suggests some areas in which more focused study may yield clinically relevant results. It is known that reduction of secondary forms of brain injury can have important effects on outcome. What we know of modifications of neural connections suggests that they will play only limited roles at least in the reconnection of distant regions. However, it appears that treatments that reduce scar tissue and promote axonal budding and growth may hold limited promise, especially in local injuries of white matter.[41-43]

Modification of synaptic function through pharmacologic treatment may provide some benefits by augmenting the naturally occurring alterations in synaptic function. To succeed, such efforts must be based on specific knowledge of the transmitter systems that have been impaired. They must also keep in mind that recovery and psychopharmacologic modifications are sometimes dissociable. In addition, a thorough investigation of which medications may have harmful effects on the recovery of specific brain systems can provide significant clinical benefit.

Clinical use of redundant neural connections rests on increased knowledge of what redundancies exist in humans, or of reasonable parallels from other species borne out by clinical research.

Functional substitution probably represents the most broadly applicable recovery mechanism for patients who are awake and able to attend to various stimuli. At present, functional substitution is usually invoked as an explanation of the observed recovery after the altered strategies have been identified. As progress is made in characterizing the processing specialties of specific brain systems, and in characterizing the processing requirements for optimal performance of specific tasks, this information may lead to more intentional application of functional substitution in rehabilitation. Thus, it may become possible, by knowing which brain regions are intact, to train patients in the type of task strategy that is best suited to the intact regions. In addition, forced-use paradigms borrowed from animal recovery research may help patients discover what impaired systems are still capable of achieving task goals.

Normal human performance is characterized by the development of automaticity with increased practice and skill. In other words, tasks come to require minimal concentration and effort as they become more skilled. This is fortunate, as concentration and effort are limited commodities. It remains to be seen to what degree *recovering* tasks can also achieve this degree of automaticity. Only if recovered functions can become relatively effortless will they truly become functional in a broad array of situations. Thus, if there is a choice of avenues to recovery that differ in their potential for automaticity, that factor should weigh heavily in treatment planning.

SUMMARY

Recovery of function following CNS damage is a remarkable and highly complex process. It consists of numerous mechanisms interacting in various combinations at various points in time. The understanding of the precise mechanisms of recovery of function is limited at present, especially in humans. The inextricable connection between mechanisms of recovery and clinical work in neurologic rehabilitation, however, necessitates an attempt to understand this field systematically. Even when the mechanisms of recovery operating in a particular patient at a particular time cannot be specified, knowledge of these potential mechanisms can be used to make predictions and develop hypotheses. In this way clinical experience becomes more focused and the chance of understanding the process of neurologic recovery is increased.

REFERENCES

1. Dail, WG et al: Responses to cortical injury. II. Widespread depression of the activity of an enzyme in cortex remote from a focal injury. Brain Res 211:79, 1981.
2. Finger, S and Stein, DG: Brain Damage and Recovery: Research and Clinical Perspectives. Academic Press, New York, 1982.
3. Schneider, GE and Jhavari, SR: Neuroanatomical correlates of spared or altered function after brain lesions in the newborn hamster. In Stein, DG, Rosen, JJ and Butters, N (eds): Plasticity and Recovery of Function in the Central Nervous System. Academic Press, New York, 1974.
4. Harvey, J and Strebnik, H: Locomotor activity and axon regeneration following spinal cord compression in rats treated with L-thyroxine. J Neuropathol Exp Neurol 26:666, 1967.
5. Isacson, O, Dunnett, SB and Bjorklund, A: Graft-induced behavioral recovery in an animal model of Huntington disease. Proc Nat Acad Sci 83:2728, 1986.
6. Field, PM: Synapse formation after injury in the adult rat brain: Failure of fimbrial axons to reinnervate the bed nucleus of the stria terminalis. Brain Res 189:91, 1980.
7. Field, PM, Coldham, DE and Raisman, G: Synapse formation after injury in the adult rat brain: Preferential reinnervation of denervated fimbrial sites by axons of the contralateral fimbria. Brain Res 189:103, 1980.
8. Goldberger, ME and Murray, M: Recovery of movement and axonal sprouting may obey some of the same laws. In Cotman C (ed): Neuronal Plasticity. Raven Press, New York, 1978.
9. Little, JW and Halar, E: Temporal course of motor recovery after Brown-Sequard spinal cord injuries. Paraplegia 23:39, 1985.
10. Kesslak, JP and Gage, FH III: Recovery of spatial alternation deficits following selective hippocampal destruction with kianic acid. Behav Neurosci 100:280, 1986.
11. Eysel, UT and Neubacher, U: Recovery of function is not associated with proliferation of retinogeniculate synapses after chronic deafferentation in the dorsal lateral geniculate nucleus of the adult cat. Neurosci Let 49:181, 1984.
12. Marshall, JF: Neural plasticity and recovery of function after brain injury. Int Rev Neurobiol 26:201, 1985.
13. Feeney, DM and Baron, JC: Diaschisis. Stroke 17:817, 1986.
14. Meyer, JS et al: Diaschisis resulting from acute unilateral cerebral infarction. Arch Neurol 23:241, 1970.
15. Robinson, RG, Bloom, FE and Battenberg, ELF: A fluorescent histochemical study of changes in noradrenergic neurons following experimental cerebral infarction in the rat. Brain Res 132:259, 1977.
16. Greenberg, LH, Brunswick, DJ and Weiss, B: Effect of age on the rate of recovery of beta-adrenergic receptors in rat brain following desmethylimipramine-induced subsensitivity. Brain Res 328:81, 1985.
17. Creese, I, Burt, D and Snyder, S: Dopamine receptor binding enhancement accompanies lesion-induced behavioral supersensitivity. Science 197:596, 1977.
18. Feeney, DM et al: Amphetamine, haloperidol, and experience interact to affect the rate of recovery after motor cortex injury. Science 217:855, 1982.
19. van Woerkom, TCAM et al: Neurotransmitters in the treatment of patients with severe head injuries. Eur Neurol 21:227, 1982.
20. Will, BE et al: Relatively brief environmental enrichment aids recovery of learning capacity and alters brain measures after postweaning brain lesions in rats. J Comp Physiol Psychol 91:33, 1977.
21. Bartus, RT et al: Selective memory loss following nucleus basalis lesions: Long term behavioral recovery despite persistent cholinergic deficiencies. Pharmacol Biochem Behav 23:125, 1985.
22. Kozlowski, MR et al: Chronic lithium administration alters behavioral recovery from nigrostriatal injury: Effects on neostriatal (^{3}H)spiroperidol binding sites. Brain Res 267:301, 1983.
23. Spear, PD and Baumann, TP: Neurophysiological mechanisms of recovery from visual cortex damage in cats: Properties of lateral suprasylvian visual area neurons following behavioral recovery. Exp Brain Res 35:177, 1979.
24. Glassman, RB: Recovery following sensorimotor cortical damage: Evoked potentials, brain stimulation, and motor control. Exp Neurol 33:16, 1971.
25. Wall, JT et al: Functional reorganization in somatosensory cortical areas 3b and 1 of adult monkeys after median nerve repair: Possible relationships to sensory recovery in humans. J Neurosci 6:218, 1986.
26. Sperry, RW: Physiological plasticity and brain circuitry theory. In Harlow, HF and Woolsey, CN (eds): Biological and Biochemical Bases of Behavior. University of Wisconsin Press, Madison, 1958.
27. Kertesz, A: Neurobiological aspects of recovery from aphasia in stroke. Int Rehabil Med 6:122, 1984.
28. Knopman, DS et al: Mechanisms of recovery from aphasia: evidence from serial xenon 133 cerebral blood flow studies. Ann Neurol 15:530, 1984.
29. Pizzamiglio, L and Mammucari, A: Evidence for sex differences in brain organization in recovery in aphasia. Brain Lang 25:213, 1985.
30. Teuber, HL, Battersby, WS and Bender, MB: Visual

Field Defects after Penetrating Missile Wounds of the Brain. Harvard University Press, Cambridge, 1960.

31. Russell, IS: Some observations on the problem of recovery of function following brain damage. Hum Neurobiol 1:68, 1982.

32. Schallert, T: Adipsia produced by lateral hypothalamic lesions: Facilitation of recovery by preoperative restriction of water intake. J Comp Physiol Psychol 96:604, 1982.

33. Bach-y-Rita, P: Sensory substitution in rehabilitation. In Illis, L, Sedgwick, M and Glanville, H (eds): Rehabilitation of the Neurological Patient. Blackwell Scientific Publications, Oxford, 1982.

34. Campbell, DC and Oxbury, JM: Recovery from unilateral visuo-spatial neglect? Cortex 12:303, 1976.

35. LeVere, NE and LeVere, TE: Recovery of function after brain damage: support for the compensation theory of the behavioral deficit. Physiol Psychol 10:165, 1982.

36. Gott, PS: Language after dominant hemispherectomy. J Neurol Neurosurg Psychiatry 36:1082, 1973.

37. Stein, DG, Finger, S and Hart, T: Brain damage and recovery: problems and perspectives. Behav Neurol Biol 37:185, 1983.

38. Gaillard, F: Recovery as a mind-brain paradigm. Int J Rehabil Res 6:331, 1983.

39. Bond, MR and Brooks, DN: Understanding the process of recovery as a basis for the investigation of rehabilitation for the brain injured. Scand J Rehabil Med 8:127, 1976.

40. Mangold, RF et al: Undernutrition and recovery from brain damage: a preliminary investigation. Brain Res 230:406, 1981.

41. Hallenbeck, JM, Jacobs, TP and Faden, AI: Combined PGI2, indomethacin, and heparin improves neurological recovery after spinal trauma in cats. J Neurosurg 58:749, 1983.

42. Kesslak, JP et al: Transplants of purified astrocytes promote behavioral recovery after frontal cortex ablation. Exp Neurol 92:377, 1986.

43. Sabel, BA, Slavin, MD and Stein, DG: GM1 ganglioside treatment facilitates behavioral recovery from bilateral brain damage. Science 225:340, 1984.

Chapter 7

Post-traumatic Epilepsy

BRYAN JENNETT, M.D.

Most of the lasting disabilities that follow head injury result from the incomplete resolution of deficits that were evident after injury. Epilepsy, by contrast, can develop months or years after injury and in a patient who has already made a good recovery. It is, however, more common after severe injuries, in patients who are also disabled to some extent in other ways. How frequently epilepsy develops after head injury depends on the severity of injury. The epilepsy rate was 2.5 percent in a study in the United States that required as evidence of head injury only that there had been some medical contact, for example, a house call or attendance at an emergency room.[1] The large United Kingdom study by Jennett[2] included only patients who had been admitted to the hospital; epilepsy occurred in 5 percent of these. After severe injuries (more than 6 hours in coma) the epilepsy rate was more than three times greater than this, and in those who were left severely disabled it was twice as great again.[3]

Any brain will generate a seizure if sufficiently stimulated—for example, with suitable drugs or by an electric current, as in electroconvulsive therapy. Whether or not epilepsy occurs with a lesser stimulus, such as injury, depends on the epileptogenic threshold of that particular individual and on the amount of brain damage. Traumatic epilepsy may occur during the first week after injury, in the phase of acutely changing pathophysiologic processes (early epilepsy); or it may begin months or years after injury, when it is assumed that the scar of the injury is acting as a focus that triggers a seizure in certain circumstances. In the context of rehabilitation it is *late* epilepsy that matters. The significance of early epilepsy is that it indicates an increased likelihood that late epilepsy will develop.

Late epilepsy is a significant disability because it is liable to persist, although the seizures may be infrequent if anticonvulsant medication is maintained. Even after a remission of 2 years, seizures often return. It is the risk of recurrence that constitutes the disability or handicap. In spite of the lessening social stigma associated with epilepsy it still imposes considerable social restrictions. The limitation that epilepsy imposes on driving affects the work and leisure activities of many people in Western society, where mobility increasingly depends on private transport. Many head injured patients are young, and their career prospects are immediately restricted by epilepsy, however infrequent the seizures are.

FEATURES OF EARLY EPILEPSY (FIRST WEEK AFTER INJURY)

Early epilepsy occurs more commonly in children under age 5, when it may follow mild injury. It seldom occurs in adults except in association with depressed fracture, intracranial hematoma, or unconsciousness lasting several hours. In 60 percent of cases, the first (and often the only) seizure occurs within the first 24 hours; in half of these cases it is within an hour of injury, often happening, therefore, in the ambulance or the emergency room. Two thirds of patients have more than one seizure, and about 10 percent have status epilepticus (which is more common in young children). About 40 percent have a generalized seizure, whereas another 40 percent have seizures that are confined to localized motor twitching (commonly the face or hand), a form of epilepsy that rarely occurs after the first week.

FEATURES OF LATE EPILEPSY

Epilepsy can take several forms and many patients have more than one type of attack. There is some focal feature, at least at the onset of the attacks, in about half the sufferers from traumatic epilepsy; in most such cases the seizures then spread to become generalized. Classic grand mal seizures without focal onset is the most disabling form of traumatic epilepsy, accounting for about half the patients. Such attacks cannot be concealed nor can avoiding action be taken when seizures occur in potentially hazardous circumstances.

About one fifth of patients have only temporal lobe attacks, and these episodes may not be immediately recognized as epileptic in nature. There are three main types of temporal lobe seizure—absences, psychic phenomena, and automatisms. In absences the flow of speech is broken, the thread of conversation lost, and for a matter of seconds the patient is out of contact; yet only an observant onlooker might notice such an event.

Psychic phenomena experienced by a patient include feelings of unexplained fear, of detachment from his or her surroundings, of déjà vu, or of olfactory hallucination. Usually there are no somatic accompaniments that someone with the patient would observe. Patients seldom volunteer information about such feelings, anticipating that they might be ridiculed or even judged to be mentally ill; it is necessary therefore to ask directly whether any of these unusual feelings have been experienced.

Automatisms comprise complex motor activities often correctly executed, but of a stereotyped nature that makes them purposeless and inappropriate in the circumstances in which they are enacted. Patients are usually unaware of what they are doing and are subsequently amnesic for the duration of the seizure. This usually lasts only seconds or minutes—time to close a door, cross a room, clap the hands, or to utter some stock phrase. Occasionally automatic behavior lasts hours, during which patients may carry out complex activities that include responding apparently normally to social cues. Some may travel across a city by public transport and then regain full consciousness in a place never visited before. Very occasionally patients have a series of such episodes lasting several days, with some clear periods in between. This may account for bizarre behavior that is interpreted as neurotic or even psychotic, and sometimes criminal acts are committed. There may be a clue to this in the form of epileptic activity in the temporal lobes on the electroencephalogram. But the best test is to give the patient anticonvulsant drugs in order to discover if they cause a dramatic improvement in behavior.

More than half the patients who develop late epilepsy have their first seizure within a year after injury. But more than one fourth begin their epilepsy more than 4 years later; focal seizures related to depressed fracture have been recorded as starting 40 years after the injury. The risk therefore never quite disappears.

PREDICTING LATE EPILEPSY

The relative infrequency of this potentially disabling complication and the delay in its appearance put a high premium on being able to identify which patients are at risk. It is then possible to take steps to minimize the risk of epilepsy by prescribing anticonvulsants, and to offer advice about work and leisure activities in the future. It used to be considered difficult to anticipate which patients would develop epilepsy, but the large-scale study by Jennett[2] has identified the few factors that influence the epilepsy rate. From a knowledge of these it is now possible to calculate soon after injury the approximate level of risk in individual patients on the basis of various clinical features of the injury and its early course.

There are three main factors that increase the likelihood that late epilepsy will develop. In order of significance, these are an acute intracranial hematoma requiring surgical evacuation within 2 weeks of injury; epilepsy in the first week after injury (early epilepsy); and a depressed fracture of the skull vault (Table 7–1).

After an intracranial hematoma has been surgically removed the risk of epilepsy in the next 4 years is about 35 percent. Epilepsy more often occurs after intradural clots (45 percent) than after extradural hematoma (22 percent).

Early epilepsy was once believed to be of little significance for the future. Certainly, it is true that three quarters of patients with early epilepsy do not have another seizure. However, the one quarter that do have seizures in the future make the overall risk of late epilepsy significantly greater than in patients who get through the first week after injury without a seizure. This increased risk applies even when there has been only a single early seizure, regardless of when during the first week the seizures occurred and whether the early seizures were focal or generalized.

Calculating the probability of late epilepsy after depressed fracture is more complicated. It depends on various combinations of other factors: whether the post-traumatic amnesia (PTA) exceeded 24 hours, whether the dura was penetrated, whether there were focal neurologic signs related to the fracture, and whether there was an early seizure. Except for early epilepsy, these are each indicators of the degree of brain damage suffered, and the more of them that occur, the greater the risk of late epilepsy. After depressed fracture this risk ranges from less than 3 percent to more than 60 percent

according to various combinations of these factors. Whereas it used to be considered that all depressed fractures were associated with an increased likelihood of epilepsy, it is now possible to reassure about 40 percent of patients that they have little chance of suffering from this delayed complication.

What are the chances that late epilepsy will develop after a head injury associated with none of the predisposing factors? For those with neither a hematoma nor a depressed fracture the risk is about 5 percent. In patients who also get through the first week without a seizure the risk is only about 1 percent; even if there is PTA of more than 24 hours the risk in such patients is still less than 2 percent. On the other hand, in these patients who have neither an acute hematoma nor a depressed fracture the occurrence of an early seizure increases the risk of late epilepsy to almost 20 percent. It is therefore in this group of patients, in whom the risk of epilepsy would otherwise be very low, that an early seizure is of the greatest significance for the future.

It has long been held that late epilepsy is a much more frequent complication of military than of civilian injuries, of missile than of nonmissile injuries. Little difference is found, however, when comparison is made between Vietnam veterans (90 percent injured by missile) and civilian injuries associated with either depressed fracture or an intracranial hematoma removed surgically within 2 weeks of injury.[4, 5] These two groups of patients constitute about 17 percent of head injuries admitted to the hospital in the United Kingdom.

The electroencephalogram (EEG) has proved disappointing in predicting the risk of epilepsy after head injury. Although patients who have already developed late epilepsy more often have an abnormal EEG than do patients without this complication, this abnormality largely reflects the degree of brain damage sustained at the time of injury. Moreover, the existence of this damage is already obvious from clinical features such as the occurrence of hematoma, different kinds of depressed fracture, the duration of PTA, or focal neurologic signs. Furthermore, a significant difference in EEG in the two groups is not evident until 2 years after injury, by which time most patients who are destined to develop epilepsy will already have had their first seizure (Table 7–2). As

Table 7–1. RISK OF LATE EPILEPSY AFTER CERTAIN TYPES OF INJURY

	n	%
Acute intracranial hematoma*	128	35
No hematoma	854	3
After early epilepsy	238	25
No early epilepsy	868	3
Depressed fracture	447	17
No depressed fracture	832	4
In patients with neither hematoma nor depressed fracture		
After early epilepsy	124	19
No early epilepsy	168	1

*Evacuated within 14 days of injury.
From Jennett,[2] with permission.

**Table 7–2. FREQUENCY OF
ABNORMAL EEG RECORDS
AT VARYING INTERVALS
AFTER INJURY**

Time Since Injury	No Late Epilepsy	Late Epilepsy	p
4 mo	76%	83%	NS
4–12 mo	59%	67%	NS
1–2 yr	64%	71%	NS
2 yr	46%	73%	< 0.001

From Jennett,[2] with permission.

a predictor the EEG therefore adds little to what is evident from clinical features.

An attempt is sometimes made to attribute the development of epilepsy to a preceding injury that was not associated with any of the epileptogenic factors already referred to. As both head injuries and epilepsy are relatively common occurrences it is inevitable that both will occur by chance not infrequently. There is a small risk that any person will develop epilepsy within the next year of his life; for adults aged 20 to 59 years the risk is 0.03 percent per year.[6] A study in Minnesota has shown no increase in the incidence of epilepsy during the 5 years after a mild head injury, defined as one without skull fracture or amnesia or unconsciousness of 30 minutes' duration.[1]

PREVENTION OF LATE EPILEPSY

There is no evidence that improved methods of treating head injuries in the acute stage in recent decades have done anything to reduce the incidence of epilepsy. The much more efficient early medical care of head injuries sustained in World War II and in successive conflicts since then, associated with dramatically reduced infection rates, has not resulted in any difference in the late epilepsy rate.[2, 4, 7] Presumably this is because epilepsy is related to the amount of brain damage sustained at the time of impact, a factor that cannot be influenced by medical intervention.

Therefore, the only course open is the judicious use of prophylactic medication for patients identified as having a high risk of epilepsy. However, a survey of American neurosurgeons revealed that many of them did not attempt to protect their post-traumatic patients.[8] The reasons they gave were that they were uncertain which patients were at risk, or that they believed that the overall risk was too low to justify medication. Now that there are reliable statistics for calculating the risk in individual patients,[2] these excuses are no longer valid. It therefore becomes a matter of deciding what level of risk justifies the prescribing of drugs to a patient who has not yet had a late seizure, and who may not have had an early seizure. Also there must be agreement regarding what drugs should be used, when they should be started, and how long they should be continued.

One reason that anticonvulsant therapy often fails to control epilepsy is that patients are not taking their drugs at all, or are doing so only irregularly, or their medication may not have been prescribed in sufficient dosage. Those involved with rehabilitation should try to ensure that patients have adequate medication and that they take their drugs regularly. Because of the mental changes after head injury, patients are often forgetful about their drugs. They may also be untruthful when questioned about how carefully they have been maintaining their medication. It is essential therefore to measure blood levels at follow-up clinics before deciding that a change of drug is needed because of failure to control seizures. Sometimes the opposite problem arises, of patients taking (or their relatives administering) too much medication in an effort to control seizures; patients may then develop signs of toxicity that the rehabilitation caregiver should be aware of. Ataxia and nystagmus are common side effects of phenytoin (Dilantin), the drug most commonly used; skin rashes and hyperplasia of the gums may also occur.

An early seizure can lead to intracranial complications, particularly in patients who are already suffering from significant brain damage. It is therefore often recommended that patients likely to develop early seizures should receive anticonvulsant therapy from the time that they are first seen after injury. This would include all patients with depressed fractures and those with intracranial hematomas requiring surgery. Perhaps all those in coma should be treated initially, discontinuing the treatment once it has become clear that no predisposing features for epilepsy have developed. This could apply also to many patients with depressed fractures who had been started on a treatment regimen before it was known whether there would be sufficient epileptogenic factors to justify continuing drug treatment.

It is certainly easier to insist on adequate treatment, with regular checks on the blood level of anticonvulsants, for 3 months than for a year or more. In patients in the high-risk groups (e.g., more than 30 percent), however, treatment should be maintained for at least a year, until there is firmer evidence to support the contention that a brief drug regimen is effective in reducing the occurrence of seizures after drugs have been discontinued. There is considerable doubt whether even a year on treatment provides any reduction in seizures occurring after this period.[9]

EPILEPSY AND DRIVING

Most countries have clear regulations that specify the conditions under which patients at risk from epilepsy may or may not drive a car or pilot an airplane. Such regulations are always more stringent for heavy goods vehicles and public service vehicles, and for commercial and military aircraft. Until recently such regulations have usually been based on a prescribed interval since the last recorded seizure, and this is commonly 2 years. However, varying degrees of discretion are allowed in some countries. More controversial is what restrictions should apply to patients who are in high-risk categories for developing epilepsy, but who have not so far had any seizures. It is now recommended in Britain that there should be a period of 6 to 12 months before such patients drive, leaving it open to decide what level risk is deemed unacceptable. However, neurosurgeons[10] and neurologists[11] vary widely in how they view these risks and how they advise their patients.

It is clearly important that those responsible for the rehabilitation of patients with brain damage should be aware of the implications of epilepsy for the future, for both private and vocational driving and flying. There is no doubt that restrictions on driving can be socially and vocationally very frustrating in Western society, and that these can pose problems for rehabilitation. But the realities of the situation have to be faced; it is essential not to set unrealistic goals for the eligibility to drive, because these may have to be abandoned.

REFERENCES

1. Annegers, JF et al: Seizures after head injury in a population study. Neurology 30:683, 1980.
2. Jennett, B: Epilepsy after Non-Missile Head Injuries, ed 2. Heinemann, London, 1975.
3. Jennett, B et al: Disability after severe head injury: Observations on the use of the Glasgow Outcome Scale. J Neurol Neurosurg Psychiatry 44:285, 1981.
4. Caveness, WF et al: The nature of post-traumatic epilepsy. J Neurosurg 50:545, 1979.
5. Jennett, B: Epilepsy after head injury and intracranial surgery. In Hopkins, AP (ed): Epilepsy. Chapman Hall, London, 1987.
6. Hauser, AE and Kurland, LT: The epidemiology of epilepsy in Rochester, Minnesota, 1935 through 1967. Epilepsia 16:1, 1975.
7. Caveness, WF, Walker, AE, and Ascroft, PB: Incidence of post-traumatic epilepsy in Korean veterans as compared with those in World War I and World War II. J Neurosurg 19:122, 1962.
8. Rappaport, RL and Penry, JK: A survey of attitudes towards the pharmacologic prophylaxis of post-traumatic epilepsy. J Neurosurg 38:159, 1973.
9. North, JB et al: Phenytoin and post-operative epilepsy. J Neurosurg 58:672, 1983.
10. Jennett, B: Anticonvulsant drugs and advice about driving after head injury and intracranial surgery. Br Med J 286:627, 1983.
11. Harvey, P and Hopkins, A: Views of British neurologists on epilepsy, driving and the law. Lancet 1:401, 1983.

Chapter 8

Neurologic Sequelae of Head Injury

RAJ K. NARAYAN, M.D.
ZIYA L. GOKASLAN, M.D.
CATHERINE F. BONTKE, M.D.
SHELDON BERROL, M.D.

In addition to the immediate primary and secondary brain insults incurred from head trauma, other neurologic injuries or delayed complications, or both, may occur. These neurologic sequelae are noteworthy in that (1) they may impede or cause deterioration of functional recovery and (2) they may be masked by the effects of the acute brain insults and thus difficult to detect.

EARLY NEUROLOGIC SEQUELAE

Cranial Nerve I

The incidence of olfactory dysfunction after head trauma has been reported as varying from 2 to 38 percent. Damage to the olfactory system occurs with great frequency in occipital blows, but the incidence is higher after frontal injury. It is the most commonly involved cranial nerve after minor head injury.[1] In testing for olfactory function, one must recognize that many substances such as camphor or peppermint are trigeminal nerve stimulants. Thus, a patient who cannot identify an odor may be able to identify the presence of a stimulus when presented with strong odors. Ammonia as a test agent should only be used to determine suspected malingering, since the tearing that accompanies its perception cannot be prevented.

Anosmia frequently is not identified until the patient has recovered from post-traumatic amnesia. Patients with dysnomia or aphasia may be incorrectly assumed to have anosmia. Testing should include absolute odor sensitivity evaluation, and odors offered should be familiar to the individual.

Additionally, head injury can produce at least a partial impairment of olfactory recognition despite relatively preserved olfactory detection. The presence of a hematoma or contusion in the frontal/temporal region is not uncommonly related to impaired olfactory recognition. Impaired olfactory recognition may result from focal and diffuse injury to the orbitofrontal and temporal regions.[2]

Animal studies have implicated a role for olfaction in the temporal lobe.[3] Temporal lobe structures have been clearly identified in emotional and motivational disturbances, and olfactory dysfunction may have a significant role in behavioral disturbance management.

Anosmia will occur in almost 50 percent of patients who sustain rhinorrhea from an anterior fossa fracture, and in about 50 percent of those who require surgical repair.[4] Spontaneous recovery of functional olfaction may occur in more than one third of patients over a period of days to 5 years after injury.[5]

Cranial Nerve II

Injury to the visual system occurs in 5 percent of all patients who sustain head trauma, regardless of severity.[6] Traumatic loss of vision may occur without overt evidence of injury to the eye. It typically results from an ipsilateral blow, usually frontal, occasionally temporal, and rarely occipital. It may occur after minor head injury.[7] Injury to the system may occur as a result of mechanical damage by shear forces, stretching, and contusion, or from local vascular insufficiency.

Crompton demonstrated evidence of ischemic necrosis and shearing lesion patterns in the anterior visual pathway in 44 percent of severely head injured patients who died of complications and in 24 percent of bilateral lesions.[8] It appears that lesions of visual pathways are often undetected clinically.

Sustained elevated ICP may produce vitreous hemorrhages that develop over time (Terson's syndrome). Serial ophthalmologic examinations are essential in head injury management.

Early Assessment of Visual System

Direct pupillary response to light is the most reliable early indicator of the extent of optic nerve injury. Ophthalmoscopic examination and roentgenologic studies are of substantially less value.[9]

Unilateral eye injury can be identified by the presence of decreased to absent pupillary reactivity to light stimulation, with preservation of the consensual reaction (Marcus-Gunn pupil). The uninvolved eye maintains a normal light reflex but impaired consensual response. These reactions indicate an afferent lesion in the pupillary light reflex pathways.

Visual evoked potentials may provide valuable objective information even during coma because patient cooperation is not essential. The procedure is more accurate than clinical examination in the early diagnosis of retrobulbar visual dysfunction.[10]

Cerebral computed tomography (CT) is of particular value in assessing the integrity of the optic canal.

As coma resolves, the patient should be evaluated for light perception. The stimulus must be presented at least to each visual quadrant, and preferably to each cardinal plane. Serial evaluations should be undertaken for the presence of visual fixation as well as for localization and tracking of stim-

uli. The visual stimulus should be sufficiently novel in intensity, density, form, and spatial representation to elicit a response; simply requesting a patient to focus on a finger or pencil may be inadequate. The optokinetic response may provide evidence of preservation of an acuity level of 20/200 in at least part of the visual field. Early assessment of visual potential allows more appropriate selection of rehabilitation intervention strategies.[11]

Spontaneous nystagmus is a principal sign of a peripheral or central visual system problem and may assist in localizing specific lesions. Spontaneous vertical nystagmus is considered a sign of mid-brain damage.[12]

Gradual deterioration in visual acuity or visual fields may be due to compression of the optic nerve by fractures about the optic canal. Serial examinations are required. Surgical decompression may be necessary. If visual loss is immediate, then surgical decompression is usually not indicated.

The term "cortical blindness" should be reserved for the patient who demonstrates amaurosis with reactive pupils, rather than including individuals who have incurred partial visual field loss. Most patients with cortical blindness will regain some limited visual capability via secondary visual pathway systems. The patient's response to high–visual intensity moving stimuli should be evaluated. The patient who is cortically blind with overt denial of the visual loss (Anton's syndrome) should be considered for early blindness training. As the state of confusion resolves, high–visual intensity moving stimuli can be introduced. It is uncommon for such patients to complain of visual hallucinations.

Cranial Nerves III, IV, and VI

Extraocular muscle dysfunction causes diplopia and may result from central or peripheral motor dysfunction. Diplopia may contribute to the confusion of the patient arousing from coma. Eye patching can abolish the double image. When the patient has the ability to suppress the second image, eye patching should be discontinued. The common practice of alternating the patch between the affected and the unaffected eye is based on the prevention of disuse amblyopia. However, as amblyopia does not occur in the adult population, we usually choose to patch the sound eye to stimulate maximal motor activity of the affected eye. During table-top cognitive tasks or computer activities, however, accuracy may be increased by allowing full use of the sound eye.

Abnormal head postures may be utilized to compensate for paretic extraocular motor function. This commonly occurs in cranial nerve IV paresis. The fourth cranial nerve is not only a depressor, but also an intorter of the eye; the patient tends to compensate by tilting the head. Attempts at "normalizing" the head position may prevent the patient from achieving binocular vision. Head tilt may also result from nystagmus because stabilizing the head against the shoulder may dampen the nystagmus.[13] Visual field deficits frequently also produce head turns in order to properly align the remaining visual field.

Spontaneous resolution of extraoculomotor (EOM) paresis occurs with considerable frequency. In cranial nerve III paresis a residual superior rectus weakness may remain. Thus the patient may complain of occasional diplopia, a symptom that requires evaluation of EOM function in all the cardinal planes. Cranial nerve IV lesions spontaneously resolve in 65 percent of unilateral involvement and in 25 percent of the bilateral cases.[14] Though some have argued that surgical correction in permanent paralysis may be merely cosmetic, Fells and Waddell[15] have demonstrated that restoration of binocularity can occur in the majority of cases. The development of appropriate criteria for patient selection is essential.

Cranial Nerve V

The patient who demonstrates an insensitive cornea, as indicated by an absent corneal reflex, in the presence of facial nerve paresis (especially if the lacrimal branch is involved) is at great risk to develop repeated neurotropic corneal ulceration, and possible loss of vision. These patients should be considered early for protective tarsorrhaphy. Protective lubricants should be used liberally as part of routine nursing.[16] Tear production, regulated by the lacrimal branch of the facial nerve, should be evaluated by the Schirmer tear test.[17]

Cranial Nerve VII

The status of the facial nerve must be documented at the initial examination. If paralysis is of immediate onset, then prompt exploration for possible decompression is essential. Generally this event results from disruption of the facial canal in the temporal bone. The facial nerve traverses a longer bony canal than does any other cranial nerve and therefore is extremely vulnerable to injury. Ten to 30 percent of longitudinal fractures of the temporal bone cause facial nerve damage. Thirty to 50 percent of transverse fractures result in facial nerve palsy.

If there is delayed development of paralysis, the prognosis is substantially better if the paralysis is not bilateral, and the patient should be followed with serial facial nerve testing. Neurophysiologic testing including nerve conduction and electromyographic studies should demonstrate some signs of recovery within 8 weeks, if recovery is to occur. In such cases, exploration is probably not necessary, as complete recovery occurs in 75 percent of the cases and partial recovery in 15 percent.[18]

Cranial Nerve VIII

The ear is the most commonly damaged sensory organ after severe head injury. Vertigo may occur as a result of vestibular apparatus damage, perilymphatic abscess, or labyrinthine concussion.

Longitudinal fractures of the petrous portion of the temporal bone are the most common fractures involved in head trauma. Hearing loss is primarily conductive as a result of ossicular chain disruption or blood in the middle ear. The ossicular chain is most often disrupted at the incudostapedial joint. Surgical intervention and prosthetic replacement of the dislocated component are essential for restoration of hearing.

Transverse fractures of the petrous portion of the temporal bone usually produce sensorineural hearing loss. The labyrinthine capsule is generally disrupted, resulting in severe vestibular and cochlear damage, including functional destruction of the semicircular canals, utricle, and saccule. Because the fracture line in transverse fractures is perpendicular to the facial nerve, both nerves are damaged in 50 percent of patients with this fracture.

The entire thickness of the petrous bone is frequently involved causing damage to both auditory and vestibular components. Thus, vertigo and nausea commonly occur with the hearing loss.

Assessment of oculovestibular responses may provide early information regarding the status of the system, and later electronystagmography may confirm end organ impairment of the vestibular nerve. No reliable diagnostic test of central vestibular nerve function is available. Brainstem auditory evoked potentials can contribute significantly to the evaluation of the integrity of auditory nerve and cochlear nucleus,[19] but provide little insight into the structure or function of the vestibular nerve component.

NEUROGENIC ALTERATIONS OF VITAL SIGNS

Sequelae of brainstem injuries producing hypertension, tachycardia and arrhythmias, respiratory problems, and hyperthermia are dealt with in Chapters 3 and 9.

LOCKED-IN SYNDROME

The terms "locked-in syndrome" and "akinetic mutism" are used synonymously.[20, 21]

Damage to the corticobulbar and corticospinal pathways in the ventral pons results in a de-efferented state characterized by tetraplegia and mutism. The patient remains aware and responsive, and higher cortical function remains unaffected.[21]

Supranuclear ocular pathways are spared so that eye movement control is at least partially preserved, usually in the vertical, and sometimes in the horizontal plane. Nonoral communication is therefore possible, either utilizing eye movements or blinking, and the use of appropriate interface systems can provide sufficient communication with which to demonstrate retained cognitive abilities. The syndrome results most often from vascular infarction and therefore is not commonly found as a result of trauma. Locked-in syndrome must be clearly differentiated from the vegetative state in which sentience is not preserved, despite a return of sleep-wake cycles and a deceptive appearance of neurologic recovery ("coma vigil") that frequently gives the patient's family and friends an unjustified sense of optimism.

SPINAL CORD INJURY

Motor vehicle accidents are responsible for the majority of both head and spinal cord injury. Impact on the skull in the presence of a flexed neck directs vector forces through the cranial contents to the cervical spine. Thus, the combination of head and spinal injury occurs in about 4 percent of patients with severe head trauma. The failure to identify acute spinal instability in the obtunded or comatose patient can have catastrophic consequences.

The brain injured patient should be treated as having a cervical spine injury until thorough evaluation rules out this possibility. The persistence of flaccidity in an extremity should raise concern for peripheral nerve or plexus injury. The persistence of flaccidity in a pattern of hemiplegia, or diplegia, should raise the suspicion of spinal cord injury. Anal reflexes should be evaluated; persistent areflexia suggests cord injury.

If there is any suspicion of cervical spine injury, a cross-table lateral roentgenogram that clearly shows all seven cervical vertebrae must be obtained. Caution to maintain the neck in neutral position is essential. Visualization of the lower vertebrae often requires downward traction of both upper extremities, or a transaxillary ("swimmer's") view.

Minor head injury is a frequent concomitant of trauma-related spinal cord injury occurring with an incidence of 25 percent to 50 percent. Any patient with a fresh spinal injury who is obtunded, confused, or disoriented should be considered as having an associated head injury. Many of the closed head injuries associated with spinal cord trauma remain undetected. Serial neuropsychologic testing should be considered. Additionally, the patient who later appears to be unmotivated, who demonstrates problems with learning, should be reassessed for cognitive status.[22]

PERIPHERAL NERVOUS SYSTEM SEQUELAE

Peripheral Neuropathies

Polyneuropathies are reported as an early complication of sepsis and other critical illnesses in up to 50 percent of patients in intensive care units.[23] This complication is occasionally recognized clinically in head injury patients. The neuropathy usually subsides as the critical illness comes under control.

Neuropathies associated with fractures can occur at the fracture site. However, compression neuropathies can result from immobility and localized pressure to a nerve over a bony prominence. Such compression most commonly affects the ulnar and peroneal nerves.

Whenever a limb remains flaccid, the possibility of neuropathy exists. In the unconscious patient, physical evaluation can be quite limited, and nerve conduction studies may be valuable.

Other Peripheral Deficits

Radiculopathies may require more detailed electrophysiologic studies and are rarely in evidence early, since spasticity masks underlying weakness. After coma resolves, the presence of neural defects with a segmental distribution indicates damage to spinal nerves or nerve roots.

Plexopathies, on the other hand, involve many muscle groups, so that tone is diminished from what would be expected. Direct injury to the shoulder or the pelvis may result in stretching, contusion, compression or laceration injuries to the brachial or lumbosacral plexus. The pattern of flaccidity in an extremity should alert one to re-evaluate the force mechanisms of the initial injury, and consider appropriate electrophysiologic studies, including nerve conduction velocities, as well as H and F reflexes. If bone fracture has occurred, the excessive callus development may result in adjacent nerve compression, with late development of nerve injury. Orthopedic-related neural injuries are further discussed in Chapter 9.

Aminoglycoside antibiotics have been implicated in causing neuromuscular junction transmission defects.[23] However, to our knowledge, this complication has not yet been reported in head injury survivors.

DELAYED NEUROLOGIC SEQUELAE

CNS injury is a dynamic process. It is generally accepted that the more severe the impact suffered, the worse the ultimate outcome is likely to be. Perhaps less well recognized is the fact that soon after the initial injury a wide variety of secondary processes come into play.[24] These sequelae can have a major impact on the patient's eventual level of recovery.[25] It is not uncommon to see two patients with similar initial injuries have widely disparate outcomes, at least partly the result of complications. Whereas certain secondary insults occur in the acute phase,[26] other complications arise, or are noticed, in the subsequent weeks and months. This section summarizes the current thinking on some of the more commonly encountered long-term neurosurgical sequelae of head injury.

Post-traumatic Hydrocephalus

DEFINITION

The syndrome of post-traumatic hydrocephalus (PTH) must be defined using both radiologic and neurologic criteria, since both features must be present to make the diagnosis. In simple terms, PTH may be described as ventricular dilatation without sulcal enlargement, associated with a clinical syndrome that may vary from deep coma to the typical picture of normal pressure hydrocephalus—dementia, ataxia, and urinary incontinence.

INCIDENCE

Although ventricular dilatation is a common finding after head injury, particularly when the injury is severe, true PTH is relatively uncommon.[27] The incidence of post-traumatic ventricular dilatation has been variously reported to be between 29 and 72 percent.[28] Obviously, differences in diagnostic methods, definition of ventricular enlargement, and patient characteristics must account for these wide differences. Kishore and coworkers[29] defined significant ventriculomegaly as a distended appearance of the anterior horn of lateral ventricles, enlargement of the temporal horns and third ventricle, and normal or absent sulci. They then prospectively followed for 1 year 100 consecutive patients who had severe head injury, with serial CT scans of the head. Twenty-nine of the 100 patients developed ventriculomegaly within the year, and 27 of that 29 developed it within the first 2 weeks.

Cordoso and Galbraith[30] reported a retrospective review of perhaps a more heterogenous group of 2374 patients with "severe" head injury. Of this group of patients (who were not scanned or followed-up according to a predetermined protocol), 17 (0.7 percent) developed symptomatic hydrocephalus. Of these 8 patients (50 percent) improved markedly, and 4 (25 percent) slightly, after shunting.

In a CT study performed at least 3 months after head injury, Gardeur and associates[31] found ventricular enlargement in 78 percent of the patients. Similarly, van Dongen and Braakman[32] reported CT evidence of cerebral atrophy in 86 percent of patients examined 1 to 4 years after closed head injury resulting in coma for at least 6 hours. Levin and coworkers[33] studied the area of the lateral ventricles on CT scans obtained at least 30 days after severe closed head injury in 32 young adults, and reported enlargement in 72 percent of the cases.

Post-traumatic hydrocephalus must be distinguished from post-traumatic cerebral atrophy. The former term denotes an active, treatable condition, which compounds existing neurologic deficits, whereas the latter represents brain parenchymal resorption secondary to diffuse tissue injury. Unfortunately, this distinction is not always readily apparent. CT scanning has certainly made the diagnosis somewhat easier to make, and interestingly, there has been a drop in the reported incidence of PTH to between 1 and 8 percent,[34-35] as compared with 21 to 36 percent in the pneumoencephalogram era.[36]

PATHOPHYSIOLOGY

It is generally believed that PTH results from an impairment in the flow and absorption of CSF. Although radiologic and pathologic evidence suggests that this blockage is usually around the cerebral convexities, it is certainly possible that blockage of the arachnoid granulations by subarachnoid blood may play a role.[37] In any case, subarachnoid hemorrhage seems to be a feature common to these two hypotheses. For a more extensive discussion of pathophysiology, the interested reader is referred to two larger reviews of PTH.[28, 38]

CLINICAL FEATURES

PTH may be manifested in a variety of ways. As reported by Kishore and colleagues,[29] 27 of the 29 patients in their series developed the syndrome within 2 weeks of injury. There is a reported case of ventricular enlargement within 7 hours of a head injury, resulting in a rapidly deteriorating level of consciousness and early herniation.[39] However, more delayed presentations are certainly possible. In fact, remote trauma is rather commonly reported in series of patients with normal pressure hydrocephalus (NPH).[40, 41]

PTH may present as classic NPH, with dementia, ataxia, and urinary incontinence. However, altered levels of consciousness and even coma may occur as part of the syndrome. Because severe head injury often results in fairly extensive neurologic dysfunction, these features may be hard to separate from the effects of brain trauma in the acute phase. Intracranial pressure (ICP) monitoring and serial CT scans can be useful in this setting. In the more chronic phase of recovery, a deteriorating level of consciousness, worsening functional capacity, or any of the features of NPH should serve as a tip-off. Some atypical manifestations such as emotional problems,[42] bilateral extensor responses, seizures, and leg spasticity have also been reported.[40]

RADIOLOGIC FEATURES

A fairly large body of data exists relating to the pneumoencephalographic diagnosis of hydrocephalus and its distinction from ex vacuo ventriculomegaly; however, these indices have essentially been rendered obsolete by CT scanning. As stated earlier, Kishore and coworkers[29] have used the following CT criteria to define hydrocephalus:

(1) distended appearance of the frontal horns of the lateral ventricles; (2) enlargement of the temporal horns and the third ventricle; (3) normal or absent sulci; and, (4) if present, enlargement of the basal cisterns and fourth ventricle. Periventricular lucency was used as an indicator of communicating hydrocephalus. Ex vacuo ventriculomegaly, or atrophy, is characterized by diffuse ventricular enlargement with prominent sulci and no periventricular lucency.

Levin and colleagues[33] used ventricular area as calculated from a CT scan to study the relationship between ventriculomegaly and neuropsychologic deficits after closed head injury. Although this technique is clearly the most accurate way of assessing ventricular size, there is no radiologic method that can reliably predict outcome from shunting.

Periventricular edema has long been recognized as a pathologic and radiologic feature of hydrocephalus. Normally, fluid from the brain parenchyma moves across the ependymal lining into the ventricles. In the presence of hydrocephalus, this normal direction of flow is reversed, and fluid moves from the ventricles into the periventricular white matter. Since T2 weighted images on magnetic resonance imaging (MRI) are very sensitive for water, it was hoped that this new imaging technique would define the population with symptomatic hydrocephalus. Unfortunately, this might not be quite so simple. Zimmerman and associates[43] reported that a review of 365 consecutive MRI studies revealed some degree of periventricular hyperintensity (PVH) in 93.5 percent of cases, regardless of diagnosis. Of the six patients in their series with NPH, two had mild nonspecific PVH and four had prominent PVH, but in all cases multiple white matter hyperintense foci (presumably representing infarctions) were also present. The degree of PVH was similar to that seen in nonhydrocephalic elderly patients and could not therefore be used as a criterion for shunting.

Selection of Patients for Shunting

There is no single clinical, radiologic, or physiologic feature that can serve as an accurate and infallible criterion for shunt placement. Needless to say, if there is severe underlying brain damage, shunting, even if indicated, may not improve functional outcome significantly. Nevertheless, every patient should be carefully evaluated and given the benefit of the doubt because in a substantial number of cases, shunting can make a difference. If a patient meets the clinical and radiologic criteria defined earlier, every effort must be made to obtain an assessment of the craniospinal axis pressure. If the patient has had an ICP monitor in place, then this information is readily available. If not, a lumbar puncture can be performed with the patient lying flat on the side and the ICP recorded when he or she is relaxed and the abdomen is not being compressed. No firm pressure guidelines are available in PTH for shunting. It stands to reason that if the lumbar CSF pressure is clearly lower than 136 mm CSF (10 mmHg) a shunt is unlikely to help, and if it is higher than 276 mm CSF (20 mmHg) it may be very useful. However, when the pressures are in between, this single reading does not provide a clear answer. Draining 20 to 30 ml of CSF may sometimes result in significant, albeit transient, clinical improvement, thus tipping the balance in favor of shunting.

When the lumbar pressure is normal, shunting may be considered if a classic picture of NPH exists. Salmon[44] found that 5 of 9 post-traumatic patients with this syndrome improved after shunting regardless of other test results. In two other studies[40, 45] a 60 to 70 percent success rate for shunting has been reported when the typical clinical features of NPH are present.

If the picture is not clear, a brief period (12 to 48 hours) of ICP monitoring may be helpful. In one study of 12 subjects,[46] patients who showed variable ICP improved following surgery, while those with consistently flat ICP tracings did not. Borgesen and coworkers,[47] however, reported that ICP data per se did not help them in a series of patients with "true" NPH who had mean ICPs not exceeding 12 mmHg. In this series they reported that conductance to CSF outflow was a much more relevant measurement. However, this method has not become widely used in clinical practice.

Cisternography has been extensively used in the past in the evaluation of patients with NPH. When radiolabeled albumin is injected into the lumbar subarachnoid space, it normally flows over the cerebral convexities and gets absorbed via the arachnoidal granulations into the major venous sinuses.

When the normal flow of CSF over the convexities is impeded, the isotope backs into the ventricles within an hour of the injection and lingers there for 24 to 72 hours. While this ventricular reflux was thought to be typical of NPH, its correlation with improvement post-shunting has been rather disappointing. Data available to date do not show any advantage of cisternography over assessments of the clinical picture and lumbar or intracranial pressures.[28]

In conclusion, a high index of suspicion for PTH must be maintained in patients with altered mentation following trauma. Serial CT scans and neurologic assessments are valuable in making the diagnosis. Lumbar or intracranial pressures may be useful in selecting patients for shunting. Other tests seem to be of little value. Approximately 50 percent of patients with ventriculomegaly will improve significantly after shunting.

Post-traumatic Epilepsy

Chapter 7 by Dr. Jennett provides an extensive and knowledgable review of the subject of post-traumatic epilepsy. We will make some additional comments on the controversial matter of the use of prophylactic anticonvulsants in patients with severe head injury.[48–50]

Prophylactic treatment with phenytoin initiated as early as possible (within 24 hours of injury) could possibly prevent the development of an epileptogenic focus; however, the randomized double-blind, placebo-controlled studies of adults by Young and associates[51] show that prophylactically administered phenytoin prevents neither early nor late post-traumatic seizures. This appeared to be true in children as well.[52] In these studies, plasma concentrations were maintained between 10 and 20 μg/ml. The authors caution that maintaining higher drug levels could have altered the study results. However, they recommend using anticonvulsants only after a patient has had a seizure. McQueen and coworkers,[53] however, point out that because of a low incidence of post-traumatic seizures (7 percent at 1 year, 10 percent at 2 years), randomized clinical trials must include about 1200 patients in order to be conclusive. If this is so, all such trials reported to date are too small (by a factor of at least six). The weight of evidence to date therefore supports the routine use of anticonvulsants in the high-risk groups, but not necessarily in all patients with head injury.

Our present practice is to use phenytoin (500 mg intravenously over 10 minutes) in the emergency room in all head injury patients who are unable to follow simple commands. This drug is then continued for 1 year. Doses are adjusted to achieve therapeutic blood levels. Based on the findings of Young and colleagues,[51, 52] aiming for higher blood levels (15 to 20 μg/ml) may be justified. The entire requirement may be taken as a single daily dose.[54] There are no hard and fast rules as to when to stop the use of anticonvulsants. Each case has to be individualized, and the risk of seizures assessed. The EEG is not generally contributory in making this decision. The drugs should be tapered off gradually rather than stopped abruptly. There is some recent evidence to suggest that carbamazepine (Tegretol) may be preferable to phenytoin for long-term use because of improved performance on tests of cognitive function.[55]

Cerebrospinal Fluid Fistulas

DEFINITION

A traumatic cerebrospinal fluid (CSF) fistula may be defined as a CSF leak occurring as a consequence of a head injury. Fistulas may present as rhinorrhea, otorrhea, or pneumocephalus.

INCIDENCE

CSF fistulas reportedly occur in 0.25 to 3.0 percent of all patients with head injury and in 5 to 11 percent of those with basal skull fractures.[56–58] It is estimated that there are 150,000 cases of traumatic rhinorrhea in the United States per year.[59] CSF otorrhea occurred in only 7 percent of 300 basal skull fractures in one report.[60] Pneumocephalus occurs in about one third of patients with rhinorrhea,[60] although this may be an isolated finding.

CSF RHINORRHEA

This condition occurs in about 25 percent of patients with anterior basal fracture. CSF may leak via the frontal sinus, through the cribriform plate or orbital plate of the frontal bone, via the sphenoid sinus, and, less frequently, via the clivus. On occasion, with a fracture of the petrous part of the temporal bone, CSF may enter the eustachian tube, and if the tympanic membrane is intact, drain from the nose. Drainage begins within 48 hours of injury in almost 80 percent of cases.[61, 62] The fluid is watery and nonmucoid, and it contains glucose. A glucose concentration of 30 mg/100 ml or greater is very suggestive of CSF.[56] Dextrostix and similar products are unreliable since normal nasal secretions may give a positive reaction.[62] Protein electrophoresis combined with immunofixation for an isoform of transferrin has been recently shown to be useful in identifying CSF.[63]

Several aspects of the management of CSF rhinorrhea remain controversial, including the use of prophylactic antibiotics, timing of surgery, and the role of lumbar drains. In general, 80 percent of fistulas will stop leaking within 1 week.[64] The patient is nursed in a position that stops or minimizes the leak. If the leak has not stopped in about 3 days, a lumbar subarachnoid drain is inserted and allowed to drain at about shoulder level for 3 to 7 days. If the leak persists at 10 to 14 days, surgery should be considered, and diagnostic testing is initiated to identify the site of the leak. Metrizamide or Omnipaque CT cisternography is currently considered to be the diagnostic test of choice.[65] In intermittent CSF leak this test may give a false-negative result. Various maneuvers such as the Trendelenberg position, Valsalva maneuver, and lumbar subarachnoid saline injection have been described to maximize the probability of detecting the site of leakage.[66]

Once the fistula site has been identified, it can be surgically repaired using an intracranial (intradural or extradural) or a transphenoidal approach, depending on the site of the leak.[64] Sense of smell may be lost as a result of the initial injury, especially with fractures of the ethmoidal bone. The incidence of anosmia may be as high as 80 percent. An intracranial frontal fossa floor repair is associated with a high incidence of anosmia, even when smell is normal preoperatively. The extradural repair may be advantageous in this regard. The size of leakage may be rather small, and the surgeon may face some difficulty in finding the dural tear. Lyophilized dura, pericranium, or fascia lata is often used to patch the defect.

CSF OTORRHEA

This condition occurs when the petrous bone is fractured, the overlying dura mater and arachnoid are torn, and the tympanic membrane is perforated.[64] Fractures of the petrous bone are classified as longitudinal or transverse, based on their relationship to the long axis of the petrous pyramid; however, most fractures are mixed. Patients with longitudinal fracture present with conductive hearing loss, otorrhea, and bleeding from the external ear. Patients with transverse fractures generally have normal tympanic membranes, and demonstrate sensorineural hearing loss from damage to the labyrinth, cochlea, or the eighth nerve within the auditory canal. Facial paresis is present in up to 50 percent of patients.[67] Longitudinal fractures are four to six times more frequent than transverse fractures, but are much less likely to cause facial nerve injury.

CSF otorrhea ceases spontaneously in the overwhelming majority of patients within a week. The incidence of meningitis in patients with otorrhea is probably about 4 percent, as compared with 17 percent with CSF rhinorrhea.[59, 64] In the rare event that it does not cease, lumbar drainage and even surgery may be undertaken.

PROPHYLACTIC ANTIBIOTICS

The role of prophylactic antibiotics in the management of CSF otorrhea or rhinorrhea remains uncertain because of a paucity of data. There is considerable variation in practice in this regard. The only prospective randomized study of the use of penicillin in patients with rhinorrhea or otorrhea was limited to 52 patients.[68] Meningitis developed in only one patient in this study, and this occurred in the placebo-treated group; that patient had an intraventricular foreign body. The authors concluded that their study did not support the routine use of prophylactic antibiotics in these cases.

Post-traumatic Vascular Complications

DEFINITION

Post-traumatic vascular complications can involve both the arterial and the venous systems, and may occur either extracranially or intracranially. They usually occur at the time of initial impact, or soon after the injury is sustained, but may not become apparent until several days or even months later.

INCIDENCE

The true incidence of vascular complications associated with head injury is uncertain because of a limited number of epidemiologic studies. Furthermore, with cerebral angiography having been virtually eliminated from the routine evaluation of head injury patients since the advent of CT scanning, this database is not likely to be improved upon. It is important therefore that clinicians maintain a high index of suspicion and obtain angiograms when the clinical picture cannot be explained by the CT or MRI scans. One study of 2000 civilian head injuries reported a 4.2 percent incidence of vascular injuries.[69]

CLASSIFICATION

Post-traumatic vascular complications may be classified as follows:

A. Arterial
  1. Cervical
    a. Direct carotid or vertebral artery transection
    b. Thromboembolic occlusion, from a traumatic nidus or intimal dissection
    c. Traumatic arterial aneurysms
    d. Traumatic arteriovenous fistulas
  2. Intracranial
    a. Thromboembolic occlusion
    b. Traumatic aneurysms
    c. Traumatic AV fistulas
    d. Carotid-cavernous fistulas
B. Venous
  1. Dural venous sinus thrombosis
C. Traumatic vasospasm

DISCUSSION

A detailed discussion of post-traumatic vascular injuries is not appropriate here, because of the relative infrequency of these complications in the rehabilitation phase of recovery. The interested reader is referred to an excellent review by Kassell and co-

workers.[70] Briefly, penetrating injuries of the neck obviously call for angiography and surgical exploration if the platysma has been penetrated. Arterial occlusion secondary to blunt neck trauma occurs infrequently, with an estimated incidence of 0.5 percent.[69] The injury is said to occur most commonly at the C2 level, with both the carotid and vertebral arteries.[70] Clinical diagnosis is often difficult and there may be a symptom-free period, usually of less than 24 hours. The patient may experience transient ischemic attacks (TIAs), form a neck hematoma, or develop Horner's syndrome. Once occlusion occurs, a focal neurologic deficit may become apparent. In cases of severe head injury, this may be hard to separate from the effects of the primary brain injury per se. The mortality rate for traumatic carotid thrombosis in the neck has been reported to be between 40 and 90 percent. Vertebral artery occlusions are less frequently documented but have a lower associated mortality—19 percent when one vertebral artery is occluded and 46 percent when both are lost. Anticoagulation may be undertaken in selected cases in which the head injury is mild and the risk of intracranial hemorrhage is low; however, the value of anticoagulation in the treatment of such patients has not been established.

Post-traumatic intracranial aneurysms are very uncommon. ElGindi's study[69] reported only seven cases among 2000 head injury patients. Furthermore, there were only two such aneurysms in more than 3000 penetrating head wounds reported from the Korean and Vietnam wars. Unlike congenital "berry" aneurysms, post-traumatic aneurysms are more likely to occur near the cortical surface and not at major arterial bifurcations. There is often no neck for clipping, but surgical exposure and clipping or wrapping remain the treatment of choice.

Intracranial traumatic AV fistulas are decidedly uncommon. They occur most often between the middle meningeal artery and a meningeal vein. They are usually associated with a penetrating head injury or a depressed skull fracture. The risk of hemorrhage from these lesions is uncertain. They can be treated by embolization via the external carotid artery or by direct surgical excision.

Carotid-cavernous (CC) fistulas are the best recognized of all post-traumatic vascular injuries. Although relatively uncommon, their characteristic features make them a well-recognized clinical entity. Sixty to 80 percent of CC fistulas are traumatic in origin; the rest presumably arise spontaneously. Spontaneous CC fistulas occur more commonly in older women, whereas the traumatic ones are found in young men. The clinical features can include proptosis, chemosis, bruit, ophthalmoplegia, visual deterioration, and headache. A bruit may be palpable and a murmur can be heard with a conventional or Doppler stethoscope. Arteriography is the diagnostic procedure of choice. The natural history of CC fistulas warrants intervention: spontaneous closure is uncommon, and the usual course is one of progressive visual loss (40 to 50 percent will develop blindness), intolerable bruit, or disfiguring proptosis. While various approaches have been used for their treatment, the current treatment of choice is occlusion of the fistula with a detachable balloon, with preservation of blood flow in the carotid artery.[71] When this is not technically possible, various alternative approaches may be used including balloon occlusion of the internal carotid artery,

packing of the posterior cavernous sinus with thrombogenic material or wire, or occlusion of the sinus by packing via the ophthalmic vein.

SUMMARY

Brain trauma may be associated with early or delayed additional insults to the central and peripheral nervous systems. These neurologic sequelae, often inconspicuous or absent in the intensive care setting, may obstruct functional improvement or induce deterioration of neurologic status. Most of the neurologic sequelae, once recognized, are responsive to treatment.

In this chapter, disorders of cranial nerves, brainstem, spinal cord, and the peripheral nervous system are identified, and principles of management outlined. Delayed CNS sequelae—hydrocephalus, epilepsy, and vascular complications—are also reviewed here, with particular emphasis on recent literature on these subjects. (Early CNS complications are considered in Chapter 3.)

REFERENCES

1. Sumner, D: On testing the sense of smell. Lancet 2:107, 1964.
2. Levin, HS, High, WM and Eisenberg, HM: Impairment of olfactory recognition after closed head injury. Brain 108:579, 1985.
3. Jennett, B and Teasdale, G: Management of Head Injuries. FA Davis, Philadelphia, 1981.
4. Brodal, A: Neurological Anatomy in Relation to Clinical Medicine, ed 3. Oxford University Press, New York, 1981.
5. Sumner, D: Post traumatic anosmia. Brain 87:107, 1964.
6. Gjerris, F: Traumatic lesions of the visual pathways. In Vinken, PJ and Bruyn, CW (eds): Handbook of Clinical Neurology. Vol. 24. North Holland Publishing, Amsterdam, 1976, p 27.
7. Kline, LB, Morawetz, RB and Swaid, SW: Indirect injury of the optic nerve. Neurosurgery 14:756, 1984.
8. Crompton, MR: Visual lesions in closed head injury. Brain 93:785, 1970.
9. Edmund, J and Godtfredsen, E: Unilateral optic atrophy following head injury. Acta Ophthalmol 41:693, 1963.
10. Greenberg, RP et al: Evaluation of brain dysfunction in severe head trauma with multimodality evoked potentials: Part II. Localization of brain dysfunction and correlation with post traumatic neurologic conditions. J Neurosurg 47:163, 1977.
11. Berrol, S: Medical Assessment. In Rosenthal, M et al (eds): Rehabilitation of the Head Injured Adult. FA Davis, Philadelphia, 1983, p 233.
12. Gay, AJ et al: Eye Movement Disorders. CV Mosby, St. Louis, 1974.
13. Kushner, BJ: Ocular causes of abnormal head postures. Ophthalmology 86:2115, 1979.
14. Sydhor, CF, Seaber, JH and Buckley, EG: Traumatic superior oblique palsies. Ophthalmology 89:134, 1982.
15. Fells, P and Waddell, E: Assessment and management of bilateral superior oblique pareses. Trans Ophthalmol Soc UK 100:485, 1980.
16. Berrol, S: Medical assessment. In Rosenthal, M et al (eds): Rehabilitation of the Head Injured Adult. FA Davis, Philadelphia, 1983, p 234.
17. Nelson, JR: Neuro-otologic aspects of head injury. In Thompson, RA and Green, JR (eds): Advances in Neurology. Vol 22. Raven Press, New York, 1979, p 107.
18. Sakai, CS and Mateer, CA: Otological and audiological sequelae of closed head trauma. Semin Hear 5:157, 1984.

19. Rappaport, M et al: Evoked brain potentials and disability in brain damaged patients. Arch Phys Med Rehabil 58:333, 1977.
20. DeJong, RN: The Neurologic Examination, ed 4. Harper and Row, Hagerstown, 1979, p 266.
21. Plum, F and Posner, JB: Diagnosis of Stupor and Coma, ed 2. FA Davis, Philadelphia, 1972.
22. Davidoff, G et al: Closed head injury in spinal cord injured patients: Retrospective study of loss of consciousness and post-traumatic amnesia. Arch Phys Med Rehabil 66:41, 1985.
23. Bolton, CF: Electrophysiologic studies of critically ill patients. Muscle Nerve 10(2):129, 1987.
24. Editorial: Preventing secondary brain damage after head injury. Lancet 2:1189, 1978.
25. Jennett, B and Carlin J: Preventable mortality and morbidity after head injury. Injury 10:31, 1979.
26. Miller, JD et al: Early insults to the injured brain. JAMA 240:439, 1978.
27. Clifton, GL et al: Neurologic course and correlated computed tomographic findings after severe closed head injury. J Neurosurg 52:611, 1980.
28. Beyerl, B, Black, P McL: Post-traumatic hydrocephalus. Neurosurgery 15:257, 1984.
29. Kishore, PRS et al: Post-traumatic hydrocephalus in patients with severe head injury. Neuroradiology 16:261, 1978.
30. Cordoso, ER and Galbraith, S: Post-traumatic hydrocephalus—a retrospective review. Surg Neurol 23:261, 1985.
31. Gardeur, D et al: Etude tomodensitometrique des lesions cerebrales post-traumatiques. J Radiol 60:79, 1979.
32. van Dongen, KJ and Braakman, R: Late computed tomography in survivors of severe head injury. Neurosurgery 7:14, 1980.
33. Levin, HS et al: Ventricular enlargement after closed head injury. Arch Neurol 38:623, 1981.
34. Gudeman, SK et al: Computed tomography in the evaluation of incidence and significance of post-trauma hydrocephalus. Radiology 141:397, 1981.
35. French, BN and Dublin, AB: The value of computerized tomography in the management of 1000 consecutive head injuries. Surg Neurol 7:171, 1977.
36. Hawkins, TD et al: Ventricular size following head injury: A clinico-radiological study. Clin Radiol 27:279, 1976.
37. Levine, JE, Povlishock, JT and Becker, DP: The morphological correlates of primate cerebrospinal fluid absorption. Brain Res 241:31, 1982.
38. Zander, E and Foroglou, G: Post-traumatic hydrocephalus. In Vinken, PJ and Bruyn, GW (eds): Handbook of Clinical Neurology. Vol. 24: Injuries of the Brain and Skull. Elsevier, New York, 1976, p 231.
39. Takagi, H et al: Rapid enlargement of ventricles within seven hours after head injury. Surg Neurol 16:103, 1981.
40. Ojemann, RG et al: Further experience with the syndrome of normal pressure hydrocephalus. J Neurosurg 31:279, 1969.
41. Guidetti, B and Gagliardi, FM: Normal pressure hydrocephalus. Acta Neurochir (Wien) 27:1, 1972.
42. Belloni, G et al: Surgical indications in normotensive hydrocephalus: A retrospective analysis of the relations of some diagnostic findings to the results of surgical treatment. Acta Neurochir (Wien) 33:1, 1976.
43. Zimmerman, RD et al: Periventricular hyperintensity as seen by magnetic resonance: Prevalence and significance. AJNR 7:13, 1986.
44. Salmon, JH: Surgical treatment of severe post-traumatic encephalopathy. Surg Gynecol Obstet 133:634, 1971.
45. Stein, SC and Langfitt, TW: Normal pressure hydrocephalus. Predicting the results of cerebrospinal fluid shunting. J Neurosurg 41:463, 1974.
46. Chawla, JC, Hulme, A and Cooper, R: Intracranial pressure in patients with dementia and communicating hydrocephalus. J Neurosurg 40:376, 1974.
47. Borgesen, SE, Gjerris, F and Sorensen, SC: Intracranial pressure and conductance to outflow of CSF in normal pressure hydrocephalus. J Neurosurg 50:489, 1979.
48. Jennett, B: Epilepsy after Non-missile Head Injuries, ed 2. Heinemann, London, 1975.
49. Rappaport, RL and Penry, JK: A survey of attitudes towards the pharmacologic prophylaxis of post-traumatic epilepsy. J Neurosurg 38:159, 1973.
50. Wohns, RW and Wyler, AR: Prophylactic phenytoin in severe head injuries. J Neurosurg 51:507, 1979.
51. Young, B et al: Failure of prophylactically administered phenytoin to prevent late post-traumatic seizures. J Neurosurg 58:236, 1983.
52. Young, B et al: Failure of prophylactically administered phenytoin to prevent post-traumatic seizures in children. Child Brain 10:185, 1983.
53. McQueen, JK et al: Low risk of post-traumatic seizures following severe head injury: Implications for clinical trials of prophylaxis. J Neurol Neurosurg Psychiatry 46:899, 1983.
54. Buchanan, RA et al: The metabolism of diphenylhydantoin following once daily administration. Neurology 26:494, 1976.
55. Andrewes, DG et al: A comparative study of the cognitive effects of phenytoin and carbamazepine in new referrals with epilepsy. Epilepsia 27:128, 1986.
56. Calcaterra, TC: Extracranial surgical repair of cerebrospinal fluid rhinorrhea. Ann Otol 89:108, 1980.
57. Lewin, W: Cerebrospinal fluid rhinorrhea in closed head injuries. Br J Surg 42:1, 1954.
58. Ommaya, AK: Cerebrospinal fluid fistula. In Wilkens, RH and Rengachari, SS (eds): Neurosurgery. McGraw-Hill, New York, 1985, p 1637.
59. MacGee, EE, Cauthen, JC and Brackett, CE: Meningitis following acute traumatic cerebrospinal fluid fistula. J Neurosurg 33:312, 1970.
60. Robinson, RG: Cerebrospinal fluid rhinorrhea, meningitis and pneumocephalus due to non-missile injuries. Aust NZ J Surg 39:328, 1970.
61. Laun, A: Traumatic CSF fistulas in the anterior and middle cranial fossae. Acta Neurochir 60:215, 1982.
62. Park, JI, Strelzow, VV and Friedman, WH: Current management of CSF rhinorrhea. Laryngoscope 93:1294, 1983.
63. Rouah, E, Rogers, BB and Buffone, GJ: Transferrin analysis by immunofixation as an aid in the diagnosis of cerebrospinal fluid otorrhea. Arch Pathol Lab Med 111:756, 1987.
64. Cooper, PR: Skull fracture and traumatic CSF fistulas. In Cooper, PR (ed): Head Injury, ed 2. Williams and Wilkins, Baltimore, 1987, p 87.

65. Ahmadi, J et al: Evaluation of CSF rhinorrhea by metrizamide CT cisternography. Neurosurgery 16: 54, 1985.

66. Naidich, TP and Moran, CJ: Precise anatomic localization of atraumatic sphenoethmoidal CSF rhinorrhea by metrizamide CT cisternography. J Neurosurg 53:222, 1980.

67. Hicks, GW, Wright, JW Jr, and Wright JW III: Cerebrospinal fluid otorrhea. Laryngoscope 90 (Suppl 25):1, 1980.

68. Klastersky, J, Sadeghi, M and Brihaye, J: Antimicrobial prophylaxis in patients with rhinorrhea or otorhea: A double blind study. Surg Neurol 6:111, 1976.

69. El Gindi, S et al: A review of 2000 patients with craniocerebral injuries with regard to intracranial hematomas and other vascular complications. Acta Neurochir 48:237, 1979.

70. Kassell, NF, Boarini, DJ and Adams, HP: Intracranial and cervical vascular injuries. In Cooper, PR (ed): Head Injury, ed 2. Williams and Wilkins, Baltimore, 1987, p 327.

71. Debrun, GM: Treatment of traumatic carotid cavernous fistula using detachable balloon catheters. AJNR 4:355, 1983.

Chapter 9

Medical and Orthopedic Complications Associated with Traumatic Brain Injury

LAWRENCE J. HORN, M.D.
DOUGLAS E. GARLAND, M.D.

During the rehabilitation of the head injured patient, the attention of the clinician is most often drawn toward the behavioral, cognitive, and neuromuscular sequelae of cerebral damage. Survivors of traumatic head injury, however, often suffer from derangements of multiple organ systems. In some cases this is secondary to associated traumatic injuries, in others from iatrogenic effects of treatment or medication, and in still others from uncommon or poorly understood manifestations of central nervous system (CNS) damage. This chapter addresses some medical and orthopedic complications encountered during the rehabilitation of head injured individuals which influence their ultimate medical and functional recovery.

MEDICAL COMPLICATIONS AFTER TRAUMATIC BRAIN INJURY

The head injured person is subject to the same maladies as the general population and the same complications seen in other disabled individuals in the rehabilitation set-ting. Many of the neurologic problems seen after trauma are discussed elsewhere in this text, and many of the special medical problems afflicting the disabled are familiar through detailed discussions in the rehabilitation literature. Therefore, the emphasis of this section is on some of those disorders that pose important or unique problems in the brain injured, with special attention directed to dysfunctions of CNS control over other organ systems. A review outline is included for the interested reader (Table 9–1). As is common for discussions of this type, the text is organized by body system.

The Skin

The head injured patient is prone to a variety of skin problems seen in other rehabilitation patients, such as decubitus ulcers and bacterial or fungal infections of the perineum which may be especially difficult to prevent or treat because of posturing or severe spasticity. Burns, lacerations, and "degloving" injuries may occur as direct results of trauma. Iatrogenic dermatologic conditions are usually secondary to medications,

**Table 9–1. MEDICAL COMPLICATIONS OF BRAIN TRAUMA
ACCORDING TO BODY SYSTEMS**

A. Skin
   1. Pressure sores
   2. Sweat disorders
   3. Drug reactions
   4. Acne
   5. Seborrhea
   6. Infections
   7. Swelling (edema)
   8. Cosmetic deformity
B. Eye
   1. Drying effect secondary to lid paralysis
   2. Infection
   3. Diplopia
   4. Movement disorders
   5. Drug reactions
   6. Injuries
   7. Visual acuity and types of blindness
C. Ear
   1. Infection
   2. Trauma
   3. Drug toxicity
   4. Hearing deficits
D. Nose
   1. Trauma
   2. Infection
   3. Anosmia
E. Throat
   1. Dental-Gingival problems
      a. Fractures
      b. Drug effects
      c. Bruxism
      d. Hygiene
      e. Dental Injuries
   2. Other dental trauma
   3. Oral infections
   4. Dysphagia
F. Larynx
   1. Cord trauma
   2. Cord paralysis
   3. Infection
G. Trachea
   1. Stenosis
   2. Erosion from intubation
   3. Tracheostomy dependence
   4. Skin fistula
   5. Infection
H. Pulmonary
   1. Emboli
   2. Pneumonias
   3. Flail chest and lung trauma
   4. Restrictive defects
   5. Recurrent pneumothoraces
   6. Hyperventilation
   7. Broncho-pleural-cutaneous fistula
   8. Adult respiratory distress syndrome
   9. Fluid overload
I. Gastrointestinal
   1. Trauma
   2. Peptic ulceration and complications

   3. Hepatitis
   4. Drug reactions
   5. Impaction
   6. Delayed emptying
   7. Incontinence
   8. Superior mesenteric artery syndrome
   9. Complications of feeding tubes
   10. Nutrition
   11. Bulimia and hyperphagia
   12. Diarrhea
   13. Infection
   14. Pancreatitis and pancreatic cysts
J. Cardiac
   1. Trauma
   2. Heart failure
   3. Arrhythmias
K. Peripheral Vascular
   1. Thrombophlebitis
   2. Hypotension
   3. Hypertension
   4. Trauma
L. Genitourinary
   1. Catheter complications
   2. Trauma
   3. Incontinence
   4. Sexual dysfunction
   5. Complications of external drainage systems
M. Gynecologic
   1. Infection
   2. Amenorrhea and oligomenorrhea
   3. Trauma
   4. Contraception
N. Metabolic-Endocrine
   1. Hypothalamic-pituitary failure
   2. Renal dysfunction
   3. Electrolyte-fluid disorders
   4. Malignant hyperthermia
O. Blood Disorders
   1. Anemias
   2. Drug toxicities
   3. Clotting defects
   4. Polycythemia
P. Musculoskeletal
   1. Osteoporosis
   2. Drug reactions-weakness
   3. Disuse weakness
   4. Contractures
   5. Heterotopic ossification
   6. Reflex sympathetic dystrophy
   7. Osteomyelitis
   8. Unrecognized fractures, soft-tissue injuries
Q. Central Nervous System
   1. Depressed sensorium
      a. Drug reactions
      b. Metabolic disorders
      c. Infection
      d. Primary brain complications

Table 9–1. *(Continued)*

(1) Recurrent or developing hematoma or hygroma	5. CNS "storm"
(2) Infection	R. Peripheral Nervous System
(3) Seizures	1. Neuropathies
(4) Hydrocephalus	a. Drug reaction
(5) CSF leak	b. Metabolic
(6) New trauma	c. Local injury
(7) Traumatic aneurysm	d. Unrecognized brachial plexopathy
2. Spasticity	S. Miscellaneous
3. Unrecognized spinal cord injury	1. Fever
4. Pain syndromes	2. Drug toxicity

Adapted from Griffith, ER: Management of Medical Problems Associated with Head Trauma in the Rehabilitation Setting. Presented at the 7th annual postgraduate course on The Rehabilitation of the Brain Injured Adult. Medical College of Virginia, Williamsburg, Va, June, 1983.

particularly antibiotics and anticonvulsants. Phenytoin and carbamazepine may produce the potentially fatal Stevens-Johnson syndrome and the clinician should be circumspect about mucosal lesions when the drugs are first instituted. Phenytoin may also produce hirsutism. Phenobarbital has been implicated as a precipitant of reflex sympathetic dystrophy,[1, 2] which is part of the differential diagnosis of extremity swelling.

Two dermatologic conditions that may be linked to CNS injury are acne and hyperhydrosis (profuse sweating). Although acne and head injury are both prevalent among teenagers and young adults, acne may first appear, or be exacerbated, with brain damage. In some cases it may be related to endocrine disturbances with relative overproduction of androgens, or from exogenous steroids. In women, it may be associated with menstrual irregularities, infertility, alopecia, and hirsutism.[3] This constellation of problems has been associated with temporal lobe lesions and epilepsy.[4] Theoretically, brain trauma could cause a disruption of normal gonadotropin pulsatile cycling, which in turn causes greater androgen production by the ovary, leading to a vicious cycle that includes amenorrhea and acne. Treatment of acne may include drying solutions (such as benzoyl peroxide), topical and oral antibiotics, and treatment of any underlying endocrine disturbance. Cyclic spironolactone blocks testosterone as well as aldosterone activity, and may be effective in eliminating the acne and restoring normal menses in women.[3]

Hyperhydrosis and anhydrosis are problems that have received little emphasis in our literature. Localized vasomotor changes may represent peripheral damage to the autonomic, usually sympathetic, nervous system secondary to trauma or reflex sympathetic dystrophy. Anhydrosis is seen in Horner's syndrome along with ipsilateral miosis and ptosis of the eye owing to injury of the cervical sympathetic nervous system. In cases of diffuse hyperhydrosis, more central disturbances of neurohumeral and autonomic function must be considered. With hypothalamic damage, other signs of autonomic dyscontrol or a hyperadrenergic state, such as tachycardia and hypertension will also be present. Flushing and sweating of the face and upper body is frequently seen in the severely injured or vegetative patient[5] and may represent disinhibition of brainstem reflex activity, such as that which mediates gustation sweating.[6] In this clinical setting, one would be obliged to evaluate the patient for occult spinal injury, given the similarity to autonomic dysreflexia. If the hyperhydrosis is secondary to central autonomic dyscontrol, it may resolve spontaneously or in response to beta-blocking medications.

Head and Neck

Trauma to the soft tissues and skeletal structures of the head and neck is common in brain injury. Ocular problems include perforation of the eye, vitreous hemorrhage, retinal detachment, and entrapment of the globe in blow-out fractures of the orbit. Peripheral or nuclear involvement of the seventh cranial nerve may lead to inadequate eyelid closure and subsequent corneal drying, abrasions, and infection. Short-term treatment consists of antibiotic ointments and "artificial tears." When recovery is not anticipated or will be delayed, tarsorraphy is recommended, whereby the outer canthus of the lids are sutured together, while still permitting unobstructed vision. The procedure is reversible.

Dislocation of the ossicles of the ear and fracture of the mandible, facial bones, or larynx require surgical intervention. Cervical strains or sprains are also common and may contribute to posturing and the development of myofascial pain with posterior headache radiating anteriorly. Fortunately, myofascial pain can be treated successfully with modalities or injection of trigger points with local anesthetic.

Iatrogenic problems include the effects of medication, and intubation. Blurred vision, tinnitus, and dizziness with or without true vertigo may be adverse reactions to many medications including anticonvulsants, cimetidine, and nonsteroidal anti-inflammatory agents.

Although subglottic stenosis may occur from direct trauma (dashboard injuries), it is usually due to prolonged or repeated endotracheal intubation, high tracheostomy placement, or tracheotomy carried out under suboptimal conditions. Tracheal stenosis is also caused by placement of endotracheal and tracheostomy tubes, and is seen at the site of the tracheotomy, at the level of the cuff or at the tip of the tube. Neither tracheal nor subglottic stenosis need be immediately symptomatic; either may become manifest weeks or months after extubation with characteristic biphasic stridor and respiratory distress, perhaps precipitated by a simple viral upper respiratory infection. Factors contributing to stenosis include direct pressure at the cuff site by positive pressure ventilation, shearing of the tracheal mucosa by the tube with inspiration and expiration, and infection, which exacerbates scarring and stenosis.[7, 8] The diagnosis can be made with soft tissue radiography or tomography, but endoscopy is the most useful procedure.

TREATMENT OF AIRWAY STENOSIS

Treatment may consist simply of observation in mild cases, especially in children where laryngeal or tracheal growth may solve the problem. Endoscopic laser therapy is a safe means of treating many cases of airway stenosis; more conventional surgical intervention may be necessary when circumferential scarring is greater than 1 cm wide, in the presence of tracheomalacia with loss of cartilage, with severe bacterial infection, or in posterior laryngeal inlet scarring with arytenoid fixation.[7] In severe cases, erosion and tracheoesophageal fistula may occur. High pressures proximal to a stenotic area may preclude decannulation or prevent closure of a tracheotomy site.

Bruxism, the rhythmic grinding of teeth, is present in 5 to 20 percent of the general population,[9, 10] in whom malocclusion, stress, and systemic disorders may be contributing causes. Its occurrence in brain injured patients is qualitatively more severe, and is frequently associated with spasticity of the muscles of mastication. If left untreated, bruxism may lead to widening of periodontal ligaments, increased alveolar bone loss, loose dentition, diffuse bone resorption of the anterior mandible, severe wearing of occlusive surfaces, and infection. Pratap-Chand[10] evaluated 20 patients in coma and noted that bruxism generally occurred as a given patient moved from one "level" of coma (based on Glasgow Coma Scale, or GCS, scores) to another, and disappeared only after significant neurologic improvement. Bruxism was present only in those patients who demonstrated sleep-wake cycles. The etiology for neurogenic bruxism is unclear, though in animal studies stimulation of the jaw region of motor cortex or limbic structures results in teeth gnashing; loss of cortical inhibition may also be important for hypothalamic lesions to cause this symptom. Pharmacologically, dopamine enhances rodent gnawing behavior, and L-dopa and amphetamine ingestions have been known to precipitate bruxism in humans.

TREATMENT OF BRUXISM

Treatment currently consists of maintenance of good oral hygiene. Use of athletic biteguards or custom fabricated splints can help prevent dental destruction, if the patient can be fitted. Theoretically, nerve blocks to the masseters could be done, but these are technically difficult. One could also consider dopamine-depleting agents, such as phenothiazines, but the undesired effects of these medications would probably outweigh their therapeutic utility. Fortunately more than half of brain injury patients with bruxism spontaneously cease tooth grinding.

Cardiovascular and Pulmonary Systems

Traumatic damage to the chest and its contents is present in 10 percent[11] of head injured patients, and up to one third of brain damaged individuals have cardiac or respiratory abnormalities.[12] Iatrogenic problems include arrhythmias which may be caused or aggravated by commonly used drugs such as anticonvulsants, cimetidine, and many major tranquilizers and antidepressants. Cardiac and respiratory complications contribute to morbidity and may further insult the injured brain through the development of hypoxemia.

The characteristic cardiovascular profile of the acutely brain injured patient consists of hypertension, tachycardia, increased cardiac output and work, with a low or normal peripheral vascular resistance.[13] When a patient postures, systolic blood pressure increases out of proportion to diastolic, and oxygen consumption increases, but the arteriovenous oxygen difference is reduced.[13-15] Contributing to this profile is a massive increase in circulating catecholamines, which occurs both as a physiologic response to stress and as a result of cerebral damage and dyscontrol. Under normal conditions limbic structures including the thalamus, septum, amygdala, orbitofrontal cortex, and hypothalamus are involved in regulation of autonomic and cardiopulmonary activity. Brainstem centers include the adrenergic cluster of the locus ceruleus, which ultimately contributes to sympathetic innervation of the heart and lungs,[16] and the dorsal vagal nucleus and nucleus ambiguous, which supply parasympathetic innervation. There is laterality of CNS cardiac regulation, with control of heart rate primarily a right-sided function, though left-sided sympathetic activity is implicated in arrhythmogenesis.[16] Animal experiments indicate that elevated intracranial pressure may increase adrenergic activity and circulating catecholamines, producing pulmonary congestion, edema, hemorrhage, and subendocardial infarction.[17] In cases of isolated head trauma, norepinephrine levels correspond to GCS scores, with levels in

comatose patients seven times those of normals.[18] Although the presence of the catecholamines is arrhythmogenic, cardiac dysrhythmias may also result from stimulation of the orbitofrontal cortex in animal experiments and fatal arrhythmias have been reported in otherwise healthy head injured patients.[19] Up to 90 percent of patients with subarachnoid hemorrhage and hypothalamic lesions develop arrhythmias and myocardial infarction.[20] Nonfatal electrocardiographic abnormalities such as nonspecific ST-T wave changes were seen in 21 percent of head injury patients in a retrospective study.[12] Therefore, brain injury with or without a hyperadrenergic state can produce potentially fatal cardiac dysfunction. Many of these cardiac and pulmonary complications can be ameliorated experimentally and clinically with adrenergic blockade.[13, 17, 19]

Hypertension is a second major cardiovascular sequela of head injury, often seen in conjunction with tachycardia, temperature abnormalities, and hyperhydrosis, implying a central autonomic dyscontrol, perhaps at a hypothalamic level.[18] It may be present in up to 11 percent of head injured patients with no premorbid history of blood pressure problems.[12] Elevations in circulating catecholamines are also implicated in the development of cerebrally mediated hypertension; norepinephrine and dopamine beta-hydroxylase levels were correlated with the degree of hypertension, tachycardia, and temperature elevation in head injured patients.[18] Decreases in cerebral blood flow are a potent stimulus to adrenal medullary release of norepinephrine[5] and elevated intracranial pressures also produce rapid sustained elevation in systemic blood pressure, which may lead to a vicious cycle of raised systemic and intracranial pressures.

In addition to these general effects of brain injury on blood pressure, focal lesions may also result in hypertension, or hypotension. A detailed account of baroreceptor and cerebral systems involved in this control mechanism may be found in a recent study by Sandel and colleagues.[5] Two structures especially vulnerable to traumatic injury are the orbitofrontal cortex, which inhibits sympathetic and promotes vagal activity, and the hypothalamus, which integrates cortical, limbic, and brainstem systems. The anterior hypothalamus normally enhances baroreceptor mediated bradycardia and lowering of blood pressure, while the posterior portion has an inhibitory effect on this system. The fine perforating vessels supplying the hypothalamus from the internal carotid, posterior, and anterior communicating arteries are especially susceptible to distortion in cases of herniation. Infarctions of the hypothalamus are seen in up to 25 percent of the fatally head injured.[21]

Other etiologies for hypertension in head injury must be investigated. These include autonomic dysreflexia from occult spinal cord injury, renal contusion or adrenal hemorrhage, which may be diagnosed by studies of renal function and computed tomography (CT) scan. Pheochromocytoma may also be studied with CT, the clonidine suppression test, in which there will be no decrement in circulating catecholamines in patients with the tumor, or with nuclear medicine studies. Iatrogenic causes include the use of major tranquilizers, phenoxybenzamine, and ephedrine.

TREATMENT OF BRAIN INJURY—
RELATED HYPERTENSION

The treatment of hypertension associated with brain injury is dependent upon blocking the effects of the hyperadrenergic state and sympathetic drive. In comparing the effects of hydralazine and propranolol for this purpose, Robertson[14] noted that hydralazine actually increased cardiac work and tachycardia because of vasodilatation and also contributed to increased intracranial pressure because of dilatation of cerebral capacitance vessels. Propranolol was preferred since in doses of 20 to 40 mg every 6 hours[22] it decreased tachycardia and cardiac index, decreased cardiac work and pulmonary venous admixture, and lowered levels of circulating catecholamines. The actions of propranolol in this situation are complex and are an aggregate of direct cardiac effects, blockage of presynaptic beta receptors in sympathetic ganglia, and possibly direct CNS activity.[14, 22] In patients with bronchospastic disease, a selective beta-1 receptor antagonist may be effective, and safer, for CNS-mediated hypertension.

Gastrointestinal System and Nutrition

Concurrent trauma to the liver or bowel occurs in 11 percent of brain injured pa-

tients.[11] The most commonly recognized gastrointestinal disorder in the rehabilitation setting is elevation of serum liver enzymes, present in up to 43 percent of patients.[12] Although trauma itself can cause this abnormality, several other etiologies merit investigation. A premorbid history of drug or alcohol abuse or of transfusions is important, and evaluation for infectious hepatitis is mandatory. Iatrogenic causes are more common, usually from medications or sometimes from the type of tubefeeding. Many drugs may elevate results of liver function tests, especially anticonvulsants and antispasticity agents. Carbamazepine and phenytoin have been associated with fulminant chemical hepatitis, but more commonly anticonvulsants produce a benign induction of microsomal enzymes and hepatocellular hypertrophy.[23] Hypersensitivity reactions generally occur in the setting of fever, rash, lymphadenopathy, hepatosplenomegaly, and eosinophilia within the first month of therapy. Evaluation consists of hepatitis screens and monitoring of the serum liver enzymes, bilirubin, albumin, and prothrombin time. In most patients with drug-induced changes, elevations of serum enzymes are modest and transient. Liver biopsy may be necessary to help diagnose the etiology and severity of persistent or marked abnormalities.

Another "iatrogenic" problem encountered in the head injured patient is the failure to recognize their extensive nutritional needs. Upon presentation to rehabilitation, the average weight loss is 29 pounds, with patients only approaching 85 percent of their ideal body weight; 31 percent have protein malnutrition on the basis of low serum albumin.[24] In acute settings, daily caloric requirements may approach 4500 kcal in decerebrating patients,[25] the mean being approximately 2400 kcal. Mean resting metabolic expenditure is 140 percent above normal, with 22 percent of caloric requirements being protein.[26] Simultaneous injury to long bones and other organs, or the presence of burns or fever, can further increase nutritional demand. Complications of malnutrition include poor wound healing and decreased resistance to infection; poor nutrition has also been implicated in the development of decubitus ulcers and gastrointestinal atrophy. Another potential problem is that total blood levels of protein-bound medications such as diphenylhydantoin may be misinterpreted as low in the presence of hypoalbuminemia, even though unbound levels are therapeutic.[27] Malnutrition contributes to morbidity and mortality in head injury[25] and even with the cost of enteral and parenteral administration, nutritional support is cost effective, especially in this era of diagnosis related groups (DRGs).[28]

There are several etiologies of this high nutritional demand in patients with head injury. Trauma results in a stress challenge with release of catecholamines and cortisol, which promote gluconeogenesis, protein catabolism, glycogenolysis, and inhibition of insulin release. Exogenous steroids probably only play a role during the first 24 to 48 hours after injury.[29] Even with immediate nutritional support, protein loss and relative malnutrition may not stabilize for several weeks,[26] although patients with head injury alone fare better in this regard than do those with multisystem injuries.[30]

Assessment of a patient's nutritional status relies on laboratory and anthropomorphic measurements. Body weight of less than 90 percent of ideal, serum albumin less than 3.5 g/dl, total lymphocyte count less than 1500/mm^3, and total protein of less than 5.4 mg/dl are all indicative of malnutrition. Anthropomorphic measurements such as triceps skinfold thickness and mid-arm circumference are useful clinical assessments. These may be supplemented by measurement of BUN, hemoglobin and transferrin levels, creatinine/height index, and total urinary nitrogen loss.

The need for nutritional support is clear, though there remains some debate as to the optimal route of its administration. Even in acute care settings there is a trend toward the axiom "if the gut works, use it," assuming at least 60 cm of functioning gastrointestinal tract. Parenteral alimentation has not proven particularly more effective than its enteral counterpart in the majority of patients, is clearly more expensive, and is probably less safe. Risks include sepsis, venous thrombosis, and a greater chance of fatty liver and hyperglycemia.[31] The enteral route is also more physiologic and may help maintain the structural integrity of the gut.[32]

There are a variety of mechanisms for providing enteral feedings. In acute, or short-term, situations (less than 2 weeks) a nasogastric tube may be used. In chronic situations it may be an irritant, contributing to agitation, increased spasticity and posturing, nasopharyngeal erosion, and gastric reflux with risk of aspiration. Nasogastric tube placement may not be possible in patients with severe respiratory failure, facial trauma, laryngotracheomalacia, or esophageal disorders. The other routes of enteral feeding are gastrostomy or jejunostomy tube placement.

The risks of surgical tube placement include wound infection, peritoneal abscess, gastric dilatation, ileus, obstruction, and hemorrhage. Jejunostomy has the benefit of a reduced risk of aspiration if recurrent gastroesophageal reflux is a problem. However, of necessity the tubes used are usually smaller in diameter than gastrostomy tubes and may clog easily with feedings or medications. For practical reasons, in the absence of documented reflux, a gastrostomy tube is preferred. A nonoperative technique for gastrostomy tube placement has been developed using endoscopy. This percutaneous approach has the advantage of lower cost, morbidity, and mortality than traditional operative placement.[33] Unfortunately, the lumens of percutaneous endoscopic gastrostomy (PEG) tubes are often small, leading to the same practical problems as those for jejunostomy.

Perhaps the most prevalent problem encountered from tube feeding is diarrhea. To control it, the type of feeding may be changed, with the simple addition of fiber often helping the problem. Administration of Lomotil syrup 10 ml/l, tincture of opium 5 drops/l, paregoric, or Kaopectate may prove useful. Morphine should be avoided because of gastric distention, and abdominal girth should be monitored carefully. In some situations, continuous feedings may eliminate diarrhea; cyclic feedings, however, are more physiologic and should be the goal. Bolus feeding is more practical, and is associated with increased visceral protein when used chronically.[31] Other etiologies for diarrhea should be investigated, including medications or infection. Stool should be cultured for *Clostridia difficile* or examined for its toxin; if present, oral vancomycin or metronidazole should be administered. Occasionally poor gastric emptying may be a problem, which, in the absence of obstruction, may be treated with metoclopramide.

Finally, the types of feedings available merit some consideration. In acute settings when fluid balance is of significant concern, one should attempt to maximize caloric intake per total volume. Tube feedings vary from 1 to 2 kcal/ml, so it is possible to virtually halve the total volume. With pancreatic or hepatic disease, fat content should be minimized, and a feeding such as Vivonex used. Elemental diets will also have less of a tendency to clog small bore tubes. In patients with pulmonary insufficiency, or who are using ventilators, the fat/carbohydrate calorie ratio becomes important as higher carbohydrate feedings may elevate V_{CO_2}. In this situation, the fat/carbohydrate ratio should be 50/50 to 70/30. Expensive solutions of high concentrations of branched-chain amino acids may be helpful in highly stressed or septic patients. In the rehabilitation setting, most standard feedings will be adequate; indeed some industrious families simply liquefy the family fare for tube feeding, resulting in tremendous cost savings.

HYPERPHAGIA

An interesting potential consequence of traumatic brain injury is the disorder of hyperphagia. Certain patients develop disinhibition of oral exploratory behaviors, putting virtually anything in their mouths, much like the experimental primates with Klüver-Bucy syndrome. Another group of patients, however, demonstrate severe, almost pressured overeating, generally confining themselves to highly palatable foodstuffs rather than the host of inanimate (and sometimes animate) objects sought by the preceding group.

The control of appetite and feeding behavior is a complex process dependent upon neurochemical and endocrine activity integrated in the hypothalamus. Afferent stimuli include those from peripheral aesthetic perceptions and from gastrointestinal, hepatic, and adipose systems. Experimental studies indicate that lesions of the ventromedial hypothalamus or nearby ascending serotonin, norepinephrine, and dopamine tracts result in hyperphagia.[34, 35] Conversely lesions of the lateral hypothalamus may lead to aphagia, which may be overcome with amphetamines, increased sensory stimulation, or presentation of highly palatable food. Bulimia from CNS lesions has been reported in trauma,[34] focal damage of the cingulum,[36] medial hypothalamus,[37] and elevated intracranial pressure.[34, 38] Associated problems may include neuroendocrine disorders and hypogonadism.[39] In animals a behavioral pattern is seen in conjunction with ventromedial hypothalamic lesions and hyperphagia: appetite is finicky, and there is decreased spontaneous activity and heightened aggressiveness.[34] Once a new adipose "setpoint" is reached, the hyperphagia ceases. Hyperinsulinemia, which precedes obesity, occurs with the hypothalamic lesions. Theoretically, ventromedial damage causes release of vagal activity and increased insulin production in response to food in the gut as well as in the basal state, leading to increased nutrient utilization and increased food-seeking behavior to prevent hypoglycemia. If hypoglycemia is controlled, or bilateral vagotomy performed, then hyperphagia can be prevented experimentally.[34]

From a neurochemical perspective, several systems participate in hypothalamic integration of feeding behavior. Endogenous opioids,[40] dopamine, and alpha-adrenergic substances promote feeding, whereas serotonin,[40, 41] beta-adrenergic agonists, and other neuropeptides (corticotropin-releasing factor, calcitonin) have been implicated in producing satiety. Theoretically, these systems could be manipulated therapeutically. Although human studies have yielded mixed results,[39] successful treatment of head injury–related hyperphagia has been reported with naltrexone,[42] an opiate antagonist. Chronic administration of opiate antagonists may not alter total caloric consumption but rather shift food preferences to fat from carbohydrates.[41] A diet high in carbohydrate and tryptophan content has also been suggested as a treatment possibility,[34, 35] as has dopamine blockade alone or with opiate antagonists.[41]

Metabolic Complications After Traumatic Brain Injury

ANTERIOR PITUITARY AND HYPOTHALAMUS

In a retrospective study,[12] only 4 percent of head injured patients were noted to have endocrine disturbances. Apparently these patients were identified because of some overt clinical symptomatology, which is characteristic of the bulk of the literature on traumatic anterior pituitary disorders.[43-46]

The diagnosis of hypothalamic or pituitary endocrinopathy in these case reports is not made until months or years after injury, raising the possibility that anterior pituitary dysfunction is an underdiagnosed phenomenon. Pathologic studies demonstrate hypothalamic or anterior pituitary lesions in 40 to 63 percent of cases of fatal head injury.[21, 47, 48] The Magee Rehabilitation Hospital pilot study[49] indicates that up to 30 percent of head injured patients experience at least transient disturbances of neuroendocrine control. Patients with these abnormalities often have associated histories of autonomic dyscontrol and facial fractures. While this work is preliminary, the apparent incidence of these disorders, coupled with their wide-ranging effects upon cognition, behavior, sexual, and general physiologic function appears to warrant at least prospective screening evaluations.

The anterior pituitary is anatomically distinct from the posterior gland and has its own blood supply largely from portal vessels descending from the median eminence along the pituitary stalk. The anterior pituitary releases hormones that influence thyroid, adrenal, and gonadal function as well as milk production by the breast (prolactin) and somatic growth (growth hormone). The anterior pituitary is regulated by the hypothalamus through its secretion of releasing and inhibiting hormones into the portal circulation. In addition to its control over the pituitary, the hypothalamus also regulates other secretory organs via the autonomic nervous system, such as the parathyroid, kidney, adrenal medulla, and pancreatic insulin and glucagon secretion. Hypothalamic endocrine activity is in turn affected by limbic and brainstem neurochemical systems. Damage to extrahypothalamic sites is implicated in post-traumatic dysinhibition of the gonadal axis, which results in precocious puberty.[46, 50] Endocrine and sexual dysfunction is also seen in a high percentage of patients with temporal lobe epilepsy, the type of disorder being related to the side and site of the epileptic focus.[4] Thus, endocrine disturbances may result from damage to multiple areas of the CNS, many of which are extrinsic to the hypothalamic nuclei and pituitary.

In pathologic studies,[21, 48] most injuries to the hypothalamus and pituitary were related to the relative immobility of the gland within the sella in relation to the rest of the brain, and its blood supply. Subarachnoid hemorrhage seeps beneath the dural covering and may produce pressure on the anterior gland. Microhemorrhages into the hypothalamus were believed secondary to shearing forces, and elevated intracranial pressure may have contributed to necrotic lesions. Infarction in the anterior pituitary was felt to be related to ischemia from vasospasm, often caused by systemic hypotension. Fracture of the sella was sometimes associated with hypothalamic and pituitary injury, and may result from extension of basilar or facial skull fractures.

Signs and symptoms of anterior pituitary dysfunction relate to the multiple target organs involved, but is often insidious. Hyperprolactinemia from loss of hypothalamic dopamine inhibition may produce gynecomastia, galactorrhea, impotence, and anovulation. Growth hormone deficiency is occult in adults, but may have dramatic effects on growth in children. ACTH deficiency is seldom life threatening, but may become manifest during stress, producing fatigue, fever, hypotension, and mental aberrations. Thyroid-stimulating hormone (TSH) deficiency, with resultant hypothyroidism, can result in mental dullness, cold intolerance, and anemia. Lack of gonadotropins will impair libido, potency, and gametogenesis with amenorrhea in females. Failure to achieve puberty may also occur.

The prospective evaluation of hypothalamic-anterior pituitary dysfunction begins with simple serum screening tests; RT_3U, T_3RIA, T_4RIA, Free T_4 index, TSH, testosterone, luteinizing hormone (LH), FSH, estradiol, DHEA (the latter two in women with amenorrhea), fasting prolactin, and A.M. and P.M. cortisol levels. If abnormalities occur, then an endocrinologist should be consulted and provocative testing undertaken.

There are numerous pitfalls in the endocrine evaluation. Obesity impairs normal growth hormone responses to provocative tests, as does diabetes. Uremia produces elevations in most pituitary hormones. Starvation elevates basal growth hormone and cortisol levels while depressing gonadal steroids. Medications also significantly interfere; exogenous steroids impair growth hormone, TSH, and LH responses to provocative testing. Anticonvulsants depress cortisol, thyroid, and gonadal hormone levels, secondary to induction of their hepatic metabolism or greater production of binding proteins. Major tranquilizers, narcotics, cimetidine, and chest wall lesions may increase serum prolactin levels.

Treatment of Traumatic Hypothalamic-Anterior Pituitary Dysfunction. Treatment of central endocrine disorders relies upon replacement of target gland hormones. Thyroid replacement should not be undertaken unless any adrenal insufficiency is treated first to avoid precipitating adrenal crisis. Amenorrhea may be effectively treated with cyclic estrogens and progesterone, but ovulation in some cases may require induction with clomiphene or other agents. In treating male gonadal dysfunction, oral testosterone preparations should be avoided as they cause severe liver disease. Elevated prolactin levels with galactorrhea or gynecomastia may be treated with bromocriptine, a dopamine agonist. Growth hormone replacement is limited to children, since its principal supply is currently from cadavers.

Prospective anterior pituitary endocrine evaluations are recommended:

1. In amenorrhea
2. For symptoms or signs of endocrine dysfunction
3. In cases of poor improvement or regression, and in all cases of severe disability in head injury
4. With a history of diabetes insipidus (DI) or syndrome of inappropriate ADH (SIADH) (see below)
5. In cases of documented basilar skull or facial fractures
6. When severe hypotension or shock is documented in the patient's history

POSTERIOR PITUITARY

Unlike anterior pituitary disorders, abnormalities in the secretion of the posterior pituitary hormone vasopressin (antidiuretic hormone, ADH) is well recognized in trauma. ADH is normally released in response to cellular dehydration from hyperosmolality of serum, in response to hemorrhage, and as part of the baroreceptor reflex in blood pressure control. When present, it acts on the kidney to increase water resorption, decreasing urine flow and increasing urine osmolality. It is estimated that 1 in 200 head injured patients have DI from lack

of vasopressin and that 30 percent of all neurosurgical patients have SIADH.[51] Onset of either disorder may be a few hours to several months after injury. The mechanism for DI appears to be a stretch or shearing injury to the posterior pituitary stalk. This disorder is transient in two thirds of patients,[52] perhaps because of regenerative sprouting or from systemic release of the hormone from a short vasopressin fiber tract to the median eminence. The mechanism for SIADH is less clear, but may represent distortion of afferent osmolar and baroreceptor stimuli or extrahypothalamic dysinhibition.

Symptoms and signs of DI include polydipsia and polyuria with normal or high serum osmolality, possible hypernatremia, and low urine osmolality. DI is often seen in conjunction with severe facial trauma but also in postconcussive states.[53] Cranial nerve disorders, especially involving the first, third, fourth, and eighth nerves are present in 40 to 65 percent of cases of DI.[53] Concurrent anterior pituitary dysfunction may also occur.[54] SIADH is associated with nausea, lethargy, seizures, and hyponatremia (less than 135 mEq/l), hypo-osmolality of serum, and concentrated urine.

The evaluation of ADH disorders relies upon plotting simultaneously obtained urine and serum osmolalities on a graph.[55] Patients with partial DI can be identified by plotting their urine and serum osmolalities after water deprivation, in which case they will show some ability to concentrate their urine. Pitfalls in this evaluation include hypothyroidism and hypoadrenalism, which mask DI. Uremia, hyperglycemia, alcohol, and radiographic contrast material all invalidate the serum/urine graph due to their hyperosmolar load. Dilantin and chlorpromazine inhibit the release of ADH, and lithium may block its action on the kidney. The use of carbamazepine, major tranquilizers, and antidepressants may produce SIADH.

Treatment of Hypothalamic-Posterior Pituitary Dysfunction. Treatment of partial ADH deficiency includes the use of chlorpropamide and clofibrate, which have a central action to increase ADH release. Hydrochlorthiazide has been used for its paradoxic effect of producing a negative salt balance with decreased fluid delivery to the distal tubule. In complete deficiency, acute fluid replacement is necessary. Subsequently, desmo-vasopressin acetate (DDAVP) via nasal insufflation every 12 hours is the optimal treatment. When cognitive or behavioral problems preclude the nasal route, intramuscular (IM) preparations may be used, but their absorption may be erratic.

Treatment of SIADH includes fluid restriction and diuretics (furosemide). Democlocycline has been used for its renal effect; unfortunately, however, it is also potentially nephrotoxic and close monitoring of renal function is recommended.[51]

ORTHOPEDIC COMPLICATIONS AFTER TRAUMATIC BRAIN INJURY

Orthopedic complications associated with traumatic head injury can be divided into three broad categories: those related to skeletal fractures and extremity injuries occurring at the time of trauma or iatrogenically, those related to heterotopic ossification, and those secondary to residual limb deformities. The latter two categories may be considered to be direct or indirect effects of cerebral injury on the musculoskeletal system. These three areas will be discussed in terms of general treatment principles so that members of the rehabilitation team may understand orthopedic concepts, assist in monitoring the patient's progress, and aid the physician in treatment decisions.

Fracture Care

Fracture care differs in many aspects from that of the general population.[56] Agitation and poor patient compliance may preclude the use of, and spasticity may cause angular and shortening deformities within, commonly used external fixation devices.[57] Traumatic heterotopic ossification may result from the initial injury or as a result of surgery for fracture reduction and fixation.[58–60]

UNRECOGNIZED INJURY

Musculoskeletal Injury. One of the most common causes of poor fracture outcome is in a sense iatrogenic—the failure to diagnose the injury. Two separate reviews have demonstrated that approximately 10 percent of patients coming to rehabilitation have unrecognized musculoskeletal inju-

ries.[56, 61] Spinal injuries should always be suspected in patients with traumatic brain injury, and cervical spine radiography should be routine during the initial evaluation. If diplegia is present, thoracic and lumbar spine radiographs should be obtained, since this neurologic sequel is extremely rare in the head injured adult. Since approximately 50 percent of upper extremity injuries occur about the shoulder girdle,[56] many injuries can be detected on routine chest radiographs, if anticipated (Fig. 9–1).

Initial radiography of the pelvis should be a relatively routine procedure.[56] Physical examination of the pelvis and hip are obscured by soft tissues, making fracture detection difficult in the comatose patient. The early diagnosis of pelvic injuries is important at the time of injury due to potential bleeding diathesis. Hip injuries require early diagnosis for appropriate treatment to ensure joint mobility. If the patient is a pedestrian victim of an automobile accident, pelvic and knee injuries should be suspected.[62]

PERIPHERAL NERVE INJURIES

Peripheral nerve injuries are frequently undetected because their diagnosis in the comatose patient is difficult, especially when they are not suspected. They may happen acutely at the time of trauma, may occur during fracture treatment, or may be delayed in onset for a variety of reasons.[61] The following are examples of how the diagnosis may be reached through early suspicion of the circumstances of the injury. Acute peroneal neuropathy should be suspected in association with a dislocated knee. When the patient thrown from a motorcycle strikes the ground, the head and shoulder may be driven in opposite directions, often causing brachial plexus palsy. The patient with a flail upper extremity—especially the motorcycle rider—has a brachial plexus injury until proven otherwise. Radial nerve injury should always be suspected in patients with humeral fractures.

Nerve palsies may also be iatrogenic and occur during fracture treatment. The agitated patient in tibial pin traction for a fractured femur may injure his or her peroneal nerve on the leg suspension apparatus, or the patient with a snug long-leg plaster cast for a tibial fracture may develop a pressure paralysis of the peroneal nerve.[63] The me-

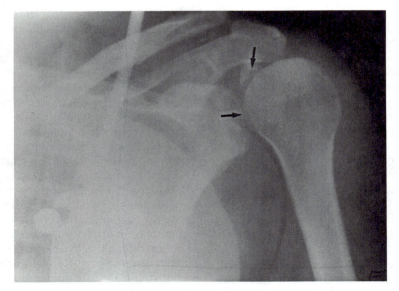

Figure 9–1. A shoulder radiograph during rehabilitation. The patient fell out of a window. On transfer for rehabilitation it was noted that external rotation of the shoulder was limited. Because spasticity of the internal rotation musculature about the shoulder is common after head injury, no other causes for this problem were sought. The radiograph demonstrates a small chip fracture in the shoulder joint and a posterior dislocation of the shoulder. The abnormality was noted on retrospect on the admission chest radiograph.

dian and ulnar nerves may be compromised from swelling while in a cast for a distal radius fracture. Late neuropathies, especially sciatic or peroneal and ulnar, may be caused by direct pressure from traumatic heterotopic ossification about the injured joint.[58]

Consequently, peripheral neuropathies must be anticipated during the entire course of rehabilitation. For example, peroneal palsy with resultant footdrop may result from a variety of causes: acute trauma with hip or knee dislocation, improper cast application for a tibial fracture or skeletal traction for a femoral fracture, or heterotopic ossification posteriorly at the hip or laterally at the knee. The diagnosis of a nerve injury will not be made without an index of suspicion and is best detected by the caregivers who see the patient daily.

TREATMENT

At times, patients are in extremis, and even though a fracture is diagnosed no treatment is initiated or is delayed. Many patients die during the first few days after a severe head injury, and another group of patients are so medically unstable their chance of survival is minimal or would be severely compromised by a major orthopedic surgi-

cal procedure. Orthopedic care is not indicated in these groups. However, most patients who have survived their head injury for 2 to 4 weeks have a good prognosis for survival and orthopedic care should proceed.[64] It is sometimes assumed that a deformity may be relatively meaningless in the neurologically handicapped. However, the contrary is frequently true because the handicapped patient with ambulatory potential may be rendered nonambulatory as the result of angular deformities or shortening of the limb (Fig. 9–2).

Recommended Treatment. In head injury patients, fracture care—and occasionally the fracture healing response—differs from that of the general population. Coma, agitation, and spasticity dictate certain treatment principles. Prolonged skeletal or skin traction have almost no role in fracture care. As a general rule, open reduction and internal fixation is the preferred treatment for long-bone fractures whenever possible (see Fig. 9–2).

Open reduction and internal fixation of hip and elbow fractures is preferred also, whenever possible, to allow early range of motion, which may be compromised by spasticity and also by the occurrence of traumatic heterotopic ossification.[58, 60] Like-

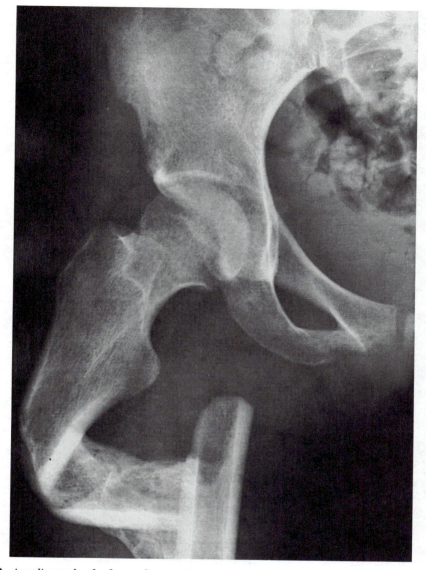

Figure 9–2. A radiograph of a femur fracture in a young patient. Because of medical instability, traction was occasionally employed as well as some splinting of the fracture. The fracture united in malposition. Six months after injury, rehabilitation was instituted. When it was deemed that ambulation was possible, open reduction and internal fixation of the fracture was performed. Limb alignment was achieved at the expense of a 1.5-inch shortening.

wise, forearm fractures have a better outcome if treated with open reduction and internal fixation.[59] Femur fractures are best treated by open reduction and internal fixation to allow knee motion and to prevent angular deformities and shortening which are caused by spasticity.[57]

COMPLICATIONS OF FRACTURES AND FRACTURE CARE

Nerve palsies, discussed earlier, require a circumspect clinician during fracture treatment. An occurrence that is uncommon in the general population, but rather commonplace in the head injured, is traumatic heterotopic ossification (HO). It may occur as a result of the initial injury or as a consequence of surgery. Traumatic HO occurs most commonly with injuries to the elbow and hip.[59, 60] Almost every elbow fracture or dislocation will develop some HO (Fig. 9–3). Hip injuries also tend to develop HO although not at the rate of injuries to the elbow.[60] Less commonly, traumatic HO may

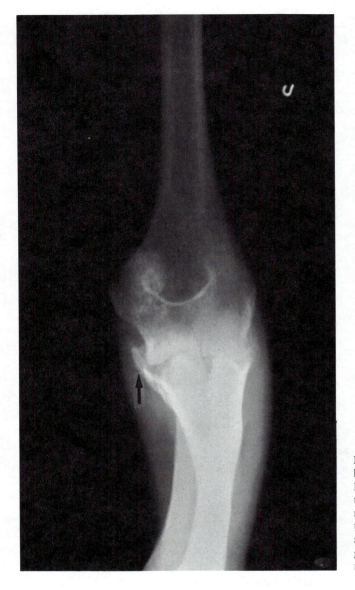

Figure 9–3. A radiograph of the elbow. The elbow has been reduced. Heterotopic ossification is forming in the vicinity of the ulnar collateral ligament. Heterotopic bone in this location elicits pain and limits motion. It also may cause swelling in the ulnar groove and be the source of tardy ulnar palsy.

occur at the shoulder and knee. The exaggerated healing response in some fractures may actually represent an iatrogenic form of HO.[57] This is noted as an increased incidence of cross-unions of operated forearm fractures and an increased incidence of HO in the operated pelvic and hip fracture.[59, 60]

Other Extremity Injuries

Extremity injuries other than fractures and dislocations are uncommon and, except for amputations, only slightly modify the rehabilitation approach. Compartment syndromes are most often the result of tibia fractures. Because the majority of this population's injuries result from high-energy accidents, the short tissues including the compartments are ruptured. Consequently, the closed compartment is unusual, as is the subsequent compartment syndrome. This is verified by the fact that more than 50 percent of tibial fractures are open.[63] A sensory deficit is the most reliable early finding of compartment syndrome followed by muscle weakness, but because many of these patients are comatose, the wick or slit catheter technique should be employed to measure pressures whenever suspicion of a compartment syndrome arises.

High-energy accidents usually cause third-degree strains of the soft tissues. Treatment is aimed at minimizing further damage to the limb and ligament. Generally, third-degree strains are treated by surgery or plaster casts. Because patients are medically and neurologically unstable, the majority of strains are treated by plaster splints. Neck strains are treated by hard or soft cervical collars. The acromioclavicular strain is treated with a sling. Reconstructive surgery is performed at a later date if the deformity is cosmetically deforming. Knee sprains are treated with splints. If an unstable knee results, reconstructive surgery will render a knee functional in the neurologically improving patient.

Joint dislocations, except for that of the hip, rarely go unrecognized owing to the obvious deformity. The most important dislocations include the glenohumeral joint, the acromioclavicular joint, the elbow joint, and the small joints of the hand. The majority are treated by plaster splints. Dislocation of the knee is associated with a 30 percent incidence of popliteal artery damage. After reduction, pulses are checked by digital examination, Doppler, and arteriography, if necessary. The knee is treated with a posterior plaster splint or knee immobilizer. The shoulder joint dislocation is common and responds to closed reduction and sling immobilization. Nerve injuries associated with shoulder dislocations are uncommon but should be sought with electromyography and nerve conduction studies in the comatose patient. The most frequent damage is to the axillary nerve.

Traumatic amputations are uncommon, and upper extremity amputations are extremely rare in this population. In the below-knee amputation, the level of amputation is usually dictated by the level of injury. Currently, any level of amputation can be fitted with an adequate prosthesis. The ideal tibial stump is 5 to 7 inches long, depending on the length of the tibia and the height of the patient. We prefer plaster cast encasement after surgery. Circular plaster protects the incision site, controls swelling, and prevents the undesirable knee flexion contracture should hamstring spasticity develop. The plaster shell is inexpensive and may be changed as often as necessary. A pylon is eventually added when gait training is initiated. The intermediate prosthesis, a pa-tellar tendon bearing (PTB) socket of fiberglass and pylon, is ordered when limb control is present with no hamstring spasticity. The definitive prosthesis is fit when limb swelling has subsided and the patient is ambulating with no difficulty in the temporary prosthesis. This may not occur until after the patient has been discharged from the rehabilitation unit.

Significant vascular injury to arteries of the leg are not common in the head injured patient. The amputation rate is directly proportional to the amount of time from the injury to an artery until that artery is repaired and blood flow is restored. A check must be made for the five P's: pulselessness, pain, paralysis, pallor, and paresthesia. All of these signs may be absent in the normal population with arterial damage and are even more difficult to assess in the head injured. Arterial spasm is so rare that it should not be considered a primary diagnosis. When signs of arterial injury are indefinite, arteriography is necessary. Once the diagnosis of vascular trauma is made, there should be no delay in moving the patient to the operating room.

Reflex sympathetic dystrophy (RSD) is a pain syndrome having varied characteristics. Signs and symptoms include severe pain out of proportion to injury, vasomotor instability, sweat disturbance, osteoporosis, and atrophy of muscles. RSD is associated with CNS injury, in which case it most commonly affects an upper extremity, but it also occurs with crush injuries to the leg, fingers, and hand or wrist; with peripheral nerve damage it may be referred to as causalgia. There are three stages of RSD. The first lasts several days to weeks and is characterized by increased superficial blood flow, erythema, warmth, edema, pain aggravated by motion, and early osteoporosis. The second phase, starting about 3 months after injury, is characterized by cool, pale skin, loss of hair, brawny edema, and limitation of joint motion. The third stage heralds intractable pain, rigid joints, skin and soft tissue atrophy, and severe osteoporosis. Prevention and treatment are most effective before 3 months. Treatment modalities include splinting, range of motion exercises, edema control through elevation and garments. A short course of high-dose oral steroids such as prednisone may be extremely helpful. Analgesics, psychotropic medication, and transcutaneous electrical nerve stimulation (TENS) units are all adjunctive modalities. Stellate ganglion blocks and occasionally dorsal sympathectomies are necessary in more refractory cases.

Heterotopic Ossification (HO)

Although the etiology of heterotopic ossification is unknown, there appears to be a relatively high prevalence in the head and spinal cord injured population suggesting a direct or indirect neurogenic cause. A genetic predisposition is also suspected. The human leukocyte antigen (HLA) system has been employed in an attempt to identify patients with a predisposition to HO formation.[65-68] Our study of 30 patients with known HO failed to demonstrate any relationship between HO and a specific HLA antigen at 68 different loci.[69]

INCIDENCE AND LOCATION

The incidence of HO varies from 11 to 75 percent, depending on the type of patients reviewed, the center involved, and whether routine skeletal surveys are performed.[70-74] Heterotopic ossification is most commonly identified 2 to 4 months after injury, with decreasing joint motion, increasing limb pain, spasticity, and swelling being the earliest signs and symptoms. Alkaline phosphatase is usually elevated, but this is not specific to HO and may be seen with liver disease and fractures. Triple-phase bone scan, if available, often confirms the diagnosis in its early stages before radiographic changes are evident.

The most common locations in brain injured patients are the shoulder, elbow, and hip, less commonly occurring at the thigh and knee. The shoulder and elbow lesions occur with similar frequency and each equals the frequency of lower extremity involvement. Heterotopic ossification occurs inferomedial to the shoulder joint, and may form anteriorly or posteriorly at the elbow (Figs. 9–3 and 9–4). Three sites of HO are noted at the hip: inferomedial, anterolateral, and posterior.[70]

TREATMENT

Treatment of HO consists of standard therapy techniques—diphosphonates, forceful joint manipulation, and surgical resection. The efficacy of diphosphonates in decreasing or preventing the occurrence and amount of HO is not known, although a recent report advocates its efficacy.[74] Diphosphonate dosage and treatment duration has been extrapolated from spinal cord injury experience.[75, 76] The consensus of opinion is that, once early diagnosis is made, most patients should be treated for 6 months at 20

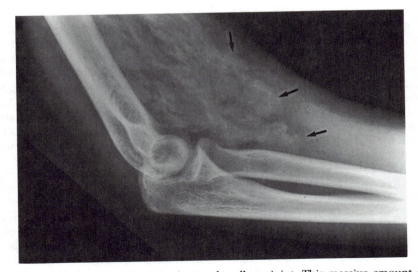

Figure 9–4. Heterotopic ossification anterior to the elbow joint. This massive amount of bone will surely produce ankylosis. If neurologic recovery occurs, resection of the bone will permit functional elbow use.

mg/kg in a single daily oral dose on an empty stomach. Diarrhea is the most common side effect but rarely mandates cessation of therapy.

Forceful joint manipulation under anesthesia is a controversial treatment modality. Some authors maintain that manipulation increases the amount of HO. Our experience indicates that manipulation does not enhance the process. Manipulation also permits differentiation of spasticity from ankylosis, positioning of a contracted limb, and maintenance or increases in joint mobility.[77]

Surgical excision of HO is not recommended less than 1½ years after injury.[78] By this time most motor recovery has occurred, an important factor in maintaining joint mobility after surgery. Although many authors feel that normal bone scans and alkaline phosphatase levels are associated with a low recurrence rate, the patient's final neurologic state may be the most important indicator of recurrence.[78] A patient with good neurologic recovery and minimal spasticity at the affected joint 1½ years after surgery will most likely gain more motion and have minimal or no recurrence when compared with the more severely neurologically compromised patient. In the minimally neurologically involved patient, good surgical outcomes can be expected regardless of the joint or the sector of the joint involved (i.e., anterior or posterior HO). In the absence of spasticity, early resection may also be successful, although many orthopedists use postoperative radiation therapy to prevent recurrence.

Residual Limb Deformity

Residual limb deformities secondary to spasticity may also be considered an indirect effect of cerebral damage on the musculoskeletal system.[79] Correction of these deformities may be safely undertaken no less than 1½ years after injury since the majority of motor recovery has taken place.[56] Surgical procedures in both the upper and lower extremities are divided into nonfunctional and functional categories.

NONFUNCTIONAL PROCEDURES

In both the upper and the lower extremities, nonfunctional procedures involve neurectomies and release of contractures in the low-level patient. The main goals of surgery are in limb placement and positioning, hygiene, and pain relief. An adducted, internally rotated shoulder may cause pain or hygiene problems. Release of shoulder internal rotator muscles followed by vigorous range-of-motion (ROM) exercises corrects the deformity. Persistent elbow spasticity is best managed by musculocutaneous neurectomy.[80] When severe wrist and finger flexor spasticity is present with no extensor tone, a flexor digitorum sublimus to flexor digitorum profundus (STP) transfer is performed.[81] The muscle bellies of the sublimi are sutured to the profundi tendons, which allows the necessary tendon lengthening while preventing extensor contractures.

Nonfunctional surgery at the hip consists of obturator neurectomy and adductor muscle release for severely adducted hips. Release of the iliopsoas muscles in the pelvis is necessary for significant hip flexion contractures. Percutaneous adductor muscle releases and release of the iliopsoas insertion are performed for mild adduction and flexion deformities. After surgery limb splinting and body proning are often necessary. Complete hamstring release, both medial and lateral, is necessary for fixed knee flexion deformities. Serial or drop-out casts are needed after surgery to gain full knee extension,[79] and to avoid stretch injury to the neurovascular bundle. Although surgery provides definitive treatment of limb deformity, appropriate use of serial casting, ROM exercises, modalities, and peripheral nerve or motor point blocks in the early stages of contracture formation may preclude the need for surgical intervention at a later date.

FUNCTIONAL SURGERY

Functional surgery allows improved limb control with or without an orthosis, and may eliminate the need for an orthosis in the higher-level patient. The most common upper extremity functional surgery occurs at the wrist, fingers, and thumb. Active hand opening is often restricted by flexor spasticity. "Fractional lengthening" of the superficial and deep finger flexor tendons and "Z" lengthenings of the wrist and thumb flexors weaken these muscles sufficiently to allow an increase in extensor control while allowing adequate flexor strength.[82, 83]

The most commonly performed functional surgery in the lower extremity is cor-

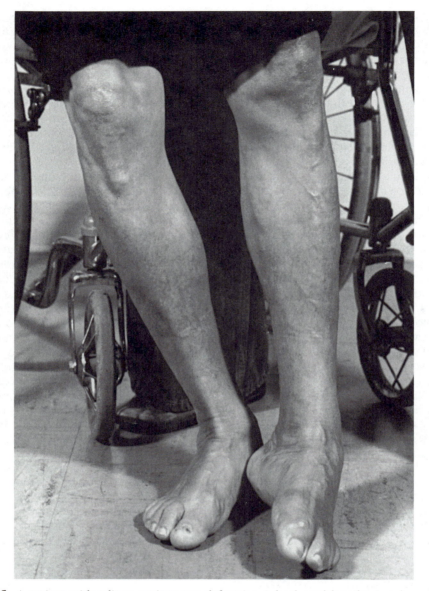

Figure 9–5. A patient with talipes equinovarus deformity. A heel cord lengthening, long toe flexor release, and split anterior tibial tendon transfer (SPLATT) will render the foot plantigrade and may allow brace-free ambulation.

rection of the talipes equinovarus deformity of the foot and ankle[84, 85] (Fig. 9–5). An Achilles tendon lengthening is combined with a split anterior tibial tendon transfer (SPLATT) to the lateral side of the foot and a toe flexor release. Approximately one third of the patients who require an orthotic device to control this deformity become brace-free after surgery,[86] and many other patients can use a lighter-weight, more cosmetic plastic brace rather than a metal ankle-foot orthosis (AFO).

CONCLUSION

Brain injured patients are commonly victims of multiple trauma, and therefore may have damage to virtually any organ system extrinsic to the CNS. In addition to injury, iatrogenic effects of medications, unrecognized traumatic damage, and various other medical and surgical manipulations may carry adverse consequences for the patient. Perhaps most important is the recognition that as the central control mechanism for the individual organism, damage to the brain alone has widespread effects on multiple other organ systems. The clinician must be aware of these potential medical and orthopedic complications, deliberately and methodically search for them, and be prepared to treat them as effectively and expeditiously as possible.

REFERENCES

1. Horton, P and Gerster, JC: Reflex sympathetic dystrophy and barbiturates. Clin Rheumatol 3:493, 1984.
2. Van der Korst, JK et al: Phenobarbital and the shoulder hand syndrome. Ann Rheum Dis 25:553, 1960.
3. Ginsberg, G et al: Androgen abnormalities in acne vulgaris. Acta Dermatol Venereol 61:431, 1981.
4. Herzog, A et al: Reproductive endocrine disorders in women with partial seizures of temporal lobe origin. Arch Neurol 43:341, 1986.
5. Sandel, ME, Abrams, P and Horn, LJ: Hypertension after brain injury: A case report. Arch Phys Med Rehabil 67:469, 1986.
6. Peterson, BW: Taste Pathways. In Netter, F: CIBA Collection of Medical Illustrations. Vol 1: The Nervous System. CIBA, 1983, p 175.
7. Friedman, E et al: Carbon dioxide laser management of subglottic stenosis and tracheal stenosis. Otolaryngol Clin North Am 16:871, 1983.
8. Sazaki, C et al: Tracheostomy-related subglottic stenosis: Bacteriologic pathogenesis. Laryngoscope 89:857, 1979.
9. Gallagher, S: Diagnosis and treatment of bruxism: A review of the literature. Gen Dentist 28:62, 1980.
10. Pratap-Chand, RP et al: Bruxism: Its significance in coma. Clin Neurol Neurosurg 87:113, 1985.
11. Rimel, R and Jane, J: Characteristics of the head injured patient. In Rosenthal, M, Griffith, E, Bond, M and Miller, J (eds): Rehabilitation of the Head Injured Adult. FA Davis, Philadelphia, 1983, p 17.
12. Kalisky, A et al: Medical problems encountered during rehabilitation of patients with head injury. Arch Phys Med Rehabil 66:25, 1985.
13. Clifton, G et al: Cardiovascular response to severe head injury. J Neurosurg 59:447, 1983.
14. Robertson, C et al: Treatment of hypertension associated with head injury. J Neurosurg 59:455, 1983.
15. Schulte am Esch, J et al: Hemodynamic changes in patients with severe head injury. Acta Neurochir 54:243, 1980.
16. Natelson, B: Neurocardiology. Arch Neurol 42:178, 1985.
17. Graf, C and Rossi, N: Catecholamine response to intracranial hypertension. J Neurosurg 49:862, 1978.
18. Clifton, G et al: Circulating catecholamines and sympathetic activity after head injury. Neurosurgery 8:10, 1981.
19. McCleod, A et al: Cardiac sequelae of acute head injury. Br Heart J 47:221, 1982.
20. Neil-Dwyer, G et al: Effects of propranolol and phentolamine on myocardial necrosis after subarachnoid hemorrhage. Br Med J 2:990, 1978.
21. Crompton, MR: Hypothalamic lesions following closed head injury. Brain 94:165, 1971.
22. Feibel, J et al: Catecholamine-associated refractory hypertension following acute intracranial hemorrhage: Control with propranolol. Ann Neurol 9:340, 1981.
23. Aiges, H et al: The effects of phenobarbital and diphenylhydantoin on liver function and morphology. J Pediatr 97:22, 1980.
24. Brooke, M and Barbour, PC: Assessment of nutritional status during rehabilitation after brain injury (abstr). Arch Phys Med Rehabil 67:634, 1986.
25. Rapp, RP et al: The favorable effect of early parenteral feeding on survival in head injured patients. J Neurosurg 58:906, 1983.
26. Clifton, G et al: Enteral hyperalimentation in head injury. J Neurosurg 62:186, 1985.
27. Bauer, LA et al: Importance of unbound phenytoin serum levels in head trauma patients. J Trauma 23:1058, 1983.
28. Schwab, G et al: The cost effectiveness of enteral nutritional support in the DRG era. Contemp Ortho 13:31, 1986.
29. Robertson, C et al: Steroid administration and nitrogen excretion in the head injured patient. J Neurosurg 63:714, 1985.
30. Fell, D et al: Metabolic profiles in patients with acute neurosurgical injuries. Crit Care Med 12:649, 1984.
31. Reilly, J (moderator): Symposium: Enteral vs parenteral hyperalimentation. Contemp Ortho 13:55, 1986.
32. Johnson, LR et al: Structural and hormonal alteration in the gastrointestinal tract of parenterally fed rats. Gastroenterology 68:1177, 1975.
33. Laucks, S et al: Percutaneous endoscopic gastrostomy. Contemp Ortho 13:11, 1986.
34. Bray, GA and Gallagher, T: Manifestations of hypothalamic obesity in man: A comprehensive investigation of eight patients and a review of the literature. Medicine 54:301, 1975.
35. Stricker, E: Hyperphagia. N Engl J Med 298:1010, 1978.
36. Angelini, L et al: Focal lesion of the right cingulum: A case report in a child. Neurol Neurosurg Psychiatry 43:355, 1980.
37. Celesia, G et al: Hyperphagia and obesity: Relationship to medial hypothalamic lesions. JAMA 246:151, 1981.
38. Krahn, D and Mitchell, J: Case report of bulimia associated with increased intracranial pressure. Am J Psychiatry 141:1099, 1984.
39. Hirsch, J: Hypothalamic control of appetite. Hosp Pract 19(2):131, 1984.
40. Levine, A et al: Opioids and consummatory behavior. Brain Res Bull 14:663, 1985.
41. Morley, J and Levine, A: Appetite regulation: Modern concepts offering food for thought. Postgrad Med 77:42, 1985.
42. Childs, A: Naltrexone in organic bulimia (abstr). Arch Phys Med Rehabil 67:667, 1986.

43. Altman, H and Pruzanski, W: Post traumatic hypopituitarism: Anterior pituitary insufficiency following skull fracture. Ann Int Med 55:149, 1961.

44. Fleisher, A et al: Hypothalamic hypothyroidism and hypogonadism in prolonged traumatic coma. J Neurosurg 49:650, 1978.

45. Klingbeil, G and Cline, P: Anterior hypopituitarism: A consequence of head injury. Arch Phys Med Rehabil 66:44, 1985.

46. Miller, W et al: Child abuse as a cause of post traumatic hypopituitarism. N Engl J Med 302:723, 1980.

47. Adams, JH, Gennarelli, T and Graham, DI: Brain damage in non-missile head injury: Observations in man and subhuman primates. In Smith, W and Cavanaugh, J (eds): Recent Advances in Neuropathology. Churchill Livingston, New York, 1982, p 182.

48. Kornblum, R and Fisher, R: Pituitary lesions in craniocerebral injuries. Arch Pathol 88:242, 1969.

49. Horn, LJ and Sandel, ME: Anterior pituitary dysfunction after traumatic brain injury: A preliminary report of 30 patients. Unpublished material, 1986.

50. Shaul, P et al: Precocious puberty following severe head trauama. Am J Dis Child 139:467, 1985.

51. Friedman, W: Head injuries. CIBA Symp 35:24, 1983.

52. Moses, A et al: Pathophysiologic and pharmacologic alterations in the release and action of ADH. Metabolism 25:697, 1976.

53. Kern, K and Meslin, H: Diabetes insipidus: Occurrence after minor head trauma. J Trauma 24:69, 1984.

54. Barreca, T et al: Evaluation of anterior pituitary function in patients with post traumatic diabetes insipidus. J Clin Endocrinol Metab 51:1279, 1980.

55. Notman, D et al: Permanent diabetes insipidus following head trauma: Observations in ten patients and an approach to diagnosis. J Trauma 20:599, 1980.

56. Garland, DE and Rhoades, ME: Orthopedic management of brain-injured adults. Clin Orthop 131:111, 1978.

57. Garland, DE, Rothi, B and Waters, RL: Femoral fractures in head-injured adults. Clin Orthop 166:219, 1982.

58. Garland, DE and O'Hollaren, RM: Fractures and dislocations about the elbow in the head-injured adult. Clin Orthop 168:38, 1982.

59. Garland, DE and Dowling. V: Forearm fractures in head-injured adults. Clin Orthop 176:219, 1983.

60. Garland, DE and Miller, G: Fractures and dislocations about the hip in head-injured adults. Clin Orthop 186:154, 1984.

61. Garland, DE and Bailey, S: Undetected injuries in head-injured adults. Clin Orthop 146:317, 1980.

62. Garland, DE, Glogovac, SV and Waters, RL: Orthopedic aspects of pedestrian victims of automobile accidents. Orthopedics 2:142, 1979.

63. Garland, DE and Toder, L: Fracture of the tibial diaphysis in adults with head injuries. Clin Orthop 150:198, 1980.

64. Heiden, JS et al: Severe head injury and outcome: A prospective study. In Popp, AJ et al (eds): Neural Trauma. Raven Press, New York, 1979, p 181.

65. Hunte, T et al: Histocompatibility antigens in patients with spinal cord injury or cerebral damage complicated by heterotopic ossification. Rheumatol Rehabil 19:97, 1980.

66. Larson, J et al: Increased prevalence of HLA-B27 in patients with ectopic ossification following traumatic spinal cord injury. Rheumatol Rehabil 20:4, 1981.

67. Minajre, P et al: Neurologic injuries, para-osteoarthropathies, and human leukocyte antigens. Arch Phys Med Rehabil 61:214, 1980.

68. Weiss, S et al: Histocompatibility (HLA antigens) in heterotopic ossification associated with neurological injury. J Rheumatol 6:88, 1979.

69. Garland, DE, Alday, B and Venos, KG: The HLA antigens and heterotopic ossification. Arch Phys Med and Rehabil 65:531, 1984.

70. Garland, DE, Blum, CE and Waters, RL: Periarticular heterotopic ossification in head-injured adults: Incidence and location. J Bone Joint Surg (Am) 62:1143, 1980.

71. Mendelson, L et al: Periarticular new bone formation in patients suffering from severe head injuries. Scand J Rehabil Med 7:141, 1975.

72. Mielants, H et al: Clinical survey of and pathogenic approach to para-articular ossifications in long-term coma. Acta Orthop Scand 46:190, 1975.

73. Sazbon, L et al: Widespread periarticular new bone formation in long-term comatose patients. J Bone Joint Surg 63B(1):120, 1981.

74. Spielman, G, Gennarrelli, ·TA and Rogers, CR: Disodium etidronate: Its role in preventing heterotopic ossification in severe head injury. Arch Phys Med Rehabil 64:539, 1983.

75. Garland, DE et al: Diphosphonate treatment for heterotopic ossification in spinal cord injury patients. Clin Orthop 176:197, 1983.

76. Stover, SL, Hahn, RH and Miller, JM: Disodium etidronate in the prevention of heterotopic ossification following spinal cord injury. Paraplegia 14:146, 1978.

77. Garland, DE, Razza, BE and Waters, RL: Forceful joint manipulation in head-injured adults with heterotopic ossification. Clin Orthop 169:133, 1982.

78. Garland, DE et al: Resection of heterotopic ossification in the adult with head trauma. J Bone Joint Surg 67A:1261, 1985.

79. Ough, JL et al: Treatment of spastic joint contractures in mentally disabled adults. Orthop Clin North Am 12:142, 1981.

80. Garland, DE, Thompson, R and Waters, RL: Musculocutaneous neurectomy for spastic elbow flexion in nonfunctional upper extremities in adults. J Bone Joint Surg 62A:108, 1980.

81. Braun, RM, Vise, GT and Roper, B: Preliminary experience with superficialis to profundus tendon transfer in the hemiplegic upper extremity. J Bone Joint Surg 56A:466, 1974.

82. Waters, RL, Garland, DE and Nickel, V: Upper extremity surgery in stroke patients. In Lamb, DW and Kuczynski, K (eds): Practice of Hand Surgery. Blackwell Scientific Publications, Edinburgh, 1981.

83. Waters, RL: Upper extremity surgery in stroke patients. Clin Orthop 131:30, 1978.

84. Waters, RL, Perry, J and Gárland, DE:·Surgical correction of gait abnormalities following stroke. Clin Orthop 131:42, 1978.

85. Waters, RL and Garland, DE: Acquired neurologic disorders of the adult foot. In Mann, RA (ed): DuVries Surgery of the Foot. St Louis, CV Mosby, 1986, p 332.

86. Keenan, MA et al: Surgical correction of spastic equinovarus deformity in the adult head trauma patient. Foot Ankle 5:35, 1984.

Chapter 10

Hypertonicity and Movement Disorders

ERNEST R. GRIFFITH, M.D.
NATHANIEL H. MAYER, M.D.

In considering the motor disorders associated with brain injury, we briefly define, classify, and describe the "pure" neurologic entities and then discuss in greater detail the more frequently occurring motor syndromes in which these entities are seen. The syndromes are often mixtures of several of the "pure" disorders. Depending on the mix—the location, extent, and severity of each component—the syndrome will have various functional consequences and treatment approaches. We will emphasize the recognition and management of functional consequences—physical and psychosocial. The presence of hypertonicity or a movement disorder is not, ipso facto, an indication for treatment.

Rigidity and spasticity are the two forms of hypertonicity.[1, 2] Rigidity states are of several types, having the common characteristic of increased involuntary contractile resistance of muscle to passive range of motion, a resistance that is independent of the velocity of movement. Although present in all muscles of an affected extremity, rigidity is usually more prominent in flexor groups.

Decorticate and decerebrate posturing are types of rigidity seen in comatose brain injured patients.[1] Decorticate posturing is the intermittent or sustained involuntary attitude of the lower limb(s) in extension synergy and of the upper limb(s) in flexion synergy. When observed as an isolated finding, the decorticate state is indicative of a lesion of cortical white matter, internal capsule, cerebral peduncle, basal ganglia, or thalamus.[3] Decerebrate posturing is the voluntary assumption of extension synergy pat-

terns for both lower and upper limb(s). Elbows may be partially flexed, forearms are pronated, and hips adducted. In its "pure" form, the decerebrate state signifies injury to the mid and upper brainstem. However, since most closed head injuries are associated with diffuse brain lesions, decorticate and decerebrate posturing often occur simultaneously or alternately.

Parkinsonian rigidity occurs much less often following head injury than does decorticate or decerebrate posturing.[2] Secondary to disorders of the nigrostriatal system, parkinsonism is associated with characteristic resting tremor, cog-wheeling, bradykinesia and hypokinesia, festinating gait, dysequilibrium, and so forth. In brain injured patients the usual bases for this syndrome probably are hypoxia,[4] or phenothiazine or butyrophenone toxicity.[5] Many of the classic signs are muted or modified by other motor abnormalities in these patients.

Also consequent to basal ganglia involvement secondary to injury or drugs, the dyskinesia group of movement disorders are associated with rigidity or hypertonicity, often fluctuating in degree.[2] The most extreme and persistent forms of rigidity are observed with dystonias. The dyskinesias will be categorized and individually described with the movement disorders.

Spasticity is that form of hypertonicity marked by increased involuntary contractile resistance of muscle to passive range of motion, resistance that is proportionate to the velocity of movement.[1, 2] The clasp-knife response is arguably uniformly present; however, it is not pathognomonic of spasticity, occurring with decerebrate rigidity as well.[3] Antigravity muscles tend to be more severely involved than their antagonists. In contradistinction to rigidity states, hyperreflexia and some degree of muscle weakness are usually present. Clonus is a unique but not constant feature. Muscle spasms and posturing may be difficult to distinguish from those of rigidity states, movement disorders, or seizures. Spasticity is the most frequently encountered form of hypertonic and movement disorders.[4, 6]

The movement disorders may be classified as follows:

A. *Ataxias*
    1. Cerebellar
    2. Noncerebellar
B. *Dyskinesias*
    1. Dystonias
    2. Tardive dyskinesia
    3. Chorea
    4. Ballisms
    5. Athetosis
C. *Tremors*
    1. Resting
    2. Action or postural
    3. Intention
D. *Myoclonus*
    1. Asterixis
E. *Akathisia*
F. *Tics*

Cerebellar ataxia is a clinical constellation of dysequilibrium, dysmetria, dyssynergia, adiadocho-kinesis, intention tremor, titubation, nystagmus, and hypotonia.[1, 2] Mild muscle weakness, fatiguability, hyporeflexia, and pendular reflexes may be additional elements. Disorders of the cerebellum or its tracts resulting from brain injury or drug toxicity produce this form of ataxia. Of the motor disorders under consideration, cerebellar ataxia is second only to spasticity in frequency among brain injured patients.[4, 6] Ataxia may be secondary to drug effects; phenytoin and diazepam are common offenders in the brain injured population.

Lesions to corticospinal tracts, posterior columns, or the vestibular apparatus can cause dysequilibrium, clumsy, incoordinate, and tremorous voluntary movements, constituting the syndrome of *noncerebellar ataxia*.[1, 2] Careful neurologic examination of these patients should allow ready differentiation from those with cerebellar ataxia.

Dyskinesias are involuntary movement disorders that may not be readily distinguishable from one another and often occur in confluent, merging fashion.[1, 2] All forms are aggravated by anxiety, excitement, or voluntary movements, and are abolished during sleep. When secondary to brain trauma they often present as focal or hemidyskinesias rather than diffuse disorders. Commonly they appear belatedly, even as preceding spasticity abates and voluntary control improves.[7] Frequently they subside spontaneously.

Dystonias are marked by sustained contorted attitudes or gyrations of torso, limbs, and face.[1, 2] These positions are the extremes of athetoid movement. Involvement of the larger axial muscles is prominent. Tonic and clonic spasms may coexist. Action dystonia is marked by inappropriate or opposing contractions during specific voluntary acts. Levodopa, phenothiazines, and butyrophenones can produce dystonias.

Tardive dyskinesia is characterized by rapid, rhythmic, automatic movements in single or generalized muscle groups, particularly in the lingual-facial-buccal-cervical area.[1, 2] Chewing, tongue protrusion, sucking, and lip-puckering are typically seen. Dystonic and choreoathetoid movements of trunk and limbs are associated findings. This disorder is induced by phenothiazines or haloperidol and is not a consequence of brain injury per se.

Chorea is manifested by abrupt, rapid, jerky, irregular, random, unsustained movements of face, torso, and limb muscles.[1, 2] These simple or elaborate motions may be incorporated into voluntary movements, investing them with a peculiar flowing dance-like quality. Hypotonia, pendular reflexes, grimacing, and grunting sounds may occur. Drugs such as anticonvulsants, CNS stimulants, antihistamines, oral contraceptives, dopaminergics, and antipsychotics can cause chorea.[5]

Ballisms are exaggerated choreiform movements, violent flingings of extremities or of the entire body.[1, 2]

Athetosis is displayed as slow, sinuous, irregular, confluent movements of trunk, limbs, face, and tongue.[1, 2] Intention spasms akin to those of parkinsonism may be present. With generalized choreoathetosis, hypotonia may be a prominent finding. Sustained athetosis may merge with dystonia.

Tremors are rhythmical, repetitive, involuntary oscillations around a fixed point, ordinarily in one plane.[1, 2] Pathologic tremors favor distal limbs, head, tongue, and jaw, whereas physiologic tremors have a generalized distribution. Furthermore, pathologic tremors are grossly visible and disappear during sleep, in contradistinction to physiologic tremors. Our further description of tremors will deal strictly with pathologic types.

Resting tremors are observed in the parkinsonian syndrome, most typically as the "pill-rolling" finger movements.[1, 2] Other manifestations include eyelid fluttering or closure, repetitive extrusion of the tongue, and alternating flexion-extension of the foot. Occurring at frequencies of 3 to 7 Hertz, these movements subside or disappear on voluntary effort and therefore generally do not interfere with functional activities.

Action or postural tremors occur throughout the entirety of voluntary movement or maintained postures, usually at frequencies of 6 to 13 Hertz.[1, 2] Tremor may be intensified by attempts at more precise movement, thus interfering with such functions. The likely site of associated lesions is the mid-brain.[8]

Intention tremors appear after the initiation of a willed act, progressing as the movement reaches its conclusion.[1, 2] Such tremors are accentuated by exacting precise movement, at times becoming violent enough to throw the afflicted individual off balance. Almost always linked with cerebellar dysfunction, intention tremors occur at frequencies of 8 to 13 Hertz. Some cerebellar outflow tremors are most evident with the arms in the "wing-beating" position. This variant has been termed "rubral" or "mid-brain" tremor.[5]

As with the dyskinesias, tremors may also be mixed, combining the features of these three types.

Myoclonus is an abrupt shocklike fine or gross involuntary movement.[1, 2, 8] When secondary to muscle contractions, the term *positive myoclonus* is applied. Contractions may be single or repetitive; focal, segmental, or generalized; rhythmic or nonrhythmic; symmetrical or asymmetrical; and synchronous or asynchronous. Contractions are usually stimulus related. When activated by voluntary movement, generally rapid, fine activities, the term *action myoclonus* is used. The causes and sites of pathologic lesions associated with myoclonus are diverse.[8] Only those forms related to brain injury are considered here.

Action myoclonus due to head injury is usually focal or segmental, confined to the body part being moved.[9] It is associated with lesions of lower brainstem and cerebellar ataxia.

Palatal myoclonus presents as a continuous rhythmic uvulopalatal movement interrupted by voluntary use of the involved muscles.[10] At times it is accompanied by an audible clicking of the eustachian tubes. The disorder may become more generalized regionally to pharynx, face, extraocular muscles, and vocal cords. Palatal myoclonus has the unique characteristic of persisting during sleep. It tends to be permanent. Focal lesions of the medulla produce this disorder.

Myoclonus can result from neurotoxicity of drugs such as L-dopa, anticonvulsants, antidepressants, antibiotics, and anesthetic agents.[11] Seizures may be associated with myoclonus.

Asterixis, a form of *negative myoclonus,* consists of arrhythmic lapses of sustained positions of limbs or body resulting from interruptions of willed contractions.[12] Gravity or muscle viscoelasticity produces the ensuing movement. This pseudotremor is often associated with corrective overshoot, creating a flapping movement. Asterixis has many causes, among which are seizures, traumatic lesions of upper brainstem, and anticonvulsant and L-dopa toxicity.

Akathisia is the state of repetitive restless movements such as foot-tapping, crossing and uncrossing of legs, patting of the scalp or face, or squirming in a chair.[2] Antipsychotic drugs and lesions of brainstem reticular activating system or thalamus can produce this syndrome.

Tics are sudden, intermittent, habitual, usually complex sequences or coordinated automatic movements.[2] Vocal tics such as coprolalia or echolalia and copropraxia are extremely common following brain injury. Tics may be induced by amphetamine or methylphenidate, especially in children.[5]

These various motor disorders may spontaneously recover over periods of time extending to 18 months or more.[4] We have witnessed examples of progressive recovery for 2 to 3 years after injury. The extent to which such improvement may be either spontaneous or the result of intensive practice or training is uncertain.

CLINICAL SYNDROMES AND THEIR MANAGEMENT

Early Posturing—Spasticity State

CLINICAL DESCRIPTION AND ASSOCIATED FINDINGS

Initial or early follow-up neurologic evaluations of the comatose patient may disclose decorticate and/or decerebrate posturing.[3, 13, 14] Either or both may appear spontaneously or in response to various stimuli; as part of the formal neurologic examination, deep pressure is the conventional stimulus applied. This early posturing may quickly disappear or it may evolve into more persisting patterns, in which one or the other form predominates.[3] The persistence of decerebrate posturing is an ominous prognostic sign.[15] Accompanying rigidity can be progressive and extreme, especially with decerebrate posturing, in which protracted torsal and nuchal extension may produce opisthotonus. Associated with the decerebrate state, hyperthermia, arterial hypertension, tachycardia and other arrhythmias, hyperventilation, diaphoresis, shivering, and extreme muscle spasm constitute the syndrome of "brainstem storm," a potential medical crisis.[3, 15] Both forms of posturing are usually sensitive to changes in head, body, and limb positioning, which invoke spinal or brainstem reflexes such as labyrinthine and tonic neck responses.[3] Moreover, both forms may be modified by a host of internal or other external stimuli. These modifications may vary greatly not only with different stimuli but also with different intensities and sites of stimulation, and with variations of body/limbs/head position upon initiation of a particular stimulus. With progressive neurologic recovery, posturing wanes over the ensuing hours, days, or weeks, and then disappears. The major exception to this course is the persistence of rigidity with the vegetative state.

Conversely, spasticity frequently is not present immediately after injury, appearing and progressing over subsequent days to weeks.[16] Depending upon its severity, and that of the pre-existing rigidity state, decorticate-decerebrate posturing may become further modified into other attitudes. Spasticity, like rigidity, is extremely sensitive to the many environmental and internal influences already mentioned.[16, 17] Further signs of spasticity may include muscle spasms, clonus, trismus, hyper-reflexia, and velocity-related resistance to passive motion.

FUNCTIONAL CONSEQUENCES

The consequences of early rigidity-spasticity include progressive musculoskeletal deformities with contractures; decubitus ulcers; trauma to skin, mouth, and other soft tissues; occasional fractures of bones or teeth; and interference with therapy and nursing care (range of motion, bed mobility, and positioning, as well as management of skin, mouth, respiratory tract, bladder, bowel, nutrition).

Brainstem or autonomic "storm" can result in dangerous elevations of blood pressure and temperature, and potentially lethal arrhythmias.[13, 15] Intracranial pressure may rise during generalized spasms or hypertensive crisis.

The psychologic effects of early rigidity-spasticity relate to the family rather than to the patient. Episodes can be frightening, and may be readily misinterpreted as seizures or conscious reactions to pain and other noxious stimuli. In contrast, milder forms of reflex activity are often perceived as voluntary movement, thereby instilling premature optimism about recovery.

MANAGEMENT

Management of this syndrome begins with preventive measures.[16, 17] External stimuli must be reduced to the barest minimum: gentle handling by caregivers, attention to details of bed positioning that will inhibit the hypertonic states, prevention of trauma, provision of a quiet environment, and early elimination of catheters and tubes. Partial flexion of the body and limbs in the prone position may reduce extensor posturing. Provision of a constant ambient temperature and prompt control of infections are further essentials of preventive management. Brainstem "storm" is controlled by hypothermia, administration of Thorazine (chlorpromazine), a benzodiazepine, and, to combat hypertension, a beta-adrenergic receptor blocking agent.[15, 18]

Gentle, passive range-of-motion and stretching exercises should be attempted in milder cases at least twice daily; however, with pronounced hypertonicity, conventional therapeutic ranging is frequently impossible, may increase the tonus, or cause injury. Therefore, movement must be sought by careful positioning and elicitation of tonic neck, labyrinthine, withdrawal, extension, or other reflexes that will either inhibit tone or provoke desired reflex movement. For example, passive stretching of toe extensors (the Marie-Foix reflex) can produce a withdrawal response of the lower extremity, thus reducing extensor posturing and briefly allowing stretching toward further flexion.[19] To facilitate these activities, cold, heat, electrical stimulation, vibration, or other physical modalities may be applied preliminarily. Splinting of the extremities may further reduce tone and sustain stretching while maintaining functional positions. For more severe degrees of hypertonicity, serial casting is indicated when no contraindications exist.[20, 21] Casting may not be possible in cases of extreme hypertonicity associated with severe spasms and posturing, complicated limb injuries, inaccessibility of limbs owing to intravenous and monitoring devices, or lack of expertise in applying and monitoring the casts. As voluntary function returns, drop-out casting can replace the full cylinder casts. Alternatively, the casts can be bivalved to provide continued splinting as hypertonicity abates and stretching proceeds toward full range of motion.

Antispastic agents occasionally have a role in the early management of spasticity, with recognition that their effect on rigidity is generally minimal.[16, 17] The side effects of these drugs are well appreciated;[22] their central effects may delay responsivity in the recovering coma patient.[17] However, as a temporary adjunctive measure, as in the management of severe spasms, these drugs can be useful in selected cases.

Selective chemical neurolysis, using phenol or alcohol, should be considered for the management of severe regional hypertonicity.[16, 17] Predominantly or wholly motor peripheral nerves may be approached by percutaneous techniques. Mixed peripheral nerves merit a more selective open technique in order to avoid injecting sensory axons.[23] Individual muscles can be approached by motor point blockade,[24] or diffuse instillation of alcohol.[25]

In the early stages of neurologic recovery, chemoneurolysis must be considered with due caution. The peripheral procedures previously described are usually completely reversible, but with repetition occasionally cause some degree of permanent weakness. Ablative surgical procedures are not indicated at this juncture of early recovery.[26]

Bilateral Hemiparesis With Spasticity

CLINICAL DESCRIPTION AND ASSOCIATED FINDINGS

Many patients emerging from coma will demonstrate tetraparesis, hyper-reflexia, positive Babinski signs, and spasticity. Findings may be asymmetrical, with one side of the body being more involved than the other; or perhaps triparesis or paraparesis predominates. Patients frequently exhibit deformities such as marked flexion of a wrist, elbow, or knee, or plantar flexion of a foot. These deformities typically develop during the period of coma when decortication or decerebration is present. Contracture, a fixed shortening of tissues, often develops in the presence of unbridled hypertonicity, and the deformity persists despite a lessening of hypertonicity when the patient emerges from coma. Spasticity combined with weakness of voluntary movement may also contribute to the observed postural deformities. Patients with bilateral hemiparesis frequently show corticobulbar tract involvement resulting in flat facies, loss of articulatory abilities, and impairment of chewing and swallowing function. Loss of head and neck control is a common finding. The patient presents with severe flexion of the neck such that the chin virtually touches the chest.

FUNCTIONAL CONSEQUENCES

Impairment of head and neck control interferes with feeding, grooming, and washing activities. Spasticity of neck flexors interferes with vertical positioning of the head which facilitates feeding, toothbrushing, and mouth care. Contracture may contribute to this deformity with or without spasticity. Weakness of cervical extension without spasticity also results in chin-to-chest posturing, but such patients are easier to position. Raising an electric bed to a 60-degree angle helps provide support for the floppy patient while he or she performs morning activities of daily living (ADL) in bed. Sitting relatively upright in a wheelchair poses a much more difficult problem: one can immobilize and support the head and neck with various wheelchair attachments or with rigid collars, but such immobilization is inimical to activities that require the patient to move the head.

Patients with bilateral hemiparesis have poor trunk control, causing major difficulty during sitting. Lower extremity spastic postures—especially thigh adduction, hip flexion, or knee extension—interfere with an adequate base of support for sitting. Some patients retain tonic postures such as scissoring of the thighs or flexion of the hips and knees. Other patients, after being placed in the wheelchair, develop phasic difficulties such as the development of a sudden extensor spasm. As limb posture changes, the patient may slip from the chair or become contorted and wedged among the various mechanical restraints created by staff to position the patient properly in the first place.

A number of factors impair wheelchair mobility when a patient has bilateral hemiparesis. Without good head and neck control, such patients cannot see where they are going and, more importantly, they cannot utilitize movement to scan the environment. Impaired trunk control will result in destabilization when patients attempt to use their limbs to operate the wheelchair. Patients who have severe posturing in the lower extremities will not have stable sitting support, a prerequisite for wheelchair operation. Those who do not have at least fair trunk control and an adequate base of support while sitting may still have difficulty operating a chair because of slowness and incoordination of upper and lower extremity movement. Asymmetry of volitional capabilities in the upper and lower extremities, obligatory movement and synergy patterns, spasticity, and contracture additionally contribute to impaired mobility function. Furthermore, impairments of motor problem solving, planning, sequencing,

taking initiative, and properly perceiving environmental cues may be superimposed, creating a highly dysfunctional patient.

Transfers and ambulation are also affected by the findings just described. Impairments in postural control impede transfers. A patient's inability to control motion between body segments such as head-on-trunk, trunk-on-hip, and thigh-on-leg movements typically requires that the patient be transferred with maximal assistance of two people. In the presence of plantar flexion contractures or spasticity, a good base of support is not available for the stand-pivot transfer. Flexion postures at the knee or hip or both foster the patient's collapse on standing because the weightline of the body's center of mass will cause further hip and knee flexion rather than the desired extension. Thus, early ambulation efforts may require maximum assistance, if they are even feasible. Although the problems are many, the neurologic picture frequently improves and, especially in young people, the source of neurophysical recovery can extend well beyond the first year following the head injury.

Patients with bilateral hemiparesis, contracture, deformity, spasticity, slowness of movement, incoordination of movement, and obligatory synergy patterns have a variety of psychosocial and communicative dysfunctions. Limb postures and deformities impair personal hygiene. Social acceptability and cosmesis are markedly reduced. Affectionate touching and handling of the patient by family members and even staff may be compromised by the stigmata of the clinical picture. Corticobulbar involvement may result in drooling and choking episodes during feeding or saliva swallowing. This is often frightening to families, friends, and hospital personnel who are not accustomed to dealing with head injured patients.

Communicative ability may often be compromised on a number of grounds. Corticobulbar involvement impairs articulation and phonation. Respiratory control necessary to provide proper breath support is also altered by the bilateral hemiparesis. The patient's ability to produce vocal speech is, therefore, distorted by severe dysarthria, dysphonia, and impairment of breath control. In such a situation, one would ordinarily use a nonvocal communication system; however, the brain injured person may have major problems with such devices. Cognitive and executive difficulties and specific language dysfunction can interfere with utilization of a nonvocal communication system. Bilateral hemiparesis with contracture deformity, spasticity, and loss of voluntary movement can severely impair the patient's mechanical operation of a nonvocal communication system.

MANAGEMENT

It is helpful to base management of postures, deformities, and movement patterns on a clinical understanding of the underlying kinesiology and pathophysiology. Impaired movement may relate to weakness of agonist muscles or inappropriate activity patterns in antagonist muscles. Clinical examination does not always provide sufficient resolution to identify contributions of agonist and antagonist to specific movements about a joint or in a limb pattern. If available, polyelectromyographic kinesiology techniques are useful in identifynig electromyographic (EMG) activity in agonist and antagonist muscles during functional movements. Severe flexion posturing of the neck may occur because of sustained or spastic contraction of neck flexors such as the sternocleidomastoid muscles, contracture or fixed shortening of these muscles with or without spasticity, or profoundly weak agonist extensor muscles. Passive extension of the neck may inform the examiner about the degree of resistance to such movement. Spastic contraction of neck flexors may be palpable, but the patient may also be voluntarily flexing the neck to splint against pain or because of confusion or misperception regarding the purpose of the examiner's actions. Resistance to passive motion may be increased because of contracture. When the examiner pulls against contractured neck flexors, pain may be induced and, as a result, the patient may resist voluntarily or spastic contractions may occur involuntarily. EMG recordings may help to sort out the contribution of various muscles during these maneuvers. In addition, EMG recordings from neck extensors may reveal whether or not the patient is able to generate active contraction in neck musculature even though little or no clinical movement is apparent. A variety of treatment approaches may be undertaken on the basis of the findings. For example, motor point blocks of the sternocleidomastoid muscle might be considered if this muscle fails to relax. If extensor volitional effort is seen on EMG, functional activities which require cervical extension such as feeding might be undertaken. If cervical extensors are extremely weak, one might utilize electrical stimulation to help strengthen neck extensors, although when this is applied it is possible for the patient to attempt to pull away and thereby strengthen flexor muscles. If EMG examination demonstrates a weak EMG pattern in cervical extensors and if the patient is cognitively and socially cooperative, then EMG feedback to extensor muscles may be considered. This would be an unusual treatment in patients emerging from coma and undergoing early recovery because of the cognitive and behavioral problems they exhibit.

Severe adduction posturing at the shoulder may be due to spasticity and contracture of the pectoralis major. Motor point blocks can be performed. Icing followed by passive stretching or contract-relax techniques may be employed, depending on the patient's cooperation. Severe flexion posturing at the elbow may be due to spasticity of the biceps and/or brachialis and/or brachioradialis. More commonly, these muscles are involved in flexor synergy patterns, and the elbow is simply not re-extended because of absent extensor patterns. Gravity becomes an ineffective elbow extensor when spasticity is present because the spastic response to extension forces at the elbow is flexion. What is important is to determine which flexor muscles are contributing to the posture. It should not be assumed automatically that a flexed elbow is due to active contraction in the biceps. We have seen cases in which brachioradialis or brachialis, or both, shows much more pronounced activity than biceps. For severe flexion posturing, short-term nerve block with anesthetic agents such as bupivacaine may be used. Passive range-of-motion (ROM) exercise should become easier after the block. Although the block typically wears off within 8 to 12 hours, the "antispastic" effect often lasts for days, thus allowing the therapy staff to range the limb more effectively. Local motor point blocks in one offending muscle can be performed, but for multiple muscles, peripheral nerve blocks are required. Blocking a nerve to a given muscle also helps the clinician determine whether a contracture is present. In the presence of contracture, serial casting can be considered if passive ROM exercise performed by staff is not producing an improvement of 5 to 10 degrees approximately every 2 weeks. Commercial splints such as the Dynasplint* are available to help provide sustained stretch.

Severe wrist flexion posturing is evaluated polyelectromyographically in a similar manner to muscle group evaluations described earlier. Median and ulnar nerve blocks at the elbow enable the clinician to discern the degree of muscle contracture. Passive stretching followed by splinting or a serial casting approach can be taken in such cases. We prefer a conservative approach to improving the range, especially in the early course of recovery. If deformity is severe and persistent over several months, surgical release may be entertained. Tendon transfers based on EMG analysis of volitional patterns would not be considered until 18 months post injury.[26] Orthopedic and neurosurgical operative procedures are usually not indicated before then. Neurologic changes may alter the results of earlier procedures. Ultimate neurologic stabilization may make such surgery unnecessary. It should be noted that all joints with contracture should undergo radiography in order to rule out bony or mechanical blocks to motion.

Finger and thumb deformities are similarly approached electromyographically. Extrinsic finger flexors and extensors as well as intrinsic muscles of the hand can be evaluated with polyelectromyographic techniques using intramuscular wire electrodes. Electromyographic examination reveals volitional effort patterns as well as passive patterns when the examiner performs passive ROM exercise on the patient during the testing. Peripheral nerve blocks can help establish the presence of contracture versus dynamic postural deformity. Therapeutic exercise, serial splinting or casting, and electrical stimulation to strengthen the agonist may be performed, if tolerated.

Indications for aggressive management in the upper extremity, as elsewhere, revolve around considerations of function. For

*Dynasplint is manufactured by Dynasplint Systems, Inc., 6655 Amberton Drive, Suite A, Baltimore, Maryland 21227.

purposes of hygiene, access to the axilla, the elbow crease, and the hand—including the interdigital spaces—is essential. Severe flexion deformities of an upper extremity also impair the patient's dressing even when performed by others. Patients will have various degrees of volitional recovery embedded within the deforming postures; therefore, an analysis of the patient's attempted activities is useful. In some cases, deformities are so severe that volitional efforts are totally masked. An electromyographic examination may clearly display the voluntary activity that is not apparent on clinical observation because of the fixed deformities. In cases when the potential for volitional muscle contraction is evident, aggressive management of deforming postures secondary to contracture or dyssynergic activity in some muscle groups can be very rewarding.

Severe flexion posturing at the hip and knee or adductor posturing of the thighs (with legs flexed or with legs extended) interferes greatly with a stable base of support for sitting (Fig. 10–1). Polyelectromyographic studies are helpful in distinguishing excessive activity between hamstrings and rectus femoris. It is difficult to record from the hip flexors but it may be possible to isolate the iliacus using wire electrodes. Frequently, the hamstrings contribute to severe knee flexion with secondary flexion posturing occurring at the hip. Sciatic nerve block can help determine the degree of fixed shortening in the hamstrings (Fig. 10–2). A program of serial casting may be tried, to stretch the hamstrings. Once the patient is casted, prone lying can help stretch the hamstrings from their points of origin.

Prior to a casting approach, we prefer to have the physical therapy staff do aggressive stretching to see if progress can be made. Hydrotherapy may be utilized as a modality during stretching. The application of ultrasound to the musculotendinous junction followed by stretching is another approach. Icing of spastic muscles followed by a contract-relax technique may be utilized as well. The program may be initiated by sciatic nerve block, which allows the therapists to stretch the hamstrings without engendering spastic resistance. In the head injured patient, behavioral considerations always play a role in the choices of therapeutic approaches. For the bilateral hemiparetic patient with spasticity of hip adductors and/or

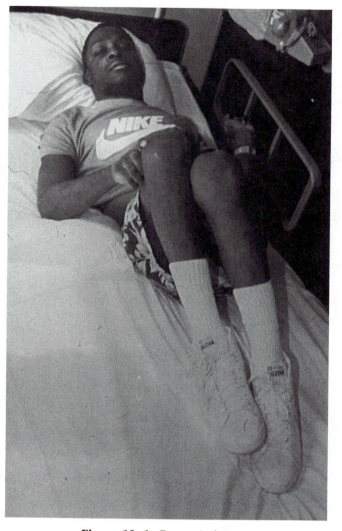

Figure 10–1. Presurgical status.

flexors, phenol application to motor branch nerves should be considered during the early course of recovery. Phenol effect is not permanent: a clinical response often lasts 2 to 6 months.

The technique we prefer involves surgical exploration to find the motor branches to the target muscles.[23] These branches are identified by using an electrical stimulator. If deformity is severe and contracture is apparent while the patient is under general anesthesia, selected tenotomies can also be performed (Fig. 10–3). If after surgical intervention range of motion is still not complete, serial casting can be performed so as to gradually increase the range of motion.

One should be aware that a contracture not only involves muscle groups, skin, and joint capsule, but also blood vessels and nerves. Therefore, a severe fixed flexion contracture at the knee of 90 degrees or more would not be treated by doing a tenotomy and then abruptly cranking out the leg to full extension. Such a maneuver is likely to cause compression of the popliteal artery and damage to or laceration of the tibial nerve. Surgical manipulations are only the beginning of treatment. Gradual physical manipulation of the deformed limb afterward is the main thrust of management.

When adductor spasticity or contracture, or both, prevent access to the perineum and

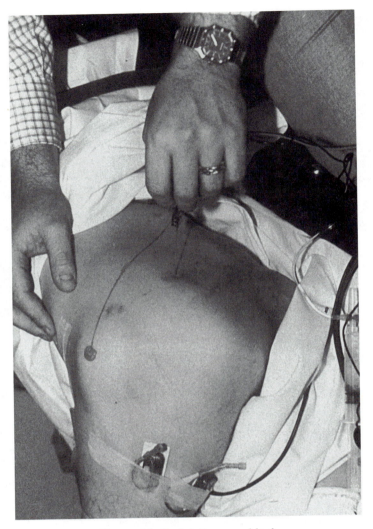

Figure 10–2. Sciatic nerve block.

impair the patient's sitting balance while in the wheelchair, obturator nerve block can help to establish the degree of contracture. With the temporary reduction in adductor muscle spasticity, the patient's subsequent sitting balance can be assessed. Abductor tenotomy and application of phenol to the obturator nerve may be done to provide access to the perineum and improve sitting balance. An additional problem relating to sitting support and balance in the wheelchair is equinus or equinovarus posturing of the ankle-foot system. If the patient is unable to place his or her feet firmly on the foot pedals of the wheelchair, sitting balance and stability of the patient in the moving chair can be altered.

The approach to evaluation is similar to what has been described previously. EMG examination of calf and anterior compartment musculature is performed. Tibial nerve block in the popliteal fossa helps to determine the degree of contracture. Aggressive stretching utilizing modalities such as ultrasound to the musculotendinous junction of the heel cord can be employed. Serial casting may be utilized. In severe cases, percutaneous tendo-Achilles lengthening may be considered, although one should be cautious with this approach since the patient may improve neurologically. If the patient becomes ambulatory at a later date, a vigorous recovery of anterior compartment muscles may result in a calcaneal

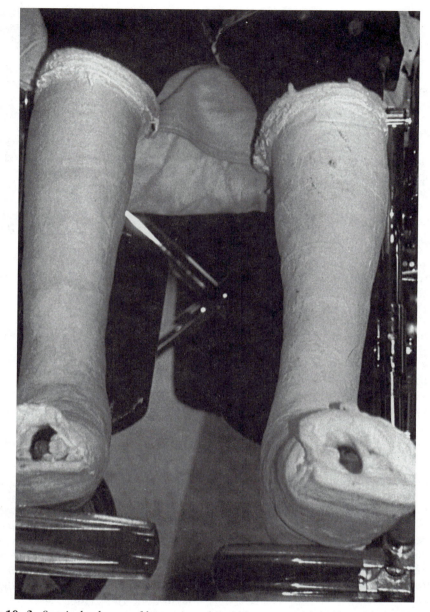

Figure 10–3. Surgical releases of hamstrings, hip adductors, and lengthening of Achilles tendon.

gait similar to the result of an overlength-ened heel cord.

Patients with bilateral upper motorneu-ron syndromes have tremendous difficulty with transfers and especially gait. In the early phase of recovery, patients may be un-able to transfer. After 6 months or more, it may be possible to develop modified stand-pivot transfer techniques, which can be taught to caregivers. These patients require considerable support if gait training is being attempted. Patients who are highly moti-

vated (and with families who "push") may persist at gait training attempts. Given that neurologic recovery can occur beyond the first year, re-evaluation and therapeutic at-tempts are introduced periodically for long-term management of such patients. The use of a variety of ambulatory aids that provide upright support by utilizing the upper ex-tremities along with lower extremity brac-ing may be part of the approach. Limb de-formities that take away a base of support or prevent limb advancement may be evaluated using the methods already described. Prognosis for functional ambulation in such patients with severe residuals of bilateral hemiparesis ranges from guarded to poor; however, the ability of the patient to transfer with progressively less assistance is observed. The burden on a caregiver, therefore, may be lessened with continuing effort on the part of the therapy staff and the patient. One should consider surgical intervention if it can facilitate transfers.

The adaptive value of movement for self-care and -mobility is equally potent for psychosocial skills. Patients and families alike express intense hopes for the recovery of movement. The paramount emphasis of the family on walking seems at times to be almost inappropriate considering the severity of brain damage during early recovery. However, movement and mobility are concrete expressions of the yearnings of family and the oriented patient for recovery of the normalcy they once knew. If mobility is recovered, then families may feel that other abnormalities will resolve similarly. Mobility provides the patient with the ability to act on and in the world rather than be acted upon in a passive fashion. Recovery of self-identity and individuality, of self-esteem and premorbid hopes for the future—these and other psychosocial factors are bound up with the overt physical features and manifestation of the brain injury. The impairment of personal appearance associated with postures, deformities, and abnormal-appearing movements has a direct bearing on the changed perception of the patient as a sexual being as well. Management of movement impairment and postural deformity has as much impact on psychosocial factors as it does on movement and mobility issues.

Depending on the degree of brain damage, relative sparing of higher cortical functions including language is possible. The means of articulatory expression, however, are highly problematic. In such cases, nonvocal communication systems may be successfully used. During the recovery phase, when confusion and maladaptive behaviors are prominent, the use of sophisticated nonvocal communication systems may not be possible. However, simple scanning systems such as yes/no cards can be employed. In some cases of severe disability even this system may not be applicable. Later on, direct-selection devices such as an alphabet board

may be attached to a wheelchair lapboard. Patients with movement disorders may benefit from a variety of electronic systems that are available to compensate for inaccuracies in target acquisition caused by the movement disorder. The Trace Center* can provide detailed information on the varieties of nonvocal communication systems that are available. In contrast to other patients with physical disability, the head injured patient must be more carefully evaluated with regard to his or her ability to comprehend and use a nonvocal communication system. In our experience, these devices come into play in later recovery (often 1 year or more following injury) rather than during the early phase. Hybridization of nonvocal communication systems with microprocessor systems (personal computers) is a current development.

Unilateral Hemiparesis

CLINICAL DESCRIPTION AND ASSOCIATED FINDINGS

Roberts examined 291 patients who were 10 or more years post–head injury.[4] In his series, the most frequently seen pattern of residual neurologic lesion was the patient with signs of a pyramidal lesion on only one side (40 percent of patients). In the majority of cases, these signs were considered to be minimal, consisting of asymmetry of tendon reflexes, mild spasticity often confined to the forearm pronators or quadriceps, and a positive Babinski's sign. These signs were usually associated with reduction in the speed of repetitive fine movements of the upper extremity or with gait disturbance. Impairment of balance, facial flatness, and some dysarthria were also noted. When hemiparesis is mild, speed and fluency of limb movement, rather than strength, are the more germane clinical concerns. Roberts found that of 115 hemiparetic patients, 109 were moderately disabled or better. Moderate disability was defined as patients with hemiparesis, spasticity, incoordination, dysarthria, or imbalance that caused difficulties with mobility or other physical ac-

*The Trace Research and Developmental Center for the Severely Communicatively Impaired, 1500 Johnson Drive, University of Wisconsin at Madison, Wisconsin 53706.

tivities in household or social life, or job. All of these patients were able to perform such activities, although they may have had obvious difficulties or limitations. Roberts attributed the majority of hemipareses with mild findings to primary traumatic injury rather than to secondary infarction.

FUNCTIONAL CONSEQUENCES

During early recovery, weakness is typically profound and very disabling for ADL. Spasticity and spreading hyper-reflexia also severely restrict function. Given the constraints of hemiplegia, how does one perform ADL under conditions of restricted capacity? This classical physical rehabilitation issue is severely compounded by cognitive and behavioral impairments that interfere with the head injured patient's ability to solve the action problems of daily skills. Impairment in the performance of feeding, bathing, dressing, grooming, toileting, transfers, and ambulation occurs in hemiparetic patients because they are physically restricted from acting in former ways of functioning and must now learn new ways of functioning, but are also learning disabled.

Functional consequences of unilateral hemiparesis with spasticity in the areas of ADL relate to the compensatory needs of the patient in these ADL. Unilateral feeding is generally achievable but if the nondominant limb is the uninvolved limb, patients initially will be awkward in their movements and require cuing and supervision. Set-up of the tray may be compromised. The opening of packets and containers becomes problematic, although many patients quickly learn to use their teeth to stabilize their performance. Cognitive confusion, poor motor planning, and poor motor problem-solving usually exacerbate faulty performance more than might be anticipated by the presence of hemiparesis alone. Dressing techniques may be impaired, particularly regarding fasteners (buttons, bra hooks, zippers, belt buckles, and shoelaces).

Transfers and gait may be impaired by limb deformity or dynamic postures in the lower extremity which alter the base of support (for example, equinovarus posturing, knee flexion contracture, or adductor scissoring). In contradistinction to the hemiparesis of stroke patients, which evolves from a hypotonic to a hypertonic clinical picture,

the head injured patient evolves into hemiparesis from a period of decerebrate or decorticate coma. Residuals from this period, which are superimposed on the motor pattern of hemiparesis, may include severe deformities of ankle-foot plantar flexion, toe flexion, knee flexion, hip flexion, or hip adduction. The upper extremity may have significant residual contractures as well. In stroke syndromes, the hypotonic phase typically precedes hypertonicity; therefore, contractures, if they do develop, are a later phenomenon. In the recovery from head injury, these coma phase phenomena superimposed on the hemiparetic syndrome complicate the functional course of recovery. It should also be noted that the so-called uninvolved side in the hemiparetic patient may, during the course of recovery, still have residuals such as contracture from the period of coma as well. Hence, although early neurologic abnormalities have disappeared on the "uninvolved" side, a remaining tight heel cord can have consequences for transfers and ambulation. Residual hip and knee flexion contractures in the lower or upper extremity limit motion and interfere with ADL and mobility training.

MANAGEMENT

Evaluation and management of weakness, spasticity, dyssynergy, and contracture follow similar lines to what was described for bilateral hemiparesis. In many cases when the neurologic picture appears to be changing relatively rapidly (cases of contusion without evidence of infarction of tissue on CT or MRI scans), aggressive physical therapy is quite satisfactory. Modalities such as heat, cold, ultrasound, and electrical stimulation can be used to reduce contracture and improve range of motion. We emphasize functional skills training as primary, with the secondary emphasis being on clinical parameters such as strength, range of motion, and so on. Bracing the patient with mild equinovarus may be necessary, to provide a solid base of support during standing or ambulation. Persistent equinovarus is not corrected orthopedically until 18 months after the injury. Stability, potential for further injury to the ankle-foot system secondary to weightbearing on the lateral border of the foot, limitations in advancement of the body over the involved limb during stance phase, and gait speed are all factors that are taken into account when considering surgical transfers such as the split anterior tibialis tendon procedure to reduce the varus tendency of the ankle-foot system.[27]

We have not found antispasticity drugs to be of much value in the spastic patient recovering from a head injury. Drugs such as Lioresal (baclofen) and diazepam have central sedating effects that can reduce arousal and responsiveness in a brain injured patient whose responsiveness has already been reduced by the diffuse brain injury he or she has sustained. The confusion experienced by the majority of head injured individuals seen early in rehabilitation centers can be worsened by such centrally acting agents. Studies of these drugs that have demonstrated effectiveness in treating spastic phenomena have been confined largely to patients with spinal cord injury and multiple sclerosis.[22] We are not aware of any studies of large series of head injury patients treated with such agents for spasticity. Dantrolene sodium can be effective in the patient who has severe episodes of persistent clonus which interferes with transfers in the lower extremity or dressing in the upper extremity.[28, 29] It is much less effective in patients with sustained or tonic spasm because the drug competes with calcium channel receptors in the sarcoplasmic reticulum.[30] In cases of sustained contraction, the sarcoplasmic reticulum is flooded with calcium and dantrolene sodium loses its effectiveness. The drug can produce liver function test abnormalities. In the patient with head injury, abdominal trauma, blood transfusions, and anticonvulsant medications may also relate to abnormal liver function tests, and the use of dantrolene sodium in such patients may aggravate hepatic dysfunction and cause confusion as to the source of the laboratory abnormalities.

A number of therapeutic techniques may be considered to help mobilize patients with bilateral hemiparesis, just as with unilateral hemiparesis. Gentle vestibular stimulation—for example, positioning and rocking body and head over a large beach ball—may help to reduce tone and facilitate trunk extension and neck extension. Elbow proning on the gym mat can facilitate extension of the neck and shoulders. Rolling activities, with emphasis on segmental rolling, are often used as preskills training for bed mo-

bility. For the patient who is unable to sit independently because of extensor hypertonicity, reduction in such posturing may be accomplished by rotating and flexing the trunk at the hips. Placing wedges on the seat of the wheelchair and on its foot pedals may assist the patient with proper positioning. Thigh bolsters and lateral trunk supports, as well as head and neck supports, can be provided as needed.

Brainstem Corticospinal and Cerebellar Pattern

CLINICAL DESCRIPTION AND ASSOCIATED FINDINGS

Twenty percent of patients in Roberts' series demonstrated evidence of associated cerebellar and pyramidal tract damage.[4] This was invariably asymmetrical. Although the pathology was believed to involve more than just the brainstem, Roberts thought that the coexistence of cerebellar and pyramidal tract damage was consistent with lesions found extensively throughout the brainstem as reported by Tomlinson.[31] These lesions were either due directly to trauma or were secondary to compression from swelling or surface compression of the brain. The cerebellar component predominated more frequently than the pyramidal. Uncal herniation compresses the brainstem, which typically produces a "blown" pupil but may also affect cerebellar and corticospinal pathways. Since the corticospinal tract decussates distal to the site of compressive uncal herniation, as the patient recovers he or she may be left with ipsilateral ataxia and contralateral spastic hemiparesis. Involvement of one or both oculomotor nerves completes the picture. Other cases may simply demonstrate mixed cerebellar and pyramidal tract findings either ipsilaterally or contralaterally.

FUNCTIONAL CONSEQUENCES

Patients with cerebellar pathway incoordination associated with the slowness and patterned movements of hemiparesis experience major difficulties in the performance of ADL, transfers, and ambulation. The clinical problem is one of poor motor control during the performance of basic skills such as feeding, dressing, grooming, and washing.

In addition, the syndrome disables the patient's expressive communications. Impairment of breath control and regulation may produce a scanning, dysphonic, and monotonous speech pattern. If self-awareness and cognitive abilities are relatively preserved (which is not likely if cerebral edema and increased intracranial pressure result in cortical herniation), the patient's self-image may be shattered by this ataxic-hemiparetic motor syndrome. Family members are highly distressed by the combination of deficits seen in this syndrome. Patients with ungainly, uncoordinated movements can be perceived as "drunk" by the lay public. Some of our patients have been turned away from public theaters because of ataxic movements and dysarthric speech; others have been questioned by the police because they appeared to be drugged or under the influence of alcohol. Patients and families are rightly distressed by these misperceptions. An identification bracelet containing medical information, along with anticipatory counseling, may be helpful.

MANAGEMENT

Patients with cerebellar ataxia and dysmetria exhibit problems in accuracy when they perform ADL. For example, when bringing a spoon to the mouth, the ataxic limb will miss its mark, producing spillage and social embarrassment. The hemiparetic limb usually has more accurate control. As long as the movement pattern available to the individual is compatible with the goals of the skill, it is probably preferable to train the hemiparetic limb for performing skilled ADL, as opposed to utilizing the ataxic limb. For instance, if the upper motor neuron limb can produce a movement pattern that can bring a spoon to the mouth, then feeding training should probably be focused on using that limb instead of the ataxic one. In some situations, it may be desirable to have the upper motor neuron limb "guide" the ataxic limb. This may have the effect of damping oscillatory ataxic movements and improving the accuracy of the ataxic limb. For example, the accuracy of transporting food to the mouth by spoon may be improved if the hemiparetic limb grasps the ataxic extremity below the wrist and helps guide the spoon in hand toward the mouth. If the upper motor neuron limb is densely

involved and provides little or no functional assistance, then one major principle of training is to keep the length of the ataxic upper extremity lever arm as short as possible during functional activities. The greater the length of a limb's lever arm about an axis of rotation, the larger the absolute magnitude of error at the target. To improve accuracy, a patient should not reach with outstretched arm but rather should move the entire body very close to the target and simply bend the elbow in order to get the index finger to touch the target. Aids have been recommended,[32] such as weighted jackets and shoes to improve walking or a weighted cap to help with feeding problems associated with poor head control of cerebellar pathway origin. A weighted cuff on the wrist may be tried routinely. In our experience, weighting is inconsistently helpful. For some patients the benefit of a weighted cuff may result from their avoidance of full-elbow extension when performing activities, in order to reduce the leverage factor of an outstretched arm with a weight at its end. The use of isoniazid and beta-adrenergic blockers[33, 34] has been reported for some cases of intentional ataxia with tremor in patients with multiple sclerosis. We have no experience with this medication in head injured patients, however.

With respect to transfers and ambulation in patients who have ataxia and hemiparesis, the key principle is to provide as stable a base as possible. If patients have equinovarus it is important to provide good bracing and, in the late stage, to consider surgical muscle transfers to provide a stable base of support during standing. These patients benefit from the use of platform walkers, which provide forearm support. We have our patients use a walker with wheels in the front so that the patient can advance the walker without having to lift it and risk losing his or her balance while doing so.

Athetoid Pseudobulbar Syndrome

CLINICAL DESCRIPTION AND ASSOCIATED FINDINGS

Roberts[4] attached the term "athetoid pseudobulbar syndrome" to patients having evidence of severe bilateral pyramidal damage with postural dystonia, striking bradykinesia, and fragmentary athetosis. The athetoid pseudobulbar pattern was seen in approximately 5 percent of patients in his long-term follow-up series. In some patients there was a remarkable discrepancy between the severity of the physical disability and the relative preservation of intellectual abilities and personality traits. Roberts suggested that dissociation between physical disabilities and preservation of intellect and personality represent focal secondary infarction rather than diffuse primary traumatic damage alone. He commented on the similarities between the athetoid pseudobulbar syndrome and many cases of congenital diplegia. Some cases he reviewed showed negligible impairment of balance despite profound, almost slothlike bradykinesia and spasticity of all four limbs—a characteristic of most patients with cerebral diplegia as well. As Roberts concluded:

> It seems possible, therefore, that cerebral perfusion failure causing widespread ischemic infarction particularly of the basal ganglia as described by Graham and Adams may be more relevant here than infarction secondary to brain stem compression.[4]

FUNCTIONAL CONSEQUENCES

In cases we have seen, severe bradykinesia and athetoid movements of the head, neck, and extremities allowed patients to participate in functional ADL without being independent in any one activity. They required assistance for transfers, and ambulation was not practical, although they could develop a gait pattern with the assistance of another person for safety. Vocal communication was extremely limited but, as in Roberts' cases, our patients showed good intellect which allowed use of an alphabet board. Although the patients were a physical burden to caretakers, their ability to read was preserved and they were not a mental and social burden.

MANAGEMENT

Drugs are not effective for athetosis. Lower extremity bracing may be considered to improve or stabilize the base of support. Contractures and postural deformities may be treated through a combination of serial casting, tendon releases, or both. Patients with true athetosis do not do well with tendon transfers, because of the constant writhing movements that are observed in various muscle groups about any one joint. Assistive devices are not always helpful because of the severe bradykinesia which can result in a fall if the patient cannot control the body's center of gravity. Corrective movements are too slow to respond to the forces that cause the fall. Nonvocal communication systems should be tried and the most suitable control site located. We found the best device for one patient to be an attachment to the patient's shoe that she could control and use as a pointer for an alphabet board. The alphabet board itself was arranged on the foot pedal of the patient's wheelchair. Generally, the patient used head movements for "yes" and "no" scanning communications, but if she had to initiate something, she used the foot pedal alphabet board with the direct selection technique. Rehabilitation engineering can frequently provide clever interfaces to enhance the motor control of individuals with disordered movements.

Ataxic Syndromes

CLINICAL DESCRIPTION AND ASSOCIATED FINDINGS

We frequently see clinical syndromes involving hemiataxia, bilateral limb ataxia, truncal ataxias, and mixed truncal and limb ataxias which entirely dominate the clinical picture whether or not soft pyramidal tract signs are present. Gerstenbrand and coworkers[35] described cerebellar syndromes as "sequelae of traumatic lesions of upper brain stem and cerebellum." They attributed nearly all of these cases to compression of the upper brainstem and tentorial herniation. In a series of patients who were decerebrate, Gerstenbrand and coworkers found asymmetrical and severe microscopic and macroscopic damage in superior cerebellar penduncles and cerebellar white matter. They favored edema and secondary infarction due to brainstem compression as the cause of these lesions. These authors indicated that the clinical presence of cerebellar findings implied a favorable prognosis for survival.

FUNCTIONAL CONSEQUENCES

Patients with hemiataxia are able to perform self-care activities but may encounter difficulties during transfers and ambulation. Generally, they are able to compensate because of the uninvolved side of the body. An assistive device such as a weighted walker may help to control balance if the hemi-ataxia is severe. Some patients who demonstrate an intention tremor can be severely dysfunctional with upper extremity ADL. These patients soon learn to ignore the involved side and use the other limb.

The patient with bilateral limb ataxia (either involving legs, arms, or all four limbs) is at extreme risk for falling. Activities of daily living that depend on upper extremity skill can be variably compromised because of the inaccuracy in movement produced by the ataxia. If severe dysmetria or intention tremor is an associated finding, clinical dysfunction can be severely exacerbated.

For patients with truncal ataxia without limb ataxia, the lower extremities can provide fairly good compensation. Typically such patients will maintain an enlarged base of support in order to allow the center of gravity to fall between the legs—that is, within the base of support. Assistive devices including "quad" canes and walkers are helpful in such cases. The worst functional cases are those in which there is truncal as well as limb ataxia. These individuals have little or no ability to compensate for their combined set of deficits.

MANAGEMENT

Patients with lower limb ataxia may require a walker with two front wheels, which improves gait stability because patients do not need to lift the walker off the ground as they advance it. Even when the walker is grounded at all times, patients with limb ataxia can suddenly fall in any direction. A platform walker may remedy this problem by allowing patients to broaden their support by leaning on the platforms with the forearms. Because the lower extremities are ataxic and foot placement therefore varies widely, it may be useful to have an extra-width walker to prevent the patient from kicking its sides. We have tried weights on the extremities, but these do not have consistent effect in all patients; in some patients, they seem to help subjectively. They may dampen intention tremor, possibly because the patient has to use more sustained muscle contraction to support the additional weight.

Patients who have dysmetria when pointing to a target (or otherwise attempting to maintain accurate spatial placement of the hand) should be taught that the longer the lever arm they are attempting to control, the greater will be the absolute excursion of their error from their target location in space. Therefore, it should be emphasized to these patients that movements and activities are best performed close to the body.

Basal Ganglia Syndrome

CLINICAL DESCRIPTION AND ASSOCIATED FINDINGS

We believe that this syndrome most usually appears as the result of secondary brain hypoxia[4] or drug toxicity.[5] Phenothiazines and haloperidol are the primary offenders. Antiseizure and dopaminergic agents, antihistamines, CNS stimulants, lithium, anticholinergics, and oral contraceptives have also been implicated. When directly related to brain injury, the syndrome often appears belatedly.[36-39] While dystonia may be the predominating form of disorder, choreoathetosis and ballisms occur, often in segmental or hemisomatic distribution. Dystonia may appear after a single dose of a neuraleptic drug. Torticollis may be present. The rigidity rarely is constant, but rather fluctuates, at times transforming to hypotonia. Anxiety, excitement, and heightened intensity of effort tend to magnify the signs and symptoms.

FUNCTIONAL CONSEQUENCES

Persons with this syndrome are prone to contracture (if associated spasticity is present), musculoskeletal deformities, and skin breakdown. If ambulation is possible, the gait may be bizarre, associated with contorsions of body and limbs that mimic functional disorders.[1] Lower extremity segments may be malpositioned; sustained plantar flexion or dorsiflexion can impair balance and gait. The swinging leg may assume a dancing (*chorea,* dance) quality, or the gait may resemble the shuffling festinations of parkinsonism. Disturbances of equilibrium and righting responses result in excessive crouching, other postural deviations, and frequent falls. Rigid "freezing," bradykinesia, and involuntary movements can restrict all forms of mobility and self-care skills. Swallowing and speech are also vulnerable. Severe dysarthrias to the point of unintelligibility occur. Other means of communication may be severely compromised because of an inability to write or manually operate a communication device. Poor oral control results in drooling, inadequate hygiene, and dental problems.

Despite the severity of physical dysfunctions, certain of these patients, whose injuries are mainly confined to infracortical brain, will have minimal or no mental deficits. In any event, psychosocial problems are predictable. Cosmetic effects, and the resultant reactions of the individual and others, are noteworthy. Self-image and sexuality are exceedingly vulnerable. Communication deficits can adversely affect interpersonal and societal relationships.

Recurrent muscle spasms can be the basis of chronic pain behavior. The physical disabilities alone may preclude employment.

TREATMENT

Any potentially offending drugs should be discontinued. With few exceptions, the syndrome will be reversible if caused by these drugs. Acute dystonic attacks secondary to drug toxicity may dramatically respond to antihistamines, anticholinergics, or diazepam.[5] Parsidol (echopropazine) or Artane (trihexiphenidyl) in massive doses sometimes alleviates dystonia.[2] Haloperidol, phenothiazines, benzodiazepines, and antiseizure drugs such as valproate, phenobarbital, and Tegretol (carbamazepine) have all been used in the effort to control choreoathetosis.[2, 5, 36–38, 40, 41] Ballisms may respond favorably to haloperidol or phenothiazine.[5] Unfortunately the effectiveness of these drugs is often quite limited. For those who display predominantly parkinsonian features, levodopa with or without carbidopa, and the centrally acting anticholinergics are the drugs of choice.[2, 5] Persisting tardive dyskinesia reportedly improves with the use of tetrabenazine.[5]

Functional approaches to therapy should include trials of relaxation and biofeedback techniques (if cognitive functions allow), attempts to reduce precipitating or aggravating environmental factors, and postural control. Kinesiologic re-education should seek to eliminate to whatever degree possible the types and speeds of movement that most profoundly aggravate the condition. As with early rigidity states, attention to head, body, and limb positioning may disclose influences on the hypertonicity. Balance and equilibrium training may prove rewarding. Ambulation and self-care training may eventually be successful in converting overly conscious movement into smoother semiautomatic engrams that better incorporate the involuntary movement. Bracing may be considered in some instances. Trials of resistive exercises, successive induction, rhythmic stabilization, joint compression, and positional sensory feedback should be considered when athetosis is the predominant disorder.[42]

Oral dysfunction may be dealt with by compensatory techniques; alternate methods of oral hygiene and dental care, head positioning to control drooling, and formal speech therapy may be indicated. Surgical reimplantation of Wharton's ducts to a more posterior location has been utilized to facilitate swallowing of saliva.[43]

Psychosocial dysfunctions are managed according to the principles of rehabilitation care: anticipation and prevention of potential problems, early identification and intervention of actual problems, and development of adaptive and coping skills toward self-fulfillment.

The principal surgical treatment of these disorders is stereotaxic thalamotomy.[44–47] This procedure should not be considered until the period of neurologic recovery is completed and other more conservative forms of treatment have been fully explored without adequate improvement. The operation is performed unilaterally, and may be repeated on the opposite side at a later date. Mortality rates are 2 percent or less. Complications include dysarthria (usually reversible) when the procedure is left sided, dysphagia, and, less commonly, hemiparesis. Pre-existing ataxia may worsen.

Stereotaxic placement of electrical stimulators into the thalamus has been performed to manage movement disorders[48] but must be considered an experimental procedure at present. Spinal cord electrical stimulation[49] must be regarded in a similar light.

Regional or local forms of rigidity may respond favorably, though temporarily, to phenol motor point neurolysis.[24]

Tremor States and Myoclonus

CLINICAL PICTURE

This syndrome frequently appears belatedly in patients with pre-existing spasticity or ataxia, or both, and may blend with the basal ganglia syndrome.[8, 9, 50] As the earlier motor disorders improve with treatment and the passage of time, tremor and myoclonus may progressively worsen. Action tremor and action myoclonus often occur together, and may be indistinguishable.[8] To further complicate matters, action myoclonus virtually always coexists with cerebellar ataxia, and so intention tremor may also be superimposed.[1] Resting tremor is more readily seen in the basal ganglia syndrome. Regional tremors are intensified by use of the noninvolved extremities. Tremor-myoclonus states may spontaneously improve in time.

FUNCTIONAL CONSEQUENCES

Mobility skills and ambulation can be profoundly compromised by intention tremors, but not greatly by other forms of tremor. Severe degrees of myoclonus in the lower extremities may disturb balance and gait. More devastating, generally, are the disturbances of upper extremity functions, particularly use of the hands. All self-care skills can be severely compromised. Feeding may be a disaster, with recurring spillage of liquids. Handwriting may be illegible. Isolated resting tremor, however, does not ordinarily impede these functions. Action myoclonus may interfere with more diffuse rapid limb movements, thus disrupting gross motor skills. Oral dysfunctions are not severe, as a rule, although palatal myoclonus can be troublesome cosmetically.

The psychosocial consequences have an impact upon cosmesis, body and self-image, sexuality, and inter-relationships in rather similar fashion to the effects of the basal ganglia syndrome. Here, too, predominantly brainstem injury occurs at times, with little or no disturbance of cognitive abilities.

TREATMENT

Action tremors sometimes respond favorably to propranolol.[51] There are several reports of beneficial effects of beta-adrenergic receptor blockers[5, 52] and isoniazid[33] on intention tremor; nevertheless this tremor is the most resistant one to drug therapy. The anticholinergic drugs used for parkinsonism are more effective in relieving resting tremor than is levodopa.[1] Action myoclonus is also resistant to drug management. Propranolol, L-tryptophan (hydroxytryptophan), Mebaral (mephobarbital), Clonopin (clonazepam), Depakene (valproate), and several other drugs[2, ,5 9, 47, 52, 53] have reportedly been of some benefit. L-tryptophan with carbidopa occasionally ameliorates palatal myoclonus. Exaggerated physiologic or pathologic tremors or tics that are secondary to CNS stimulants usually disappear with removal of the drug. Tics may respond to clonidine or tetrabenazine.[5]

Functional approaches to management should explore the modalities and techniques discussed in the preceding syndrome: biofeedback-relaxation techniques, kinesiologic modifications, and ADL-mobility training to achieve semiautomaticity.

Adaptive aids and substitute methods for ADL and upper extremity activities deserve consideration. Weighted resistance may improve intention tremor.

Management of the psychologic aspects adheres to the principles noted for the basal ganglia syndrome.

The merits of stereotaxic thalamotomy should be weighed according to the criteria and complications previously listed. Recent neurosurgical publications are enthusiastic concerning the efficacy of the procedure for the dyskinesias, tremor states, and myoclonus.[44–47, 54] However, few of these reports detail the long-term or functional results in brain trauma subjects.

SUMMARY AND CONCLUSIONS

Disorders of muscle tone and movement may compromise physical and psychosocial functions and cause secondary complications in survivors of brain injury. Evaluation and management should be oriented to these functional consequences. The disorders need not be treated routinely; they may not reduce function and may spontaneously improve or disappear as part of the process of neurologic recovery.

The spectrum of hypertonic, dyskinetic,

and related states of movement disorders is categorized and described. In the brain injured population these states are frequently clustered as syndromes such as early posturing-spasticity, bilateral hemiparesis with spasticity, unilateral hemiparesis, brainstem-cerebellar pattern, ataxic syndromes, basal ganglia syndrome, and tremor-myoclonus. The clinical picture, functional consequences, and management of each of these syndromes is presented.

A judicious admixture of medical, rehabilitative, and surgical techniques can provide a comprehensive approach that will enable many of these patients to improve their functional capacities and minimize complications. Drug therapy remains, in most of these syndromes, a secondary and often disappointing adjunctive measure. For selective cases of severe and resistive disorders, neurosurgical procedures such as stereotaxic thalamotomy or implantation of electrical stimulators are a final therapeutic consideration. Detailed long-term functional outcomes of these procedures have not yet been educed.

Some of the syndromes, particularly the variants of cerebellar ataxia, may significantly improve over several years. Even after spontaneous neurologic improvement has ceased, continued or belated rehabilitative efforts may achieve still further functional recovery in patients with these disorders.

REFERENCES

1. Adams, R and Victor, M: Principles of Neurology, ed 3. McGraw-Hill, New York, 1985.
2. Rowland, LP (ed): Merritt's Textbook of Neurology, ed 7. Lea and Febiger, Philadelphia, 1984.
3. Davis, RA and Davis, L: Decerebrate rigidity in humans. Neurosurgery 10(5):635, 1982.
4. Roberts, AH: Severe Accidental Head Injury: An Assessment of Long-Term Prognosis. The Macmillan Press Ltd., London and Basingstroke, 1979, p 38.
5. Appel, SA (ed): Movement disorders. Neurol Clin 3(2), 1981.
6. Thomsen, IV: Late outcome of very severe blunt head trauma: A 10–15 year second follow up. J Neurol Neurosurg Psychiatry 47(3):260, 1984.
7. Adams, JH: The neuropathy of head injuries. In Viken, PJ and Bruyn, GW (eds): Handbook of Clinical Neurology. Vol 23: Injuries of the Brain and Skull. Elsevier, Amsterdam, 1975.
8. Fahn, S, Marsden, CD and Van Woert, M: Definition and classification of myoclonus. In Fahn, S, Marsden, CD and Van Woert, M (eds): Advances in Neurology. Vol 43: Myoclonus. Raven Press, New York, 1986, p 1.
9. Starosta-Rubinstein S, et al: Post-traumatic intention myoclonus. Surg Neurol 20:131, 1983.
10. Lapresle, J: Palatal myoclonus. In Fahn, S, Marsden, CD and Van Woert, M (eds): Advances in Neurology. Vol 43: Myoclonus. Raven Press, New York, 1986, p 265.
11. Klawans, H et al: Drug induced myoclonus. In Fahn, S, Marsden, CD and Van Woert, M (eds): Advances in Neurology. Vol 43: Myoclonus. Raven Press, New York, 1986, p 251.
12. Young, R and Shahani, B: Asterixis—One Type of Negative Myoclonus. In Fahn, S, Marsden, CD and Van Woert, M (eds): Advances in Neurology. Vol. 43: Myoclonus. Raven Press, New York, 1986, p 137.
13. Klug, N et al: Decerebrate rigidity and vegetation signs in the acute midbrain syndrome with special regard to motor activity and intracranial pressure. Acta Neurochir (Wein) 72(3–4):219, 1984.
14. Jabre, A, Sawaya, R and Arthur, S: Decerebrate posturing with the syndrome of inappropriate secretion of antidiuretic hormone. Surg Neurol 23(1):56, 1985.
15. Jennett, B and Teasdale, G: Management of Head Injuries. FA Davis, Philadelphia, 1981, p 236.
16. Griffith, ER: Spasticity. In Rosenthal, M et al (eds): Rehabilitation of the Adult with Head Injury. FA Davis, Philadelphia, 1983.
17. Glenn, MB and Rosenthal, M: Rehabilitation following severe traumatic brain injury. Sem Neurol 5:(3):233, 1985.
18. Sandel, ME, Abrams, PL and Horn, LJ: Hypertension after brain injury: Case report. Arch Phys Med Rehabil 67(7):469, 1986.
19. Matthews, DJ: Inhibitive Casting in Pediatric Head Injury. Presented at 10th annual post-graduate course on Rehabilitation of the Brain Injured Adult and Child. Williamsburg, Virginia, June, 1986.
20. Barnard, P et al: Reduction of hypertonicity by early casting in a comatose head-injured individual. A case report. Phys Ther 64(10):1540, 1984.
21. Booth, BJ, Doyle, M and Montgomery, J: Serial casting for the management of spasticity in the head-injured adult. Phys Ther 63(12):1960, 1983.
22. Young, RR and Delwaide, PJ: Drug therapy-spasticity (two parts). N Engl J Med 304(1,2):28, 96, 1981.
23. Garland, DE, Luch, RS and Waters, RL: Current uses of open phenol nerve block for adult acquired spasticity. Clin Orthop 165:217, 1982.
24. Halpern, D and Meelhuysen, FE: Phenol motor point block in management of muscular hypotonia. Arch Phys Med Rehabil 47:659, 1966.
25. Carpenter, EB and Seitz, DG: Intramuscular alcohol as an aid in the management of spastic cerebral palsy. Dev Med Child Neurol 22:497, 1980.
26. Garland, DE and Keenan MA: Orthopedic strategies in the management of the adult head-injured patient. Phys Ther 63(12): 2004, 1983.
27. Hoffer, MM et al: The split anterior tibial tendon transfer in the treatment of spastic varus hindfoot

of childhood. Orthop Clin North Am 5(1):31, 1974.

28. Herman, R, Mayer, N and McComber, SA: Clinical pharmaco-physiology of dantrolene sodium Am J Phys Med 51(6):296, 1972.

29. Mayer, N, McComber, SA and Herman, R: Treatment of spasticity with dantrolene sodium. Am J Phys Med 52(1):18, 1973.

30. Herman, R, Freedman, W and Mayer, N: Neurophysiologic mechanisms of hemiplegic and paraplegic spasticity: Implications for therapy. Arch Phys Med Rehabil 55(8):338, 1974.

31. Tomlinson, BE: Brain stem lesions after head injury. J Clin Pathol: 23(Suppl 4): 154, 1970.

32. Rodineau, J et al: Long term motor prognosis in patients with severe cranial trauma. Ann Med Phys 13:25, 1970.

33. Koller, KC: Pharmacological trials in the treatment of cerebellar tremor. Arch Neurol 41:280, 1984.

34. Edwards, RV: Nadolol use for cerebellar tremor. Am J Psychiatry 139(11):1522, 1982.

35. Gerstenbrand, F et al: Cerebellar symptoms as sequelae of traumatic lesions of upper brainstem and cerebellum. Int J Neurol 7:271, 1970.

36. Pettigrew, LC and Jankovic J: Hemidystonia: A report of 22 patients and a review of the literature. J Neurol Neurosurg Psychiatry 48(1):650, 1985.

37. Sandyk, R: Hemichorea—A late sequel of an extradural haematoma. Postgrad Med J 59(693):462, 1983.

38. Burke, RE, Fahn, S and Gold, AP: Delayed onset dystonia in patients with "static" encephalopathy. J Neurol Neurosurg Psychiatry 43:789, 1980.

39. Brett, EM: Progressive hemidystonia due to focal basal ganglia lesion after mild head injury. J Neurol Neurosurg Psychiatry 44:460, 1981.

40. Chandra, V, Spunt, AL and Rusinowitz, MS: Treatment of post-traumatic choreo-athetosis with sodium valproate (letter). J Neurol Neurosurg Psychiatry 46(10):963, 1983.

41. Robin, JJ: Paroxysmal choreo-athetosis following head injury. Ann Neurol 2:447, 1977.

42. Harris, FA: Facilitative technique and technological adjuncts in therapeutic exercise. In Basmajian, JV (ed): Therapeutic Exercise, ed 4. Williams and Wilkins, Baltimore, 1984.

43. Diamant, H: The salivary apparatus. In Hinchcliffe, R and Harrison, D (eds): Scientific Foundations of Otolaryngology. Year Book Medical Publishers, Chicago, 1976.

44. Andrew, J: Surgery for involuntary movements. Br J Hosp Med 26(5):522, 1981.

45. Andrew, J, Fowler, CJ and Harrison, MJG: Hemidystonia due to focal basal ganglia lesion after head injury and improved by stereotaxic thalamotomy. J Neurol Neurosurg Psychiatry 45:276, 1982.

46. Niizuma, H et al: Stereotaxic thalamotomy for postapoplectic and posttraumatic involuntary movements. Appl Neurophysiol 45(3):295, 1982.

47. Bullard, DE and Nashold, BS Jr: Stereotaxic thalamotomy for treatment of post-traumatic movement disorders. J Neurosurg 61(2):316, 1984.

48. Rosenberg, DB and Nelson, M: Reduction of dystonia and spasticity following deep brain electrode implantation: Correlation with somatosensory evoked potential studies. Poster presentation at American Academy of Physical Medicine and Rehabilitation and American Congress of Rehabilitation Medicine annual meetings, Baltimore, October, 1986.

49. Waltz, JM, Reynolds, LO and Riklan, M: Multi-lead spinal cord stimulation for control of motor disorders. Appl Neurophysiol 44(4):244, 1981.

50. Eiras, J and Garcia-Cosmalion, J: Post-traumatic myoclonic syndrome, effectiveness of the thalamic lesions on the action myoclonus. Arch Neurobiol (Madr) 43(1):17, 1980.

51. Ellison, PH: Propranolol for severe post-head injury action tremor. Neurology 28(2):197, 1978.

52. Obeso, JA and Narbona, J: Post-traumatic tremor and myoclonic jerkings (letter). J Neurol Neurosurg Psychiatry 46(8):788, 1983.

53. Lance, JW: Action myoclonus, Ramsey Hunt syndrome and other cerebellar myoclonic disorders. In Fahn, S, Marsden, CD and Van Woert, M (eds): Advances in Neurology. Vol. 43: Myoclonus. Raven Press, New York, 1986, p 33.

54. Andrew, J, Fowler, CJ and Harrison, MJ: Tremor after head injury and its treatment by stereotaxic surgery. J Neurol Neurosurg Psychiatry 45(9):815, 1982.

Chapter 11

Communication Disorders in Adults

MICHAEL E. GROHER, Ph.D.

Loss of the ability to communicate effectively can be a frequent finding secondary to severe head trauma. Only in the past decade has the importance of speech and language come to the fore as a crucial determinant of the patient's acute and future health status. As Najenson and colleagues[1] have pointed out, communication may play the pivotal role in determining the quality of survival.

Most of the literature has dealt only with the medical management of the patient, treating communication and its role in total rehabilitation in an accessory manner. The importance of speech and language deficits after head trauma has been minimized, partly from failure to agree on an accepted terminology that accurately describes the deficits, partly from the lack of empirical data relative to the treatment of communication disorders, and partly from the failure to believe that communication deficits secondary to head trauma deserve special attention because they represent a unique speech and language symptomatology.

The difficulty in describing the exact nature of the speech and language deficits is in part due to the variability in the acute communication symptomatology and in the eventual course and outcome of recovery. Patients who are rendered unconscious or who are semicomatose rarely are able to communicate. Less severe injuries may produce clinically normal speech and language skills, but the patient may not be aware of the events that transpired immediately before or after the accident. Between these two extremes, there may be any manner of deficit in the patient's communication skills. The patient's communication status may de-

pend on when the examiner completes the assessment. Failure to state when communication measures are made during the course of recovery is part of the reason much of the earlier literature[2–5] relative to communication deficits after trauma lacked agreement as to the exact nature of the pathology and its progression over time. Patients clearly manifest a different set of communication deficits at different stages in their recovery. The problem of accurate description is compounded by the failure of many investigators to use either a repeatable or a standardized testing procedure, thus creating gaps and irregularities in the interpretation of the accumulated data. To report that a patient evidenced a naming deficit or a problem with auditory comprehension, without knowing the level of severity or complexity, opened the door for different interpretations of the patient's communicative abilities and led to subsequent confusion over the nature of the deficit.

Further difficulty in understanding the nature of the communication deficits after head trauma arises from the inconsistencies in the terminology used to describe the disorder. Early reports[2, 3] focused on the issue of post-traumatic amnesia and the accompanying loss of memory as the primary mechanism to explain poor communication skills. Russell and Espir[6] stated that these severe losses of memory that may be part of post-traumatic amnesia often amount to a mild form of aphasia. London[7] described communication losses as changes in intellectual functioning due to forgetfulness, poor concentration, and slow wits. Luria[8] felt those communication deficits after head trauma definitely were consistent with a pattern of confused language that was clearly different from that of patients who had aphasia secondary to etiologies other than trauma. After investigating a sample of 14 patients with closed head trauma, Groher[9] concluded that the patients evidenced both elements of aphasic and confused language disturbance in the acute stages of recovery, but that the specific aphasic component quickly resolved, leaving the patient with what Halpern and coworkers[10] termed "the language of confusion." After examining 69 patients who were at least 1 year after injury Sarno and associates[11] found that they could be divided into three groups: those with classic aphasia including all subtypes; those with dysarthria and linguistic deficits; and those with "subclinical aphasia" characterized by language processing disorders during testing but without impressive clinical manifestation of aphasia. Hagen and colleagues[12] have taken the stance that language impairments after head trauma should be diagnosed and treated as part of an underlying cognitive disorganization. Stern and Stern[13] conceptualized the disorder as one of disruption in thought processing whose pattern is dictated by levels of abstraction and complexity.

These seemingly apparent differences in the use of descriptive terminology lead one to question whether or not investigators are describing truly identical groups of patients, whether or not different descriptions arise because of when the observations were made, or whether, as Hagen[14] notes, their wide "variability is their only commonality." That is, to study this population as a homogeneous group is very difficult.

Descriptions of communication disorders after trauma may be at odds because of several often ignored methodologic considerations. Answers to some of the following questions may help eliminate some of these discrepancies. First, one must consider the nature of the traumatizing act. Did it produce an open or a closed head injury? Missile wounds, for instance, are more likely to produce open head injuries, whereas automobile accidents typically produce closed head injuries. If there is a communication deficit secondary to the traumatizing act, is there a difference between these two groups?

Second, are age and a previously positive neurologic history important in determining the effects of trauma on communication? Unfortunately, many of these patients are eliminated from group studies.

Third, has the investigator selected patients who were comatose or not comatose following trauma? Does this affect recovery? What radiographic and/or neurologic evidence is presented? That is, do the patients have focal, multifocal, or diffuse disease? Was there extracerebral hematoma or intracerebral hemorrhage? Did they have extensive neurosurgical intervention, and were there complications? At what point in the patient's recovery were observations of communication skills made, or were observations gathered longitudinally?

Finally, are patients who present with communication disorders secondary to trauma appropriately grouped, or were they studied as part of a sample of patients with communication dysfunction secondary to vascular disease? Attention to parameters of patient selection and methods of observation should assist the clinician in interpreting the variability that exists among studies of patients with communication disorders following head injury.

OPEN VERSUS CLOSED HEAD TRAUMA

Most of the early literature that discussed communication disorders and head trauma dealt with patients who had suffered open head injury, usually from fragment penetration during war.[8, 15, 16] These descriptions usually sought to connect a particular speech or language disorder to a specific lesion site in the central nervous system. Invariably, postmortem analysis revealed that these penetrating lesions producing speech and language disorders were generally confined to the frontal, temporal, and parietal lobes of the left cerebral hemisphere. Patients were then divided into groups using typologic systems for classifying aphasia. Dresser and associates[17] concluded that in left hemisphere lesions, the deeper the penetration, the poorer the eventual outcome of communication skills. In a large series of World War II veterans with penetrating head injuries, Walker and Jablon[18] found that in one-third of the patients studied, language recovered after 9 months. After 7 to

8 years, one half of this group remained aphasic. Mohr and coworkers[19] supported these data in a study of Vietnam veterans, concluding that linguistic recovery, if it were to occur, would take place within 1 year. Aphasic symptomatology in the group of patients studied was more associated with periods of unconsciousness following injury. Salazar and associates[20] studied the language and cognition 5 years after trauma in 15 Vietnam veterans suffering basal forebrain lesions. They found only minimal deviations in performance when compared with normal control subjects; however, these patients did perform poorer on tasks involving recent memory, probably related to their accompanying involvement of the hippocampus. After reviewing the linguistic profiles of patients with penetrating injuries, Newcombe[21] concluded that most had nonfluent disorders with outcomes most similar to those of patients with linguistic disorders secondary to vascular insult.

Luria's work[8] remains the only investigation that sought to compare the speech and language deficits of open and closed head trauma patients. After reviewing 800 cases, Luria concluded that there did not appear to be any significant differences in the language capabilities of both groups immediately after trauma; the two groups did differ, however, after a period of 1 to 3 months. Incidence of aphasic disturbance following trauma to the left cerebral hemisphere decreased from 75 to 38 percent in closed head injuries, whereas they declined from 88 to 68 percent in open head injuries. Open head injury patients also displayed aphasic symptomatology longer than did closed head trauma patients. In addition, closed head injury patients in the initial period suffered fewer communication deficits as a group than did the penetrating wound patients. The implication from Luria's work is that patients with closed head injuries and communication deficits not only improved more following trauma than did patients with open head injuries, but also improvement occurred at a faster rate.

Hagen and coworkers[12] have suggested there may be clinical differences in communication symptomatology between open and closed lesions because of the varying nature of the pathology. They chose to divide trauma patients into four categories: closed head trauma, depressed skull fracture, pene-

trating wounds, and brainstem/cerebellar pathology, all of which have the potential of creating different and varying effects on communication. In some cases, the resultant deficits may overlap among groups.

The incidence of communication disorders in large groups of patients with open head trauma ranges from 14 to 23 percent, with a median of 20 percent.[22–24] Variation in incidence of communication dysfunction in unselected groups of patients with closed head trauma appears to depend on whether or not the patient was rendered unconscious and on how one defines the resultant communication deficit. For instance, in a study of 125 closed head injured patients consecutively admitted to a rehabilitation medicine center with histories of coma ranging from 10 minutes to 6 months, all patients had disorders of communication efficiency.[11] Thirty-seven percent of this group met the criterion to be classified as aphasic, while the remainder experienced subclinical aphasic symptomatology with and without dysarthria. Thomsen[25] found that 50 percent of consecutively admitted patients with unconsciousness and closed head injury had aphasia by observation 4 months after the trauma. A similar figure was reported by Najenson and associates[1] in a mixed group of open and closed head injured patients. After administering the Multilingual and Neurosensory Examination for Aphasia to a consecutive series of 50 patients with and without periods of unconsciousness, Levin and associates[26] found that 16 percent could be classified as aphasic, while one half had deficits in naming that presumably compromised communication skills. Writing to dictation also was a common deficit.

DURATION OF UNCONSCIOUSNESS

In general, even short periods of unconsciousness following closed head injury will impact negatively on communication skills.[9, 11, 27] Experience is conflicting as to whether or not the duration of coma can be correlated with the severity of the communication disorder. After reviewing the data of 125 patients tested at a median of 26 weeks following injury with durations of coma ranging from 10 minutes to 6 months,

Sarno and associates[11] could not find a direct correlation between coma length and severity of linguistic impairment. Although they did not provide evidence to support correlative significance, Najenson and co-workers[1] did find that even after prolonged coma, communication recovery was possible. Arts and associates[28] reported on the dramatic recovery of an 18-year-old girl who was in vegetative state for 2½ years who recovered communication skills 6 years following her severe head injury. Groher[9] measured the relationship between language and memory test scores for 5 consecutive months, and the number of days unconscious in 14 patients who had suffered closed head trauma. He concluded that a positive relationship did exist for those patients who were unconscious for 6 or fewer days and for 32 or more days; that is, patients who were unconscious for fewer than 6 days had better initial and final language and memory skills than other patients, and patients who were unconscious for more than 32 days had the poorest communication immediately following insult and 6 months later. After studying 50 patients with closed head injury, Levin and associates[29] found a positive correlation between coma and specific aspects of linguistic performance—particularly visual naming skills, word associations, and oral and written language comprehension. No correlations were found on sentence repetition and the Token Test. With the exception of the work of Sarno and her associates,[11] the small number of patients in these studies and the lack of other empirical evidence relative to communication deficits and the length of unconsciousness make it difficult to be sure that the duration of unconsciousness plays a direct role in either the initial communication deficits or their eventual outcome.

EFFECTS OF FOCAL AND DIFFUSE DAMAGE ON COMMUNICATION

Trauma to the skull is capable of producing focal, multifocal, and diffuse effects in any part of the central nervous system at any particular level with varying degrees of decompensation of communication. Usually, the location and extent of the lesion, together with the patient's age and premorbid medical history, will dictate the accompanying speech and language deficits. However, because head trauma can produce lesions at the trauma site, opposite it, and anywhere in between, it may be difficult initially, as Wertz pointed out,[30] to classify the resultant symptoms. Luria[8] suggested that it was too difficult to localize the pathology immediately after the trauma (both open and closed) but that localizable signs could be forthcoming after a 1-month period when brain edema had subsided.

It is generally accepted that closed head injuries tend to produce more diffuse or multifocal neurologic symptoms,[30, 31] whereas penetrating injuries produce more focal pathology[12, 17] that may be similar in outcome to that of patients with focal injury from vascular etiology.[27] Luria[8] found that specific localization of pathology from focal or diffuse effects was easier in closed head injury because the dura remained intact. Understanding the implications for diagnosis and treatment of whether or not a patient has a communication disorder secondary to closed (diffuse or multifocal) or open (focal) head injury is important in prognosis and rehabilitative approach. Focal left cortical pathology usually results in disorders of language, right focal cortical pathology in disturbances of perception and visual integration, and diffuse impairment in disturbance of cognition including awareness, attention, memory, abstractive skills, and orientation, of which specific deficits of language and perception are a part.

APHASIA SECONDARY TO TRAUMATIC AND VASCULAR ORIGINS

Many investigations of aphasia in the past 30 years have selected their subjects without regard to whether the etiologic factor producing the aphasia was vascular or traumatic. In those patients who had suffered closed head trauma, there usually is no neurologic evidence to support a unilateral focal lesion. In light of the present knowledge about the effects of trauma on communication, the wisdom of grouping trauma and vascular patients with communication disorders into one empirical investigation is highly suspect.

Alajouanine and associates[32] argued that

traumatic language problems did not differ from those of vascular etiology because both had localizable damage; however, their prognoses may be different because trauma patients tended to be younger. It was not clear in this study whether or not Alajouanine meant closed or open head trauma. In their discussion of recovery, Kertesz and McCabe[33] acknowledged the uniqueness of trauma patients by providing a separate analysis of their recovery, noting that their recovery was better and faster than that of patients with vascular disease and communication disorders. They also alluded to the young age of the typical trauma patient as a variable that may play an important role in recovery.

One of the first studies to separate patients whose aphasia was secondary to vascular insults from those whose aphasia was due to trauma was completed by Heilman and colleagues[34] in 1971. It was one of the first efforts to study systematically a group of patients, all of whom evidenced speech and language pathology secondary to closed head trauma. Although their evaluation of the patients selected focused on types of aphasia, the authors did note that the most common form of aphasia in this group (anomia) was often associated with other higher cortical functions.

The differences between the types of speech and language performance of trauma patients and patients with vascular disease were also a part of the investigation by Halpern and coworkers.[10] They tested a group of 40 patients with neurologic involvement, using 10 parameters of speech and language performance. The pattern of performance in the trauma group was clearly different from that of the group of patients who suffered impairment from vascular etiologies. They felt that the pattern of performance by the trauma patients was most consistent with confused language, wherein patients evidenced specific language impairment (not as severe as those with vascular insults) and a generalized disorientation that affects the structure and relevancy of language.

Use of the term "aphasia" to classify the language disorder following head trauma has important clinical manifestations for recovery and prognosis of communication. First, aphasia is the result of focal (usually left hemisphere) disease, implying a specific linguistic deficit with all other cognitive functions remaining relatively unimpaired. Treatment would focus on strengthening linguistic skills utilizing other intact cognitive modalities as systems for input. Behavioral disorders that might interfere with learning are minimal.

Levin and coworkers[29] evaluated the linguistic recovery in 21 patients with traumatic head injury with different levels of initial severity and pathologic sequelae. Nine patients totally recovered. Of the remaining 12, 6 had specific linguistic deficits associated with mild diffuse and left focal pathology. The remaining 6 had expressive and receptive deficits together with cognitive impairment associated with severe diffuse injury. Implicit in this division is the use of the term "aphasia" to describe focal pathology and recognition of the fact that some patients evidence additional deficits not unlike those described by other investigators.[9, 10, 12, 30] Luria[8] also found that he could divide a large number of both open and closed head injured patients into three groups: (1) those with total aphasia with loss of basic cognitive skills, (2) those with aphasia not accompanied by deficits in cognition, and (3) those with subtle language impairment only seen on more difficult linguistic tasks.

After studying the communication disorders of 125 patients with closed head injury, Sarno and coworkers[11] found that the group could be divided into three subgroups: (1) those with classic aphasia, N = 37; (2) those with dysarthria and subclinical aphasia, N = 43; and (3) those with subclinical aphasia, N = 45. Subclinical aphasia was defined as those patients with deficits in linguistic processing during testing who did not evidence deficits clinically. Using a test battery administered at a median 26 weeks after injury that tapped both functional and confrontational language skills, they found significant differences between the group with classic aphasia and the one with subclinical aphasia. The designation of a separate group of classic aphasic subjects from a population of traumatically injured patients supports the findings and conclusions of other investigators.[8, 26, 29] Of interest was that while *all* patients in their study admittedly "evidenced linguistic impairment which was only apparent on testing, not in conversation," Sarno and coworkers described in their classic aphasia group 13 patients with nonfluent aphasia and 5 with global aphasia. It is difficult to imagine that those two subgroups did not evidence linguistic impairment in conversation, since the former group (even those with mild impairment) usually show obvious expressive struggle and agrammatism, while the latter group rarely comprehends or can participate in conversation. Perhaps if followed for a longer period of time the classic aphasia group's linguistic profile would approximate that of the subclinical aphasia group. Then, the only distinguishing factor would be those with linguistic (high-level) deficit with or without dysarthria. Groher[9] found support for use of the term "aphasia" only for the acute stages following trauma. Thomsen[35] used "aphasia" to describe the linguistic deficits of her subjects but concluded that "it (was) not possible in this series to consider aphasia as an isolated disorder, since impaired language was part of a neuropsychological syndrome in which residual deficits of general memory often dominated."

Hagen and associates[12] and more recently Hagen[14] have acknowledged the presence of a specific linguistic disorder in the traumatically injured, but argue that such impairments do not stand alone and are part of an underlying cognitive disorganization that is characterized by poor memory, poor judgment, disorientation, and perceptual disturbances—all of which will have an impact on the patients' use of language. The residual language impairments of the traumatically injured are part of an underlying cognitive disorganization and are, therefore, distinct from other language disturbance secondary to neurologic causative factors.[12] Moss[36] has summarized the cognitive approach to diagnosis and treatment by noting that what have been damaged are the supportive processes for communication, of which speech and language are just one part. The theoretical underpinnings of the cognitive approach in understanding the communication deficits of trauma patients are most useful because they allow one not only to explain specific speech and language deficits, but also to link these deficits to the oft-observed disorders of memory, orientation,

and perception, and abnormal psychosocial behavior, which receive special attention in other sections of this book.

SPECIFIC SPEECH AND LANGUAGE DEFICITS

Luria[8] divided the aphasic symptomatology of both open and closed trauma, left hemispheric lesions into three major categories: (1) total aphasia, which was a severe loss in the powers of expression and reception of language and was accompanied by loss of ability to attend (this form usually lasted for the first 2 to 3 weeks); (2) typical aphasic symptomatology, including disorders of auditory comprehension, naming, word-finding, and reading and writing disturbances, not accompanied by other disorders of cognitive function such as attention, perception, or memory; and (3) subtle and slight loss of language in which expressive output was less smooth, articulation impairment on difficult or more unusual words, and poor comprehension of more difficult grammatical constructions, all of which were not equally apparent at all times, especially during patient fatigue.

Leischner,[5] in a group of 55 patients with open head trauma, found that the majority evidenced deficits in both the expression and reception of language secondary to lesions in the left parietal and temporoparietal lobes. The second most common finding was an expressive aphasia, followed by sensory aphasia and anomias. In addition, most patients evidenced agraphias, alexias, finger agnosia, constructive disorders, and apraxias. Mohr and colleagues[19] found that most patients with penetrating injuries had nonfluent disorders associated with parietal lobe damage. Patients with nonfluent aphasia showed the most improvement, whereas three fourths of those with Wernicke's aphasia did not.

Heilman and coworkers[34] studied 13 patients with closed head trauma and aphasia. Using the Boston Test for Aphasia, they divided their subjects into two major groupings based on expressive and receptive language scores. Nine of the 13 patients demonstrated anomic dysphasia that was characterized by mostly fluent speech with verbal paraphasias and circumlocutions. Evidence for a large number of patients with naming disorders has been supported by other investigators.[10, 27] An overall preponderance of fluent rather than nonfluent disorders as residual deficits following closed head injury has been a consistent finding among investigators.[9, 11, 25, 27, 37] Of those patients described as aphasic by Sarno and associates,[11] most were classified as demonstrating Wernicke's aphasia, while those with deficits ascribed to subclinical aphasia had high test scores in overall fluency with particular difficulty noted on sentence repetition tasks.

Adamovich and Henderson[37] sought to compare the linguistic capabilities of normal control subjects with those of patients with traumatic injury both prior to and at 6 months after injury, utilizing a battery of 39 selected diagnostic subtests. Both trauma groups demonstrated poorer verbal and visual recall scores than did the normal control group. The less-than-6-month trauma group had no consistent pattern of errors, but had more difficulty with reading, verbal and graphic naming, verbal absurdities, and describing differences than the group that was 6 months postinjury, although the latter group also had deficits in tasks of sequencing, problem-solving, and insight.

Five of the 10 patients studied by Halpern and coworkers[10] who evidenced confused language skills were patients suffering from trauma of less than 3 months' duration. Those patients were measured in 10 categories of intellectual and language functioning. Confused patients evidenced deficits in all 10 categories. The highest percentage of impairment for this group was in arithmetic, followed by reading comprehension, writing to dictation, and relevance. The least affected areas were fluency, auditory retention, naming, and syntax. The category of language relevance separated this group from those with aphasia, general intellectual impairment, and apraxia. The authors also commented that these patients gave bizarre responses to the testing stimuli, leading them to conclude that clarity in thought process and accuracy of memory were impaired. Such irrelevance in their responses was not evident to the patients, and they made no attempts to correct them. Lack of relevance in language output has been frequently mentioned by other investigators as one of the hallmarks of patients suffering from head trauma.[9, 12, 38]

Using the Porch Index of Communicative Ability (PICA), Groher[9] measured the speech and language characteristics of 14 closed head trauma patients immediately after regaining consciousness and at monthly intervals up to 6 months after injury. Patients initially showed a marked reduction in all language modalities when compared with other aphasics. Verbal skills were the strongest (33rd percentile), while graphic (12th percentile) and gestural (6th percentile) skills lagged behind. Most difficulty on the PICA was noted on subtests II and III, which require the patient to show the examiner what to do with common environmental objects. In addition, comprehension of reading material was poor, a finding both Heilman[34] and Halpern[10] and their colleagues reported. All subjects initially had a marked anomia, with both literal and nominal paraphasic errors during production. Patients were unable to write the names of objects and could not write to dictation. By the end of the fifth month, all language skills were at the 70th percentile level. Patients were able to make their needs known verbally and could sustain an informal conversation. In fact, most observers felt that their communication skills were normal, which was consistent with the findings of Sarno and associates.[11] However, standardized testing revealed that patients continued to show delays in simple and complex auditory processing tasks, irrelevance in language output, and difficulty in spelling and sentence construction.

Hagen and coworkers[12] list some of the more typical language problems that usually occur at some time during the patient's recovery: word retrieval problems, decreased auditory comprehension, poor visual and reading comprehension, expressive language that may be characterized as jargon, linguistically intact statements that lack relevancy, confabulation, circumlocution, tangential expressions, failure to inhibit the flow of language, and problems with verbal and graphic syntax.

In his characterization of confused language skills of patients suffering from presumably chronic closed head injury, Hagen[14] found that most patients retain the basic phonologic, syntactic, and semantic

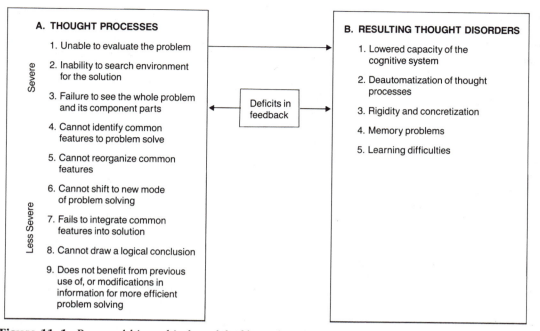

Figure 11–1. Proposed hierarchical model of how disordered levels of thought processes (problem-solving skills) contribute to resultant thought disorders. The model is particularly applicable in identifying levels of processing disorders as a method in understanding the problem-solving deficits associated with traumatic brain injury. (Adapted from Stern and Stern.[13])

relationships in language, yet have difficulty in communication because responses are irrelevant, confabulatory, circumlocutory, and tangential, often lacking a logicosequential relationship between thoughts. Summarized by Holland,[39] their residual deficits are one of communication competence in the face of good linguistic skills.

Stern and Stern[13] sought to theoretically conceptualize the linguistic deficits of the traumatically injured as part of a neuropsychologic model explaining the relationship between language and thinking (Fig. 11–1). Such a model is similar to the conceptualizations by Hagen,[14] implying that communication deficits secondary to traumatic injury represent problems in thought processes that lead to thought disorders or problems in using language to solve problems. The preponderance of irrelevancy, confabulation, circumlocutory, and tangential responses in language noted by Hagen[14] are natural consequences of disordered thought processes. Patients who are unable to recognize, analyze, and synthesize the use of language to draw conclusions and make inferences will quite naturally confabulate and

circumlocute as they attempt to solve a problem. Failure to process thoughts logically will give rise to irrelevancy and tangentiality while attempting to sequence relationships between thoughts, all of which will distort the message, decompensating communication effectiveness.

RECOVERY OF COMMUNICATION

In the acute stages of recovery from head trauma, maintenance of vital life functions is the primary concern of the medical staff. As the patient achieves medical stability, attention is focused on the evaluation of motor and sensory systems and failure to communicate with the environment. Establishing a viable communication system between patient and staff greatly enhances the ease with which medical care can be provided. Communication can become an important barometer for assessing change in the patient's acute medical status. Therefore, it can help provide a valuable dimension in the physician's prognostic statements to the family. As the patient improves, documentation of positive change in communication may be most important in determining the quality of survival, many times dictating future social and vocational goals.

As previously noted, patients who remain in comatose or vegetative states for long periods of time tend to have poorer prognoses for communication recovery than do those with a shorter duration of unconsciousness. While some may indeed show return of communicative function, the amount of recovery across all linguistic modalities will not be as great as for patients who do not remain comatose for extended periods.

Recognizing the need to describe communication recovery from comatose states to states of more awareness and participation in the communicative act, Hagen and associates[40] developed eight descriptive categories that aid in describing communicative recovery. This categorization is important because it links communication recovery with cognitive recovery. Therefore, it relies not only on charting the patient's communication skills but also on observation of behaviors other than communication that are important prerequisites for meaningful communication. The scale ranges from level one (no response), in which patients are unaware of any external input; through level four (confused-agitated), in which patients respond primarily to their own internal confusion with inappropriate verbalizations and confabulation; to level eight (purposeful and appropriate), in which patients are finally able to communicate effectively by integrating recent and past events (although social, emotional, and intellectual capacities may still be reduced in situations involving the use of more complex and abstract language strategies).

Ideally, information on the recovery of communicative function in trauma patients should include not only the amounts and kinds of functions recovered, but also data on how fast the recovery occurred. In general, investigators have found that patients with communication disorders secondary to head trauma recover more communicative skills at a faster rate than do patients with vascular etiologies. Additionally, recovery can continue for a longer period of time[41, 42] than the 1-year period most aphasiologists generally agree on for those suffering communication deficits secondary to cerebral vascular disease. Return of comprehension often precedes verbalization, but both skills quickly parallel one another in recovery. Patients frequently attain good conversational skills after 6 months,[11] but residual deficits are elicited easily[34, 41] with confrontational linguistic tasks,[11] and on tasks that force the patient to use their language to solve problems.[9, 11, 25, 37, 41] Residual deficits in more abstract reading and writing skills are common and persistent.[25]

Benton[43] reported that verbal skills for traumatically injured as measured with the Wechsler Adult Intelligence Scale typically peaked at 18 months, whereas recovery on the performance subtests continued to improve for several years.

Kriendler and coworkers[44] studied verbal fluency in eight closed trauma and 12 open trauma patients immediately after suffering the insult and 1 to 3 months later. Compared with the speaking rate of normal persons, theirs was slower in 10 cases and normal in 9, one patient having complete speech loss. Re-evaluation of speaking rate showed the rate had increased in 18 patients. The speaking time and the number of utterances also had risen significantly by 3 months postinjury.

Najenson and associates[45] studied the cognitive deficits of 40 closed and open head trauma patients at 6 months postonset. All had been rendered unconscious, but had regained consciousness within 3 months. Their initial language evaluations revealed that 20 of the 40 were aphasic. At 6 months, 6 of that 20 no longer could be classified as aphasic based on scores obtained with the Functional Communication Profile (FCP); the other 14 remained aphasic. During the 6-month period, they observed a great deal of variability in recovery of functions, although patterns of recovery did exist. All subjects showed progressive improvement, more in listening and reading skills than in oral expression and writing. After 6 months, most of the language difficulty involved high-level reading tasks and narrative writing. After 6 months no patient remained in the "severe" category of impairment on the FCP.

Najenson and associates[1] studied the recovery pattern of another group of 15 patients, mostly with closed head injuries. The mean age was 33, and none of the 15 underwent craniectomy. None functionally recovered, and six remained vegetative. Recovery of this group was similar to that of the first group. Visual and auditory comprehension returned first, followed by oral expression; however, this group showed later recovery of reading and writing skills. The first sign of recovery occurred from 3 weeks to 5 months after regaining consciousness, with complete recovery ranging from 4 to 9 months. The authors noted that communication recovery paralleled locomotor recovery.

Those investigators who sought to classify the linguistic deficits by aphasia type have noted a consistent pattern of recovery, from global involvement to disorders of naming.[34, 41, 46] The pattern of recovery from global involvement to disorders of fluency is atypical when compared to recovery patterns of aphasics with cerebrovascular disease. Those with cerebrovascular disease and global aphasia resolve into disorders of nonfluency (Broca's, isolation, and transcortical motor aphasia). Although disorders of nonfluency are described,[8–11] they do not predominate. Typical of fluent disorders, verbalizations are marked by paraphasic output and deficits in auditory monitoring.

Using the PICA, Groher[9] measured the speech and language characteristics of patients with closed head trauma immediately after regaining consciousness (mean time 9 days) and each month for a period of 5 months. All subjects were male veterans, and their mean age was 31. Unlike the recovery patterns reported by Najensen and associates,[1, 45] verbal skills were the first to return and were superior to comprehension capabilities up to the first month. Significant improvement in comprehension, verbal, and graphic skills was noted at 2 months after onset. Verbal skills improved significantly up to the fourth month. After 4 months, comprehension abilities were as good as verbal skills. Writing performance was just becoming functional after 4 months. As language improved, so did negative behavior patterns such as striking out during care and uncooperative behavior during therapeutic rehabilitation sessions. All patients were capable of making their needs known verbally after 5 months but still evidenced signs of aphasia characterized by processing delays and word-finding difficulty. After 6 months, patients scored well on most standardized measurements for aphasia but still evidenced problems of relevancy, inhibition of verbal output, and sequential organization of ideas into logical outcomes. After 6 months, six of the 14 patients returned to work. All six had difficulty with job assignments, primarily related to continued ineffective problem-solving using communication, poor memory, and poor judgment.

Reporting on their experience with 2000 head trauma patients over a 17-year period Hagen and coworkers[12] found that recovery of communication skills was closely allied to, and even dependent upon, the patient's cognitive recovery. Levels of cognitive function during recovery served as important determinates of communication recovery. It is their contention that cognitive (and, therefore, communication) recovery is hierarchical, beginning with the recovery of attention mechanisms (both internal and external), discrimination, seriation, memory, categorization, association, and finally skills involving analysis and synthesis of input and output.

Kaplan and associates[47] followed six patients with closed head trauma for a period of 2 to 6 months, rating their cognitive function upon hospital admission and at discharge. Part of this assessment included general communication status, oral expression, reading, writing, and evaluation of dysarthria. Other aspects of cognition that were tested included memory and perception. Patients had impairments on all language tasks ranging from moderate to severe. After discharge, most patients had mild reading and moderate writing disturbance. Four of the patients' overall communication dysfunctions were judged as moderate impairment, while the remaining three patients evidenced mild impairment. None of the seven reached the communication level of minimal impairment.

Six of the seven trauma patients presented by Kertesz and McCabe[33] had achieved aphasia quotient scores of 90 and above on the Western Aphasia Battery after 3 months. Initial aphasia quotient scores ranged from below 30 to 88. One patient continued to show improvement after 2 years. Porch[48] also has presented data suggesting that recovery of trauma patients can continue past 2 years. He found that their recovery pattern was characterized by a series of recovery spurts followed by plateaus. Gradual improvement was seen up to 32 months after onset.

Thomsen[41] did a 10- to 15-year follow-up study on 50 patients, 19 of whom had been initially aphasic. Sixteen were aphasic after 2½ years and four remained aphasic after a 10- to 15-year period; 10 patients were lost to follow-up. However, more than four patients continued to complain of memory disorders and had problems with auditory analysis with frequent occurrences of forgetting what they wanted to say. Nonetheless, these data provide numerical support to the view that linguistic recovery can continue past 3 years.

Scherzer's data[42] support the notion that visual information processing can continue to recover with training, although verbal processing did not show significant change. His patients entered a 30-week training program with an average postcoma interval of 59 months.

Groher[9] reported that although patients at 6 months postinjury could not be described as typically aphasic, they were still unable to use their language to solve problems at home and at work. Malkmus[38] confirms this impression, commenting that most patients at 6 months have intact language skills as tested by standardized aphasia test batteries; however, their language capabilities are only sufficient for more concrete and simple tasks. For instance, auditory and graphic retention of material beyond one sentence may be difficult, especially if the requirement is to focus on one specific bit of information. In general, the retention and integration of auditory and graphic information become poorer as the amount and complexity increases. Malkmus[38] found that expressive language skills after 6 months are intact for most daily conversational needs but, when patients are asked to formulate specific responses, begin to deteriorate. Patients often continue to evidence ideational perseveration, with difficulty shifting from topic to topic, continued word-retrieval problems, disorganization of thought content with incompleteness of expression, and reduced abstract verbal reasoning capacity. It is these language characteristics that led Thomsen to the conclusion that it is not language per se but the ineffective use of it that

may be a part of failure to socially adjust.[42] Errors of relevancy, perseveration, and incompleteness, coupled with a failure to recognize such errors, make social successes difficult. Such errors clearly are the result of organicity, but because patients evidence seemingly normal linguistic competencies they will be viewed as personality deviations, forcing many undesirable behavioral compensations. Sarno and coworkers[11] noted that in two thirds of 125 traumatically injured patients, discrepancies between seemingly normal linguistic skills and their deficits could easily lead to unrealistic expectations resulting in failure, hopelessness, and a sense of frustration.

Difficulty with higher-level language skills past 6 months also was noted by Thomsen.[25] In a follow-up study of 12 patients with aphasia secondary to closed head trauma, Thomsen found that four had no characteristics of aphasia but had aphasic traits like poor verbal learning. Patients also showed continued difficulty on language problems involving analysis of synonyms, antonyms, metaphors, and picture descriptions.

Groswasser and colleagues[49] studied a group of 20 patients with closed and open head trauma with aphasia, at admission, at 6 months, and at 30 months after onset. After 6 months, 14 of the 20 remained aphasic; at 30 months, nine remained aphasic, with the majority of scores on the Functional Communication Profile ranging between 31 and 74.

In a 15-year follow-up of 864 open and closed trauma patients, Dresser and associates[17] found that 53 of the 88 who were aphasic were now employed, implying that their communication deficits did not significantly interfere with their employment. In comparison with the group without aphasia, these authors felt that the presence of aphasia was a significant predictor of unemployment.

THE PROBLEM OF SPEECH PRODUCTION

Early consequences of severe traumatic injury may leave the patient unable to relate to his or her environment, especially through expressive modalities. Differentiation among early expressive disorders seen in the vegetative state, in the locked-in syndrome, in akinetic mutism, and in mutism is important if one is to establish a viable communication system. While some of these disorders such as dysarthria can be said to be pure motor disorders, others such as akinetic mutism can be associated with motor production and linguistic processing deficits.

Patients who are considered to be in the vegetative state show little or no perceptible interaction with the environment. Clearly, input channels are involved and expressive language may be compromised by linguistic and motor production disorders. Patients who are locked-in suffer from whole body motor de-efferentiation that compromises motor speech. Some linguistic skills remain intact as the patient is able to communicate with eyeblinks that are appropriate to incoming stimuli and in some cases show evidence of minimal comprehension and make attempts at sound production, although speech is never well formed. Involvement of both motor and linguistic expressive systems is presumed. Levin and associates[50] described mutism as the abolition of speech not attributable to cranial nerve involvement wherein the patient can understand simple commands and communication through nonvocal channels. In a prospective study of patients with mutism, Levin and coworkers[50] found that 3 percent of 350 consecutive brain injury admissions were mute. Further study of the nine patients who were mute revealed that most were under 20 years old and that cortical and subcortical pathology could both be associated with mutism. Those with diffuse cortical injury had prolonged mutism, while those with focal basal ganglia lesions had the best prognosis. Bricolo and colleagues[51] found that the return of comprehension preceded that of expression in patients who were initially mute.

The incidence and type of dysarthria following head trauma are not well known. In general, the type and its effect on speech intelligibility will be reflected by the locus of damage in the central nervous system. Diffuse upper motor neuron involvement produces pseudobulbar effects, whereas brainstem contusions produce ataxic or flaccid effects. During the acute stages of recovery, multiple systems may be involved. Currently there are no data documenting the incidence of dysarthria without accompanying linguistic disorders. The data that Sarno and associates[11] presented suggest that even those patients suspected of having dysarthria alone had accompanying linguistic deficits. In general, it appears that dysarthria is a frequent accompaniment of traumatic injury, although the extent that it compromises speech intelligibility is not well documented. Once identified it appears that the problem persists over time. In longitudinal group studies no data on response to treatment have been reported.

Rusk and coworkers[4] reported that in a group of 93 trauma patients approximately one third (30) evidenced dysarthria in their acute illness. In follow-up studies between 5 and 15 years, 35 patients were unchanged, while 14 patients had significantly improved. Specific measures of improvement were not discussed. Dresser and associates[17] reported that eight continued to show signs of dysarthria after 15 years. Hagen and associates[12] acknowledge the presence of dysarthria in trauma patients, secondary to both neurologic system damage and cognitive (failure to monitor articulation) deficits. They reported such symptomatology as articulatory imprecision, reduced or accelerated rates, reduced audibility, and monopitch and monoloudness, which they feel is part of "the language of confusion." Najenson and coworkers[1] also have noted the prevalence of the harsh and monotonous voice quality with reduced breath support. They found that the dysarthric symptomatology continued to be present after language skills had approached normal levels. Malkmus[38] has estimated that 20 percent of her patients with language deficits also evidenced either mixed, flaccid, or spastic forms of dysarthria, which initially produce severe intelligibility problems; however, her experience suggests that good intelligibility returns after 12 months. All 14 of the closed head trauma patients studied by Groher[9] evidenced dysarthria after regaining consciousness. Nine of the 14 had spastic (pseudobulbar-type) dysarthrias and five had spastic-ataxic involvement. Six of the nine patients with spastic dysarthria completely resolved within 6 months, while the remaining eight continued to evidence only minimal intelligibility problems, none of which significantly interfered with communication. Kaplan and coworkers[47] reported similar improvement in their patients, noting that all seven patients initially had dysarthria ranging from severe to moderate, while the majority had only mild effects at discharge 2 to 6 months later.

Thomsen[25, 41] documented the presence of aphasia and dysarthria in 50 traumatically injured patients at 2½ and at 10 to 15 years post-trauma. All 15 patients who had dysarthria immediately after coma continued to have dysarthria 10 to 15 years later, although intelligibility scores were not reported. During this period, linguistic skills improved. From a group of 125 closed head injured patients, Sarno and colleagues[11] found 13 patients with dysarthria (median 26 weeks postinjury) accompanied by linguistic deficits. The dysarthria ranged from mild to completely unintelligible. Presumably their reduced verbal test scores in comparison to a group with linguistic deficits and no dysarthria were negatively influenced by the presence of motor incompetency.

SUMMARY

The study of communication disorders secondary to head trauma is only in its initial stages. The importance of the communication act in the rehabilitative process cannot be underestimated, as the constructs of language are closely tied with other cognitive dimensions such as perception, memory, orientation, attention, and psychosocial behavior—all of which are frequently impaired. Because of the frequent involvement of more than one cognitive system, the treatment of specific language, perceptual, or memory deficits should be interdependent, thus placing the responsibility on all professionals of the rehabilitation team to coordinate their efforts. Prerequisite behavior for successful communication— including environment awareness, selective attention, and auditory and visual discrimination—often are acutely impaired and need to receive the special attention of the speech/language pathologist. Patients must be directed through these early stages of recovery if they are to receive the maximum benefits from communicative remediation efforts.

The evidence presented suggests that communication disorders that result from head trauma are different from those whose etiology may be vascular, neoplastic, or metabolic. Trauma patients with communication disorders tend to be younger, display multiple cognitive system involvement, recover more language at a faster rate, improve for a longer period of time, and have the opportunity to return to some type of work setting more often than do patients with vascular disease and aphasia. These differences suggest that the approach to treatment of trauma patients may be different from that used with other aphasic patients. Although more traditional aphasia rehabilitative techniques may be used at some point in the patient's recovery, other types of treatment strategies also must be initiated. These include structuring the patient's environment to aid in orientation and communication; providing constant organized language inputs at appropriate levels of complexity; providing tests that develop selective attention and discrimination of incoming stimuli; developing environments that allow the patient to respond in his or her strongest expressive modality; and eventually providing treatment to assist the patient in solving life's everyday problems that depend on language.

Even though most patients recover basic language skills by 1 year, they continue to show deficits in the analysis and synthesis of receptive and expressive language skills. These skills are necessary for any successful communication beyond more automatic and social conversational levels, in the performance of job assignments, and in the learning of new information. Patients need continued speech and language evaluation and rehabilitation even though their performance may appear normal to most observers. Remediation should be directed toward helping the patient retain specific bits of critical information gathered from larger pieces (auditorily and graphically), analysis and/or summarization and categorization of language inputs, organization of expressive outputs into logical sequences, and concentration on shifting topics without significant delay. All tasks should be oriented toward focusing the patient to perform in a way that is relevant to the stimulus input, whether self- or environment-stimulated. Success in job performance and in psychosocial adjustment will depend on how well the patient is able to perform these more abstract tasks of language use.

REFERENCES

1. Najenson, T et al: Recovery of communication function after prolonged coma. Scand J Rehabil Med 10:15, 1978.
2. Russell, WR: Cerebral involvement in head injury: A study based on the examination of 200 cases. Brain 55:549, 1932.
3. Glaser, MA and Shafer, FP: Skull and brain trauma; their sequelae: Review of 255 cases. JAMA 98:271, 1932.
4. Rusk, HA, Block, JM and Lowman, EW: Rehabilitation of the brain-injured patient: A report of 157 cases with long term follow-up of 118. In Walker, E, Caveness, W and Critchley, M (eds): The Late Effects of Head Injury. Charles C Thomas, Springfield, IL, 1969, p 202.
5. Leischner, A: The pathological brain syndrome in the brain injured. In Walker, E, Caveness, W and Critchley, M (eds): The Late Effects of Head Injury. Charles C Thomas, Springfield, IL, 1969, p 364.
6. Russell, WR and Espir, MLE: Traumatic Asphasia: A Study in War Wounds of the Brain. Oxford University Press, London, 1961, p 111.
7. London, PS: Some observations on the course of events after severe injury of the head. Ann Roy Coll Surg Engl 41:460, 1967.
8. Luria, AR: Traumatic Asphasia: Its Syndromes, Psychology and Treatment. Mouton, The Hague, 1970, p 39.
9. Groher, M: Language and memory disorders following closed head trauma. J Speech Hear Res 20:212, 1977.
10. Halpern, H, Darley, FL and Brown, JR: Differential language and neurologic characteristics in cerebral involvement. J Speech Hear Disord 38:162, 1973.
11. Sarno, MT, Buonaguro, A and Levita, E: Characteristics of verbal impairment in closed head injured patients. Arch Phys Med Rehabil 67:400, 1986.
12. Hagen, C, Malkmus, D and Burditt, G: Intervention Strategies for Language Disorders Secondary to Head Trauma: Short Course. American Speech-Language and Hearing Association, Atlanta, 1979.
13. Stern, B, and Stern, JM: Neuropsychological outcome during late stage of recovery from brain injury: A proposal. Scand J Rehab Med Suppl 12:27, 1985.
14. Hagen, C: Language disorders in head trauma. In Holland, AL (ed): Language Disorders in Adults. College-Hill Press, San Diego, 1982, p 260.
15. Goldstein, K: After-Effects of Brain Injuries in War: Their Evaluation and Treatment. Grune & Stratton, New York, 1942, p 87.
16. Hook, O: Comments on rehabilitation of the brain injured. In Walker, E, Caveness, W and Critchley, M (eds): The Late Effects of Head Injury. Charles C Thomas, Springfield, IL, 1969, p 179.
17. Dresser, AC et al: Gainful employment following head injury: Prognostic factors. Arch Neurol 73:111, 1973.
18. Walker, AE and Jablon, S: A follow-up study of head wounds in WW II. VA Medical Monograph, 1961.
19. Mohr, JP et al: Language and motor deficits following penetrating head injury in Viet Nam. Neurology 30:1273, 1980.
20. Salazar, AM et al: Penetrating war injuries of the basal forebrain: Neurology and cognition. Neurology 36:459, 1986.
21. Newcombe, F: Missile Wounds of the Brain. London, Oxford University Press, 1969, p 161.
22. Pense, F: Diagnosis and therapie der neurosen bei hir neurletzten. In Rehwaldied, E (ed): Das Himtrauma. G. Thieme Verlag, Stuttgart, 1956, p 107.
23. Hillbom, E: Delayed effects of traumatic brain injuries, neurological remarks. Acta Psychiatr Scand 137:7, 1959.
24. Teuber, HL: Recovery of function after brain injury in man. In Outcome of Severe Damage of the Central Nervous System. CIBA Foundation Symposium. Elsevier-North Holland, New York, 1975, p 13.
25. Thomsen, IV: The patient with severe head injury and his family. Scand J Rehabil Med 6:180, 1974.
26. Levin, HS, Grossman, RG and Kelly, PJ: Aphasic disorder in patients with closed head injury. J Neurol Neurosurg Psychiatry 39:1062, 1976.
27. Levin, HS: Aphasia in closed head injury. In Sarno, MT (ed): Acquired Aphasia. Academic Press, New York, 1981, p 427.
28. Arts, WFM et al: Unexpected improvement after prolonged post-traumatic vegetative state. J Neurol Neurosurg Psychiatry 48:1300, 1985.
29. Levin, HS et al: Linguistic recovery after closed head injury. Brain Lang 12:360, 1981.
30. Wertz, R: Neuropathologies of speech and language: An introduction to patient management. In Johns, DF (ed): Clinical Management of Neurogenic Communicative Disorders. Little, Brown, Boston, 1978, p 78.
31. Brookshire, R: An Introduction to Aphasia. BRK Publishers, Minneapolis, 1973, p 84.
32. Alajouanine, T et al: Etude de 43 cas d'aphasie post traumatique. Encephale 46:1, 1957.
33. Kertesz, A and McCabe, P: Recovery patterns and prognosis in aphasia. Brain 100:1, 1977.
34. Heilman, K, Safron, A and Geschwind, N: Closed head trauma and aphasia. J Neurol Neurosurg Psychiatry 34:265, 1971.
35. Thomsen, IV: Evaluation and outcome of aphasia in patients with severe closed head trauma. J Neurol Neurosurg Psychiatry 38:713, 1975.
36. Moss, C: Unpublished master's thesis, 1980.
37. Adamovich, BB and Henderson, JA: Cognitive deficits post-traumatic head injury: Diagnostic and treatment implications. Paper presented at American Speech-Language Hearing Association Annual Convention, Cincinnati, November, 1983.
38. Malkmus, D: Personal communication, 1980.
39. Holland, AL: When is aphasia, aphasia? The problem of closed head injury. In Brookshire, RH (ed): Clinical Aphasiology Conference Proceedings. BRK Publishers, Minnesota, 1982, p 345.
40. Hagen, C, Malkmus, D and Durham, P: Levels of cognitive functioning. In Rehabilitation of the Head Injured Adult. Professional Staff Association, Downey, CA, 1979, p 27.
41. Thomsen, IV: Late outcome of very severe blunt head trauma: A 10–15 year second follow-up. J Neurol Neurosurg Psychiatry 47:260, 1984.

42. Scherzer, BP: Rehabilitation following severe head trauma: Results of a three year program. Arch Phys Med Rehabil 67:366, 1986.

43. Benton, A: Behavioral consequences of closed head injury. In Odom, GL (ed): Central Nervous System Trauma Research Status Report. National Institute of Neurological and Communication Disorders and Stroke, Bethesda, MD, 1979, p 49.

44. Kriendler, A, Michailescu, L and Fradis, A: Speech fluency in aphasics, Brain Lang 9:199, 1980.

45. Najenson, T et al: Prognostic factors in rehabilitation after severe head injury: Assessment six months after trauma. Scand J Rehabil Med 7:101, 1975.

46. Thomsen, IV: Evaluation and outcome of traumatic aphasia in patients with severe verified focal lesions. Folia Phoniatri (Basel) 28:362, 1976.

47. Kaplan, P, Phillip, P and Halper, A: Recovery of self-care activities in patients with traumatic brain damage. Presented at the 3rd Annual Postgraduate Course on the Rehabilitation of the Traumatic Brain-Injured Adult, Williamsburg, VA, 1979.

48. Porch, B: Recovery from Aphasia. PICA Workshop, Albuquerque, NM, 1976.

49. Groswasser, Z et al: Re-evaluation of prognostic factors in rehabilitation after severe head injury: Assessment thirty months after trauma. Scand J Rehabil Med 9:147, 1977.

50. Levin, HS et al: Mutism after closed head injury. Arch Neurol 40:601, 1983.

51. Bricolo, A, Turazzi, S and Ferriotti, G: Prolonged post-traumatic unconsciousness. J Neurosurg 52: 625, 1980.

Chapter 12

Cognitive Deficits

D. NEIL BROOKS, Ph.D.

After severe head injury, cognitive deficits are the rule. The early deficits (confusion, disorientation, prolonged retrograde amnesia) are associated with an impairment in conscious level and reflect the effects of diffuse and limbic brain damage.[1] Most patients who do not die early after injury eventually recover consciousness, and regain full orientation, when they may show a wide range of severities and chronicities of cognitive deficit. These have been documented extensively in the last 15 years, and this chapter therefore concentrates mainly on the post-1980 literature and will deal with issues that dominate the literature (the nature, prediction, evolution, variability, and functional consequences of cognitive deficits). The remaining dominating issue (remediation) is dealt with elsewhere in the book.

This chapter begins with a discussion of the nature, prediction, evolution, and variability of cognitive deficits, before moving on to deal with functional consequences. An underlying philosophy is that, whereas general rules concerning prediction can readily be derived, they are of little value in guiding management of the individual patient. As in any branch of clinical medicine, patient management remains an art as well as a clinical science.

THE NATURE OF COGNITIVE DEFICITS

A wide variety of deficits has been reported, including disorders of intellect, learning and memory, language, perceptual-motor function, goal selection, and planning. These have been summarized extensively, and the reader is referred to recent texts.[2–5]

In view of the variety of deficits, researchers have attempted classifications ranging from simple lists of different deficits[5] to aggregations of deficits under broad functional headings.[6] Prigatano's classification (Table 12–1) is useful.[6] It may be difficult to separate disorders or attention and concentration from disorders of speed of processing (as Prigatano has done) or initiation and planning from judgment and perception, but the classification is nevertheless a useful aide memoire. Furthermore, it can be seen that any one psychologic measure (e.g., an intelligence test) will not address all these post-traumatic cognitive issues. Unless measures sensitive to head injury are used, deficits will be missed.

As a way of structuring the rest of the section, Prigatano's broad headings are used,[6] but aggregated under the three following headings:

1. Disorders of learning and memory
2. Disorders of complex information processing (incorporating speed, planning, and so on)
3. Disorders of perception and communication

Disorders of Learning and Memory

Learning and memory disorders occur as a rule after severe brain injury. Memory complaints are made frequently by patients and corroborated by relatives (Table 12–2). The complaints range from trivial forgetfulness to a profound and temporary[7] or permanent amnesia. The deficits result in such widespread problems that an intriguing research problem consists of finding memory procedures on which head injured patients can perform within normal limits.

Table 12–1. CONDENSED VERSION OF PRIGATANO'S CLASSIFICATION OF COGNITIVE DEFICITS[6]

Attention and concentration
Initiation and goal direction
Judgment and perception
Learning and memory
Speed of information processing
Communication

IMMEDIATE MEMORY

Compared with more complex procedures, those relying on immediate memory are in general relatively spared in most patients. Even when impaired, the impairment is usually minor, unless the injury was of extreme severity or there has been a specific language impairment such as conduction aphasia. However, when the tasks become more prolonged or complex, deficits will certainly be found, particularly early after injury or during post-traumatic amnesia.[2, 8]

LONG-TERM MEMORY

With increasing task complexity or more prolonged storage of information, head injured patients begin to have marked difficulties.[9–12] The difficulties are likely no matter what the nature of the task (new learning, relearning, recall, recognition, or remote memory). While the existence of severe learning and memory deficits has been recognized for many decades, the underlying nature of the deficit is not well understood.

UNDERLYING DEFICITS

Usually it is assumed that the memory deficits necessarily result directly from brain damage diffusely distributed throughout the cortex, and more specifically within limbic structures.[13] Nevertheless, any clinician has seen the motivationally impaired patient who does not care about learning; or the frontally damaged patient who cannot make appropriate action plans for efficient learning; or the attentionally impaired patient who cannot sustain attention long enough for effective information encoding. In each case, the end result is poor performance on a test of learning and memory, but a poor performance achieved by diverse routes. Only a carefully chosen procedure administered and interpreted with clinical skill will enable specification of the mechanisms of cognitive breakdown.

In view of the problems in interpreting memory test performance, it is worth considering the broad processes involved in memory and learning (encoding, storage, and subsequent retrieval of information), to try to specify where breakdown has occurred. There may, of course, be disorders of all three broad stages resulting simply from a slowness in information processing.[14] Such a slowness is the rule after severe head injury (33 percent of Van Zomeren and Van den Berg's patients reported slowness at 2 years postinjury,[15] and 67 percent of Brooks and coworkers' cases at 5 years postinjury).[16]

Evidence that slowness may be one determinant of poor learning comes from Miller's pilot study of spatial learning.[17] Head injured patient performance was characterized by poor initial levels of learning but a substantial degree of subsequent learning which showed transfer to a similar task. However, caution must be used in interpretation of spatial and motor learning, as even in patients with severe amnesia or dementia such learning may be relatively well preserved.[18, 19]

A number of studies have attempted to identify specific disorders of encoding, or storage or retrieval,[2, 20–24] but a clear consensus is difficult to find. Certainly initial

Table 12–2. FREQUENCY OF COMPLAINTS OF MEMORY DISTURBANCE

Study	Complainant	Time after Injury	Frequency
Haramburu and coworkers[10]	Patient	Various	60%
Van Zomeren and Van den Berg[15]	Patient	2 years	54%
Sichez-Auclair and Sichez[67]	Patient	1 year	72%
Brooks and coworkers[16]	Relative	5 years	67%

storage of information is impaired,[2] but attempts to identify specific deficits (e.g., in encoding) have been thwarted by very small effects,[21] great variability,[24, 25] or a head injury performance that, though quantitatively below normal, is not qualitatively different.[22, 25] The study by Vakil and Tweedy[24] is particularly interesting in its attempt to separate automatic from effortful encoding of information, showing that head injured patients do have problems in encoding information of a type that is normally coded automatically (information such as frequencies of occurrence, temporal order, spatial locations).

In summary, the exact nature of memory disturbances has proved difficult to unravel. The memory deficit is so pervasive and insensitive to experimental manipulation that it has to be concluded that most or all underlying cognitive processes are impaired (encoding, storage, retrieval), or that some other processes (speed of information processing, formulation of cognitive plans, intention to learn) may be at least partly responsible. While, on balance, it is likely that for most patients the underlying disturbance does indeed reflect specific memory impairments associated with damage to limbic structures,[1, 13] the influence of other cognitive deficits must not be underestimated, nor must the influence of other factors such as low motivation, poor morale, and depression.

Disorders of Complex Information Processing

Although few studies have discussed this issue per se, many have addressed it tangentially by studying intellectual functioning. The most commonly used intellectual instrument has been the Wechsler scale—initially the Wechsler-Bellevue, then the WAIS, and finally the WAIS-R. Despite disadvantages of these procedures (long, multifactorial, sensitive to practice effects), their undoubted advantages have kept them in frequent use. These advantages include the profile of abilities gained, the opportunities for rich clinical observation on qualitative aspects of test performance, and the huge clinical folklore built up about performance on the scales.

On the Wechsler measures, results are easily summarized. Head injured patients have deficits. These are maximal on measures demanding learning, perceptuomotor response, and psychomotor speed. More "crystalized," overlearned functions are relatively well preserved, unless there is left hemisphere damage interfering with semantic processing. More "fluid" aspects of function involving here-and-now responses to new situations are much more vulnerable. This pattern of relatively preserved crystalized and relatively damaged fluid intellectual abilities has been known for many years as a consequence of any kind of acute or chronic diffuse damage, and its existence after severe head injury should be no surprise.[2, 5, 27–29] Why should there be such deficits? Attempts to answer this have appeared since the 1930s and have often indicated that speed of cognitive performance or keeping up a sustained effort may be primary problems.

In a further attempt to tease out the nature of the intellectual deficit, Mandleberg and Brooks[30] speculated that the reason underlying the relative vulnerability of "performance" compared with "verbal" intellectual items may be the more complex nature of the former. Performance items demand the integration of a number of functions (learning, perception, speed, cross-modal integration), and deficits of any of these could be manifested as a performance intelligence quotient (IQ) deficit.

A much more detailed "micro" analysis of the cognitive consequences of severe brain injury has come from psychologists working within an information-processing framework, and addressing issues of attention, speed of information processing, and distractibility.[31–35] Indeed Van Zomeren and colleagues[35] refer to the "riddles of selectivity, speed, and alertness" after head injury, suggesting that any of these processes could be damaged independently. "Selectivity" refers to focused arousal, the ability to concentrate and ignore distraction. "Speed" refers to speed of overall information processing, and "alertness" to arousal or level of activation. Each area is reviewed both conceptually and clinically by Van Zomeren and coworkers,[35] who show that on visual choice reaction time (assessing selectivity and speed) there was a highly deleterious effect of irrelevant information on the performance of head injured patients compared with controls. The mechanism of deficit appeared to be response interference, resulting from a deficit in speed of processing rather than focused attention per se.

The initial Dutch results concerning speed of processing are clear.[32, 33] On both simple and four-choice reaction time tasks, severely head injured patients performed poorly, but disproportionately so on the four-choice task. As the complexity of the information demand increased, so did the magnitude of the deficit. The earlier study involved patients seen at 3 to 4 months postinjury. At 2-year follow-up, most patients had normal results on simple reaction time, but showed continuing impairment on the four-choice task. The "complexity effect" was found even at the late follow-up. However, replication of this complexity effect has not been easy. Brouwer's recent study[34] failed to replicate, and he speculated that the complexity effect may be found only in patients with very severe injury. Similarly, Bennett-Levy,[14] using a much simpler test of speed of processing, failed to find a complexity effect.

The final area of attention investigated by the Dutch group is alertness. In the normal person, an expectation of performance demands (e.g., a warning signal) will trigger an electroencephalograph (EEG) pattern known as the contingent negative variation (CNV, or expectancy wave). Studies in head injury showed a decreased or absent CNV, suggesting a deficit in tonic alertness.[36, 37]

The ability of head injured patients to keep up a sustained effort has only recently been investigated in detail. On an examination of sustained effort and attention, as well as vigilance and EEG arousal,[34, 38] both head injured (8 patients tested early after injury) and control subjects showed a normal response decrement over time, with no evidence of a differential deficit in head injured patients.

In terms of drowsiness and attention lapses, the results were contrary to expectation; controls rather than head injured patients showed an increasing number of drowsy episodes over time. There was no evidence of a differentially greater tendency to attention lapses in head injury—if anything, the reverse pattern was found. Why head injured patients should show *less* drowsiness than normals is not certain. It may simply be that this small group of patients was unrepresentative of the severely injured population as a whole. A further possibility is contained in the compensation or coping hypothesis, which asserts that the cognitive deficits after head injury (e.g., memory, slowed information processing) will have marked effects on daily life, for which the patient may compensate, at least over a short time, by making greater efforts. With chronically raised levels of effort, the patient may begin to show secondary symptoms of stress (e.g., anxiety).

An alternative approach to the study of information processing has been carried out in New Zealand by Gronwall and coworkers.[39-42] She has made extensive use of the Paced Auditory Serial Addition Test (PASAT). In this demanding test, the patient hears a series of random digits. The second must be added to the first, the third to the second, and so on. In its requirement for constantly attending to and processing new information, while discarding the results of previous computations, this test can cause severe problems for head injured patients. Gronwall's initial results showed that even mildly head injured patients performed poorly on this task, particularly at fast presentation speed.

Within the attention and information-processing literature, some consistent results may be found. Head injured patients are slower at almost every aspect of cognitive performance from initial understanding of the task to planning strategies for solution and acting on those plans. As the complexity of information processing increases, the performance of head injured patients drops, but so does that of noninjured controls. Early work by the Dutch group reported a complexity effect in which increasing information-processing demands had a disproportionate effect on head injury performance; however, this effect has proved difficult to replicate, and it may simply have been a function of the initial severity of injury.

Deficits in Perception and Communication

The classic "focal" perceptual and constructional impairments found in stroke patients are not as a rule seen in patients with head injury, except very early when almost any stroke phenomenon can be seen. Later on in recovery, the "focality" of the deficits reduces greatly.

To some extent perceptual and communication deficits (particularly perceptual deficits) have been addressed already in the discussion of the effects of head injury on complex intellectual tasks, and in the discussion of studies such as those of Stokx and Gaillard[25] which have manipulated perceptual aspects of cognitive processing. For example, Stokx and Gaillard[25] examined encoding of information by presenting increasingly degraded visual stimuli. Degradation increased reaction time significantly in head injured patients, but it did the same, and to the same degree in noninjured control subjects. No specific disproportionate perceptual deficit was found here, although the finding of increased threshold for perceptual recognition has been noted by others.[43, 44]

On a more complex task (facial recognition) clear deficits were found.[12] Disordered facial recognition was common, being found in more than one quarter of severely injured patients. This reinforces the reports of family members early after injury that the injured patient appeared not to recognize them—another indication of the "focality" of the picture found early rather than late after injury.

Exactly why visual perceptual deficits are found is not certain. It may be that the early deficits (e.g., in facial recognition) may simply reflect the pervasive effects of cognitive confusion.[2] Alternatively, focal pathology such as hematoma may be to blame, but the important pathophysiologic mechanism of diffuse shearing should not be underestimated as a possible cause of visual disturbances. In postmortem studies ischemic and shearing lesions of the optic nerve and visual pathways can be found.[45] The former were particularly associated with diffuse damage, and it is quite possible that these could underlie at least some of the visual perceptual disturbances found late after injury. An alternative hypothesis is that visual perceptual deficits simply result from cognitive slowing so that time limitations prevent adequate analysis of information.

Just as perceptual deficits (particularly auditory deficits) have been relatively neglected, disorders of communication have been under-researched. Many workers included measures of language as part of a wider cognitive battery,[27, 28, 46] but until recently few have investigated language specifically. For exceptions see the work of Levin and coworkers,[47, 48] Najenson and associates,[49] Groher,[50] Thomsen,[51–53] and Sarno.[54, 55]

Language disturbances have been investigated indirectly by researchers using the Halstead-Reitan Battery,[29] or measures of semantic processing[27] or comprehension.[27] Verbal fluency deficits are certainly found, but it is a moot point whether such disorders should be called language deficits or deficits of complex processing, as the failure to make an adequate choice of retrieval strategy could underlie a poor performance here, as could simple slowness. Severe auditory comprehension deficits are rare.[27]

Levin's detailed study of language showed deficits on visual naming, word fluency (word association), and language comprehension (the token test).[48] Brooks and Aughton's results replicated those of Levin for fluency but not comprehension,[27] and this discrepancy may reflect the very early testing of many of Levin's patients, as Brooks and Aughton did find significant comprehension deficits 3 months after injury, but not thereafter.

Further examinations of aphasic impairment have come from Israel,[49] Scandinavia,[51–53] and the United States.[54, 55] Najenson[49] showed "complete recovery" in "semantic functions" in six of the 15 patients studied, and persisting aphasia in three patients. A much greater impediment to communication was dysarthria shown by a very large proportion of patients who recovered consciousness. The most vulnerable aspect of language was therefore the "motor aspect of speech," resulting in dysarthria, or amnestic or expressive aphasia.

Thomsen[51–53] has studied both early and later language performance, and found that dysarthria and residual language problems were very common; the latter including difficulties in word finding, word and phrase repetition, and difficulties in complex skills such as use of metaphor or complex descriptions. The deficits tended to be expressive rather than receptive (similar to the Israeli results), with only one patient (with a slow-wave EEG focus in the dominant parieto-occipital region) showing a comprehension disorder.

Sarno's detailed studies[54, 55] showed that within the first year of injury "no patient was spared some degree of verbal impairment, however mild or apparent." Thirty-nine of her 56 cases (70 percent) had either aphasia only or dysarthria with some clinical aphasia. The deficits were often substantial, and the pattern of performance was frequently that of the classic focal aphasia, with seven fluent; seven nonfluent; two anomic, and two global aphasics.

In summary, classic "focal" deficits may be seen with great frequency very early after injury, but as the patient recovers the focality of the deficits reduce. Nevertheless, subtle deficits in language and perceptual functioning are often present even late after injury, and may well be severe enough to cause difficulties in the patient's everyday functioning.

THE PREDICTION AND VARIABILITY OF COGNITIVE DEFICIT

Heterogeneity of cognitive performance is the rule after severe head injury, and this has become an emerging focus in the literature.[56–58] Studies of large groups of severely injured patients show a range of severities from quite unimpaired to devastated, and many workers have used indices of both focal and diffuse brain damage to try to predict cognitive performance.

Diffuse Damage

In view of the pathophysiology of head injury (e.g., primary brain damage resulting from diffuse neuronal shearing), there have been many attempts to assess the impact of diffuse damage on cognitive performance. Indices of diffuse damage have included coma duration (reflecting diffuse or left basal forebrain damage)[1] and post-traumatic amnesia (PTA). Both coma and PTA relate to more general aspects of outcome.[59–61] For assessing more focal damage, neurologic indices have included the presence of a hematoma, or of contusional or ischemic damage assessed by neuroimaging using computed tomography (CT) or magnetic resonance imaging (MRI).

As far as coma and PTA are concerned there are statistically significant relationships between increasing durations of either measure and increasingly impaired cognitive performance.[2, 5, 11, 13, 15, 32, 42, 62] Rather than laboriously summarizing each study, an attempt will be made to give an overview.

When correlations are performed between coma or PTA duration and cognitive outcome, they are usually statistically significant, but small, leaving much variance unexplained. When an analysis of variance rather than correlational approach is taken the results are usually significant:[62] for instance, a step-wise deterioration in memory performance when patients with PTA of short (0 to 7 days'), medium (8 to 27 days'), and long (more than 27 days') duration were compared. Variances were high, however: some patients with very long-duration PTA performed well and others with PTA of short duration performed badly.

An examination of the PTA studies suggests that there may be a threshold effect: patients who have PTAs of 2 weeks or less show great variability of performance, but as PTA increases, the predictability of cognitive deficit increases considerably.[14, 15] Very long PTAs (over a month) are very likely to result in poor cognitive performance. Shorter PTAs (2 weeks or less) may or may not be associated with good cognitive performance. Nevertheless, a coping, resourceful personality, high drive, and supporting social milieu may compensate for even a very long PTA.

Although there is a broad relationship between PTA/coma duration and cognitive performance, the relationship is by no means linear, and some workers have attempted to find limiting factors in the relationship. There is increasing evidence that PTA relates much more strongly to cognitive performance early rather than late after injury.[30, 57, 60, 63] Mandleberg and Brooks' study[30] of very severely injured patients found that PTA was a good predictor of more verbal aspects of intelligence up to 6 months after injury only, and performance aspects up to 12 months only. Surprisingly, Groher[50] found no significant relationship between duration of unconsciousness and language or memory skills either early (as soon as consciousness was regained) or late (120 days after injury).[50]

The Mandleberg and Brooks study[30] raises a further interesting point about predictors such as PTA, and this is that the predictive value may depend upon the cognitive task under consideration. Highly overlearned skills are much less vulnerable to injury,[29] and to that extent may show a much less clear relationship with severity of injury.

Even within highly overlearned skills, there are differences in the extent to which severity of injury predicts performance. For example, in the study by Levin and colleagues,[48] there was a significant relationship between coma and some but not all language functions. Significant associations were found for reading comprehension, visual naming, word fluency, and language comprehension, but not for sentence repetition or the token test—a result replicated using PTA as a predictor of token test performance.[62] Similarly, in Gronwall and Wrightson's study,[42] PTA correlated significantly with scores on an attention task but not with scores on visual sequential memory. On the Buschke Selective Reminding procedure, PTA correlated significantly with the mean number of words recalled on each trial, the cumulative number of words recalled on each trial, and the cumulative number of words in memory (long-term memory storage)—but not with long-term retrieval.

An unusual approach to the identification of the etiology of cognitive deficit has been reported by Ewing and associates,[64] who took groups of mildly head injured patients and noninjured control subjects and, by means of a hyperbaric chamber, tested them at a simulated altitude of 3800 m, high enough to cause mild hypoxia. The head injured patients' cognitive performance deteriorated under hypoxia, particularly so on vigilance and memory, unlike that of the controls. Hypoxic stress provoked a cognitive deficit almost certainly of an organic cognitive nature.

An alternative approach to the study of the relationship between diffuse damage and cognitive function has been to examine correlates rather than predictors of cognitive function. A correlate is a measure that can be taken at the same time as the cognitive examination, but that relates clearly to the severity of diffuse damage. Such a correlate would be a general outcome measure, e.g., the Glasgow Outcome Scale (GOS),[65] which divides conscious survival into three rating levels (severe disability, moderate disability, and good recovery).

At least four studies have addressed explicitly the relationship between Glasgow Outcome Scale categorization and cognitive status.[59, 60, 66, 67] These studies show that there is a much greater likelihood of continuing cognitive deficit in patients in the "severe disability" category when compared with those in the "good recovery" or "moderate disability" category. Usually patients with "severe disability" are quite disproportionately worse than those in the other two categories, although the distribution of cognitive scores of those in the "moderate disability" category overlap considerably with those in the remaining two categories. This overlap may be illustrated by the results of Sichez-Auclair and Sichez,[67] who showed that two of the 20 patients with severe memory deficit were in the GOS "good recovery" category and 10 were in the "severe disability" category. Seventeen of the 18 patients with minimal/absent memory deficits were in the "good recovery" category, and the remaining patient had "moderate disability." For those patients with a moderate memory deficit, 15 were in the "good," 10 in the "moderate," and one in the "severe" GOS category.

In view of a possible interaction of severity measures with time (e.g., the apparently increased efficiency of PTA as an early, rather than a late, predictor), the analyses of variance in the Brooks and coworkers study[60] were recalculated separately for patients seen early (within 3 months of injury) and those seen later. For the "early" patients, eight of the nine F ratios were significant comparing cognitive scores across three outcome categories, but for the "Late" group only two were significant. Pair-wise comparison showed that the significant F ratios arose from the particularly poor cognitive performance of the severe disability group. It may be that during the early period, outcome scale categorization and cognitive performance are heavily dependent on severity of injury, whereas later, both psychologic test performance and outcome scale categorization become much more multidetermined, with factors such as injury severity, focal neurologic deficit, affective, social, and behavioral status of the patient all contributing to the categorization.[60]

Focal Damage

The advent of high-resolution tomographic imaging of the brain has allowed other measures of brain damage (focal and diffuse) to be used in predicting later outcome. The study by Callum and Bigler[29] assessed the relationship between neuropsychologic performance and CT, using computerized techniques to estimate ventricular volume (VV), and the degree of cortical atrophy (ATVOL). The VVs were used to determine a volumetric ventricular-brain ratio (VBR). An examination of the VBR showed no significant findings in relation to verbal IQ (crystalized intelligence) but "robust negative correlations" with performance IQ. The memory quotient correlated significantly negatively with a variety of VBR measures (both left and right hemisphere). The degree of overall atrophy showed a significant relationship with WAIS performance (but not verbal) IQ, and the significant performance IQ correlation appeared to arise largely from left frontal atrophy. This study is particularly interesting, not only because of its meticulous use of volumetric CT data, but also because of its findings that fluid aspects of intelligence (rather than crystalized) relate to the degree of cerebral atrophy, and because of the finding of a relationship between cognitive performance and atrophy in the frontal regions. The role of frontal damage in cognitive deficits will be addressed in more detail toward the end of this section.

Other more focal predictors have been reported including the site or side of skull fracture; the site of initial impact, and the presence of a hematoma. Recent reviews[2, 5] have indicated that despite the overwhelmingly diffuse nature of the initial pathology in head trauma, focal cognitive effects can be found. For example, traumatic aphasic patients, although selected initially on simple severity of injury, nevertheless showed slow-wave EEG disturbance in the dominant temporal lobe or in both temporal lobes.[52] The pattern of cognitive disturbance in the Cullum and Bigler studies[29, 68] broadly reflected the lateralization of CT imaged brain damage.

An intracerebral hematoma is an obvious possible predictor of cognitive disturbance; patients with an evacuated subdural hematoma tended to perform worse on language measures than those without a hematoma.[28, 68] On memory performance, hematoma cases were found to be worse than those without. However, the various measures of brain damage are not independent. Patients with a hematoma tend to have larger ventricles and more cortical atrophy, just as those with a skull fracture tend to have a higher incidence of hematoma. Furthermore, in one study the patients with CT-verified intracranial lesions ("focal intracranial hemorrhage or mass effect") had a poor cognitive outcome after rehabilitation.[69] However, they also had very long comas and permanent motor disabilities compared with patients without such focal lesions.

This interaction between focal effects and severity of diffuse damage is not always in the expected direction.[62] When patients with a hematoma were compared with those without, they proved to be significantly better on a variety of cognitive measures. This was almost certainly because of a selection bias in the sample of cases and because results were not analyzed as a function of the locus of hematoma (e.g., epidural, subdural).

The classic "lateralized" cognitive deficits have been found to be associated with CT or positron emission tomographic (PET) or other evidence of lateralized lesions.[70, 71] However, a number of workers[2, 52] have found that increasing cognitive impairment is related not only (or even largely) to the pattern of lateralized damage, but to the position of damage in the neuraxis (the lower the damage the worse the cognitive deficit).[8, 66, 67, 72] For example, Levin and co-workers[66] found that early oculovestibular deficit predicted neuropsychologic impairment and did so independently of overall severity; and Sichez-Auclair and Sichez[67] found increasing severity of memory and intellectual deficit with lesions deeper in the neuraxis. (Patients with diencephalic lesions performed less badly cognitively than those with mesencephalopontine lesions.) Presumably damage to the upper brainstem of the type that results in oculovestibular disturbance in Levin's study also causes severe and diffuse damage to the white matter along the neuraxis toward the cortex, despite Levin's failure to find a relationship between the presence of oculovestibular deficit and longer durations of coma.

Although researchers such as Cullum and Bigler[29, 68] have reported interesting results on cognitive performance in relation to anatomic information, unequivocal interpretation of such data—particularly CT data— may be difficult. The difficulties are particularly pronounced when attempts are made to interpret the significance of lack of evidence (lack of signs of hemispheric damage). This point has been brought into focus recently by work in Glasgow that showed that MRI detected twice as many lesions following head injury as did CT.[73] For example, deep white matter lesions were detected in 30 percent of MRI images, but only 2 percent of CT images. Neuropsychologic testing in the same study[73] showed neuropsychologic deficits (particularly on learning and memory) in patients who had normal CTs but abnormal MRIs, indicating that the MRI lesions were indeed of functional significance.

That there should be at least some relationship between the pattern of focal or lateral abnormality of cerebral tissue and the pattern of cognitive deficit is not surprising, as the functional anatomy of the cerebral cortex in terms of cognition has been known for many years. What is surprising is that the relationship persists in blunt head injury, with its essentially diffuse primary damage. It is likely that focal and lateral predictors of cognitive deficit have been relatively underplayed, until at least the late 1970s, and the development of brain-imaging tools of increasing resolution is now changing this. Nevertheless, a word of caution is necessary. There is a broad correlation between the laterality of the cognitive deficit and the laterality of focal lesions, but many patients do not fit this trend. For example, Levin and associates[48] found that only seven of the 15 patients with predominant involvement of the left hemisphere were impaired on a least one language test, whereas six of the 10 patients with "greater injury of the right hemisphere" showed such an impairment.

Organic and Other Predictors

In view of the dramatic nature of severe head injury—loss of consciousness and life-threatening, severe, and prolonged disability in many cases—it is to be expected that researchers should assume that any cognitive deficits seen after injury result solely from the effects of brain damage. This assumption is increasingly difficult to justify. The nature of the head injury population (young risk

takers who may not have had a particularly impressive educational history before injury) and the more general effects of injury (loss of work, loss of friends, reduction in self-esteem) may all contribute to the final observed pattern of poor cognitive performance. To some extent careful matching of head injured patients and control subjects can account for the premorbid factors, but the pervasive noncognitive effects of head injury are difficult to replicate in a control group.

The work reviewed in this chapter has concentrated until now exclusively on organic predictors, and has found convincing evidence of dose-response relationships with indices such as coma and PTA. Nevertheless, there is a growing literature concerned with nonorganic predictors of cognitive deficit, particularly predictors relating to the patient's preinjury status. The most detailed recent study is that by Grafman and his colleagues.[74] This study concerned patients who had suffered predominantly missile injuries in the Vietnam conflict, and assessed the relationship between preinjury intelligence and lesion location and severity. The specific locus of injury proved to be more important than the volume of tissue loss when predicting specific cognitive impairments (e.g., verbal test impairment related to lesions of the left frontal and temporal cortex and underlying white matter), and impairment on tasks such as block design related to right hemisphere lesions, particularly to deep white matter. As far as more general cognitive functions are concerned (e.g., Wechsler IQ measures) total volume of brain tissue loss was of some value as a predictor of deficit in left hemisphere lesion patients, but much less so in those with right hemisphere lesions. The best predictor of persistence of cognitive deficits was preinjury intellectual or educational level. Nonorganic factors may be of considerable importance in predicting post-trauma cognitive performance, and such factors will set real limits on expectations of recovery. The rehabilitation implications of these findings are obvious.

Grafman and his colleagues are not the only ones to examine premorbid factors. Cullum and Bigler[29] noted the relationship between premorbid educational level and post-traumatic IQ, and Haramburu[10] and Brooks[75] and their coworkers found that patients who achieved successful vocational outcome following severe injury were those with a higher educational or occupational level before injury. Similarly, Sichez-Auclair and Sichez[67] found that premorbid factors were very important in predicting post-traumatic intellectual level. Before injury 19 percent of their 103 cases had deficient scholastic records, and 49 percent had premorbid sociocultural deprivation. Indeed, the researchers very kindly suggested that the negative premorbid features we noted,[30] (features such as heavy drinking and petty crime) were "pas un phenomene purement Britannique." A rough translation would suggest that such factors are not specifically British.

It appears therefore that two broad categories of variables predict the patient's post-traumatic cognitive status. The first is the severity of brain damage, and its relative distribution between the hemispheres and between cortical and subcortical structures. The second is the premorbid intellectual and social status. Naturally the preinjury and injury variables interact to give the final clinical picture. A further predictor of final cognitive status is likely to be the nature of the noncognitive changes suffered by the patient. These include impulsivity, motivational impairment, and lack of insight and drive. There appears to be little published information on these factors as predictors of cognitive outcome.

One type of change in the patient which falls somewhere between behavioral and cognitive is the so-called frontal pattern(s) of behavior, described so graphically and accurately by Harlow[76, 77] in his report of Phineas Gage.

Although the changes described were behavioral rather than cognitive, their impact upon cognition would be obvious and dramatic. It is now increasingly realized that the disorganization of behavior seen after frontal lobe damage will underlie deficits on many cognitive functions. One of the best recent clinical accounts of the clinical impact of frontal change after head injury is found in Walsh.[4] This text, which is strongly recommended, uses a brief literature review and an analysis of individual patients to show the range of deficits (in conceptual behaviour, perseveration, planning, executive functions) that may be found after frontal damage.

Broadly speaking, the frontal cortex may be divided functionally into dorsolateral, basal or basomedial, and medial zones. There is some evidence that the nature of the deficit varies according to the primary pattern of damage, so that dorsolateral lesions are likely to result in severe impairment in planning and a resulting deficit in learning. A very good example of this is found in the performance of such patients on maze tasks. Typically they show poor learning because they consistently break the rules and appear not to benefit from repeated performance, making the same error again and again in a perseverative fashion. This lack of the normal coupling between observation of error and subsequent change of performance will cause problems on many tasks including conceptual thinking, problem solving, and so forth.

Lesions of the basal or basomedial cortex may result in the classic frontal personality change of disinhibition—described so clearly by Harlow in his report on Phineas Gage. Such patients will have great difficulty in suppressing a previously learned or customary mode of responding. With lesions of the medial cortex (found rather less frequently after head injury than lesions in the other frontal areas), the deficits appear to be largely in the function of drive and/or arousal so that the patient shows poor self-direction and reduced levels of drive and activation, and presents a passive and lethargic picture. Again, the cognitive impact of such a behavior change is obvious. For further accounts of the effects of frontal damage, the reader is referred to Lishman,[78] Lezak,[3] Stuss and Benson,[79] and Stuss and co-workers.[80]

Medication

This section has reviewed the influence of organic, pretrauma, and post-trauma behavioral deficits on cognitive function after injury, and the interactions among these features. There remains one further variable that may have a major impact on cognitive performance, but on which there is somewhat less documentation. The factor is the medication that the patient may be taking. Many patients will be receiving anticonvulsants, either because of seizure disorder or prophylactically. Not only are anticonvulsants used commonly, but also other psycho-active drugs such as anxiolytics and major tranquilizers are used, both of which have documented deleterious cognitive effects.

In view of the high usage of anticonvulsants after head injury, it is this group of drugs that should be examined most closely. A number of different anticonvulsants are used after head injury, and their cognitive toxicity varies very dramatically. This issue has been studied recently by Trimble and his group,[81] who have shown that anticonvulsant drugs do impair cognitive function but to quite different degrees. Four drugs examined (phenytoin, carbamazepine, sodium valproate, and clobazam) resulted in significant deficits in performance even when serum levels were within conventional therapeutic ranges. However, the magnitude of the deficits varied widely. The most marked changes were with phenytoin. Sodium valproate and clobazam appeared to result in a slowing of mental processing speed, particularly so as the information processing demands of the task increased. Carbamazepine, on the other hand, appeared to result in a motor rather than mental slowing. Studies of epileptic patients showed that a change from polytherapy to monotherapy resulted in cognitive improvement, particularly if monotherapy was by carbamazepine. Even with monotherapy, cognitive function related to serum levels of the drug. These results are particularly important, in view of the widespread nature of anticonvulsant treatment after head injury. The head injured patient is likely to show not only cognitive deficits resulting from the initial brain damage (and the other factors described), but also additional deficits unless the pharmacologic status is kept under close review.

EVOLUTION AND RECOVERY OF COGNITIVE DEFICITS

Cognitive recovery studies have been reported since the 1930s. The studies have varied in the nature of the patient population, the intensity and duration of follow-up, and the cognitive functions under investigation. General intellectual functions, memory,[27, ,30, 82, 89] language,[49–53] and attention,[32, 40, 90] have all been reported. The vari-

ability referred to at the beginning of this section makes clear interpretation difficult, as do the unique problems raised by recovery studies.[58]

Intellectual Recovery

Even the earliest studies of intellectual recovery showed that the more complex, multifactorial, and intellectually demanding the procedure, the slower the recovery.[43, 82] Studies with more prolonged follow-up and more severely injured patients have involved the Wechsler Adult Intelligence Scale (WAIS)[30, 84, 85, 91] and Progressive Matrices and Mill Hill Vocabulary Scale.[92–95] The Mandleberg and Brooks data[30, 84, 85] showed marked improvement over time, particularly for the performance items. These items, however, showed the greatest deficits early after injury, and this finding both of differential sensitivity to injury, *and* a more prolonged recovery period for performance than verbal functions is also reported elsewhere.[87, 91] The Mandleberg and Brooks study incorporated a "comparison group" of 40 nonhead injured males who had been referred for a psychiatric consultation. At first administration all WAIS subtest results other than "Similarities" were significantly lower in the head injured group, but by the 5-month administration four of the verbal subtest results were essentially normal—unlike the performance items, all of which were significantly low. A more recent study[87] involved a small group of severely head injured patients, first very early and then a year later. It is difficult to know exactly how early after injury patients were tested, as this was described only as "shortly after the patient was considered testable, and testing could be arranged." Significant improvements were found on all subtests other than digit span. The authors suggest that because the verbal IQ–performance IQ discrepancy, apparent at the first testing had diminished by the second testing, the performance measures may be more sensitive to brain damage in the acute stage but become less so as time goes on. A further interpretation is that the discrepancy disappeared because of the differentially greater sensitivity to practice of the performance subtests.

Language and Memory Recovery

Language recovery was reviewed by Brooks[5] and by Levin.[2, 48] The studies of Thomsen[51] showed that on a re-examination 29 months after very severe injury there were still severe deficits involving amnestic and perseverative errors. Global aphasics tended toward sensory aphasia, often with severe dysnomia, a finding partly replicated by Kertesz.[96] A further analysis of a single patient[53] seen over a 10-year period showed enormous improvement from the 2-year picture of severely impaired semantic analysis, severe amnestic aphasia, and other difficulties, to mild or absent language problems at 12 years.

The important Israeli study[49] involved patients with prolonged coma and showed not only that functions may recover at different rates (visual and auditory comprehension improving before oral expression, reading, and writing), but also that different individual patients recover at very different rates. In some patients no improvement in language performance was seen until many weeks or even as many as 5 to 7 months after injury, although dysarthria remained a problem for many patients. This study is particularly valuable because of its close attention to an individual analysis of patients, the severe nature of the population studied, and the documentation of very late changes.

The final language study to be reviewed[50] involved small numbers of patients of considerable severity. The patients were tested five times on the Porch Index of Communicative Ability (PICA). Although there were language improvements over time, inspection of the data suggests that improvement was greatest early after injury between the first and second tests. In terms of the order of recovery, verbal skills continued to improve significantly up to the fourth assessment, whereas gesture and graphic skills improved significantly only up to the second assessment, indicating that although the recovery rate was high for these skills, the ultimate level reached was rather low. This would accord with Thomsen's[51] results that despite improvements, none of the 12 patients studied had a completely normal language function by 3 years after injury.

The more recent studies of memory recovery[88, 89, 97] give results similar to those reported in early studies.[31, 43, 82] Memory recovery appears to be slower than that of many other functions, and even 3 years after injury, many patients are achieving below-average scores on memory.[88] The Scottish and Dutch data[58] showed slow recovery over the first year, although with a marked improvement on verbal learning from the third test at 6 months to the fourth at 12 months. Nevertheless, the 12-month performance was still not normal.

A number of the studies have reported recovery curves giving mean scores at different time intervals when patients have been tested and retested. Unfortunately, although standard deviations or variances may be reported, individual performance rarely is. When individual reports are given (as, for example, in the Israeli study of language), there is great variability. The Israeli data suggested that once improvement had started it was maintained, but Glasgow data[94] suggest that over the first 5 years after injury patients may show many different patterns of performance—with some remaining largely the same for long periods, some improving, and others deteriorating, at least as far as test performance is concerned. The predictors of these changes and their functional significance are not yet known.

FUNCTIONAL IMPACT OF COGNITIVE IMPAIRMENT

Neuropsychologic tests are not the only, nor necessarily the most effective, way of assessing outcome following severe brain injury.[94] Psychologic tests may have the limitations already referred to in this chapter (e.g., susceptibility to practice), and they may not relate clearly to other aspects of outcome. The problem becomes as much one of defining outcome as of assessing the functional impact of cognitive deficits, whether measured by neuropsychologic tests or other means.

Very general aspects of outcome have been reported frequently, and researchers have related such general aspects to neuropsychologic performance. Studies examining neuropsychologic performance in relation to the Glasgow Outcome Scale have already been reviewed in this chapter, showing that the severely disabled cases perform conspicuously badly neuropsychologically. This should be no surprise in view of the nature of the GOS. To be placed in the "severe" category, patients must be conscious but must nevertheless need assistance from others for at least some activities of daily living every day. These patients are conscious but dependent.

The Israeli group[49] have assessed functional recovery and found that although many patients show continuing intellectual improvement in terms of IQ scores, they may nevertheless fail to perform at a level consistent with their assessed capacity. For example, 64 percent of those deemed capable of sheltered work and 36 percent of those able to do simple work were not employed at follow-up. The authors comment that this may reflect a lack of ability on the patient's part to accept his or her change in status, as well as an inability of the family and community to understand and accept the behavior and other changes resulting from severe head injury.

Recent French studies have reported functional outcome in large groups of cases (103 cases in the Sichez-Auclair and Sichez study[67] and 102 in the study by Haramburu and coworkers.[10] The Haramburu study[10] was concerned particularly with the impact of memory disturbance on functional rehabilitation. There proved to be a highly significant relationship between memory performance and the likelihood of returning to work (either at the same or a reduced level), but further inspection of the data showed that this relationship was particularly strong for patients under age 30. This study, like that by Sichez-Auclair and Sichez[67] contains much rich clinical information that cannot adequately be conveyed here.

Sichez-Auclair and Sichez,[67] like Brooks and associates,[16] concluded that simple outcome categorizations are inadequate to indicate the range and quality of recovery. Furthermore, they discuss the important divergence between neuropsychologic test results and socio-professional or scholastic recovery. In an analysis of individual patients, they identify 9 out of 64 who appear to have made a complete cognitive recovery but who nevertheless were not "reinserted" professionally or scholastically at 1 year postinjury, whereas 2 out of 20 patients with severe memory disturbance and 2 of 14 with severe disturbance of intellectual efficiency were "reinserted" favorably. Just as for the relationship between cognitive deficit and organic measures such as PTA,

there is a broad statistical relationship between general outcome and cognitive test performance, but one that frequently breaks down in individual patients.

The relationship between memory deficit and functional outcome has been studied by Sunderland and his colleagues.[95, 98] Patient and relatives each filled out a memory questionnaire and checklist over a period of 1 week. The 65 patients were seen early (a mean of 11 weeks after discharge from hospital) or late (2 to 8 years postinjury), and were compared with orthopedic controls. The absolute frequency of reported memory failure was rather low for all subject groups. Nevertheless, when total memory scores (on cognitive tests) were examined, the mean total for the relatives' questionnaire and diary or checklist did show significantly more frequent memory failure for head injured patients than for control subjects. Interestingly, the relatives' measures "generally failed to show any significant difference between head injured and control groups." Sunderland then assessed the correlations between the memory test scores and the questionnaires and checklists, finding the highest correlations in the "late" group. Here the relatives' questionnaires showed significant correlations with six of the 14 memory tests, but the patients' questionnaires showed no correlations significant at $p < 0.01$.

The same issue has been addressed in Glasgow by correlating memory test performance and reports by relatives and patients of memory failures in the patient. The correlations were typically of the order of 0.3 to 0.6, indicating statistically significant but weak relationships. When an alternative approach was used by comparing cognitive test performance in the patient across three subgroups classified in terms of the relatives' assessment of whether the patient's overall memory deficit was mild, moderate, or severe in its functional consequences, there were consistent trends for the patients with severe deficits to have the lowest memory performance. These results did not, however, reach significance. Furthermore, the conceptual problems in attempting to obtain reports of memory impairment from patients with a memory impairment are obvious and serious.

In summary, there is a broad relationship between cognitive disturbance as assessed by test, and functional impairment in everyday life assessed in a variety of ways. Nevertheless, the relationship is a general one, and breaks down readily in individual cases.

SUMMARY AND CONCLUSIONS

The basic cognitive consequences of head injury were clearly identified in the early studies in the 1930s and 1940s. These consequences include learning and memory deficits, disturbance of thinking and complex perceptual skills, and a slowness in information processing. During the last 20 years investigators have confirmed the accuracy of these early results and have attempted to understand why the deficits occur, both in terms of psychologic (e.g., encoding, retrieval) and pathophysiologic (e.g., effects of diffuse versus focal damage) processes. Gains have been made here, but there are still many areas of ignorance.

When a fractionation of performance (particularly memory performance) in terms of separate psychologic processes is attempted, head injured patients often seem to perform much like normal subjects but at

a lower level, suggesting a disturbance of fundamental attentional processes or simply a basic slowness or inefficiency in all aspects of information processing. However, general rules such as this always have exceptions, and it has become increasingly evident that performance varies immensely from patient to patient.

Furthermore, there is a growing realization of the importance of frontal deficits, both as crucial deficits in their own right and as deficits underlying poor performance on a very wide variety of cognitive tests.

Not only is performance variable, but so is the rate and extent of recovery. As a result, prediction of the rate of recovery or extent of final outcome is difficult. Indeed, it is difficult to say with any confidence exactly when outcome should be considered final. In a situation like this, there is a scientific and moral obligation of clinicians dealing with head injured patients to assume that change is possible unless the contrary evidence is overwhelming (e.g., devastating severity of brain damage). This rule, like every other, will break down, but if it does, the breakdown is in the patient's favor rather than the reverse.

REFERENCES

1. Salazar, AM et al: Consciousness and amnesia after penetrating head injury: Neurology and anatomy. Neurology 36:178, 1986.
2. Levin, HS, Benton, L and Grossman, RG: Neurobehavioural Consequences of Closed Head Injury. Oxford University Press, New York, 1982.
3. Lezak, M: Neurological Assessment. Oxford University Press, New York, 1983.
4. Walsh, K: Understanding Brain Damage: A Primer of Neuropsychological Evaluation. Churchill Livingstone, Edinburgh, 1985.
5. Brooks, DN (ed): Closed Head Injury: Psychological, Social and Family Consequences. Oxford University Press, New York, 1984.
6. Prigatano, G et al: Neuropsychological Rehabilitation After Brain Injury. Johns Hopkins University Press, Baltimore, 1986.
7. Haas, DC and Ross, GS: Transient global amnesia triggered by mild head trauma. Brain 109:251, 1986.
8. Wilson, JTL et al: Early and late magnetic resonance imaging and neuropsychological outcome after head injury. J Neurol Neurosurg Psychiatry 51:391, 1988.
9. Brooks, DN: Disorders of memory. In Rosenthal, M et al (eds): Rehabilitation of the Head Injured Adult. FA Davis, Philadelphia, 1983.
10. Haramburu, Ph et al: Troubles mnesiques, reinsertion sociale a et professionnelle chez les traumatises

cranio-encephaliques graves. Annales de Readaption et de Medicine Physique 26:271, 1984.
11. Schacter, DL and Crovitz, HF: Memory function after closed head injury: A review of the quantitative literature. Cortex 13:150, 1977.
12. Levin, HS, Grossman, RG and Kelly, PJ: Impairment of facial recognition after closed head injuries of varying severity. Cortex 13:119, 1977.
13. Teasdale, G and Brooks, N: Traumatic amnesia. In Fredriks, JAM (ed): Handbook of Clinical Neurology. Vol 1 (45): Clinical Neuropsychology. Elsevier, Amsterdam, 1984.
14. Bennett-Levy, JM: Long term effects of severe closed head injury on memory: Evidence from a consecutive series of young adults. Acta Neurol Scand 70:285, 1984.
15. Van Zomeren, AH and Van den Burg, W: Residual complaints of patients two years after severe head injury. J Neurol Neurosurg Psychiatry 48:21, 1985.
16. Brooks, DN, Campsie L, Symington, C, Beattie, A. and McKinlay, W: The five year outcome of severe blunt head injury—a relative's view. J Neurol Neurosurg Psychiatry 49:764, 1986.
17. Miller, E: The training characteristics of severely head-injured patients: A preliminary study. J Neurol Neurosurg Psychiatry 43:525, 1980.
18. Brooks, DN and Baddeley, A: What can amnesics learn? Neuropsychologia, 14:111, 1976.
19. Eslinger, PJ and Damasio, AR: Preserved motor

learning in Alzheimer's Disease: Implications for anatomy and behaviour. J Neurosci 6:3006, 1986.

20. Buschke, H and Fuld, PA: Evaluating storage retention and retrieval in disordered memory and learning. Neurology 24:1019, 1974.

21. Richardson, JTE and Snape, W: The effects of closed head injury upon human memory: An experimental analysis. Cognitive Neuropsychology 1(3):217, 1984.

22. Maring, W, Deelman, BG, and Brouwer, WH: Deficient memory in closed head injury patients: The impact of variations in (study) time, organisation instructions and word characteristics. Paper presented at Seventh European Conference of the International Neuropsychological Society, Aachen, W. Germany, June, 1984.

23. Brooks, DN: Long and short term memory in head injured patients. Cortex 11:329, 1975.

24. Vakil, E and Tweedy, JR: Encoding of frequency of occurrence, temporal order, and spatial location information by closed head injured and elderly subjects: Is it automatic? Paper presented at Meeting of International Neuropsychological Society, San Diego, February 1985.

25. Stokx, LC and Gaillard, WK: Task and driving performance of patients with a severe concussion of the brain. J Clin Exp Neuropsychol 8:421, 1986.

26. Hasher, L and Zacks, RT: Automatic and effortful processes in memory. J Exp Psychol (General) 108:356, 1979.

27. Brooks, DN and Aughton, ME: Psychological consequences of blunt head injury. Int Rehabil Med: 1:160, 1979.

28. Klove, H and Cleeland, CS: The relationship of neuropsychological impairment to other indices of severity of head injury. Scand J Rehabil Med 4:55, 1972.

29. Cullum, CM and Bigler, ED: Ventricle size, cortical atrophy and the relationship with neuropsychological status in closed head injury: A quantitative analysis. J Clin Exp Neuropsychol 8:437, 1986.

30. Mandleberg, IA and Brooks, DN: Cognitive recovery after severe head injury. 1. Serial testing on the Wechsler Adult Intelligence Scale. J Neurol Neurosurg Psychiatry 38:1121, 1975.

31. Van Zomeren, AH and Deelman, BG: Differential effects of simple and choice reaction after closed head injury. Clin Neurol Neurosurg 79:81, 1976.

32. Van Zomeren, AH and Deelman, BG: Long-term recovery of visual reaction time after closed head injury. J Neurol Neurosurg Psychiatry 41:452, 1978.

33. Van Zomeren, AH: Reaction Time and Attention After Closed Head Injury. Swets and Zeitlinger, Lisse, Holland, 1981.

34. Brouwer, W: Limitations of Attention After Closed Head Injury. Ph.D. Dissertation, University of Groningen, The Netherlands, 1985.

35. Van Zomeren, AH, Brouwer, EH and Deelman, BG: Attention deficits: The riddles of selectivity, speed and alertness. In Brooks, N (ed): Closed Head Injury: Psychological, Social and Family Consequences. Oxford University Press, Oxford, 1984.

36. Rizzo, PA et al: A CNV study in a group of patients with traumatic head injuries. Electroencephalogr Clin Neurophysiol 45:281, 1978.

37. Currie, SH: Event-related potentials as indicants of structural and functional damage in closed head injury. Prog Brain Res 54:507, 1981.

38. Brouwer, WH and Van Wolffelaar, PC: Sustained attention and sustained effort after closed head injury: Detection and 0.10 Hz heart rate variability in a low event rate vigilance task. Cortex 21:111, 1985.

39. Gronwall, D and Sampson, H: The Psychological Effects of Concussion. Oxford University Press, Auckland, New Zealand, 1974.

40. Gronwall, D and Wrightson, P: Delayed recovery of intellectual function after minor head injury. Lancet 2:605, 1974.

41. Gronwall, D and Wrightson, P: Cumulative effect of concussion. Lancet 2:995, 1974.

42. Gronwall, D and Wrightson, P: Memory and information processing capacity after closed head injury. J Neurol Neurosurg Psychiatry 44:889, 1981.

43. Ruesch, J: Intellectual impairment in head injuries. Am J Psychiatry 100:480, 1944.

44. Hannay, HJ, Levin, HS and Kay, M: Tachistoscopic visual perception after closed head injury. J Clin Neuropsychol 4:117, 1982.

45. Crompton, MR: Visual lesions in closed head injury. Brain 93:785, 1970.

46. Dye, OA, Milby, JB and Saxon, SA: Effects of early neurological problems following head trauma on subsequent neuropsychological performance. Acta Neurol Scand 59:10, 1979.

47. Levin, HA: Aphasia in closed head injury. In Sarno, AB (ed): Acquired Aphasia. Academic Press, London, 1981, p 427.

48. Levin, HS, Grossman, RG and Kelly, PJ: Aphasic disorder in patients with closed head injury. J Neurol Psychiatry 39:1062, 1976.

49. Najenson, T et al: Recovery of communicative functions after prolonged traumatic coma. Scand J Rehabil Med 10:15, 1978.

50. Groher, M: Language and memory disorders following closed head trauma. J Speech Hear Res 20:212, 1972.

51. Thomsen, IV: Evaluation and outcome of aphasia in patients with severe closed head trauma. J Neurol Neurosurg Psychiatry 38:713, 1975.

52. Thomsen, IV: Evaluation and outcome of traumatic aphasia in patients with severe verified focal lesions. Folia Phoniatrica 28:362, 1976.

53. Thomsen, IV: Neuropsychological treatment and longtime follow-up in an aphasic patient with very severe head trauma. J Clin Neuropsychol 3:43, 1981.

54. Sarno, MT: The nature of verbal impairment after closed head injury. J Nerv Ment Dis 168:685, 1980.

55. Sarno, MT: Verbal impairment after closed head injury. J Nerv Ment Dis 172:475, 1984.

56. Lezak, M and Gray, DK: Sampling problems and nonparametric solutions in clinical neuropsychological research. J Clin Neuropsychol 6:101, 1984.

57. Brooks, N et al: The effects of severe head injury upon patient and relative within seven years of injury. J Head Trauma Rehabil 2(3):1, 1987.

58. Brooks, DN et al: Problems in measuring cognitive recovery after acute brain injury. J Clin Neuropsychol 6:71, 1984.

59. Jennett, B et al: Disability after severe head injury: observations on the use of the Glasgow Outcome Scale. J Neurol Neurosurg Psychiatry 44:285, 1981.

60. Brooks, DN et al: Cognitive sequelae of severe head injury in relation to the Glasgow Outcome Scale. J Neurol Neurosurg Psychiatry 49:549, 1986.

61. Clifton, GL et al: Neurological course and correlated computerized tomography findings after se-

vere closed head injury. J Neurosurg 52:611, 1980.

62. Brooks, DN et al: Cognitive sequelae in relation to early indices of severity of brain damage after severe blunt head injury. J Neurol Neurosurg Psychiatry 43:529, 1980.
63. McLean, A et al: The behavioral sequelae of head injury. J Clin Neuropsychol 5:361, 1983.
64. Ewing, R et al: Persisting effects of minor head injury observable during hypoxic stress. J Clin Neuropsychol 2:147, 1980.
65. Jennett, B and Bond, MR: Assessment of outcome after severe brain damage. Lancet 1:480, 1975.
66. Levin, HS et al: Long term neuropsychological outcome of closed head injury. J Neurosurg 50:412, 1979.
67. Sichez-Auclair, N and Sichez, JP: Profils neuropsychologiques et mentaux dans les lesions encephaliques diffuses post-traumatiques severes. Neurochirurgie 32:63, 1986.
68. Cullum, M and Bigler, ED: Late effects of haematoma on brain morphology and memory in closed head injury. Int J Neurosci 28:279, 1985.
69. Timming, R, Orrison, WW and Mikula, JA: Computerized tomography and rehabilitation outcome after severe head trauma. Arch Phys Med Rehabil 63:156, 1982.
70. Uzzell, BP et al: Lateralised psychological impairment associated with CT lesions in head injured patients. Cortex 15:391, 1979.
71. Rao, N et al: 18F positron emission computed tomography in closed head injury. Arch Phys Med Rehabil 65:780, 1984.
72. Hadley, DM et al: A follow-up study of head injured patients by MRI and neuropsychological examination. Paper presented at 5th Annual Meeting of Society of Magnetic Resonance in Medicine, Montreal, August 18–22, 1986.
73. Jenkins, A et al: Brain lesions detected by magnetic resonance imaging in mild and severe head injury. Lancet 2:445, 8504, 1986.
74. Grafman, J et al: The relationship of brain tissue loss volume and lesion location to cognitive deficit. J Neurosci 6:301, 1986.
75. Brooks, N et al: Return to work within the first seven years of severe head injury. Brain Injury 1:5, 1987.
76. Harlow, J: Passage of an iron rod through the head. Boston Med Surg J 39:389, 1848.
77. Harlow, J: Recovery from the passage of an iron bar through the head. Mass Med Soc Publ 2:329, 1866–1868.
78. Lishman, A: Organic Psychiatry. Blackwell, Oxford, 1980, p 217.
79. Stuss, DT and Benson, DF: Neuropsychological studies of the frontal lobes. Psychol Bull 95:3, 1984.
80. Stuss, DT, Delgado, M and Guzman, DA: Verbal regulation in the control of motor impersistence: A proposed rehabilitation procedure. J Neurol Rehabil 1:19, 1987.

81. Trimble, MR and Thompson, PJ: Anticonvulsant drugs, cognitive function, and behaviour. Epilepsia (Suppl 1) 24:555, 1983.
82. Conkey, RC: Psychological changes associated with head injuries. Arch Psychol 232:1, 1938.
83. Ruesch, J and Moore, BE: Measurement of intellectual functions in the acute stage of head injury. Arch Neurol Psychiatry 50:165, 1943.
84. Mandleberg, IA: Cognitive recovery after severe head injury. 2. Wechsler Adult Intelligence Scale during post-traumatic amnesia. J Neurol Neurosurg Psychiatry 38:1127, 1975.
85. Mandleberg, IA: Cognitive recovery after severe head injury. 3. WAIS verbal and performance I.Q.'s as a function of post traumatic amnesia duration and time from injury. J Neurol Neurosurg Psychiatry 39:1001, 1976.
86. Becker, B: Intelligence changes after closed head injury. J Clin Psychol 31:307, 1975.
87. Drudge, OW et al: Recovery from severe closed head injuries: repeat testings with the Halstead-Reitan Neuropsychological Battery. J Clin Psychol 40:259, 1984.
88. Lezak, MD: Recovery of memory and learning function following traumatic brain injury. Cortex 15:63, 1979.
89. Parker, SA and Serrats, AFL: Memory recovery after traumatic coma. Acta Neurochir 34:71, 1976.
90. MacFlynn, G et al: Measurement of reaction time following minor head injury. J Neurol Neurosurg Psychiatry 47:1326, 1984.
91. Vigouroux, RP et al: A series of patients with craniocerebral injuries, studied neurologically, psychometrically, electroencephalographically, and socially. In Head Injuries: Proceedings of an International Symposium held in Edinburgh and Madrid. Churchill Livingstone, Edinburgh, 1971, p 335.
92. Raven, JC: Guide to the Standard Progressive Matrices. HK Lewis, London, 1960.
93. Raven, JC: Extended Guide to the Mill Hill Vocabulary Scales. HK Lewis, London, 1962.
94. Brooks, DN: Measuring neuropsychological and functional recovery. In Levin, HS et al (eds): Neurobehavioural Recovery From Head Injury. Oxford University Press, New York, 1987.
95. Sunderland, A, Harris, JE and Baddeley, AD: Do laboratory tests predict everyday memory? A neuropsychological study. J Verb Learn Verb Behav 22:341, 1983.
96. Kertesz, A and McCabe, P: Recovery patterns and prognosis in aphasia. Brain 100:1, 1977.
97. Brooks, DN and Aughton, ME: Cognitive recovery during the first year after severe blunt head injury. Int Rehabil Med 1:166, 1979.
98. Sunderland, A, Harris, JE and Gleave, JG: Memory failures in everyday life following severe head injury. J Clin Neuropsychol 6:127, 1984.

Chapter 13

Behavioral and Psychiatric Sequelae

MITCHELL ROSENTHAL, Ph.D.
MICHAEL R. BOND, M.D., Ph.D.

The enduring behavioral and psychiatric consequences of closed head injury pose the greatest challenge for health care professionals and family members engaged in the process of facilitating community reintegration and long-term adaptation. The nature, variety, and duration of these difficulties are sometimes predictable, based on knowledge of the individual's neuropathology, but more often than not are uncertain because of the uniqueness of each head injured individual. It is clear, however, that ultimate restitution of social roles is dependent on the capacity of caregivers to fully understand and treat these troublesome sequelae.

To understand the nature of behavior dysfunction, it is first necessary to state an operational definition of it. For the purpose of the present discussion, behavior dysfunction means "those overt actions (behaviors) that result in socially maladaptive interactions between the patient and the environment." Such behaviors may be "respondent" in that they are reflexive in nature and occur as a result of direct activity within the nervous system (e.g., episodic dyscontrol), which has its basis in an abnormality in brain function, possibly epileptic in nature, caused by injury. Knowledge of the behavioral changes of the respondent type is important because some may be reduced by psychopharmacologic intervention. More commonly, behavioral disturbances are "operant" and can be viewed as actions of people which elicit a response from the environment. This class of behaviors is sensitive to such responses, and they are often amenable to change.[1] For example, they may be reinforced by a positive and supportive response; however, if no response or an aversive response is offered, the chance of the operant behavior being repeated is diminished. In this case, operant behaviors may be amenable to change through behavioral interventions (see Chapter 28).

Consideration of a further psychologic dimension based on changes in emotion and personality helps in understanding the range of behavior and emotional changes that occur in the various phases of recovery after severe head injury. It utilizes the psychiatric frame of reference which defines organic disorders of brain dysfunction (organic brain syndromes) in the Diagnostic and Statistical Manual of the American Psychiatric Association, Third Edition, Revised (DSM-III-R).[2] The definitions of the various states concerned, to be described later, include references to associated cognitive dysfunction, though not the whole range of cognitive disorders that may follow head injury (i.e., defects in thinking, information processing, learning ability, memory, visual perception, and the like). Such deficits do, however, play a part in the creation of maladaptive operant behaviors. (For further discussion of the nature of cognitive dysfunction, see Chapter 12.)

The following discussion presents a description of key etiologic factors that may be responsible for behavioral dysfunction after head injury, a perspective on the course and presentation of these disturbances, a scheme based on DSM-III-R for classifying these disorders, and a description of characteristic secondary emotional and behavioral dysfunctions that arise in the course of adapting to the disability. The chapter does not specifically address those behavioral disturbances (commonly known collectively as the "postconcussional syndrome") that follow minor head injury (for further discussion of those behavioral disturbances, refer to Chapter 17).

DETERMINANTS OF BEHAVIORAL DYSFUNCTION

The variety and complexity of behavior disorders following head injury have stimulated some debate regarding to what extent specific etiologic factors are responsible for personality disturbance after traumatic brain injury. Prigatano[3] notes two guiding conceptualizations—namely, (1) that disturbances of thinking, judgment, and perception are at the root of psychiatric disturbances; and (2) that psychosocial factors are a greater determinant of psychiatric disturbances than the severity of brain injury itself. Lishman[4] lists a number of etiologic factors including mental constitution, premorbid personality, emotional impact of injury, emotional repercussions of injury, environmental factors, compensation/litigation, response to intellectual impairment, development of epilepsy, amount of brain damage incurred, and location of brain damage. The factors that may play a part in determining post-traumatic behaviors following severe brain injury are listed in Table 13–1.

Though no definitive answer has yet been given as to which factor or sets of factors is responsible for personality disturbances after head injury, a reasonable working assumption is that behavior disturbances after head injury are multifactorial in etiology; that is to say, their roots lie in an interaction between several factors, as depicted here:

$$\text{Behavior} = f\,(\text{function})$$
$$\text{Person} \times \text{Organism} \times \text{Environment}$$

The formula devised by Cronholm[5] may be reconceptualized as follows:

Coping behavior = The product of the interaction of

Person's preinjury intellect personality & social behavior

× The physical, cognitive & emotional/ behavioral effects of injury

× The nature of the social environment

To the working clinician, such a formulation has a great deal of face validity. It is so often the case that families will describe preinjury personality characteristics that often appear as exacerbations in the observable behavior after head injury. For example, the patient with a history of asocial behavior, impulsivity, impaired interpersonal relationships, and a chaotic family life may be expected to exhibit marked behavioral disturbances in-

---

Table 13–1. FACTORS THAT SIGNIFICANTLY INFLUENCE THE BEHAVIORAL CONSEQUENCES OF SEVERE BRAIN INJURY

Pretraumatic Factors
1. Personality and social competence
2. Personal and family material resources

Factors Relating Directly to Brain Trauma
1. Age: the state of cerebral maturity or decay
2. Extent of injury and sites of major areas of damage; the nature of primary deficits in cognition, personality, and behavior determined by site and severity
3. Epilepsy, if psychomotor it is of major psychiatric significance
4. Secondary emotional reactions to primary physical and mental deficits

Social factors
1. Post-traumatic interpersonal relations with family and friends
2. Post-traumatic social resources
3. The presence or absence of proceedings for compensation

dependent of the specific lesion; yet, the presence of a prefrontal lesion will likely loosen inhibitions and create an even more maladaptive behavior pattern. Thus, instead of rigidly adhering to a framework whereby one category of variable is largely or totally responsible for a given behavior disturbance, the astute clinician should carefully and exhaustively analyze each of these variables before arriving at a definitive diagnosis and treatment plan.

Premorbid Factors

A detailed analysis of premorbid history should include data obtained from both patient and family and encompass many different types of information. As stated earlier, the nature of cognitive dysfunction following head injury often plays a role in the determination of behavioral disturbances. Therefore, a clear understanding of the *cognitive* strengths and weaknesses existing prior to the injury would be critical. This is often obtained by examining school records and standardized test results or from interviewing family members. It is not uncommon for head injured patients to have a premorbid history of learning disability or other cognitive disabilities, as well as a history of antisocial behavior (e.g., alcohol or drug abuse, public misconduct).

Several researchers have noted a high frequency of preinjury *behavior disorders*[6-8] among head injured adults and children. Inquiry should be made as to the nature of preinjury behavior disorders—specifically antisocial behavior, alcohol and/or substance abuse, hyperactivity, depression, and so forth. Such information can be directly obtained from family members, but they may be reluctant to divulge it as it may be perceived to have a negative bearing on the patient's rehabilitation or on continuing legal proceedings. Another method by which this information may be obtained is through the administration of rating scales, such as the Neurobehavioral Rating Scale[9] or the Katz Adjustment Scale.[10]

Family dynamics is another important area for investigation. Premorbid problems in marital, family, and parent-child relationships often are noted by the relatives of the head injured patient. Schaffer and coworkers[11] suggested that high preinjury levels of family distress often led to a greater degree of psychiatric disturbance in the families of head injured children. Similar observations were reported by the Glasgow Group,[12] who noted that there was a significant relationship between a measure of the level of emotionality shown by relations and their reports of emotional/behavioral changes in the head injured patient's family members. Therefore, it does appear that a relative's personality is related to the reports he or she gives of behavior changes in the brain injured adult. Similarly, Evans and associates[13] studied the preinjury family interactions of stroke patients and found a significant relationship to long-term psychosocial adaptation. In this study, the McMaster Family Assessment Device was found to be a reliable and valid tool for measuring preinjury levels of family functioning.

Finally, another factor that would certainly influence the behavioral sequelae of head injury is the presence of pre-existing *neurologic conditions.* Among the significant conditions would be a history of previous head injury, presence of epilepsy, brain tumor, and history of dementia or cerebrovascular accident. In these instances, it is imperative that previous medical records be obtained so as to carefully document the nature of prior behavioral dysfunction owing to preinjury neurologic dysfunction. As Symonds[14] noted:

> The later effects of head injury can only be properly understood in the light of a full psychiatric study of the individual patient, and in particular, his constitution. It is not only the kind of injury that matters, but the kind of head (p.1092).

In sum, these are some of the major areas of premorbid function that may contribute to behavior and personality dysfunction after head injury. Other areas of inquiry that may have direct or indirect effect include previous occupational history, past history of dealing with stress, and relationships with significant others beyond the immediate family.

Site of Lesion

Advances in neurodiagnostic techniques and neuroscience research have allowed investigators to visualize lesions after head injury more accurately and thereby to correlate the presence of specific lesions with subsequent behavioral manifestations. There is a wide consensus among investigators that damage to the frontal lobes and its limbic connections (especially the temporal lobes and hypothalamus), which is extremely common in closed head injury, often results in a variety of striking personality disturbances, including lack of goal-directed behavior, adynamia (loss of drive), anhedonia (loss of sense of pleasure), disinhibition of sexual and aggressive impulses, and dull or flattened affect. The well-known case of Phineas Gage, who suffered a penetrating head injury as result of an explosion that catapulted a tamping iron (a type of crowbar) through his frontal lobe, illustrates some components of frontal lobe–damage behavior. Though he was considered to be a well-balanced, socially appropriate individual before his injury, the effects of it left him with intact formal intellect but great changes in his personality:

> He is fitful, irreverent, indulging in the grossest profanity, manifesting little deference for fellows, impatient of restraints or advice . . . . a child in his intellectual capacity and manifestations, he has the animal passions of a strong man. . . .[15]

In addition, there is an impairment in "executive functions," which encompass the capacities to plan, carry out, and monitor activities and social interactions.[16] These deficits, if persistent, are likely to greatly diminish the likelihood of such an individual returning to gainful employment. The head injured patient may appear to be without a sense of identity, as he exhibits little aim or ambition. These patients may behave as a 3- or 4-year-old child in that they live from moment to moment and fail to appreciate the consequences of their actions.

The behavioral changes described are due not only to damage to the prefrontal part of the brain itself, but also to white matter lesions which disrupt the connections between the frontal lobes and other structures such as the hypothalamus, amygdala, and dorsal medial nucleus of the thalamus.[17]

Damage to the medial surfaces of the temporal lobe and the limbic system has often been cited as a primary factor for the appearance of sexual and aggressive disinhibition in brain-damaged patients.[18, 19] This type of behavior is often seen in patients with temporal lobe epilepsy and although post-traumatic epilepsy does occur, the statistical percentage (5 percent) is quite small and may not need be a necessary condition to evoke such behavioral disturbance.

Environmental Factors

Within the past 5 years, organized rehabilitation efforts have extended beyond the acute and subacute hospitalization phases into a phase termed "community re-entry." There has been a realization that the long-term behavioral residua of brain injury may be positively or adversely affected by the nature of the postdischarge environment.

As mentioned earlier in this volume, the entire family system and social network is greatly affected by the presence of a brain injured relative (see Chapter 16 on effects on the family system). Family members may experience high levels of burden in the day-to-day management difficulties associated with personality changes.[20] The manner in which the family (often spouses or parents) respond to these personality changes can create conditions that maintain dysfunctional behavior or result in secondary behavioral disturbances. Such reactions may in themselves reflect preaccident psychologic or emotional problems with the relatives and between the relatives and the patient. This is perhaps a major reason why family members are routinely incorporated into both acute and community re-entry programs, so as to optimize their adjustment to the situation and provide them with the appropriate strategies to manage their relatives' behavior.

It is not just the immediate or even the extended family that is affected by brain injury. Kozloff[21] and Livingston and colleagues[22] recently demonstrated that the social network of the head injured patient most often disintegrates after approximately 6 months postinjury. In addition, Kozloff pointed out that families view social support as a major factor in long-term adaptation. As most head injured are within the young adult age group, loss of peer support can have devastating consequences. Clearly, the oft-reported social withdrawal of the head injured and their families is likely in reponse to their feelings of a disintegrated social network.

Socioenvironmental factors also include

financial resources. Though some of the head injured have pending litigation (which may eventually provide financial security), many are without immediate and adequate economic resources. It is often the case that vocational rehabilitation cannot be achieved for several years and economic hardship is the norm. Lack of meaningful vocational or avocational activity can lead to much unproductive, unstructured, unsatisfying experiences. A consequence of this may be the resumption of maladaptive preinjury behavior patterns such as substance and/or alcohol abuse, law-breaking, or exacerbation of post-traumatic behavior patterns.

ORGANIC BRAIN SYNDROMES OCCURRING DURING STAGES OF RECOVERY FROM SEVERE HEAD INJURY

The process of recovery from severe head injury may be arbitrarily divided into three stages, each of which has specific physical,

mental, and social characteristics.[23] These are shown in Table 13–2.

The first stage of recovery begins with the initial coma produced by the injury and continues through the period of altered consciousness that constitutes the phase of post-traumatic amnesia. The termination of the latter can be assessed quite simply by using a scale such as the Galveston Orientation and Attention Test.[24] Having emerged from PTA, the patient continues in a period of rapid physical and psychologic improvement. During this phase various behaviors, some adaptive and some maladaptive, together with variations in emotion, are frequently the source of concern to relatives, the professionals dealing with the process of rehabilitation, and often the patient also. The process of rapid recovery begins to slow between 6 and 12 months postinjury, after which a prolonged period of adjustment occurs at a more leisurely pace. During this stage, patients continue their attempts to reintegrate with their family and the community. Reactive emotional problems and associated behaviors develop dur-

Table 13–2. RECOVERY FROM SEVERE HEAD INJURY

Average Duration	Neurologic State	Mental State	Management Priorities
	Stage 1		
Days	Intense physical reactions to injury to brain	Unconscious	Intensive physical care
	Maximum neurologic deficit	Beginning emergence from coma	Behavioral mangement
	Stage 2		
2A: days–3 months	Physical reaction to injury slow	Organization of mental events serving full consciousness	Continued physical care and rehabilitation
		Acute behavioral disturbances commence	
2B: 3–6 months	Continued recovery of processes basic to physical recovery	Full consciousness achieved; continued rapid recovery of processes basic to higher mental functions	Introduction of psychologic and social methods of rehabilitation*
	Stage 3		
6–12 months	Level of physical disability more or less established	Recovery of cognitive disability established to significant, but further recovery occurs	Psychologic and social rehabilitation
	Further recovery slight and rate of recovery slow	Longer-term complex behavioral responses to injury emerging	

*Speculative.

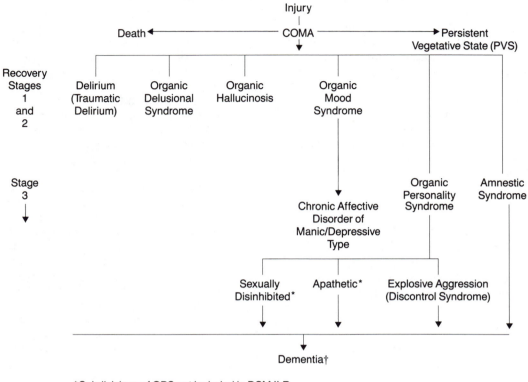

ORGANIC BRAIN SYNDROMES (Adapted from DSM III-R)

*Subdivisions of OPS *not* included in DSM II-R

† If dementia develops it may be mild, moderate or severe

Figure 13–1. Organic brain syndromes. (Adapted from DSM-III-R.)

ing this stage and often require rehabilitation involving both medical and psychologic strategies.

As mentioned earlier, it is convenient from a diagnostic viewpoint to have a framework such as that provided by DSM-III-R, which allows a systematic description of the wide range of post-traumatic changes occurring in the mental state after brain injury as the patient passes through the stages of recovery mentioned briefly here. In DSM-III-R, which provides such a framework, organic brain syndromes are grouped into six categories, three of which are relevant to recovery from severe brain injury:

Stage 1—Delirium, organic delusional syndrome, organic mood syndrome, and organic hallucinosis

Stage 2—Organic delusional syndrome, organic hallucinosis, amnestic syndrome, and organic personality syndrome

Stage 3—Amnestic syndrome, organic personality syndrome, and dementia.

Several syndromes are of relatively short duration (delirium, organic hallucinosis, organic delusional syndrome) and tend to occur as indicated in the first or second stages of recovery. The extent to which behavioral changes occur and their nature varies among the syndromes and the individuals who exhibit them. The relationship between organic syndromes and recovery from coma is shown in Figure 13–1, which has been extended beyond the framework given in DSM-III-R as indicated. All may ultimately be associated with post-traumatic dementia, though use of this diagnosis should be delayed for many months or even years, given the fact that considerable improvement in various aspects of cognition, mood, and behavior occur over a long period of time in many patients.

DISORDERS COMMONLY ASSOCIATED WITH STAGES 1 AND 2

Delirium

Delirium is an acute disturbance of consciousness classically associated with metabolic dysfunction rather than structural damage to the brain, although head injured patients may have a combination of both. Therefore, some patients pass into a traumatic delirium upon recovering from coma. There are distinct mental and behavioral abnormalities in delirium, including disorientation for time, place, and person; disturbed attention span with distractibility; impaired memory; and decreased capacity for abstract thinking (Table 13–3). Patients often exhibit a fearful or suspicious mood but on occasion may be withdrawn and apathetic. They misidentify those around them; hallucinations (usually visual) and delusions (almost always of the paranoid type) often occur. Restlessness, irritability, fatiguability, and a reversed sleep pattern are also features of the state. During the course of this phase of disturbed consciousness, delusions or less often hallucinations may be the predominant feature, in which case the patient is said to have either a traumatic organic delusional syndrome or traumatic organic hallucinosis. When patients exhibit the symptoms and behavior described, a search should be made for evidence of infection (chest or urine) or for hypoxia (chest infection or injury, or anemia). Given the wide extent of injury to the brain following severe head trauma, the usual characteristics of delirium are not always present in the "pure" form associated solely with a metabolic problem. Elements of the syndromes—for example, the amnestic syndrome or personality disorder, both of which become fully obvious only later in recovery—may distort the clinical picture.

ORGANIC DELUSIONAL SYNDROME AND HALLUCINOSIS

The diagnostic features of these two syndromes are given in Table 13–4.

Delusions and hallucinations usually develop within the period of disturbed consciousness represented by PTA. As mentioned earlier, the delusions tend to be of the paranoid type and they are thought to be the consequence of a long period of partial and disordered consciousness with grossly distorted perception and orientation. These disorders of thought and perception may persist after the patient has moved into clear consciousness, and it is obvious that such symptoms are a continuation of the earlier process. Recovery is usually spontaneous but, on occasion, an agitated and paranoid patient requires medication, preferably with a phenothiazine such as fluphenazine, which has a low seizure potential.

Complex hallucinatory states other than those occurring as part of delirium are rare and usually self-limiting. Both paranoid delusions and hallucinations (auditory, visual, or gustatory), especially when occurring later in recovery, may indicate the presence of temporal lobe epilepsy. Treatment is primarily by means of anticonvulsant drugs,

---

Table 13–3. DIAGNOSTIC CRITERIA FOR DELIRIUM

A. Reduced ability to maintain attention to external stimuli
B. Disorganized thinking
C. At least two of the following:
   1. Reduced level of consciousness
   2. Perceptual disturbances
   3. Disturbed sleep-wake cycle
   4. Increased or decreased psychomotor activity
   5. Disorientation to time, place or person
   6. Memory impairment
D. Clinical features develop over a short period of time (usually hours to days) and tend to fluctuate over the course of a day
E. Evidence of a specific organic factor (or factors) judged to be etiologically related to the disturbance

**Table 13–4. DSM III-R CRITERIA FOR ORGANIC DELUSIONAL
SYNDROME AND HALLUCINOSES**

Organic Delusional Syndrome	Hallucinoses
Prominent delusions	Prominent persistent or recurrent halluci- nations
Evidence from the history, physical examina- tion, or laboratory tests of a specific organic factor judged to be etiologically related to the disturbance	Evidence from the history, physical examina- tion, or laboratory tests of a specific organic factor judged to be etiologically related to the disturbance
Not occurring exclusively during the course of delirium	Not occurring exclusively during the course of delirium

the first choice being carbamazepine, but behavioral techniques may be required to enhance the patient's social control.

Apart from the occasional continuation of delusions into clear consciousness during the second stage of recovery, the major problems occurring at this time are the organic personality syndrome and the amnestic syndrome, with the organic mood syndrome being a relatively uncommon problem.

Organic Personality Syndrome

Of the group of syndromes described in DSM-III-R, this is the most common of those that persist after the immediate recovery from disordered consciousness. Therefore, its variants are of considerable importance because they form the basis of much of the

workload for rehabilitation units dealing with behaviorally disturbed patients.

To make the diagnosis, the criteria shown in Table 13–5 must be present. It is possible for more than one of the sets of conditions in A to be present at the same time (A2 and A4) and the episodic dyscontrol syndrome, characterized by sudden and unexpected outbursts of an aggressive nature, may occur with any or all of the characteristics mentioned under A1, A2, and A4.

As far as head injured patients are concerned, the chief alternative diagnosis is that of dementia in which loss of intellectual abilities predominates. It is clear that a number of well-recognized states are covered by the term "organic personality syndrome," including the various aspects of the so-called frontal syndrome and the episodic dyscontrol syndrome (organic personality syndrome—explosive type) mentioned elsewhere in this chapter.

**Table 13–5. DIAGNOSTIC CRITERIA FOR ORGANIC
PERSONALITY SYNDROME**

A. A persistent personality disturbance, either lifelong or representing a change or accentuation of a previously characteristic trait, involving at least one of the following:
1. Affective instability (e.g., marked shifts from normal mood to depression, irritability, or anxiety)
2. Recurrent outbursts of aggression or rage that are grossly out of proportion to any precipitating psychosocial stressors
3. Markedly impaired social judgment (e.g., sexual indiscretions)
4. Marked apathy and indifference
5. Suspiciousness or paranoid ideation
B. Evidence from the history, physical examination, or laboratory tests of a specific organic factor (or factors) judged to be etiologically related to the disturbance
C. This diagnosis is not given to a child or adolescent if the clinical picture is limited to the features that characterize attention deficit hyperactivity disorder.
D. Not occurring exclusively during the course of delirium and not meeting the criteria for dementia.

Specify explosive type if outbursts of aggression or rage are the predominant feature.

For convenience, it is suggested that the patients with behavioral problems occurring as manifestations of the organic personality syndrome be divided into two groups. The first should include those in whom the most obvious behavioral characteristic is apathy. Such individuals show no drive or spontaneity. They may make limited plans but do not act upon them. Their mood is neutral, thereby differentiating them from patients who are depressed. Psychologic testing reveals a poor overall performance, with grossly impaired attention and concentration.

The second group consists of patients who show evidence of impaired behavioral control, which may be experienced as generalized disinhibition with loosened control of many aspects of social behavior or in a more focused way. In the latter case, the behaviors that give rise to concern may be predominantly aggressive or sexual or a combination of both. Patients with organic personality syndrome often reveal exaggeration of pretraumatic traits in their behavior. Behavioral changes of the apathetic or disinterested type pose a particularly difficult challenge for rehabilitation professionals, but severe cases of the aggressive–sexually disinhibited type can also be sources of great concern for relatives and therapists alike.

Affective Changes Following Severe Head Injury

Affective instability is often first detected early in the process of recovery from severe head injury, though the diagnosis of an organic mood syndrome should not be made if the patient exhibits clouded consciousness (Table 13–6).

Experience with the head injured reveals that occasionally during the latter half of the second or in the third stage of recovery, symptoms of mania occur and may persist if not treated with appropriate medication. The presence of hallucinations or delusions should not overshadow the mood change and may be present as part of the altered mood state. In addition to being overactive with an impaired sleep pattern, patients with a manic disorder are often irritable and aggressive, but may be noisily cheerful and irresponsible.

Table 13–6. DSM-III CRITERIA FOR ORGANIC MOOD SYNDROME

A. Prominent and persistent depressed, elevated, or expansive mood
B. Evidence from history, physical examination, or laboratory tests of a specific organic factor (or factors) judged to be etiologically related to the disturbance
C. Not occurring exclusively during the course of delirium

Affective instability is usually self-limiting, though treatment with medications such as haloperidol may be required for the manic or hypermanic patient. An antidepressant such as Trazadone or L-tryptophan may be used for the persistently depressed patient, although the development of major depressive illness is, in the authors' experience, usually delayed many months or years after the injury, probably being a reaction to the physical, mental, and social problems caused by the injury.

Apart from the specific syndromes mentioned earlier, other behavioral changes occur during the second stage of recovery from injury. For example, the patient may show perseverative responses, either verbal or motor, and appear to be stimulus bound—that is, unable or unwilling to adapt to minor changes in the daily schedule or in the environment. Family members are often surprised to observe the childlike dependence that begins to show at this point, and the patient may reveal an extraordinary attachment to relatives and friends and become easily upset when they leave the hospital or rehabilitation unit. Another manifestation of this dependency may be seen in the number of telephone calls made by the patient on a daily basis to home, much to the consternation of staff members and friends. This childlike state of dependence may continue for a period of many months, although its intensity rarely persists unless reinforced by the family.

STAGE THREE

As mentioned previously, during the first 6 to 9 months after injury a rapid recovery in the patient's physical and mental health takes place and it is during this stage that evidence for a severe and persistent disorder of memory begins to emerge, becoming established as the process of recovery begins to slow.

The third phase of recovery is often associated with the time when a patient is transferred to a long-term rehabilitation unit or to the family home. The patient becomes increasingly aware of physical limitations and of some of the mental deficits caused by injury. Because impulsive behavior tends to diminish at this time, less intense supervision of daily activities is required; however, irritability and a low level of tolerance for frustration are often preserved in patients for a considerable time. The patient's denial of disability is manifested in statements such as "I am as good as I ever was before; why won't you let me go home or return to school?" This feeling of a return to normality is often reinforced by the frequent appearance of physical integrity, the ability to move about independently, and the capacity to perform most daily activities. During this stage, which continues indefinitely, head injured patients have to come to terms with their new identity, which is invariably less desirable than their previous one. Often they are confused and upset by the restrictions placed on their behavior. When full acceptance of disability occurs, anxiety, depression, and anger may develop. Patients express fears about the permanence of brain damage and its implications. Rejection by peers or family members is often perceived, and one of the unfortunate consequences of adapting to head injury is the upsetting appreciation that the remainder of life will be difficult and a struggle.

Disorders Commonly Associated With Stage 3

AMNESTIC SYNDROME

Injuries that lead to severe damage to both medial and temporal regions of the brain produce a disorder known as the amnestic syndrome, in which a profound disturbance of memory occurs (Table 13–7). It is manifested as a total loss of recall, except for partial recollections of the events preceding the injury. Confabulation—that is, the unconscious manufacture of facts to fill an otherwise empty memory—is frequently seen at an early stage, though this tends to disappear fairly quickly. The fact that most patients retain insight into their abnormality produces considerable unhappiness and depression among them. However, over a period of years the repetition of simple acts of daily life (e.g., recognition of friends seen frequently, ability to find rooms in the home) may develop. Indeed, it has been shown by psychologic testing that such patients may retain certain types of memory capacity (a geographic memory) and so learn, or relearn, tasks without being fully conscious of doing so. Management of patients with the amnestic syndrome is chiefly by careful environmental cueing and constant repetition of simple but necessary tasks (e.g., finding and putting on clothes, using the toilet).

DEMENTIA

Many conditions that affect the brain are progressive (e.g., Alzheimer's disease, multiple sclerosis, and Parkinson's disease) with a

Table 13–7. DIAGNOSTIC CRITERIA FOR AMNESTIC SYNDROME

A. Demonstrable evidence of impairment in both short- and long-term memory—with regard to long-term memory, very remote events are remembered better than more recent events; its impairment (inability to remember information that was known in the past) may be indicated by inability to remember past personal information (e.g., United States past presidents, well-known dates); short-term memory impairment (inability to learn new information) may be indicated by inability to remember three objects after 5 minutes

B. Not occurring exclusively during the course of delirium, and not meeting criteria for dementia (i.e., no impairment in abstract thinking or judgment, no other disturbances of higher cortical function, and no personality change)

C. Evidence from the history, physical examination, or laboratory tests of a specific organic factor (or factors) judged to be etiologically related to the disturbance gradual and predictable decline in brain function and associated behavior being observed until the state of dementia is reached, which in turn ultimately leads to death. However, following acute insults to the brain (stroke, infections, trauma) there is a prolonged period of recovery and unless the damage is such that a very profound disturbance of function occurs that is incompatible with more than a very limited recovery, the diagnosis of dementia should not be made (although it may be predicted in some cases). Working practice indicates that those involved with the severely brain injured tend to set more stringent criteria for the diagnosis of dementia than those working in other fields. This may be because the use of the term "dementia" carries a connotation of hopelessness and as such is rejected for a long time by both professionals and relatives. The essential features of dementia are shown in Table 13–8. Difficulties with an all-or-none approach might well

be solved by using the DSM-III-R criteria for the severity of dementia given in this table.

LONG-TERM EMOTIONAL AND BEHAVIORAL CONSEQUENCES OF SEVERE BRAIN INJURY

There is very little reliable statistical information dealing with the long-term emotional reactions to severe brain injury. The Glasgow group[25] and Thomsen[26] in Denmark have revealed a general picture of deterioration in emotion and behavior in a significantly high number of patients assessed 5 to 15 years after injury. Predominant among the Glasgow observations were increasing aggressiveness, threats of violence, raised levels of alcohol consumption, and threats of suicide. Danish studies show increasing social isolation and withdrawal from activity over a longer time period, which seems to

Table 13–8. DIAGNOSTIC CRITERIA FOR DEMENTIA

A. Demonstrable evidence of impairment in short- and long-term memory. Short-term memory impairment (inability to learn new information) may be indicated by inability to remember three objects after 5 minutes. Long-term memory impairment (inability to remember past personal information [e.g., what happened yesterday, birthplace, occupation] or facts of common knowledge [e.g., United States past presidents, well-known dates])
B. At least one of the following:
  1. Impairment in abstract thinking
  2. Impaired judgment
  3. Other disturbances of higher cortical function, such as aphasia (disorder of language), apraxia (inability to carry out motor activities despite intact comprehension and motor function), agnosia (failure to recognize or identify objects despite intact sensory function), and "constructional difficulty" (e.g., inability to copy 3-dimensional figures, assemble blocks, or arrange sticks in specific designs)
  4. Personality change
C. The disturbance in A and B significantly interferes with work or usual social activities or relationships with others
D. Not occurring exclusively during the course of delirium
E. Either (1) or (2):
  1. There is evidence of a specific organic factor (or factors) judged to be etiologically related to the disturbance
  2. In the absence of such evidence, an etiologic organic factor can be presumed if the disturbance cannot be accounted for by any nonorganic mental disorder (e.g., major depression accounting for cognitive impairment)

Criteria for Severity of Dementia
  Mild: Although work or social activities are significantly impaired, the capacity for independent living remains, with adequate personal hygiene and relatively intact judgment
  Moderate: Independent living is hazardous, and some degree of supervision is necessary
  Severe: Activities of daily living are so impaired that continual supervision is required (e.g., patient is unable to maintain minimal personal hygiene; largely incoherent or mute)

be related to loss of close family figures, particularly parents. In terms of conventional psychiatric diagnoses little has been written about the specific neurotic developments in the severely brain injured, although there is a certain amount of information about psychotic disorders and suicide rates.

Anxiety

Marked anxiety with a loss of self-confidence occurs in many of the brain injured. Probably only when disinhibition predominates is anxiety lacking, although even among the disinhibited, tension, anxiety, and aggression may occur briefly. The anxiety experienced by head injured patients may amount to panic at times, especially if the person is left alone or finds himself or herself in an unfamiliar environment. In fact, some patients become so dependent on their relatives that they cannot be separated from them for more than a few minutes at a time. It is possible to reduce such anxiety and to increase self-confidence by intensive psychologic treatment based on cognitive/behavioral therapy that aims to provide a structured daily routine for patients, which, once mastered, restores feelings of self-control and confidence. Even those with lesser degrees of injury experience anxiety in relation to returning to work and dealing with novel situations. Treatment by counseling and psychologic treatment techniques are preferred, and the use of benzodiazepines as an anxiolytic is not indicated.

Depression

A report by Dikmen and Reitan,[27] who assessed patients using the Minnesota Multiphasic Personality Inventory (MMPI), revealed that patients with significant deficits on neuropsychologic tests showed evidence of increased depression and hypochondriasis 18 months after a moderate head injury. Brooks and colleagues[25] found that reports by relatives of depression and threats of violence in the injured were significantly greater at 5 years, compared with 1 year after severe brain injury. Studies of suicide among head injured men who had been soldiers in World War II revealed a higher incidence than would be expected and they accounted for 14 percent of all deaths among the men studied.[28, 29] Clearly, the risk of suicide increases with time, reaching a peak about 15 to 20 years after injury.

Depression and suicide are often the result of financial difficulties, marital and family problems, and, in many cases, excessive drinking. The change in personality caused by injury is a significant factor in many cases of suicide, and almost half of those who kill themselves do so when severely depressed. Those involved in the care of the severely brain injured should be on the lookout for signs of depressive illness late in recovery and, when present, treatment with antidepressant drugs, such as trazodone or amitriptyline in full doses, should be commenced.

Obsessional Disorders

Obsessional symptoms arise in two distinct contexts following severe brain injury. A number of patients become excessively concerned about tidiness and are distressed if their daily routine and personal possessions are disturbed by others. It has been suggested that this is a behavioral response to the threat of internal chaos caused by the cognitive emotional and perceptual and emotional consequences of injury and that the new behavior serves to establish order and structure in everyday life. Developments of this type may well be related to an individual's premorbid tendency to obsessional traits.

A second and quite different origin for obsessional symptoms has been described by McKeon and coworkers,[30] who reported that after moderate to severe injuries a small number of patients developed full symptoms of an obsessional neurosis within a matter of days of injury and in the absence of premorbid obsessional personality characteristics. In these cases it would appear that injury to the brain was primarily responsible for the onset of symptoms. In the former group, reduction of tension may be achieved by accepting the need for a reasonably rigid daily schedule but excessive preoccupation with rituals should be modified by behavioral techniques. Cases of sudden onset of a full-blown obsessional neurosis are very rare, and treatment should be based on the usual behavioral and pharmacologic treatments used for this condition.

Conversion Disorder/Hysterical Disorder

There appears to be an inverse relationship between the severity of brain injury and the tendency to develop conversion disorders. Therefore, mild to moderate injuries are most often associated with this form of abnormality. Patients so afflicted may exhibit neurologic signs that do not have an obvious physical basis such as a hemiparesis, sensory changes in the limbs, or pseudoseizures (which, on occasion, may be mixed with true, organically determined seizures). Ganser's syndrome is a rare condition that is included in this category. It is characterized by a history of mild to moderate injury and a period of good recovery, which is followed by a depression of mood and then withdrawal into a monosyllabic state. The way questions are answered indicates that the patient understands what is asked, but the reply is nevertheless not quite correct. The outcome of post–head injury hysterical disorders varies considerably, but it is said that Ganser's syndrome disappears abruptly once the underlying source of conflict causing it has been resolved. In most instances this is found to be the pursuit of compensation for injury, and we have experienced at least two cases in which the disorder disappeared within a month of settlement of the litigation. Patients who do not have Ganser's syndrome require expert psychiatric attention and are often treated by a combination of psychotherapy and behavioral management.

CONCLUSION

Research and clinical experience have clearly established that the behavioral disorders are the most enduring and socially disabling of any of the dysfunctions commonly seen after traumatic brain injury. These alterations in personality and social behavior limit the capacity for successful return to work or school, independent living, and the re-establishment of social relationships with peers and family members. The accurate diagnosis and treatment of these disorders is essential but often can elude experienced rehabilitation clinicians.

In this chapter, a schema for classifying behavioral and psychiatric disorders, derived from DSM-III-R, is introduced. In the context of the "typical" recovery process, it is possible to identify patterns of behavior that are consistent with various forms of organic brain syndromes, as well as neurotic states, which are often viewed as a long-term emotional reaction to the brain injury rather than primarily related to a specific pattern of brain damage.

To adequately understand and diagnose behavioral and psychiatric disorders in traumatic brain injury, one must look beyond simple presentation of symptoms and not apply a diagnostic schema in a "cookbook" manner. It is essential that both premorbid constitution and posthospital environment be carefully considered. Recognizing premorbid problems such as attention deficit disorder, learning disability, substance abuse, prior history of head injury or other neurologic disease, family dysfunction, depression, or antisocial behavior may alter behavioral management strategies. The presence of any of these premorbid conditions can be exacerbated by the type of brain damage commonly seen in patients who have suffered traumatic brain injury. Similarly, in the post–hospital discharge phase, ineffective family coping strategies, dissolution of the social network, financial hardship, and inability to access outpatient rehabilitation services can all greatly modify the nature and severity of personality disturbances.

Therefore, the current challenge for caregivers is to resist simple formulations of complex behavioral changes. Though some forms of behavioral disturbance fit neatly into the categories described in this chapter, the process of recovery from traumatic brain injury is dynamic and is influenced not only by the site of lesion and by preinjury and postinjury factors, but also by the preconceptions of staff who treat these patients. Failure to appreciate the multiple possible explanations for observed behavioral disturbance will result in an even greater handicap for those who struggle to manage these problems effectively.

REFERENCES

1. Wood, R: Brain Injury Rehabilitation: A Neurobehavioral Approach. Aspen Publ, Rockville, MD, 1987.
2. American Psychiatric Association: Diagnostic and Statistical Manual of Mental Disorders—Revised, ed 3. Washington, DC, APA, 1987.
3. Prigatano, GP: Neuropsychological Rehabilitation after Brain Injury. Johns Hopkins Press, Baltimore, MD, 1986.
4. Lishman, WA: Psychiatric sequelae of head injuries: problems in diagnosis. Journal of the Irish Medical Association 71:306, 1978.
5. Cronholm, B: Evaluation of mental disturbances after head injury. Scand J Rehabil Med 4:35, 1972.
6. Tobis, JS, Pure, K and Sheridan, J: Rehabilitation of severely brain injured patients. Paper presented at the American Congress of Rehabilitation Medicine Annual Meeting, San Diego, CA, 1976.
7. Rutter, M: Psychological sequelae of brain damage in children. Am J Psychiatry 138(12):1523, 1981.
8. Fahy, TJ, Irving, MH and Millag, P: Severe Head Injuries: A six-year follow-up. Lancet 2:475, 1967.
9. Levin, HS et al: The neurobehavioral rating scale: Assessment of behavioral sequelae of head injury by the clinician. J Neurol Neurosurg Psychiatry 50:183, 1987.
10. Katz, MM and Lyerly, SB: Methods for measuring adjustment and social behavior in the community. Psychol Rep 13:503, 1963.
11. Schaffer, D, Chadwick, O and Rutter, M: Psychiatric outcome of localized head injury in children. In CIBA Foundation Symposium, Vol 34, Outcome of Severe Damage to Central Nervous System. Elsevier–North Holland Publ, New York, 1975.
12. McKinlay, WW and Brooks, DN: Methodological problems in assessing psychosocial recovery following severe head injury. J Clin Neuropsychol 6(1):87, 1984.
13. Evans, RL et al: Pre-stroke family interaction as a predictor of stroke outcome. Arch Phys Med Rehabil 68(8):508, 1987.
14. Symonds, CP: Mental disorder following head injury. Proc R Soc Med 30:1081, 1937.
15. Harlow, JM: Recovery from the passage of an iron bar through the head. Publications of the Massachusetts Medical Society, 1868.
16. Lezak, M: Relationships between personality disorders social disturbances and physical disability following traumatic brain injury. J Head Trauma Rehabil 2(1):57, 1987.
17. Alexander, M: The role of neurobehavioral syndromes in the rehabilitation and outcome from head injury. In Levin, HS et al (eds): Neurobehavioral Recovery from Head Injury. Oxford University Press, Oxford, 1987, p 191.
18. Bear, DM and Fedio, P: Quantitative analysis of interictal behviour in temporal lobe epilepsy. Arch Neurol 34:454, 1977.
19. Lishman, WA: Brain damage in relation to psychiatric disability after head injury. Br J Psychiatry 114:373, 1968.
20. McKinlay, WW et al: The short-term outcome of severe blunt head injury as reported by relatives of the injured persons. J Neurol Neurosurg Psychiatry 44:527, 1981.
21. Kozloff, R: Networks of social support and the outcome from severe head injury. J Head Trauma Rehabil 2(3):14, 1987.
22. Livingston, MG, Brooks, DN and Bond, MR: Three months after severe head injury: psychiatric and social impact on relatives. J Neurol Neurosurg Psychiatry 48:876, 1985.
23. Bond, MR and Brooks, DN: Understanding the process of recovery as a basis for the investigation of rehabilitation for the brain injured. Scand J Rehabil Med 8:127, 1976.
24. Levin, HS et al: Long-term neuropsychological outcome of closed head injury. J Neurosurg 50:412, 1979.
25. Brooks, DN et al: The five year outcome of severe blunt head injury: A relative's view. J Neurosurg Psychiatry 49:764, 1986.
26. Thomsen, IV: Late outcome of very severe blunt head trauma: A 10–15 year second follow-up. J Neurol Neurosurg Psychiatry 48:870, 1984.
27. Dikmen, S and Reitan, RM: Emotional sequelae of head injury. Ann Neurol 2:492, 1977.
28. Vauhkonen, K: Suicide among the male disabled with war injuries to the brain. Acta Psychiatr Neurol Scand (Suppl) 137:90, 1959.
29. Achte, KA and Anttinen, EE: Suizide bei Hirngeschadigten des Krieges in Finland. Fortschr Neurol Psychiatr 31:645, 1963.
30. McKeon, J, McGuffin, P and Robinson, P: Obsessive-compulsive neurosis following head injury. A report of 4 cases. Br J Psychiatry 144:190, 1984.

Chapter 14

Deficits in Activities of Daily Living

ROBIN McNENY, O.T.R.

Activities of daily living (ADL) are those tasks necessary for an individual's day-to-day functioning. These activities can range from the most basic (i.e., dressing and feeding) to the intensely complex (i.e., financial management and driving). The pursuit and completion of these activities satisfies the needs of the individual as well as those dependent upon him while also maintaining their quality of life.

The occurrence of a head injury has a devastating effect on an individual's ability to perform activities of daily living independently and effectively. The recovery process following head injury is quite lengthy and involves extended periods of partial or total dependence on others. Often, despite the efforts of the rehabilitation team, full independence in daily living skills cannot be achieved.

The process of retraining the daily living skills of a head injured patient should be approached with the patient's premorbid life tasks, interests, and social roles in mind. Family input and involvement are critical and often vital to the success of the program. The rehabilitation team must work as a unit to maximize consistency and carryover.

EVALUATION OF DAILY LIVING SKILLS

Many assessment scales exist to evaluate both basic and advanced daily living skills. The Functional Life Scale,[1] the Functional Capacity Evaluation,[2] the Burke Stroke Time-Oriented Profile,[3] the Klein-Bell Scale,[4] the Kenny Self Care Evaluation,[5] the Barthel Index,[6] and the Comprehensive Evaluation of Basic Living Skills,[7] as well as dozens of nonstandardized evaluations are available for clinicians. Each head injury team needs to determine which functional evaluation best suits its program and patients.

Regardless of the type of evaluation used, however, therapists should analyze the patient's performance and determine those factors that limit independence. Careful analysis will reveal whether the patient's performance is limited by a physical, perceptual, cognitive, and/or behavioral problem. In addition, evaluation can help the therapist recognize whether the patient is ready for training in a particular skill area. A state of readiness is essential to successful retraining. Finally, a thorough evaluation will aid the therapist in determining which subskills of a daily living task need to be practiced before embarking on formal training in activities of daily living.

Re-evaluation should occur at intervals, perhaps every 3 to 4 weeks. The results will help the team, the patient, and the family determine the rate of progress in retraining ADL. While some patients will progress rapidly from dependence to near-independence, other patients will move at a slower rate. Nevertheless, patients exhibiting steady progress, no matter how slow, should continue to be challenged toward greater independence.

DAILY LIVING SKILLS

Feeding

Immediately following head injury, a patient's nutritional needs are often met through a feeding tube of some sort; for example, a nasogastric tube. However, as the medical status stabilizes and the level of cognition improves, the attention of the rehabilitation staff turns to the feasibility of oral feeding.

In assessing readiness for oral feeding and self-feeding, three factors should be considered: oral-motor ability, physical skills, and cognitive/behavioral skills. Deficits in any or all of these areas can greatly limit the safety and success of oral feeding.

ORAL-MOTOR SKILLS

Dysphagia, drooling, and oral-motor weakness are common sequelae to head injury.[8] A team approach to their evaluation should be made prior to the onset of oral feeding and often it is led by a speech pathologist. Assessment should include an examination of the following:

1. The strength and quality of oral structures
2. The quality of swallowing ability
3. The quality of the patient's oral sensory receptors
4. The patient's ability to manage liquids and a variety of food textures

Once the evaluation has been completed, recommendations regarding oral feeding can be made. These should include the following:

1. The type of diet the patient should have (i.e., pureed, soft, minced, regular)
2. The type of liquid the patient should have, if any (i.e., thick versus thin, cold versus room temperature)
3. The methodology for feeding (i.e., whether feeding should be done only in therapy, as part of the feeding program, or in the dining room)

Obviously, the determination of these recommendations involves a variety of professionals, including the speech pathologist, occupational therapist, nurse, physician, and dietitian. It is vital that family be included in the process as well, so that they reinforce these guidelines.

It is unfortunate that not every patient with oral-motor deficits progresses to eating a completely normal diet. Nevertheless, the goal of treatment should be to normalize the patient's level of skill as much as possible to allow reintegration into family and social dining. Careful monitoring by the rehabilitation team makes it possible to determine the types of food with which the patient is successful, strategies to improve oral management of food, and techniques for food preparation necessary for the patient's particular needs.

PHYSICAL SKILLS

Many physical components are combined in the process of self-feeding. Severe head injury may impair one or more areas of physical function which, in turn, may impact on the patient's self-feeding skills.

Deficits in upper extremity function are common. Hemiplegia, contractures, peripheral nerve injury, sensory deficits, incoordination, spasticity, and weakness all limit effective use of utensils. Poor head control and impaired balance are frequently seen with the low-level patient. Jaw and facial fractures often occur and interfere with feeding. Visual disturbances such as blindness or ptosis will create problems in self-feeding. Rarely are these physical deficits seen in isolation; rather it is likely that several of them will be seen in a single patient.

In most rehabilitation programs, physical limitations are well addressed by the professional team. The physical therapist is concerned with motor control, range of motion, strength, and balance. In occupational therapy, the patient works on fine motor control, head control, and sensory retraining. Splints or positioning aids might be prescribed; adaptive aids might be employed. The rehabilitation nurse reinforces and applies positioning and adaptive techniques. The concomitant use of a variety of therapeutic interventions designed to hasten physical recovery is important in the success of a feeding program.

As the patient's abilities are assessed and appropriate aids are utilized, the therapist is able to delineate specific physical guidelines for feeding. To be considered in these guidelines are the following components:

1. The types of feeding surface the patient requires (i.e., lapboard, raised table, regular table)
2. The specific positioning needs of the patient
3. The aids required by the patient

4. The amount of assistance required from another individual

5. The patient's level of endurance (i.e., easily fatigued patients should be restricted to self-feeding for only a small portion of the meal and then receive assistance with the remainder)

It is critical to keep the expectations of staff and family consistent from meal to meal in order to avoid frustration. Asking the patient to perform beyond his or her capability will lead to a sense of failure and a slower rate of progress.

BEHAVIORAL, COGNITIVE, AND
PERCEPTUAL PROBLEMS

The head injured adult typically suffers from multiple problems in behavior, perception, and cognition. These deficits can impact on feeding skills and limit progress toward independence and reintegration into social dining situations.

The agitated patient finds it difficult to attend to meals as well as to instruction and feedback offered by therapists. The lethargic patient lacks sufficient endurance and attention to complete a meal without assistance. Behaviorally based feeding problems have also been observed in which patients spit out food and liquids, hold food in their mouths for extended periods of time refusing to chew or swallow, or reject food totally. Impulsive and disorganized individuals tend to eat too rapidly, fail to chew properly, and leave their place in the dining room in disarray.

For these patients, special approaches are required to maximize success. A calm, quiet environment will be of benefit to the agitated individual. On the other hand, lethargic feeders might profit from the use of cool washcloths to the neck and face, stimulating physical activity prior to eating; the introduction of cold, spicy, or sour food; and maximum cueing throughout the meal.

The behavior problems mentioned in regard to feeding are perplexing. Seemingly, no simple solutions to these problems exist. It is generally agreed, though, that staff and family should not push feeding. Making food available at mealtimes is a favored approach. Efforts should be directed toward maintaining a casual, inviting environment during meals. These behavioral problems usually come to an end without special intervention.

Patients suffering from impaired attention and heightened distractibility find the normal feeding environment too stimulating. With the sounds of clanging dishes and utensils, multiple conversations, and perhaps a television in the background, they experience difficulty filtering stimuli and focusing on the task of eating. Effective feeding is further complicated if the patient is also disoriented. These individuals definitely benefit from a structured environment that has a minimum of distractions and close supervision.

Perceptual dysfunction also greatly limits a head injured individual's ability to self-feed. The presence of a neglect or homonymous hemianopsia will cause such patients to perceive only half of their tray. Depth perception deficits are manifested by the patient overshooting when reaching for food or drink. Impairment of body schema may interfere with the process of bringing food from plate to mouth or the patient's skill in using utensils.

The hemianopsic patient must be taught to compensate for the field deficit in feeding as in other activities. Having food confined to specific boundaries (for example, on a plate, serving tray, or placemat) offers a consistent cue to the patient. Initially frequent cues from staff may be required to remind patients to look to their neglected or visually deficient side; however, with careful environmental structure and repetition, cueing should become less necessary.

Depth perception deficits may improve spontaneously. If diplopia is causing the deficits in depth perception, a consultation with the physician regarding modalities designed to reduce the double vision is in order. Weighted cups and cup holders can also help prevent spilling.

Apraxia may be a significant problem for patients learning feeding. Often even the simplest component of feeding such as picking up the spoon will be nearly an impossible task. Apraxic patients have particular difficulty with the process of bringing food from plate to mouth. Cutting food and pouring liquids are just as puzzling.

When a patient has trouble feeding because of apraxia, brief structured treatment sessions are helpful initially. Physically guiding patients through feeding also improves their performance. Every new aspect of feeding encountered will require this intensive treatment. On the positive side, however, due to the repetitive nature of feeding and the frequency with which patients eat, apraxia typically resolves fairly quickly.

A FEEDING PROGRAM AS A MODEL FOR TREATMENT

Head injured patients can benefit from a feeding program that supplies intensive intervention by a team of staff professionals. In this model, the oral-motor, physical and behavioral, cognitive, and perceptual dysfunctions affecting feeding are addressed. There is a focus on safe, effective feeding at a level of maximum independence that provides excellent nutrition and hydration for the patient. The skills of all team members are well utilized by this approach.

The team involved in the feeding program should include the occupational therapist, the speech pathologist, the nurse, and the dietitian. Naturally, family education, involvement, and support are crucial to the program's success. All meals taken by an individual are included in the feeding program with intensive training being provided by different team members. For example, the speech pathologist will work with the patient individually at breakfast. Then the patient is involved in the lunchtime feeding group, where the occupational therapist concentrates on the mechanics of self-feeding. At dinner, a trained family member assists under the supervision of a nurse.

Determination of appropriateness for the feeding program should be based upon these criteria and should be a team decision:

1. The patient's oral-motor status
2. The patient's ability to physically manage self-feeding and the potential for improvement
3. The patient's endurance and tolerance for feeding

The patient's ability to take sufficient food and liquid orally is one of the criteria, as often food taken at meals is viewed as supplementary to tube feeding. Careful calorie counts as well as input/output records are maintained to assist in decision making. Once oral intake of both food and liquids is sufficient to meet the patient's needs, the dietitian and nurse will recommend the removal of feeding tubes and the cessation of tube feeding.

After the patient is placed in the feeding program, an interdisciplinary approach in retraining of feeding begins. Oral-motor training will focus on the process of chewing, swallowing, and lip closure, and as improvements occur, the consistency of the diet will be upgraded. The team will retrain patients in their ability to identify food and drink before them as well as their ability to bring food and drink to the mouth. Throughout meals, appropriate table behavior is emphasized. Family style dining is ideal for the retraining of social skills associated with eating. Neatness, use of napkins, and polite conversation are encouraged.

Initially the highly distractable and disoriented patient may be isolated from the group dining situation but a quiet environment helps him or her to focus on food, feeding skills, and behavior. Gradually, patients are introduced into the noisier and more normal dining setting, where cueing provided by staff assists them in remaining on the task.

Performance in the feeding program is evaluated weekly to determine change, and the nature of components involved in self-feeding are rated. Improvements indicate a need for continued involvement in the feeding program; failure to make improvements needs to be evaluated to determine the cause. Among the factors frequently contributing to lack of progress are a change in the patient's medical status, a medication change, the onset of a problematic behavior, and of course the attainment of maximum benefit from the feeding program. Depending on the factor or factors responsible for lack of progress, the team should decide whether the feeding program should be continued.

Learning to feed oneself is a self-reinforcing activity. Improved skills allow for the removal of nasogastric, gastrostomy, and jejunostomy tubes. In addition, the variety of food available to the patient is increased, and the social interaction so closely interwoven with eating is reinstated.

Dressing

Problems with dressing following head injury are typically associated with impaired physical skills and cognitive and/or perceptual deficits. The head injured patient newly admitted to the rehabilitation unit usually is not immediately ready for a formal dressing retraining program. Therefore, it is advisable that a state of readiness be achieved prior to the onset of retraining, thus maximizing the program's success.

Hemiplegia, impaired balance, poor coordination, generalized weakness, and decreased endurance interfere with dressing. Usually, although these deficits may slow patients' progress toward independence, they do not generally prevent it. In fact, physical deficits will lessen with practice sessions, instruction in and learning of adaptive techniques, and the use of adaptive aids.

More often, it is perceptual and cognitive problems that limit independence. Deficits in visual field, visual attention, praxis, body schema, right-left orientation, figure-ground perception, and depth perception will lead to problems in locating and identifying clothing and parts of garments, orienting garments to body parts, completing dressing of all body parts, and following adaptive techniques. Though some perceptual deficits improve, it is the effects of those that fail to respond to intervention that create the greatest problems.

The cognitive deficits that accompany severe head injury complicate the relearning of dressing. Attention to task is critical to dressing, as is some level of orientation to the environment and to time. The individual with deficits in problem solving, organization, sequencing, and generalization will find independent dressing difficult; every dressing experience will pose its own set of new problems and challenges, which this type of patient will find very hard to meet. Impaired memory will limit carryover and the retention of new techniques. However, providing cue cards and lots of repetition during the dressing program may facilitate independence.

Naturally, patients with poor initiation will require someone present to keep them on task, and those patients who are unable to manage frustration may have outbursts if they run into problems. Patients with impaired judgment skills may attempt aspects of dressing that are unsafe or beyond their skill level, without calling for help. Poor quality control may be evident in the individual who fails to achieve a neat, well-coordinated appearance. Unless a change in these behaviors can be achieved through a dressing program, patients with impaired initiation, frustration tolerance, judgment, and quality control will require another person present if only to monitor their performance and ensure their safety.

The dressing program should begin when the patient has achieved readiness. Prior to the initiation of a full, formalized retraining program, many head injured patients benefit from training in predressing skills. This includes brief sessions involving the relearning of components of dressing (i.e., putting on a shirt, practicing buttoning, or learning the use of an adaptive aid). Once the components have been practiced and some mastery achieved, promotion to the total retraining program may be indicated. Though determination of readiness varies from person to person, some basic factors can be considered:

1. The patient's level of alertness and attention: ability to maintain attention 15 minutes with minimal to moderate redirection
2. The patient's physical status: balance, head control, and ability to manage extremities
3. The patient's medical condition: the status of wounds and fractures
4. The patient's success in the predressing program

A team effort among occupational therapy, nursing, and the family is critical to success. All techniques recommended by the occupational therapists must be taught to the family and staff. Throughout the process of retraining, several principles should be practiced by those involved:

1. All dressing should be done in a consistent manner. Written cue cards may facilitate this.
2. Independence should be encouraged. All staff and family should avoid and discourage the manipulative patient's attempt to solicit more help than he or she actually needs. Cue cards should clearly designate those areas in which assistance is allowed.
3. Maintain the atmosphere of retraining. Aid patients in problem solving rather than simply providing them with assistance to get them out of difficulties.
4. Neatness should be reinforced. Guide

the patient as clothing is selected, offering advice about coordinating garments. Provide cues to aid the patient in reviewing his or her appearance (i.e., to button buttons, tuck in shirt tails, and pull up socks)

There is a logical progression for head injured patients as they relearn dressing. Beginning with total dependence, the patient moves to partial dependence in a structured environment. From there, patients regain skill allowing them independence in that structured environment. It is hoped that the improvements will continue, enabling patients to progress to a less structured environment. The ultimate goal is total independence performed within a reasonable period of time in a normal environment. It is the function of the dressing program to help the patient achieve the highest possible level of function.

Hygiene Skills

It is our external appearance that creates others' first impressions of us. Therefore, most people consider it critical to their social success to maintain a pleasing appearance.

Following head injury, deficits in hygiene maintenance are typically quite obvious to those interacting with the individual. There appears to be an unawareness and unconcern for the appearance early on. Then later, as awareness increases, often the multiple areas of deficit limit the patient's ability to correct his or her deficient hygiene and grooming. Because of the association between an individual's appearance and others' acceptance of him or her, it is advisable that instruction in basic hygiene skills begin as early as possible.

As with other aspects of self-care, physical, perceptual, and behavioral/cognitive problems will limit independence in hygiene. When physical limitations impair performance, frequently adaptive aids can provide the needed assistance. Built-up handles for toothbrushes, shaver holders, and implements with suction-cup bases are often useful. Often, patients' low level of endurance limits their ability to complete all components of a task, but a gradual increase in the level of performance expected of them will usually increase their tolerance for activity.

It is more often the perceptual, behavioral, and cognitive deficits that limit independence. Disorientation and a lack of motivation and initiative inhibit the natural drive to be attractive and neat. The patient with impaired organizational and sequencing skills will find it difficult to manage independently the multistep process of self-grooming. In addition, patients may find it impossible to make time in their schedule for needed personal hygiene, and will therefore require assistance from staff and family. Memory deficits will limit carryover and retention. Impulsive individuals will require cues to achieve a quality result from their efforts.

There are several options for treating deficits in hygiene. Regardless of the method chosen, readiness for training should be established. Patients who are capable of relearning hygiene skills should meet these criteria:

1. They should have some level of orientation and some awareness of themselves and their environment.

2. They should possess sufficient physical skills to engage in the task with assistance. Clearly, the totally physically dependent patient is not ready for retraining.

3. They should demonstrate an attention span of a minimum of 5 minutes.

Obviously, motivation to improve their appearance will be an asset in the retraining process.

With most head injured patients, the initial training sessions should be individualized and should focus on only one skill area. The nurses and family should then incorporate new skills into the daily routine of care. Some clinicians utilize group hygiene sessions to teach specific skills. However, because hygiene and grooming involve such personal tasks, the group approach may meet with little enthusiasm from some patients.

The key to later independence in hygiene is to incorporate the learned skills into the patient's routine while still hospitalized. A schedule of activities that includes time for grooming posted at bedside is the best way to ensure inclusion of necessary hygiene tasks in the patient's day. Family, staff, and patient should all tune in to the schedule and follow it because it is most likely to succeed if all are included in its development.

Some patients who find it difficult to organize activities will benefit from increased environmental structure (e.g., keeping all bathing and hair care supplies in a basket to carry to the shower). Checklists and cue cards can provide needed assistance with sequencing and memory impairment.

The level of independence achieved will vary from patient to patient. Nevertheless, the rehabilitation staff needs to attend to hygiene deficits early in rehabilitation to maximize function. Recovery of these skills should not be left to nature, time, or chance.

Transfers

Motor deficits, perceptual deficits, and cognitive impairment can hamper an individual's independence in transfers. On any given head injury unit, one will see the lethargic patient with impaired balance and poor head control sitting slumped forward and sliding out of the wheelchair. Next to this patient one might see the restless and impulsive patient struggling with restraints and attempting to stand up without help. It is likely both of these individuals require assistance with transfers; however, their needs and the kind of assistance required may be quite different.

The critical components in teaching the head injured patient transfers are the same for all transfers to all surfaces for all patients. Regardless of the patient's status or the type of transfer, these guidelines are critical to the success of teaching independent transfers to the head injured patient:

1. Establish early the amount of assistance, if any, required for transfers and communicate this to all staff. Signs hung at bedside plus discussion in care conferences will reinforce this information for staff and family. Because head injured patients are notably unreliable and unsafe, they should not be relied upon to communicate the status of their transfers to others.

2. All transfers should be done the same way every time. Staff and family should offer the appropriate amount of assistance—no more, no less. Families should be taught the sequence of safe transfers by staff and be cleared to do transfers without staff supervision or assistance.

3. The routine followed for transfers should be verbalized throughout the process for the patient's benefit. Hearing the steps repeated frequently and matching this to performance should enhance carryover.

4. Changes in the level of performance for transfers should be communicated immediately to ensure consistency and carryover.

5. Transfers should be performed slowly. Give the patient time to process and respond to instructions. This will improve performance and learning.

6. Delineate specifically those components of the transfer the patient should perform without assistance and/or cues. For example, locking brakes and/or pivoting to sit. Consistency in this area will provide the patient with building blocks toward increased independence.

7. Set clear limits if necessary. Some patients will need to be told they can perform transfers only after requesting help. If strict limit-setting is not effective and patients pose a hazard to themselves, then use restraints as needed to ensure safety. Unfortunately, it is often the case that patients' level of mobility does not match their level of cognition, necessitating artificial restraints.

By using these guidelines, the goal of maximizing independence while providing safety is met. Consistency and repetition enhance learning and is best accomplished through an interdisciplinary approach to transfers.

ADVANCED LIVING SKILLS

Advanced living skills include a wide range of activities that require high-level skills and are essential to independent living. However, the recovery of full independence in these areas typically takes a considerable amount of time and creates alterations within the family unit.

As part of the rehabilitation program, advanced living skills should be addressed. Unfortunately for some head injury adults, the possibility of performing advanced living skills seems quite remote because of the severity of their injury. For others, however, the picture is much brighter.

Not every advanced life skill is crucial to a satisfied lifestyle for every patient. The high school student needs to master writing and interpersonal skills, whereas the young mother of two needs to practice cooking, homemaking, and parenting. Likewise, the middle-aged man may be most interested in driving and relearning financial management skills so he can resume his family duties. It is vital, therefore, that goals be set with the patient and family, taking into consideration the patient's premorbid life roles in order to provide meaningful and relevant therapy.

Communication Skills

Most people communicate daily by writing, typing, and/or using the telephone. After head injury, these tasks, so taken for granted prior to the injury, become very difficult—if not impossible—for the patient to perform. Intervention is required, therefore, to improve function.

Writing skills may be limited by incoordination, weakness, loss of function in the dominant hand, impulsivity, apraxia, poor quality control, visual field cut, visual inattention, perseveration, and various language disorders. While the speech pathologist addresses dysfunction in language, the occupational therapist can provide treatment for the physical, perceptual, and cognitive deficits limiting writing.

In cooperation with physical therapy, a program should be designed to maximize physical skills. Activities to improve praxis, dominance, fine motor coordination, and attention should be introduced. To decrease the effects of field cuts and perseveration, compensation techniques should be taught. Though initially quality control will be provided by the therapist, the patient should be taught to decrease speed and improve concentration to minimize errors.

Reinforcement of newly relearned writing skills can be provided by having the patient record daily events in a journal or by writing out his or her own schedule. Games such as "Hangman" or "Tic Tac Toe" challenge writing indirectly.

Effective use of the telephone is another important aspect of communication; therefore, phone retraining should be included in the program at some point. Physical impediments to phone use are generally manageable through adaptive aids. Phone companies offer a variety of options for handicapped customers, which may be explored. Good visual perception, sequencing, and attentional skills are necessary to successful dialing. Practice using the phone should lead to improvements in accuracy and independence.

Appropriate phone behavior can be incorporated in social skills training. Role-playing phone conversations will allow practice; taping these practice sessions and playing them back for the patients can be useful. Emphasis should be placed on knowing how to use a phone in an emergency. If deemed necessary, cue cards can be provided to assist patients in phone use. A review of the use of the phone directory should be part of the treatment program. Again, sequencing skills, problem solving, and attentional and organizational skills are important for success.

Homemaking Skills

The need for some level of skill in homemaking is becoming increasingly important for all adults, as both men and women share the cooking, cleaning, and laundry responsibilities. While physical impairments can pose significant obstacles to the performance of these tasks, it is typically the individual's significant cognitive problems that limit his or her ability to do homemaking chores safely and judiciously.

Cooking activities should begin at a simple level with intensive supervision. Prior to beginning kitchen activities, the patient should be reasonably oriented and able to follow instructions. Safety, judgment, organizational skills, impulse control, and quality control can all be challenged and assessed during cooking. The therapist should offer patients feedback and assist them in problem solving and error recognition.

Some therapists find the use of cooking groups beneficial. This allows patients to benefit from each other's assets, experiences, and observations. Group planning and problem solving is encouraged. Group sessions also allow greater frequency of practice in the kitchen.

Frequent exposure to cooking experiences is beneficial for head injured patients. Repetition appears to enhance learning and competency. Families should be involved if possible. Allowing families to observe while the therapist teaches the patient provides an opportunity for modeling appropriate coaching and feedback. When the patient and family are ready, cooking should be practiced during weekend therapeutic leave.

Other aspects of homemaking should be addressed as appropriate for each patient. Setting aside a time weekly when patients can do their laundry may prove helpful. As proficiency increases, the responsibility for laundry can be shifted to the patient with cues from the family or nurses. Ironing, bedmaking, vacuuming, washing dishes, and dusting can be practiced as indicated. The same tasks can then be assigned as "homework" during weekend leave.

The keys to retraining homemaking skills are a thorough evaluation and determination of competency through the use of practice sessions in the hospital and at home. By critically analyzing the patient's performance, the therapist is able to determine the following:

1. The patient's level of safety
2. The patient's competency and potential for gains
3. The quality of the patient's judgment skills
4. The necessity for supervision during the performance of these tasks

Because the kinds of deficits posed by head injury are unique to these individuals and pose such an array of implications, careful evaluation and good family education are vital.

Interpersonal Skills and Social Roles

Most head injured individuals bring with them to the rehabilitation unit a concerned and loving family. However, as a result of the head injury, the patient frequently has difficulty maintaining relationships within the family and close circle of friends. The treatment team must attend to this problem and begin intervention.

Several strategies are suggested for dealing with changes in interpersonal skills and social roles. First, the family and close friends of the head injured adult should be active in rehabilitation from the beginning, if at all possible. If they seem unable to generate and sustain activities and conversations with the patient, then team members should suggest a repertoire of suitable activities. Family education should be ongoing and should include practical tips on techniques to use to reinforce appropriate behavior and conversation. Often it is the informal discussions with family regarding a recent occurrence that are most meaningful.

Second, team members should model appropriate interaction with the patient. Some families tend to "baby" their loved ones; others give in to every request made by the patient, no matter how absurd or unreasonable; still others are immobilized by the fear of saying or doing the wrong thing. By demonstrating the correct way to interact with the patient, the team helps alleviate the families' fears and maladaptive responses.

Family members have to learn the importance of reestablishing their personal lives. Frequently spouses, parents, siblings, and children keep a vigil at the bedside of the head injured patient from the moment of hospitalization; in fact, the hospital and the patient become the center of their existence. However, upon transfer of the patient to the rehabilitation facility, families should be strongly encouraged to re-establish some of their normal daily routines. While their participation in therapy is important, it is usually unnecessary for them to be present at the hospital throughout the entire day. If there is a cooperative air among the staff and family, convenient schedules for the latter can be arranged by therapists and nurses. As appropriate, family members can be advised to return to work or school, to take "days off" from the hospital and to visit only at select times of the day or evening. By assuming responsibility for limiting family visits, the rehabilitation team relieves families of any guilt they might feel when they must be away from the hospital because of illness, vacation, or business.

Naturally, in every family, someone must assume some of the roles of the injured person, at least temporarily. The stress created by this is often difficult for family members to handle. If some normality can be established in their lives, often the burden of taking on the "jobs" of the head injured adult are easier to manage.

A fourth strategy involves social skills training. A formal group approach designed to improve social skills is beneficial for head ıred adults. When coupled with video-ping, this technique allows the patients to interact, then to view and evaluate themselves. Techniques discussed in the group can be shared with family and other team members to encourage reinforcement and carryover.

A final strategy is to challenge social skills behavior by involving the patient in group activities and weekend leave. Head injury units offer a range of group activities ranging from a physical activities group to orientation group to recreation group. In all of these settings, the head injured patient is expected to behave appropriately and as a group member. This involves inhibiting certain behavior and verbalization, behaving cooperatively with others in the group, switching roles from leader to follower, and providing support and feedback. Throughout these changes, staff members can provide cues and assistance.

On weekend leave, the family must assume responsibility for monitoring the patient's social skills, providing needed cueing and giving feedback to the staff following the leave. In the more familiar environment of home, it is noted that social interaction seems more appropriate and functional. Therefore, during the leave, the opportunities to practice the wide range of social skills should be available.

Throughout the process of re-establishing appropriate interpersonal and social behavior, it is crucial that the patient receives praise and encouragement for the use of appropriate skills. Likewise, cueing should be offered when less desirable behavior is displayed. Suggestions for improved responses should be discussed with the patient because although the family and treatment team might overlook or excuse an unsuitable phrase or behavior, the rest of society will not be so forgiving.

Time Management

Every normal individual possesses some ability to manage time, to prioritize activities, and to meet deadlines, but the head injured adult typically loses the ability to do so. It is the goal of the rehabilitation team to help the patient regain independence in time management. The process begins with the establishment of a daily schedule into which are incorporated self-maintenance tasks, therapies, and social activities.

Initially, decisions about the timing of items in the schedule come from the rehabilitation team. However, as the patient's cognition improves, his or her input is solicited; for example, a rest period or a favorite television show might be worked into the day. Patients should have a copy of the schedule available to them; attaching schedules to wheelchairs can be very helpful as well.

Utilization of a written schedule is in part based upon a knowledge of the time of day at any given moment. For this reason, clocks should be placed generously throughout the unit and the patient should wear a watch if possible.

For a considerable time after injury, individuals suffering from head injury may have difficulty structuring their free time. Evening and weekend hours may be the most troublesome. Typically, when individuals do not have a scheduled activity they can be found asleep, wandering aimlessly, or watching television; but for most adults these do not represent the most ideal use of leisure time.

The patient's daily schedule should run until bedtime and include a variety of activities. Therapists should assign homework to be completed outside therapy. Recreational programs and supplies for lesiure activities should be available. Families should be encouraged to take the patient to the cafeteria for supper or out on the grounds. A comfortable area conducive to socialization should be designed on the unit. Magazines should be available to patients. Whenever possible, bedtime should be delayed to a normal hour—i.e., 10 o'clock rather than 7 o'clock which some head injury units designate as bedtime. Making family members aware of the patient's difficulty managing time early in the program will prepare them for similar problems at discharge. Their help during the in-patient stay is vital.

Financial Management

Prior to head injury most of the patients in a rehabilitation unit probably managed their own finances; suddenly, with their injury, this function is severely impaired. Impaired alertness, poor judgment, impulsivity, and illogical thinking, coupled with deficits in mathematics, contribute to this situation. Although often a guardian is named for the patient early in the recovery process, the goal of therapy should be the achievement of independence in the management of his or her financial affairs.

For the physically impaired patient who finds handling money, writing checks, and using a calculator difficult, sessions to practice these skills should be planned. Adaptive aids may prove helpful. The perceptually impaired individual may find it difficult to discriminate coins (size discrimination), locate specific coins from among a group of coins (figure-ground perception), locate money in their purse or pocket (stereognosis), find money on one side of them (field of vision), or read prices on a price list (tracking).

The cognitively impaired patient experiences multiple areas of deficit that impair money management. These include poor memory, attention, and concentration; impulsivity; decreased organizational skills; impaired problem solving and decision making; and poor reasoning.

In therapy, the retraining process should focus on specific skill areas:

1. Recognition of and assignment of value to coinage and bills
2. Simple computation of coins and bills
3. Use of money to purchase needs
4. Change-making
5. Budgeting (this includes a sound knowledge of needs versus wants and savings programs)
6. Banking skills, i.e., writing checks and balancing a checkbook

Community experiences are particularly helpful in allowing the patient to practice opportunities in a real environment with supervision. These experiences can be built into the program during recreational and leisure pursuits—for example, shopping or dining out. In addition, therapeutic leave should include community activities under family supervision.

Driving

A high level of recovery must be achieved before most head injured adults are permitted to resume driving.[9] For some victims of head injury, their impairments are too severe and persistent to ever allow driving. The decision regarding an individual's ability to return to driving should not be made casually or too early in the recovery process.

The presence of certain specific conditions should prevent driving. These include uncontrolled seizures and severe motor impairment that limits vehicle control. Individuals should not drive if they take medication that significantly slows response time or impairs consciousness. The presence of poor judgment and disorientation, severe perceptual deficits, and visual deficits also tend to make driving unsafe.

However, should a patient be free of these problems, driving may be appropriate. The initial step should be a thorough review of recent perceptual and neuropsychologic tests, visual tests, and a physical assessment followed by referral to a driving evaluator, preferably a health care professional familiar with head injury.

The evaluation performed by the evaluator should include several areas:

1. Physical skills
   a. Physical management of the vehicle
   b. Need for adaptations to the controls
   c. Endurance
2. Visual skills
   a. Peripheral vision
   b. Visual scanning
   c. Visual discrimination
   d. Visual acuity
3. Perceptual skills
   a. Depth and distance perception
   b. Spatial relations and orientation
   c. Traffic sign recognition
   d. Right/left orientation
4. Speed of motor responses
   a. Braking time
   b. Shifts in lane position
   c. Reaction to emergency situations
5. Judgment
   a. Decision-making skills
   b. Quality control

Once the comprehensive evaluation is completed, a determination of driving eligibility can be made. Without careful and professional evaluation of their skills and performance, it is quite difficult to predict whether head injured persons can safely return to driving.

Community Skills

For the head injured patient, it is often the transition from dependence on others to meet their community-based needs to independent performance of these skills that is so very hard to achieve. Because of the nature of head injury, it is most frequently the cognitive and behavioral sequelae that limit their community reintegration. Nevertheless, rehabilitation should address independent living skills—specifically shopping, transportation, and recreation.

Many rehabilitation facilities address these needs by developing a training program for patients. Neistadt[10] describes a program that addresses these areas as well as others and involves multidisciplinary team members. A syllabus of lectures has been developed for this program, which patients are expected to attend. The patients complete homework and also participate in sessions designed to practice skills.

Shopping for clothing, food, gifts, and personal needs involves several components: recognition of the need, organization of the shopping trip and execution of the purchase including transportation, selection, and management of money. Head injured adults may have trouble with any or all of these areas. For this reason, training should focus on the deficit areas while building the areas of strength. For example, a patient may recognize the need to do grocery shopping and be physically able to perform the task but lack the organizational skills to make a list prior to leaving home. The same patient may be able to handle money well enough to purchase food but always overspends the allotted budget. If appropriate, some of the more subtle, though important, aspects of shopping should be addressed. Comparative shopping, selection of quality merchandise; and social skills pertinent to shopping should be discussed as a group, and then put into practice.[7]

Because a significant number of head injured adults cannot safely drive, it is important to teach them how to use public transportation effectively. Strategies such as writing the transit company's number by the phone or a cue card to help the individual locate the correct change for the bus may prove useful. Staff members should take patients for practice sessions on city buses or in taxis, allowing increasing amounts of independence. As with other skills, a routine for use of public transportation should enhance performance. Always boarding and disembarking at the same time or place reduces confusion. Keeping bus money in the same pocket daily makes boarding smoother, and having a backup procedure written down and tucked away in a pocket or wallet will help alleviate fears and confusion for some individuals when there is a disruption in the usual routine.

Planning for and constructive use of leisure time is a skill with which many head injured adults have difficulty. Prolonged periods of in-patient hospitalization, dependence on others for a majority of needs, and decreased cognitive skills all have an impact on the individual's ability to pursue recreation. In addition, premorbid leisure interests may be precluded by physical deficits, cognitive problems, lack of opportunity, and lack of money.

The intervention of therapeutic recreation is invaluable for people with such problems. Leisure counseling can help them improve their use of leisure time and offer a direction for retraining. Community outings can provide opportunities to test new skills and practice social skills. All team members should be involved in the outings in order to see their patients in the real world. During retraining, recreation appropriate for groups and solitary time should be reviewed. Self-esteem and confidence are bolstered by exposure to therapeutic recreation. Families should be involved in fun time with patients and experience laughter and excitement. Creativity and planning by the recreation therapist are crucial, as is a good sense of the impairment associated with head injury.

CONCLUSION

While the process of training daily living skills usually begins during the in-patient hospitalization, it continues for months, even years, after discharge. Often retraining is delayed because the patient is not ready. For this reason, the rehabilitation team must be vigilant and provide good follow-up care in order to detect signs of readiness during follow-up.

All too often, the head injured adult is unable to achieve full independence in all areas of function. This places a burden on the family, who find it their job to aid the patient. This may come in the form of physical or cognitive help and may well continue for many years. The restrictions this places on families are tremendous and cause constant stress to the family unit.

To meet the demand for such assistance on the part of patients and their families, more and more programs are being developed to handle the needs of head injured adults who, even years after injury, remain dependent on others to some extent. Day hospitals, day care, respite care, transitional living, group homes, sheltered work environments, residential facilities, and home care assistance are examples of some of the options.

The challenge to rehabilitation professionals is to approach deficits in daily living skills innovatively and enthusiastically, with the goal of maximizing the head injured adult's potential and ability to live independently. Because of the nature of head injury, extra dedication and creativity are often required to approach the achievement of this goal. There is also the relentless battle against frustration that springs up in the patient, family, and professional as attempts fall short of the goal and techniques fail. Nevertheless, optimism must prevail and all eyes focus on the ultimate goal of a return to a satisfying lifestyle filled with the pursuit of work, play, and friendship.

REFERENCES

1. Sarno, JE, Sarno, MT and Levita, E: The functional life scale. Arch Phys Med Rehabil 54:214, 1973.
2. Jette, AM: Functional capacity evaluation: An empirical approach. Arch Phys Med Rehabil 61:85, 1980.
3. Feigenson, J et al: Burke stroke time-oriented profile: An overview. Arch Phys Med Rehabil 60:508, 1979.
4. Klein, RM and Bell, BJ: Self care skills: Behavioral measurement with the Klein-Bell ADL scale. Arch Phys Med Rehabil 63:335, 1982.
5. Iverson, IA et al: Revised Kenny Self Care Evaluation. Rehab Pub. 722, Minneapolis, Sister Kenny Inst.
6. Mahoney, F and Barthel, D: Functional evaluation: The Barthel index. MD State Med J 14:61, 1965.
7. Casanova, JS and Ferber, J: Comprehensive evaluation of basic living skills. AJOT 76:101, 1976.
8. Logemann, J: Evaluation and treatment of swallowing disorders. College-Hill Press, San Diego, 1983.
9. Jones, R, Giddens, H and Croft, D: Assessment and training of brain-damaged drivers. AJOT 37:754, 1983.
10. Neistadt, ME and Marques, K: An independent living skills training program. AJOT 38:671, 1984.

BIBLIOGRAPHY

Bardach, J: Psychological factors in the handicapped driver. Arch Phys Med Rehabil 52:328, 1971.
Baum, B: Relationship between constructional praxis and dressing in the head-injured adult. AJOT 35:438, 1981.
DeTienne, S: Long term care dining challenge—adequate nutrition and maximum independence. OT Forum 2:17, 1986.
Griffin, KM: Swallowing training for dysphagic patients. Arch Phys Med Rehabil 55:467, 1974.
Hunter, J: Swallowing disorders: the hidden danger. OT Forum 1:1, 1986.
Kreutzer, J et al: A glossary of cognitive rehabilitation terminology. Cog Rehabil 4:10, 1986.
Lezak, MD: Living with the characterologically altered brain injured patient. J Clin Psychiatry 39:592, 1978.
Oddy, M, Humphrey, M and Uttley, D: Stresses upon relatives of head injured patients. Br J Psychiatry 133:507, 1978.
Panikoff, L: Recovery trends of functional skills in the head injured adult. AJOT 37:735, 1983.
Sivak, M et al: Improved driving performance following perceptual training in persons with brain damage. Arch Phys Med Rehabil 65:163, 1984.
Sivak, M et al: Driving and perceptual/cognitive skills: behavioral consequences of brain damage. Arch Phys Med Rehabil 62:476, 1981.

Chapter 15

Sexuality and Sexual Dysfunction

ERNEST R. GRIFFITH, M.D.
SANDRA COLE, A.A.S.E.C.T., C.S.E., C.S.C.
THEODORE M. COLE, M.D.

Human sexuality conceptually embraces the composite of those factors that result in our capacity to love and procreate. A related aspect of sexuality is the individual's perception and expression of "womanliness" or "manliness." By these terms, it is predictable that a catastrophic event such as brain injury will almost ineluctably affect the sexuality of the survivor. Sexual disabilities may include disturbances of any of the component functions of sexuality: sexual drive, interests, beliefs, attitudes, behaviors, identity, activities, responses, and fertility.

For purposes of evaluation and treatment it is useful to classify sexual dysfunctions according to their causative factors.[1] Those disabilities resulting from physical or organic factors are termed primary dysfunctions. This classification requires further elucidation in those dysfunctions ensuing from brain diseases or injuries, since organic factors may result in changes in mental functions, which, in turn, may produce sexual dysfunctions. We will consider that primary sexual dysfunctions resulting directly from brain injury are neural or endocrine disorders influencing sexual interest, activity, and reponses, as well as fertility.

Secondary sexual dysfunctions resulting from brain trauma are those disturbances of psychosocial abilities or sexual responses due to the mental deficits and psychologic reactions consequent to the injury. Secondary sexual dysfunctions may arise in the partner, if one exists, as the consequences of reactions to the disabled person and the altered life situation. Both primary and secondary sexual disabilities may have existed in either the brain injured person or the partner before the injury.

Current evidence indicates that secondary factors account for the great majority of sexual dysfunctions in brain injured subjects. However, more recent data suggest that primary factors may be less rare than previously surmised.[2, 3]

A survey of the existing scientific literature on this subject is rather unrewarding, with some notable exceptions. In contrast to the growing body of general information on psychosocial aspects of brain trauma, very little has been written about sexuality. We are indebted to Romano,[4] Lezak,[5] Bond,[6] Brooks,[7] and Rosenbaum and Najenson[8] for providing extensive insight into the relationship of brain injured people with their partners. Secondary sexual dysfunctions of the partners are revealed and their origins derived in several of these studies. Furthermore, the long-term psychosocial sequelae of the injured, with some of their sexual implications, are explored. Other recent contributions include hypothalamic-pituitary axis disruptions, which sometimes alter gonadal function,[2, 3, 9, 10] and a series of 40 cases of Klüver-Bucy syndrome.[11] Berrol's contribution on sexuality in head injured adults[12] may have been the only existing chapter on that subject in a medical textbook until now.

Much of the earlier literature consists of case reports of unusual brain syndromes causing sexually aberrant behaviors. Two more extensive surveys, those of Meyer[13] and Walker and Jablon[14] provide some conflicting data. Walker and Jablon's study of 739 men disclosed that 8.1 percent experienced decreased potency that was related to the severity but not the locus of injury. Meyer's report of 100 men disclosed that 81 percent experienced a reduction of erections, which was related to severity and site of injury. Only Walker[15] and Panting and Merry[16] provide data concerning divorce rates. Walker cites a figure of 11 percent, whereas the British investigators, reporting in the same year (1972), found that figure to be 40 percent.

Weinstein[17] and others,[18, 19] describe focal traumatic lesions of frontal, temporal, and limbic areas which sometimes produce distinctive syndromes such as Klüver-Bucy or temporal lobe seizures that have sexual components. These authors confirm that such syndromes are most often marked by decreased sexual interest and activity.

From this cursory review, it should be evident that there are many significant gaps in our information. Perforce we have bridged some of the gaps by dint of clinical experiences, communications with colleagues, and applications of methods that have proved useful in other disability states. Nevertheless, these alternatives will not entirely substitute for the further information to be derived from more extensive research.

DESCRIPTION OF SEXUAL DYSFUNCTION

Primary (Organic) Dysfunctions

Sexual responses—erection, vaginal lubrication, ejaculation, orgasm, and fertility—are not altered as a direct consequence of brain injury unless the hypothalamic-pituitary function has been disturbed or disrupted. The resulting endocrinopathies have received increasing attention, with recognition that testicular and ovarian hypofunction can occur.[2, 3, 9, 10] Some women with mesial temporal lobe foci of seizures have recently been reported to have hypogonadotropic hypogonadism.[20] Women often become temporarily amenorrheic following severe trauma, but menses should ordinarily resume within 4 to 6 months. Persistent amenorrhea should alert the clinician to the possibility of pituitary dysfunction. Similarly, men frequently have transient impotence, but the ability to achieve an erection should reappear after several months. Testicular or ovarian failure, resulting in infertility and loss of secondary sexual characteristics or failure to undergo puberty, evidently is an extremely rare event. In children, precocious puberty has been reported in association with temporal lobe injuries.[21] Chapter 9 on medical and orthopedic complications includes a more detailed discussion of endocrinopathies.

Sexual activities may be altered or inhibited by a number of motor or sensory disorders resulting from brain trauma. The various hypertonicity states and movement disorders described in Chapter 10 can interfere with preparations for or participation in lovemaking to varying degrees. Not only may intercourse be unachievable, but the brain injured person or partner also may experience discomfort or even trauma in the attempt. Conversely, because of syndromes of apraxia and abulia, there may be inability to initiate sexual activity. Seizures occurring during sex acts are disruptive and frightening experiences; they may be precipitated by hyperventilation during sexual excitement.[22] Hemisensory deficits, hyperesthesias, thalamic pain syndrome, and a variety of perceptual deficits occasionally are the major source of dysfunction.

Coexisting injuries at times produce sexual disabilities that may not be readily recognized. Neurologic deficits affecting sexual acts and responses occur after spinal cord injury, pelvic injuries from which lumbosacral plexopathies ensue, radiculopathies, and peripheral nerve injuries (see Chapter 7). Trauma to the craniofacial area, primary or secondary sexual organs, and orthopedic injuries resulting in amputation, contractures, deformities, and chronic pain are potential sources of dysfunction. Pelvic fractures may result in deformities causing dyspareunia or cephalopelvic disproportion. Abdominal or pelvic vascular injuries can compromise circulation to the genitalia, producing impotence or other alterations in sexual responses.

Recurrent medical complications, sustained bed rest, and inactivity with its many consequences cause deconditioning and other effects that impinge upon sexual activity. A multitude of drugs produce side effects that influence sexual acts and responses (Table 15–1).[23, 24] Polyneuropathies, excessive sedation, impotence, or its equivalent; inadequate or absent vaginal lubrication and clitoral responsiveness, ataxia, and other movement disorders, hormonal disorders, and teratogenesis in pregnancy are some of the iatrogenic disturbances. Of further concern is the extreme physical and psychic intolerance of the brain injured person to alcohol, marijuana, and other "street" drugs.

Finally, pre-existing disorders may become additive factors contributing to primary sexual dysfunction. Cardiac, vascular, pulmonary, or other types of diseases may already have compromised sexual function of the elderly before injury. Drug abuse and previous injuries are prominent sources of sexual dysfunction in the younger age groups.

Secondary Sexual Dysfunctions

PREMORBID PSYCHOSOCIAL SEXUAL DYSFUNCTION

The head injured person may have had little or no social opportunity to develop an intimate relationship. It is central to identify at what time in his or her life the incident occurred. This provides a perspective on whether the person was still in the process of developing a sexual role or whether an established role was interrupted. A stable sexual role relies on experiences, habits, and expectations in pursuing and maintaining intimate relationships. If this process is interrupted, then the ability to use these human aspects in relationships—the person's ability and effectiveness to manage the relationship—is interrupted as well. In addition, the inappropriate spontaneous behavior frequently manifested by a traumatic brain injured person will only serve to amplify these deficits. It is well recognized that in the able-bodied population there is a high incidence of natural sexual dysfunction such as anorgasmia, dyspareunia, vaginismus, erectile disorders, premature ejaculation, and sexual aversion. These may also appear following the incidence and stress of traumatic head injury.[25]

It is also necessary to determine whether or not the individual has received information about sex education and/or understands the information accurately. In addition, a youth may have had limited social experience such as dating or courtship. The individual may also have had only one partner experience in "casual sex" or "exploring" situations. He or she may not have been looking for a permanent partner and, therefore, the experience may have been on a superficial level.

Awareness of premorbid values and expectations is useful so that the professional can assess what a traumatic brain injury will mean in terms of psychosocial sexual loss or change.

Table 15–1. DRUG CAUSES OF ORGANIC IMPOTENCE

Major tranquilizers
  Phenothiazines
  Butyrophenones
  Thioxanthines
Antidepressants
  Tricyclics
  MAO inhibitors
Minor tranquilizers
  Benzodiazepines
  Mephenesin-like drugs
Sedatives and hypnotics
Anticholinergic drugs
  Antispasmodics
  Antiparkinsonian drugs
  Antihistamines
  Muscle relaxants
  Antiarrhythmic (disopyramide)
Antihypertensives
  Diuretics
  Vasodilators (questionable)
  Central sympatholytics
  Neurotransmitter depleters
  Alpha- and beta-adrenergic blockers
Drugs with abuse potential
Miscellaneous
  Cimetidine
  Clofibrate
  Cyproterone
  Estrogens
  Progestins
  Digoxin
  Indomethacin
  Lithium
  Methylsergide
  Metoclopramide
  Metronidazole
  Phenytoin

Adapted from Van Arsdalen, et al.[23]

There is a high incidence of alcohol abuse and a predictable increase of interpersonal problems within relationships after head injury. In addition, legal imbroglios create a strain on families. There are likely to be educational difficulties experienced by this population which make instructing, correcting, or learning new things more of a challenge.[4, 5, 26]

A head injured person may have had a lifestyle, family, or social life situation that did not include the opportunity or availability of a partner. Also the person may not have identified himself or herself in terms of sexual orientation by the time of the injury. In addition, if a brain injured person's sexual orientation is homosexual, this fact may not yet have been disclosed to the public or even fully comprehended by the person himself or herself. Conversely, the injured person may have had multiple partners, may have had unusual or deviant early sexual experiences (rape, molestation, or incest), may have been promiscuous, or may have experienced neglect or physical abuse as a child.

If an existing relationship has been interrupted by the traumatic brain injury, it will be important to identify if there were previous marital or relationship difficulties, sexual dysfunctions common to intimate relationships or general communication difficulties.[5]

Risk-taking behavior can be the cause of traumatic brain injury. It also can indicate the difficulty experienced in structured social situations and can lead to problems with law enforcement personnel, drugs, alcohol, and chemical abuse. These types of difficulties may have been present before the injury as well and may already have had a negative effect on an existing partner or family relationship, resulting in residual feelings of anger and frustration of the family member or partner.

History of sexual dysfunction prior to brain injury can predict target areas of increased sexual difficulties for the injured person or the partner, or both. For example, if prior to the injury to her partner, an able-bodied woman has had difficulty achieving satisfactory orgasm during sexual intercourse or other activities, it is predictable that she may experience increased problems obtaining orgasm. The overwhelming impact of brain injury may create changes in the accustomed physical and mental behavior of her partner, and thereby potentially discourage, frustrate, anger, or repulse her during postinjury activities. Again, she may experience common sexual dysfunctions such as anorgasmia, dyspareunia, or vaginismus.

Similarly significant changes in intimate behavior of a brain injured woman can amplify existing problems of erectile function of her able-bodied male partner. All aspects of the partner's customary sexual function can be affected by the traumatic brain injury. The injury imposes more stress on intimacy, which may already be strained, constrained, embarrassing, dysfunctional, abusive, or mistrusting.

SECONDARY DYSFUNCTION RELATED TO MENTAL SEQUELAE OF INJURY

Perhaps the most disabling forms of secondary dysfunction result from the mental sequelae of brain injury. The manifold deficits of cognition, so often associated with behavioral and emotional problems, alter social and interpersonal skills, sexual drive, and sexual interest, even attitudes and beliefs that are the very foundation of sexuality. The nature and variety of those mental sequelae are thoroughly documented elsewhere in this text as well as in publications of Brooks,[7] Levin and coworkers,[27] Lezak,[5] and others.[6, 28, 29] Resultant sexual dysfunctions range widely from the less frequently occurring hypersexuality syndromes to total apathy and inactivity.

Certain of these syndromes merit further description. Injuries to the limbic system at times provoke a constellation of increased sexual interest; provocative, seductive, yet childish behavior; solicitations; exhibitionism; and occasionally increased sexual activity.[17] More often, however, despite the interest and importuning behavior, sexual activity is minimal. Bilateral temporal lobe injury has created the Klüver-Bucy syndrome, a combination of indiscriminate placement of objects into the mouth, bulimia, hypersexual behavior, psychic blindness, and docility.[11, 30] The syndrome, often partial and reversible, is less rare than originally thought. Temporal lobe seizures may produce automatic behaviors, sexual arousal, orgastic sensations, and stereotypic sexual activity.[22, 31] The preictal and postictal conditions of these individuals are usually states of reduced sex drive and interest. Frontal lobe syndromes range from such extremes as "akinetic mutism," seen with lesions of the dorsolateral area, to hyperkinetic rage, including sexual violence, associated with orbitomedial injuries.[32] Most frequently, with diffuse frontal trauma, there are mixes of flattened affect, selfishness, lack of empathy or profound feeling for others, childishness, deficient executive skills, slovenliness, and disinhibition without accompanying guilt. Some of these people have reduced sex drive, interest, and impotency. Many will act out their disinhibition with solicitation and acts to inappropriate people at injudicious times and places. Deficient memory and perseverative behavior may abet increased interest to the point of constant demands for sexual activity, whether or not it can be consummated. Coprolalia, exposure, masturbation, and indiscriminate approaches to relatives, staff, and other patients (members of either sex) are often observed. These performances are associated with indifference to or even enjoyment of the discomfort, remonstrations, or other reactions of onlookers.[33] Having had a premorbid Victorian upbringing does not exempt one from these sorts of outrageous behaviors. When seen in the early phase of progressive recovery from coma, and especially with a pre-existing conservative sexual ethic, such behavior may become reduced or disappear.

Occipital and parietal lobe lesions, in addition to the usual perceptual difficulties, can be associated with more exotic disorders such as proposagnosia or genital hallucinatory sensations.[34]

Postconcussion syndrome includes headaches (often aggravated by sexual acts) and impotency.[35] Both of these symptoms usually disappear with time.

Communication, the essence of loving relationships, may be impaired by aphasia (although these are less severe with brain injury than with stroke), dysarthria, and aphonia, but most severely by the reduction of language and ideation ensuing from severe cognitive deficits.

Closely related are the ravaged interpersonal and social skills that cripple dating, courting, and other mutually rewarding and sustaining interchanges.

SECONDARY DYSFUNCTIONS RELATED TO POSTINJURY REACTIONS

Reactions of Family and Partner. The family will experience a convolution and subsequent redefinition of roles. These changes will evolve initially around the events of the trauma and general response to the crisis. Of great importance is the need to recognize the vulnerabilities in the family system and to perceive and understand the changes the family is experiencing and will continue to experience.

Most families will have had a hierarchical order and all persons an implicit or explicit role prior to the injury.[4] When these interpersonal roles are suddenly and dramatically changed as a result of deficits and losses, the affectionate communication in the family may also change. Loving and caring behavior may be replaced with anxiety, avoidance, revulsion, or embarrassment.[5, 8]

Families, including the injured person's spouse, identify many common problems and complaints that seem to burden them both physically and psychologically. These problems are ones that seem to occur with high frequency among such families. The patient's complaints often include tiredness and difficulty remembering. The family's perception of the patient is often that he or she shows loss of physical and psychological endurance, a loss of concentration, emotional indifference, and so on. The family members commonly experience fatigue, isolation, loneliness, lack of communication, and revulsion for the patient.[7, 36]

A study conducted in Israel concerning changes in mood and behavior among wives of severely brain injured soldiers indicated greater sexual difficulties, feelings of desertion of friends, and sexual aversion to the partner.[8] Frustration with sexual needs and affection can also impact on the spouse. The patient may make excessive or inappropriate sexual demands on his or her partner.

The spouse can also feel trapped in the situation, unable to be fulfilled emotionally and intellectually, while at the same time unable to find another partner with whom to interact. He or she often reports feelings of guilt and oppression.

Children frequently become the recipient of the larger family problems. The spouse may take out his or her frustrations on the child, who mistakenly believes himself or herself to be responsible for the family's overwhelming dilemma. The injured parent may ignore the children, and the healthy parent may neglect them. Young children suffer from these dynamics more directly than do older children, who tend to act out their own frustrations by running away, truancy, and the like.[5]

The able-bodied partner may experience his own difficulty with role changes and feel imposed upon, isolated, or resentful. In addition, society often does not support the partner's grief. These understandable situations can produce feelings of physical and emotional fatigue at a crucial time when the brain injured person may especially need love and tenderness. The caretaking role can be problematic for any family member, particularly the sexual partner.[15]

Reactions of the Brain Injured Patient. The brain injured individual and the partner or spouse may experience and react to these changes differently. A common reaction of the partner is the loss of feelings of physical attractiveness toward the injured person at the same time as the partner may be responding with inappropriate sexual behavior, language, or personal grooming deficits that are not acceptable to the other.[5] The resultant conflict needs to be recognized as a natural set of events that can be addressed openly by the professionals working with the clinical situation.

Religious convictions and cultural beliefs may be transgressed in such circumstances and may cause anxiety and further sexual and communication difficulties, particularly if the injured person makes "inappropriate" and "new" demands on the partner that conflict with earlier beliefs.

The brain injured person may recognize some of the changes in his or her own appearance, functional capacities, behavior, and ability to communicate and to be consistently in control in sensitive sexual activity. This can result in feelings of lowered self-esteem, depression, sadness, or despondency for the injured person. Recognition that another person is providing personal intimate care and hygiene can lead to feelings of infantilization with attendant desexualization.

If the brain injured person experiences anxiety, rejection, impatience, embarrass-

ment, anger, and avoidance, his or her self-esteem and sense of masculinity or femininity will be affected. Careful attention must be given to addressing family communication, expectations, and education to the subtle and specific changes in the person's overall personality. Often the most difficult events experienced by the family are situations in which inappropriate sexual language or behavior occur.

Reactions of Professional Staff. Hostile behavior and general vulnerability of a brain injured person are apt to be confusing to an inexperienced staff. Inconsistent behavior from the brain injured person can lead to frustration for all concerned.

Therefore, in sexual matters, the staff will best facilitate the patient's environment by responding in a consistent, firm, encouraging, and respectful manner (i.e., the same as they would for a "nonsexual" issue).

Spontaneous and inappropriate touching, exposing of self in public, and inappropriate language can serve to provoke even the most understanding staff. The injured person's inability to differentiate between public and private behavior and between appropriate and inappropriate touch are predictable stress-producing situations for the staff.

There is a parallel between developmental disabilities and traumatic brain injury deficits. The need to learn appropriate behavior and to limit offensive and variant behavior will be major tasks. Uniquely with brain injury, the deficits and inappropriate behaviors will change from time to time and are often inconsistent. This leads to frustration. The staff, as well as the family, must try to understand and not judge the injured person harshly. Instead, all efforts should be made to facilitate appropriate behavior. In some cases, staff members may have difficulty even perceiving the brain injured adult as a sexual person because of manifested deficits and thereby in subtle ways may inadvertently treat the individual as asexual, further compounding the problem.

Community Response. Society will respond with rejection, punishment, ridicule, and hostility to sexually inappropriate behavior in public places. Both the brain injured person and the family can benefit from discussion and further preparation for such situations. The resultant conflict needs to be recognized as a natural set of events that can be addressed openly by the professionals working with the clinical situations. Families, associates, friends, and the community can learn new ways to respond to such behavior.

Self-confidence can improve for the brain injured person and/or the partner when any existing primary and secondary sexual dysfunctions are addressed by the health care team. Providing assistance to adapt to the changes will have long-lasting benefits for both the brain injured person and the partner or family. Skills relating to sexual competency, which include communication and managing appropriate behavior, will ultimately benefit the entire family system or couple. It will be essential that the brain injured person be assisted in acquiring and maintaining appropriate social behavior when possible and be assisted in acquiring skills in effective and appropriate communication in order to maintain an existing relationship (if indeed that is a realistic goal).

Re-entry into society is challenging for the entire family, and this additional stress will be felt by the sexual partner in conflicting ways. For avoiding sustained discouragement about all of these changes, each aspect of sexual dysfunction can be carefully identified and discussed with realistic goals for possible change and recovery of both emotional and sexual intimacy for the future. Discussion about the future should contain realistic expectations for the partner and family, recognizing that they will be in an active state of grieving.

METHODS OF ASSESSMENT

Getting information about sexual function is difficult. Societal taboos, personal discomfort, stylistic awkwardness, language blocks, and information inadequacies all may combine to yield a situation in which it may be difficult to ask, to give, and to receive information. Added to these are the additional difficulties produced by the brain injury itself—memory and other cognitive losses, emotional ability, distractibility, reduction of executive skills and judgment, inappropriate behavior, to cite several. When necessary, appropriate relevant information may be obtained more reliably from the spouse, significant other, sexual partner, or family member of the brain injured person. A closely attuned professional staff can contribute further information concerning the nature and circumstances of current sexual behaviors.

Even when theory is understood, importance is accepted, and need is apparent, the practitioner often has difficulty getting started. An excellent way to begin is to be specific and to use the familiar medical model. What is the patient's chief complaint? The practitioner should individualize his or her approach because each person is distinct. By asking specifically about the individual's problem, you may be allowed into the discussion that is necessary. Directness also helps the patient know that you are seriously interested in being helpful with his or her particular problem.

There is no more understandable place to begin than with questions about genital function. For example, when talking with a man, ask about penile erection and techniques for sexual intercourse that the person has tried or would like to try. Remember that erections during sleep occur cyclically and help differentiate functional problems in men who do not have erections during the daytime or under erotic conditions. The presence of nocturnal erections establishes that the neurologic pathways and vascular mechanisms are present and functioning. It is reasonable to ask the patient or partner to investigate for the presence of erection when one wakes at night for other reasons. Ask if ejaculation and orgasm *both* occur. Is the ejaculation anterograde or retrograde? Is the semen volume unusual?

For women, ask about vaginal lubrication, pain on attempted intercourse, and sexual arousal. Vaginal lubrication is the counterpart of penile erection in the male. Lubrication occurs during sexual arousal just as does penile erection. The woman can investigate its presence by digital examination of the vagina. Information about the character of orgasm may lead to helpful information about sexual activity, since a painful or unpleasant orgasm may inhibit sexual activity. For some, orgasm may not be of great importance; but to those for whom it is important, advice on helping achieve it will be greatly appreciated.

Information about masturbation is part of a complete history. Is it done alone or is it incorporated into the sexual activities of the couple? The practitioner must be aware that sexual mores will determine whether or not masturbation or sexual pleasuring is attempted or, if attempted, is considered acceptable. Answers to questions about masturbation may guide the investigator to information about freedom of sexual expression as well as to specific information about the characteristics of penile erection or vaginal lubrication.

Gaining a description of attempts at sexual intercourse may lead to specific suggestions. In addition to intercourse, other sexual activities or desires should be considered. The use of manual or oral stimulation or the use of mechanical devices such as vibrators can be sensitively discussed. In private and with sensitivity, one may also seek information about other sexual partners or sexual orientation. The practitioner may erroneously assume that a married person has no sexual partner other than the spouse or that an individual is heterosexual.

Associated medical issues such as venereal or other genital diseases should also be explored. Medication history, use or abuse of alcohol or drugs, or other tests and treatments that have been carried out should be identified. It is also important to ask about the importance which the patient or partner attaches to the sexual concern: it may be of paramount or of relatively incidental importance, but the practitioner should not make assumptions without specific inquiry.

Other injuries associated with the event that produced the brain injury may by themselves produce sexual dysfunction, or at least sexual concerns. The frequency of facial injuries should raise obvious issues.[37] There may occur functional or cosmetic derangements of structures that are extremely personal and vital to one's self-image or to a partner's acceptance. For example, dysarthria or oropharyngeal trauma, or both, may change the quality of one's voice. Damage to teeth, lips, or palate may produce articulatory disturbances or interfere with oral hygiene such as eating or controlling saliva. Tracheostomies limit phonation outright or at least change the essentials of conversation so important to intimacy. Fractures, at least for a period of time, may limit mobility of extremities, which results in loss of the ability to embrace, touch, or simply be close. The effects of pelvic fractures, spinal

cord, root, lumbosacral plexus, injuries, and medications have already been mentioned in this chapter.

Just as the aforementioned inquiries can and should be asked of the brain injured individual, they can and should also be asked of the partner. Beliefs, concerns, desires, and information for one may be different for the other. Often it is useful to interview the partner privately as well as in the presence of the patient. The answers may differ in the two situations. When the couple is at hand, information about their relationship may set a course for further action. The duration and strength of the relationship are vital as are the communication habits established within the relationship. Also important are previous patterns of sexual activity; for example, which partner initiates and with what frequency; a past history of sexual abuse, rape, or incest; and issues of desire, fear, fertility, and pregnancy. All may play a role in current sexual attitudes and practices.

The medical model also includes a mechanism for inquiring about other organ systems and a social history, which may lead to important information about sexual function. Understandably living arrangements will affect privacy. Issues of dependency and independence may bear on sexual interest and activities.

A careful examination of the genitourinary system will complement the historic information. Physiologic or organic dysfunctions of the genitourinary tract must be identified as part of the evaluation of sexual function. However, the practitioner must not forget that alterations or dysfunctions of the genitals are not necessarily synonymous with sexual dysfunction. Erotic and therefore sexual parts of the body are abundant and available for use by willing and interested people. The key here is to think of sexuality more broadly than genital function and sexual expression more broadly than sexual intercourse.

The following five areas deserve special inclusion in the physical examination.

1. *The Motor System.* Problems with spasticity, mobility, strength, or coordination can affect choices of sexual expression. They should be evaluated and the identified impairments incorporated into medical advice. In individuals who are limited in mo-

bility, strength, or coordination, there are still many remaining options both for giving and for receiving sexual pleasure.

2. *Somatic Sensation.* Somatic sensory dysfunction may also pose important issues in sexuality. Anesthesia or hypesthesia of body parts may require adaptive methods. Almost anywhere the body is capable of being eroticized. The skin is the largest sexual organ in the body, and a disabled person may wish to use a "whole body" approach to sexuality. Dyesthesias and painful syndromes can occur after traumatic brain injury and may pose additional problems for the patient or couple as well as for the practitioner. However, dealing with pain that interferes with sexual function is fundamentally no different than pain interfering with any other important function. Approaches may be employed that alleviate pain or alter pain behavior.

3. *Special Sensory Organs.* Sexual activity frequently involves the body's organs of special sensation (e.g., sight, sound, olfaction, and taste). If one or more of these modalities is impaired from traumatic brain injury, adapting to the remaining sensations is desirable. Again the fundamental approach to sexuality in this regard is no different than any other adaptive strategy in the presence of a physical disability that interferes with function.

4. *Amputations and Cosmesis.* Traumatic brain injury is sometimes associated with alterations or loss of body parts. Traumatic amputation can interfere with function, and disfiguring injuries can produce cosmetic problems. Obviously, both situations can adversely affect sexual function. Counseling, adaptive strategies, or similar remediations may be helpful. Patients and their partners may benefit from frank discussions and recommendations that may not otherwise have occurred to them. Just as in the rehabilitation of other physical disabilities, the practitioner has choices among remedial exercises and compensatory strategies that can be applied to the individual or his or her environment. Creativity and openness of discussion will go far toward solving sexual problems following traumatic brain injury.

5. *Cognition and Perception.* Cognition and perception are vital components to sexual communications. Dysfunctions can be approached in a systematic and therapeutic fashion. Foresight, pacing, judgment, control, appropriateness, concentration, and focusing are all important to satisfactory sexual activities. When they are impaired following brain injury, their remediation should improve sexual communication and satisfaction in the same way that nonsexual functions are benefited.

One can also gain important information about the patient's sexuality during the physical examination by observing communicative, intellectual, and social skills. Speech control, emotional content, and information transfer all relate directly to sexuality issues. Memory and the ability to use executive skills may be evident during the physical examination. Body language, appropriate behavior, social skills, hygiene, modesty, and pacing will also be useful adjuncts to an overall impression of the patient's sexuality.

After completing a history and physical examination, the clinician must judge whether or not an identified sexual dysfunction is related to the traumatic brain injury. Sexual dysfunction may have predated the head injury or may have been brought into focus by the injury. One may be misled into attributing the sexual dysfunction to the obvious head injury rather than recognizing that it may be tangentially related or perhaps not related at all.

The evaluation may be complemented by selective diagnostic procedures.[23] An endocrinologic survey may be indicated (see Chapter 9). Urologic procedures are often necessary, and may be especially useful in evaluating associated sexual dysfunctions. Cystourethrometrography and visual inspection of the bladder may help differentiate between organic and functional sexual problems. Nocturnal penile tumescense monitoring is of further value in the differentiation of erectile problems. Electrodiagnostic studies may include needle electromyography of sacral muscles, nerve conduction studies of the lower extremities, the bulbo cavernosus reflex,[38] and pudendal nerve somatosensory evoked potentials.[39] These extensions of the neurologic examination may facilitate localization of previously identified motor and sensory losses. Vascular studies such as Doppler stethoscopy of the penile arteries or angiography may help identify localized circulatory problems related to the patient's reports of erectile or lubrication dysfunctions.[23]

Finally, it is important for the practitioner to accomplish an additional step when evaluating for sexual function. One must educate the patient about the meaning of the questions asked, the studies done, and the findings. Not to do so may leave the individual or couple feeling very anxious about interpretations or, worse still, misinterpretations. Patient education is, of course, critical to all aspects of health care but in the area of sexual health care is of prime importance.

TREATMENT APPROACHES

Educational

A structured approach to social skill training, including sex education and setting of realistic sexual behavior goals, is best integrated as part of the overall treatment strategy. Early sex education and counseling of the family in the intensive care unit (ICU) should be stressed as a way of setting expectations and beginning an ongoing dialogue with the treatment team. Feelings of helplessness, fear of survival versus death, loss of privacy, and frustration over the inability to communicate with the comatose patient can be overwhelming to the family members. It seems to be effective to initiate discussion of sensitive matters as a way of bridging some of the frustrations and fears.

It is also helpful to acknowledge that in the medical setting there is minimal privacy. This decreases the ability to caress and otherwise express affection in intimate ways, particularly during times of stress. This situation, coupled with the inability to participate in the care of the patient in the ICU, can affect the family member or partner significantly. Empathic discussion will begin to facilitate the family and team to work together with the challenges ahead. Families can, to some extent, be involved in levels of patient care—even in the ICU. In addition, they can be encouraged to express affection and to talk to the patient. A certain degree of privacy may be provided in some situations.

Social skill training includes all social skills, oral motor praxis, eye contact and movement, cosmesis, discretion, modulation or pacing, logic, and sequence. Privacy issues of behavior and sexual activity by oneself or with a partner or spouse will be integrated into social skill training. The brain injured person and/or partner will need assistance in re-establishing their relationship. Appropriate use of touch and its importance in health care can be included at this time. Attention to the self-image concept will include grooming, cosmetic appearance, and appropriate behavior.

SPOUSES, PARTNERS, AND FAMILY

Education about strategies to reacquire communication skills should focus on three components of language:

1. Ability to normalize speech
2. Ability to recognize feelings and innuendos in speech
3. Information passing

Conversation rules can be reviewed to include closeness, situation-appropriate behavior, and body language. Here, practice with feedback in a consistent manner will be an effective approach.

Sexual expectations may change for all persons involved. Situations may arise where inappropriate touch is experienced and the family member, spouse, or partner may experience times of intense reluctance to touch or respond. Privacy needs for the family or the couple will be included in discussion of the home living situation. Extended stays in a medical care facility may generate increasing needs for privacy for the individual and partner. The health care team can be assistive and sensitive to these needs, perhaps making arrangements for privacy in the health care setting.

Changes in personality, creating mood swings and unpredictable behavior in the brain injured person, is essential to discuss. Early counseling in the ICU can help the family anticipate and prepare for emerging behaviors in the awakening patient. Expectations will need to be modified based on these changes. In addition, physical limitations of the brain injury may result in other environmental modifications that may have an impact on the previous living patterns of the individual and family. These things can include physical modifications in the home, special equipment, presence of an attendant, and physically therapeutic activities that may interrupt a previous established lifestyle.

As indicated earlier, changes in sexual response may be present. A review of normal sexual function, both male and female, is helpful in describing some of the sexual changes experienced in relationship to a disability. There may also be practical changes in physical activity as well as different behaviors and responses to social situations in comparison to earlier experiences.[25]

Self-image changes, particularly negative ones, are better understood when discussed openly by the health care team. Often, guilt is accompanied by negative perceptions from the partner or family about some of the dramatic changes the individual may be experiencing. This negative feedback can be picked up by the brain injured person and further influence negative self-image. Limitations in mobility could affect sexual activity and be discussed in creative conversations about alternative suggestions. Many times support groups and peer advocates are helpful in discussing the silent and private feelings family members may be experiencing. Supportive reading material can also be of assistance. Family members, spouses, and partners will all be concerned with issues of dignity, respect, and self-esteem. A sensitive health care team will anticipate and respond to these needs (see Suggested Reading).

Counseling

SPOUSES, PARTNERS, AND FAMILY

With all of the changes experienced with traumatic brain injury there is apt to be emerging concern about sexual role reversal or role confusion for all. This sometimes can lead to emotional dysfunction. The sexual partner can experience conflict between the roles of caretaker and lover. All persons are concerned for the future of the brain injured individual, for themselves, and for their relationship. Limitations on mobility can result in isolation and all of the frustrations surrounding a sense of being deprived. Past relationships may be dramatically altered if not severed, and difficulties may be experienced in establishing new relationships. These situations can at times seem overwhelming to the partner or family members.[4]

The sexual partner of the brain injured person may have to deal with mechanical needs or require assistance in preparing for sexual expression if there are other physical limitations that create embarrassment and reduce desire. A discussion of earlier memories may help the partner to recognize the impact of these experiences. At times, the partner may feel the desire to abandon the brain injured person, or may be frustrated or overwhelmed by the challenges facing him or her. Religious beliefs and cultural expectations can strongly influence a person's ability to handle this level of stress. Counseling to relieve stress and anxiety can be provided on such topics as guilt about feelings, embarrassment, or shock about sexual talk or behavior (coprolalia, autism, echolalia, masturbation, exhibitionism, and attempted physical advances). The treatment team and family can discuss and plan the behavioral techniques to assist in dealing with some of these behaviors.

Instruction about sexual changes should include direct conversation about medication and its side effects. A thorough discussion with a sexual partner should always include a past history to discover any unforeseen problems.

COUNSELING THE BRAIN INJURED INDIVIDUAL

Counseling the brain injured person will include discussion about feelings of infantilization. Assessing memory or memory loss can also include awareness of previous sexual behavior if the person has a partner. Discussion of appropriate sexual activities can be initiated with the brain injured person as well as the partner. As mentioned earlier, communication abilities must be assessed to anticipate the brain injured person's ability to experience closeness, comfort, and intimacy. Observation about physical behavior will be helpful in making recommendations for sexual activity. Physical care assessment includes ability to dress and perform basic hygiene functions. This information will help determine what is independently possible for the injured person in sexual activity. Counseling should also include self-responsibility skills (i.e., manners and social skills). Essential to all counseling on sexual activity is discussion of birth control, if appropriate; the possible addition of enrichment aids to assist in sexual expression (vibrators); and practical suggestions concerning physical positioning.

The professional-patient relationship may readily be misperceived by the latter as an erotic attachment. Anticipation of that eventuality will facilitate early recognition and effective, sensitive dealing with the situation.

Medical-Surgical Approaches

Treatment of primary sexual disabilities frequently entails the use of pharmacologic or surgical modalities. Endocrinopathies are responsive to hormonal replacement. Disabling spasticity may require neurolysis, neurosurgical, or orthopedic procedures, as described in Chapter 10. Some of the movement disorders may be amenable to drugs or stereotactic thalamotomy. Depending on their etiology, pain syndromes may respond to analgesics or anti-inflammatory drugs. Tegretol (carbamazepine) or Dilantin (phenytoin) have been beneficial in the treatment of neuritic pain. Reflex dystrophies may improve with physiotherapy, usage of adrenergic blocking agents, antidepressants, anticonvulsant agents, corticosteroids, anesthetic regional or sympathetic blockade, sympathectomy, or dorsal column electrical stimulation.[40] Orthopedic deformities may require surgical correction. Heterotopic ossification merits consideration of Didronel (etifronate disodium) and surgical excision. Vasculogenic or neurogenic impotence that persists and is unresponsive to other forms of treatment is a possible indication for penile implantation.[41] Vascular reconstructive surgery can restore genital circulation and function. Drugs whose side effects produce sexual dysfunctions can be discontinued, reduced in dosage, or substituted for by other drugs. Meticulous treatment of associated or pre-existing diseases may allow sufficient stabilization to restore partial or considerable sexual function. Seizures are generally well controlled by anticonvulsant drugs.

Secondary sexual disabilities occasionally necessitate concomitant medical and psychologic management. Antidepressant drugs must be considered in managing the various depressive states. Paradoxically, this class of drugs is used to reduce agitated, violent behavior. The use of pharmacologic agents in the treatment of behavioral and emotional disorders is detailed in Chapter 28. Craniofacial and other cosmetic deformities may be improved or corrected by plastic surgery. Excessive salivation or drooling may be treated by anticholinergic drugs or by surgical rerouting of Wharton's ducts more posteriorly so as to facilitate swallowing of saliva.[42] The contraceptive armamentarium of female hormones, spermatocides, diaphragms, tubal ligation, and so forth, should be available for routine purposes or for the protection of vulnerable disinhibited females. Sexually violent males have been treated with Depo-provera (medroxiprogesterone) or cytoproterone inhibitors of testosterone.[43] Methadone substitution, tranquilizers, and massive vitamin supplementation are among the component forms of treatment of heroin, alcohol, and other addictions. A reminder: The partner may also have sexual dysfunctions that are amenable to medical or surgical interventions.

Functional Retraining

Regardless of the setting where a rehabilitation program is initiated, the team should consider sexuality as an indispensable component of its assessment-management plan to maximize life functions. Thus, all disciplines must share concern and responsibility for sexual rehabilitation. Sexual training is largely an extension, a further refinement of knowledge and skills taught by each discipline. We will illustrate the application of such training with some salient examples in each major functional area.

Physical functions of mobility and self-care skills can readily be extended to sexual activities. Proper support and positioning may reduce drooling, spasticity, pain, and the activity of movement disorders. They may facilitate mobility, comfort, accessibility, and tactile sensibility. Instruction in transfers and mobility usually complements this phase of training. As part of preparation for sexual activity, hygienic and cosmetic skills such as oral and skin care and bowel and bladder preparation need attention. Dressing and undressing may require further instruction or modifications in clothing. Remembrance and capability in using contraceptive devices may be compromised. Spasticity and movement disorders may be subdued by relaxation, biofeedback, or positional changes.

Sensory and perceptual retraining could include identifying regions of intact sensation for purposes of tactile exploration or erotic stimulation, fantasy techniques are unlikely to be effective in those with severe cognitive deficits.

Cognitive training can encompass many aspects of sexuality. Early body orientation should include the sexual apparatus; those organs may be among the earliest to be rediscovered upon arousal from coma. The process of providing sexual information can proceed, geared to the changing level of attention, memory, and other mental abilities. Memory deficits relative to sexual activity may be circumvented by extending the diary or ledger to include notations of when menses, sexual acts, and the like, last occurred.

Behavioral-emotional interventions can be directed specifically at sexual concerns.[44] Applicable behavior modification techniques include social reinforcement, token economies of delayed reinforcements, time-out, aversive reinforcement, overlearning, and enforced "practice" of undesired behaviors. Teaching acceptable sexual behaviors may require focus upon appropriate time and places for sexual activities. Practice in the behaviors of loving can facilitate patience and skill in touching, caressing, and kissing; refinement of sensibility to responses of the partner; and development of judgment as to whether these expressions should or should not proceed to explicit sexual acts.

Communications and language training may deal with verbal and nonverbal expressions of affection, love, and desire. The discreteness and appropriateness of such communications usually demands attention. A limiting factor in training may be the severity of cognitive loss and attendant poverty of thought. The speech-language pathologist is a source of additional expertise in dealing with problems such as tongue-lip control and drooling.

Social skills training should include allowing ease and confidence in communicating with partner, family, and others. Community and leisure skills can be directed toward dating activities.

Therapeutic exercise and physical modalities are further adjuncts to the training program. Reconditioning through strengthening and endurance activities; training for motor control, coordination, and balance; modalities to modulate spasticity or pain, to facilitate stretching of adaptive aids; and modification of the environment (the bedroom) are examples of these applications.

A private place within the rehabilitation facility is mandatory for the teaching and practice of much of this training.[45] The "place" serves a number of purposes: it is a locus for the professional to educate, train, and counsel patient and partner in privacy. It allows confidential communications and privacy for patient and family or partner. It serves as a quiet site for intimacy of any type for patients with or without their partners. Thus, it may be a laboratory for experimentation and practice, or simply a place for solace and seclusion; it is not, however, a substitute for the practice that should occur during therapeutic passes.

What if no partner is available for the training program? Does the team provide a surrogate sexual partner? If so, whom? A member of the team? A trained individual? A prostitute? All of these options have been explored in sexual therapy.[46] There are no generalizations that suffice to answer these questions, other than to state that the beliefs and attitudes of the patient (if not greatly distorted by the disability), family or guardian, and, of course, the surrogate partner must be heeded. The ethical and legal implications of surrogate training are a source of continuing controversy.

The danger of transmission of the virus producing the autoimmune deficiency syndrome (AIDS) by either partner is an additional concern. Head injured patients are particularly vulnerable to AIDS. Some have contracted the virus via blood transfusions before the era of screening of donors. Others are susceptible because of drug or sexual practices.

As with other aspects of rehabilitation, sexual training often continues at an intensive level after hospital discharge. The emphasis of this training usually shifts more heavily to psychosocial and communication aspects, which may early require frequent revisions. Therefore, continued training and follow-up assessment should be incorporated into the comprehensive rehabilitation plan. Changes of sexual function with time, critical stresses, and changes in family and marital interrelationships must be antici-pated. Just as the rehabilitation and mainte-nance of life functions is a lifetime process, so it is with sexual function.

CHILDREN: SPECIAL CONSIDERATIONS

Psychosexual Growth and Development

All children develop sexually from in-fancy to adulthood. This development re-sults in physical attributes and feelings re-lated to sexual characteristics of children as they grow and are reflected in physical, in-tellectual, and emotional stages. Not all chil-dren mature at the same rate, nor do they respond in the same manner emotionally to each other, parents, and other adults.

It is essential that parents and adults be available for questioning so that children will naturally feel that they can ask sensitive questions or receive needed information. Consistency, basic information, support, and affirmation are essential components to sex-ual health. Equally important is the ability to anticipate future problems and issues the child will experience and be available to provide guidance.

From birth to 5 years of age, it is natural for children to explore through touch. They are also learning boy/girl sex roles and try-ing to understand adult behavior. They ac-quire language and learn to understand touch. The majority of children ask ques-tions, sometimes incessantly, and generally learn by exploration, curiosity, and trial and error. They learn boundaries of responsibil-ity and a sense of value and are basically cu-rious and accepting. Toward the end of this stage a child might become shy, more so-cially aware, ask fewer questions, and realize that sexuality is "different."

From the ages of 5 to 10, children are aware of the "good" and "bad" aspects of normal body functions and body parts. They may experience anxiety or general discom-fort regarding topics of sexual nature. Gen-erally, children are impressionable and inquisitive, particularly about their bodies. Most children explore masturbation as a natural curiosity. During these years, chil-dren tend to play with peers of the same sex. Children may also appear to be disin-terested or disgusted about sex, and re-spond more readily to brief, spontaneous exchanges of information and guidance. They are aware that touching feels good and are learning about appropriate responses and the difference between public and pri-vate behavior.

Puberty is a time for confusion, embar-rassment, self-consciousness, and difficulty in asking for information. At this time, chil-dren are very vulnerable, particularly in seeking assistance. Their decision-making skills and cognitive abilities are still de-veloping and they are still identifying social-sexual roles. Some may even become sex-ually active at this time, often without ade-quate understanding of the responsibilities and maturity that go along with these be-haviors.

It is important to recognize that many children have been sexually abused, ex-ploited, or molested by the time they reach adolescence. This can have a lifelong impact of guilt and shame on the child if the offense is not detected and stopped, and appropri-ate help provided. Many children may have experienced molestation or abuse from per-sons known to them. Handicapped children in particular may not have had enough basic information even to recognize that inappro-priate sexual things have been done to them by adults. Physical and mental deficits make these children especially vulnerable to sex-ual abuse. Because of their desire to please and their often low-self-esteem, they may readily accede to abuse or even aggressively pursue indiscriminate sexual activity.[48]

The following case history illustrates some of these points:

A 17-year-old girl about 3 months post–severe closed head injury was brought for emergency medical evaluation and counsel-ing by her mother, after learning that she had repeatedly granted sexual favors to a group of construction workers. Recently discharged from a hospital rehabilitation program, she was now living at home with her parents. A mild left hemiparetic, she was fully mobile and physically indepen-dent. However, moderate cognitive, emo-tional, and behavioral problems persisted. She was childish, injudicious, rather "flat" emotionally, openly seductive, and uninhib-ited about sexual thoughts and activities. The girl casually revealed to her mother that she had on several occasions, while walking about the neighborhood, heeded the requests of a small group of on-the-job workers to join them. She further related that she had consented to engage in sexual acts with each of the men. Although she had no concerns about the consequences of these events, her parents were frantic. They confessed that she had been somewhat sexually permissive premorbidly, but had never displayed the flagrantly irresponsible behavior now unveiled.

Hormonal contraception was initiated after determining that she was not pregnant. Patient and parental counseling was begun. The parents consulted an attorney. They informed the foreman of the construction crew of the situation and of the girl's circumstances. No additional legal measures were taken. With further counseling, full activation of an outpatient rehabilitation program, and gradual improvement of psychologic functions, no further sexually indiscriminate behaviors were reported.

Adolescence is a time for experimentation, conflict, breaking away from the family, becoming emotionally and socially adult, and practicing decision-making skills. Thoughts about sexuality occupy a major part of adolescents' lives at this time. Sexual activity is viewed as part of identity and possibly as reserved for adults. Children of this age appear defensive when confronted or threatened. To others, they appear sophisticated about sexual issues even though they may not be. Fashion, grooming, friends, and self-confidence are central ingredients necessary for development of their adult sexual roles.

Parents of brain injured children can experience frustration by some of the inevitable sexual changes in their children. They may also experience difficulty in managing some of the predictable behavioral changes resulting from the brain injury. An affectionate parent may be the target of seductive or frankly sexual behavior by a undiscriminating child.

Together these changes compound the challenge for parents and other adults who care for brain injured children. It is likely to be difficult in many situations to determine which of the behaviors may be normal growth and development issues, which are the result of the injury, and which are a combination of both. During these situations, children and parents alike need to feel support and understanding as they work with these events that may at times feel overwhelming.

Parents have the ability to influence and encourage the brain injured child in all aspects of life, including communication, social skill cueing, and education. They have the opportunity to teach limitations of behavior, teach communication to monitor behavior, and intervene or validate when appropriate. The caretaking role is a consuming experience for many parents. Emphasis can effectively be placed on the importance of the family sharing in these role-modeling responsibilities. Frequently this job falls to the mother, without previous negotiations.[4]

Siblings of the brain injured child need to be educated fully about the nature of brain injury and its outcome. It is important for siblings to be told, to feel, and to believe that they have their own individual lives to live and that their lives and life experiences are not secondary to those of their injured sibling. If they are able to maintain their role in the family and have enough personal freedom, although these may be somewhat altered, they will be able to relate positively to the injured sibling. They will need to be taught how to interact with the injured person and how to give feedback, retrain, and encourage the sibling. If there is any possibility of normal sexual exploration among siblings, strong consideration should be given to recommending avoidance of such spontaneous exploration because the brain injured child would not have the ability to experience this common kind of sexual exploration in an incidental manner. It may be mistaken for affectionate behavior and could result in sexual exploitation.

Peers of the brain injured child need to be educated about brain injury as well. Stigma and rejection may be common reactions for friends and playmates. Peers need to be able to set realistic expectations for communication, play, and risk-taking activities as they attempt to re-establish a relationship with the brain injured individual. There also may be some reluctance to include the brain injured child in group play. Consistent information and encouragement through peers can generate respect, concern, and positive interaction without guilt, fear, or resentment.

Education: Role of the School

Teachers and administrators in the schools will need to be educated regarding brain injury as they will need to interact with the medical team and the family in an ongoing manner. They must be encouraged to set realistic goals and expectations. Teachers should be knowledgeable about sexuality in general so that they are aware of the increased communication demands for traumatic brain injury and will be able to look for consistent behavior outcomes from the brain injured person. They will be more able to intervene in a positive way if they are confronted with inappropriate behavior, particularly with sexual acting-out behavior. If they can be alerted to the problems, then they can be creative in preventing them.

TRAINING AND EDUCATING TRAINERS

The trainer must be able to teach about different models of interaction and have an ability to discuss specific sexual behaviors and subjects, which can often generate resistance from the staff. Frequently this resistance is a result of general lack of exposure to sexuality education of any sort; therefore, it is understandable that predictable staff difficulties relating to issues of sexuality and traumatic brain injury can occur.

PLISSIT Model

The PLISSIT model of interaction, designed by Annon,[49] is particularly effective in creating opportunities for different levels of interaction:

P	Permission Giving
LI	Limited Information
SS	Specific Suggestions
IT	Intensive Therapy

This allows the professional to initiate discussion about sexuality reflecting his or her own level of competence as well as awareness of what level the situation requires. For example:

The Permission level reflects a willingness to discuss matters of privacy and intimacy with the patient or family member.

Limited Information involves an awareness and ability to discuss and provide practical information on changes and expectations for sexual behavior and attitudes concerning the brain injured person.

Specific Suggestions implies counseling skills in making recommendations in conjunction with the partner or family and having direct conversation with the brain injured person. The "specific suggestion" level is an advocacy role requiring counseling and diagnostic skills.

Intensive Therapy requires sophisticated training and intervention in situations where the injured person or family feels out of control, overwhelmed or in crisis. These skills involve assuming responsibility as an intervener and making decisions that will change the difficult situation. This is an advanced level and is usually provided by a trained specialist.

Health care staff will be most responsive to training in sexuality if they can focus on a clinical situation that creates a common basis for communication. This gives them an opportunity to respond with their feelings. They need to work toward a goal of feeling comfortable with themselves, toward gaining skills in conducting a sex-related discussion, and in problem-solving; and toward developing a facilitative style.

Acquisition of Skills

Assessment skills for the health professional include the ability to take a sexual history and to determine the nature of the impact of head injury on an existing lifestyle. Advanced skills include an ability to assess the family attitudes toward sexuality and toward disability. These attitudes will influence how the present situation is handled. Also important to assess are attitudes toward masculinity, femininity, sexual expectations, and hygiene (bowel, bladder), and, perhaps more importantly, the family attitudes toward being different or viewed as not fitting into the norms of society. This information will provide useful material in assisting the brain injured person and family members as they adjust to the result of trauma.

General topics to evaluate in the patient include those previously mentioned in this chapter such as social skills, body image, impact of loss, self-esteem, risk-taking personality, neurophysiology, interpersonal issues, psychologic issues, clinical issues (sensory, mobility, bowel and bladder, deconditioning, pain), communication problems, cognitive deficits, medication, fertility changes, depression, body changes, and function changes.

An effective method of training the staff is in difficult case presentations using an in-service model. Peer education increases dialogue, comfort with the topic and awareness of skills that are effective in dealing with difficult situations. Conferences on brain injury routinely address issues of sexuality. Journal articles, book chapters, and articles in the lay literature may also be helpful. Sexual history-taking skills should be practiced and refined and a sexual history should be included in all assessments.[50]

Sexual Attitude Reassessment Seminar (SAR)

This intensive seminar provides a professional with an opportunity to deal with his or her own sexual feelings and knowledge, in view of the wide range of sexual behavior. It provides opportunity for reassessment of one's personal values regarding sexual behavior as well as the opportunity to listen to peers describe their perceptions. A basic premise of this type of training acknowledges that information presented with an opportunity to discuss increases the professional's awareness and comfort. This, in turn, increases professionals' skills and abilities to conduct sex-related discussions in meaningful and sensitive ways. When the intensive training seminars are focused to include special situations such as traumatic brain injury, professionals can more readily recognize the wide range of concerns and potentially profound impact the disability will have on existing relationships and intimacy of all affected persons.[51]

SUMMARY AND CONCLUSIONS

The subject of sexuality has found a proper place in the considerations of rehabilitation of the brain injured person. Although research-generated information is scanty, there is need to share those data as well as the information gained by a growing clinical experience. Certainly the majority of sexual disabilities stem from the cognitive, personality, emotional, and behavioral sequelae of brain injury. However, closer scrutiny may uncover a larger number of primary sexual dysfunctions, particularly those related to endocrinopathies or non-cranial injuries.

The management of sexuality and sexual dysfunction should commence in the very early postinjury period, dealing with family and professional staff once survival seems assured. An interdisciplinary rehabilitation approach to the assessment, treatment, and long-term follow-up care of sexual functions is recommended, using the PLISSIT model of Annon. When a partner is available, that person becomes an integral part of the management process. At times, however, the needs and problems of the partner may be at variance with those of the disabled person. Brain injured children require an approach that recognizes the factors that distinguish childhood or adolescent sexuality from that of the adult. A sexuality treatment team can evolve by processes of education, training, and experience that enable its members to practice with expertise, comfort, and compassion.

REFERENCES

1. Griffith, ER and Trieschmann, R: Sexual dysfunction in the physically ill and disabled. In Nadelson, C and Marcott, D (eds): Treatment Interventions in Human Sexuality. Plenum Press, New York and London, 1983, p 241.
2. Horn, LJ and Sandel, ME: Anterior pituitary dysfunction after traumatic brain injury—a preliminary report of 30 patients. Presented at 10th An-
nual Post-Graduate Course on Rehabilitation of the Brain Injured Adult and Child. Williamsburg, VA, June, 1986.
3. Klingbeil, GE and Cline, P: Anterior hypopituitarism: a consequence of head injury. Arch Phys Med Rehabil 66:44, 1985.
4. Romano, M: Family response to traumatic head injury. Scand J Rehabil Med 6:1, 1974.

5. Lezak, M: Living with the characterologically altered brain injured patient. J Clin Psychiatry 39(7):592, 1978.

6. Bond, MR: Assessment of the psychological outcome of severe head injury. Acta Neurochirurgica 34:57, 1976.

7. Brooks, N (ed): Closed Head Injury—Psychological, Social and Family Consequences. Oxford University Press, New York, 1984.

8. Rosenbaum, M and Najenson, T: Changes in life patterns and symptoms of low mood as reported by wives of severely brain-injured soldiers. J Consult Clin Psychol 44:6, 881, 1976.

9. Kosteljanetz, M et al: Sexual and hypothalamic dysfunction in the post-concussion syndrome. Acta Neurol Scand 63:169, 1981.

10. Barreca, T et al: Evaluation of anterior pituitary function in patients with post-traumatic diabetes insipidus. J Clin Endocrinol Metab 51:1279, 1980.

11. Gerstenbrand, F et al: Kluver-Bucy syndrome in man: experience with post-traumatic cases. Neurosci Biobehav Rev 7(3):413, 1983.

12. Berrol, S: Issue of sexuality in head injured adults. In Bullard, D and Knight, S (eds): Sexuality and Disability, Personal Perspectives. St Louis, CV Mosby, 1981, p 203.

13. Meyer, J: Sexual disturbances after cerebral injuries. J Neurovis Rel Suppl X:519, 1971.

14. Walker, AE and Jablon, S: A followup of head injured men of World War II. J Neurosurg 16:600, 1959.

15. Walker, AE: Long term evaluation of the social and family adjustment to head injuries. Scand J Rehabil Med 4:5, 1972.

16. Panting, A and Merry, P: The long term rehabilitation of severe head injuries with particular reference to the need for social and medical support for the patient's family. J Rehabil 38:33, 1972.

17. Weinstein, E: Sexual disturbances after brain injury. Medical Aspects of Human Sexuality 8(10):10, 1974.

18. Hierons, R and Saunders, M: Impotence in patients with temporal-lobe lesions. Lancet 2:761, 1966.

19. Boller, F and Frank, E: Sexual dysfunction. In Neurological Disorders: Diagnosis, Management and Rehabilitation. Raven Press, New York, 1982, p 50.

20. Herzog, A et al: Reproductive endocrine disorders in women with partial seizures of temporal lobe origin. Arch Neurol 43:341, 1986.

21. Shaul, P et al: Precocious puberty following severe head trauma. AJDC 139:467, 1985.

22. Adams, R and Victor, M: Principles of Neurology, ed 3. McGraw-Hill, New York, 1985.

23. Van Arsdalen, KN, Malloy, TR and Wein, AJ: Erectile physiology dysfunction and evaluation. II. Etiology and evaluation of erectile dysfunction. Monogr Urol 4:5, 1983.

24. Griffin, JE and Wilson, JD: The testis. In Bondy, P and Rosenberg, L (eds): Metabolic Control and Disease, ed 8. WB Saunders, Philadelphia, 1980, p 1560.

25. Kaplan, HS: The New Sex Therapy. Brunner/Mazel, New York, 1974.

26. Hackler, E and Tobis, J: Reintegration into the community. In Rosenthal, M et al (eds): Rehabilitation of the Head Injured Adult. FA Davis, Philadelphia, 1983, p 421.

27. Levin, H, Benton, A and Grossman, R: Neurobehav-

ioral consequences of closed head injury. Oxford University Press, 1982.

28. Prigatano, GP et al: Neuropsychological rehabilitation after brain injury. Johns Hopkins University Press, Baltimore, 1986.

29. Ben-Yishay, Y et al: Working approaches to remediation of cognitive deficits in brain damaged. NYU Medical Center Monographs, Nos., 59–61, 1978–1981.

30. Lilly, R et al: The human Kluver-Bucy syndrome. Neurology 33:1141, 1983.

31. Remillard, G et al: Sexual ictal manifestations predominate in women with temporal lobe epilepsy: a finding suggesting dimorphism in the human brain. Neurology 33:323, 1983.

32. Stuss, DT and Benson, DF: Frontal lobe lesions and behavior. In Kertesz, A (ed): Localization in Neuropsychology. Academic Press, New York, 1983, p 429.

33. Evans, CD: Rehabilitation After Severe Head Injury. Churchill Livingstone, Edinburgh, New York, 1981.

34. Smith, B and Khatic A: Cortical localization of sexual feeling. Psychosomatics 20(11):771, 1979.

35. Cartlidge, NEF and Shaw, DA: Head injury. WB Saunders, London, 1981, p 145.

36. Brooks, DN et al: Five year outcome of severe blunt head injury: a relative's view. J Neurol Neurosurg Psychol 49:764, 1986.

37. Davidoff, G et al: The spectrum of closed head injuries in facial trauma victims: incidence and impact. Ann Emerg Med, 17(1):6, 1988.

38. Mehta, A et al: Peripheral nerve conduction studies and bulbocavernous reflex in the investigation of impotence. Arch Phys Med Rehabil 67(5):332, 1986.

39. Haldeman S, et al: Pudendal evoked responses. Arch Neurol 39:280, 1982.

40. Escobar, P: Reflex sympathetic dystrophy. Orthoped Rev 15(10):646, 1986.

41. Wein, A, Malloy, T and Shrom, S: Surgical treatment of impotence. In Lief, HI: Sexual Problems in Medical Practice. AMA, 1981.

42. Diamant, H: The salivary apparatus. In Hinchliffe, R and Harrison, D: Scientific Foundations of Otolaryngology. Year Book Medical Publishers, Chicago, 1976.

43. Renshaw, DC and Lief, HI: Partner surrogates. In Sexual Problems in Medical Practice. AMA, 1981.

44. Eames, P et al: Rehabilitation after severe head injury: a followup study of a behavior modification program. J Neurol Neurosurg Psychol 48(7):613, 1985.

45. Griffith, ER and Trieschmann, R: Use of a private hospital room in restoring sexual function to the physically disabled. Sex Disabil 1:179, 1978.

46. Laschet, V: Antiandrogens in the treatment of sex offenders. In Zubin, J and Money, J (eds): Contemporary Sexual Behavior: Critical issues in the 1970's. Johns Hopkins University Press, Baltimore, 1973, p 203.

47. Planned Parenthood of Mid Central Illinois: Sex Education in the Family Series, 1980.

48. Cole, S: Facing the challenges of sexual abuse in persons with disabilities, J Sex Disabil 7(3):71, 1987.

49. Annon, JS: Behavioral Treatment of Sexual Problems. Harper and Row, New York, 1976.

50. Glasgow, M and Williams, R: Talking About Sex/

Taking A Sexual History (study guide accompanying video, "Taking A Sexual History"). Available through Sun-Rose Associates, Cambridge, 1986.

51. Cole, TM and Cole, SS: Sexual attitude reassessment programs for spinal cord injured adults, their partners and health care professionals. In Sha' Ked, A (ed): Human Sexuality and Rehabilitation Medicine: Sexual Functioning Following Spinal Cord Injury. Williams and Wilkins, Baltimore, 1981, p 80.

SUGGESTED READING

Barbach, L: For Yourself: The Fulfillment of Female Sexuality. Doubleday, New York, 1975.

Zilbergeld, B: Male Sexuality. Bantam Books, New York, 1978.

Kolodny, RC, Masters, WH and Johnson, VE: Textbook of Sexual Medicine. Little, Brown, Boston, 1979.

Chapter 16

Effects on the Family System

M. G. LIVINGSTON, M.D.

When people with serious illness are discharged home from the hospital, a burden of care is likely to fall on the family, particularly if the patients have handicaps or deficits. Indeed, many patients are discharged home only by virtue of the fact that a caring relative is present. Often this relative is a woman, possibly with young children and other dependent relatives in the family. In such situations, finance may be limited, and relatives may find that they face their burdens alone.

Attempts at measuring the impact of illness on family members have begun to appear in the literature.[1] Severe head injury is particularly common in young men from lower socioeconomic groups.[2] Associated with the injury are a constellation of factors, such as heavy alcohol consumption, risk taking, and assault, which almost form a stereotypic picture. As a result of such injuries, approximately 1500 people a year are rendered severely disabled in the United Kingdom;[3] this figure is much higher in the United States, where head injury is more common. Many individuals suffer physical incapacity such that they have difficulty walking, speaking, seeing, hearing, and smelling. They complain of a number of physical symptoms, such as headache, fatigue, and speech difficulty, and may have problems in coping with skills of everyday living, be unable to work, and have intellectual impairment and behavioral and emotional changes. It would not, therefore, be surprising if relatives were to find themselves overwhelmed by the dependency needs of patients who have multiple handicaps.

The aim of this chapter is to review research on the impact of severe head injury on patients' relatives. If knowledge can be gained of the nature of the maladaptive response found in some relatives, then this may facilitate the design of rehabilitation programs in which patients and relatives participate. Particular emphasis will be placed on studies in which a replicable methodology is described.

PROBLEMS DESCRIBED BY RELATIVES

Romano[4] observed the responses of 13 families in which a relative had suffered severe head injury. The families only had contact with the social worker when survival seemed likely, and Romano felt that families often became locked in denial and were unable to advance beyond this point in adjusting to their loss. Denial prevents relatives from making appropriate decisions; Romano quotes the example of a family who refused to consider contraception for a promiscuous woman who, on discharge, subsequently became pregnant. Relatives who had been faced with the patient's possible death were simply relieved that the individual was alive, at the cost of accepting the true loss in terms of the person's personality. Denial may result in relatives being unable to accept that either death or disability may be an inevitable consequence of severe head injury. Such families may be tempted to search out the elusive expert who will be able to cure their relative. More productively, relatives may channel their energies

225

**Table 16–1. EFFECTS OF HEAD INJURY ON PERSONALITY
AND BEHAVIOR**

Personality or Behavioral Construct	Changes Caused by Head Injury
Capacity for social perceptiveness	Self-centered behavior Diminution or total loss of self-criticism Loss of ability to show empathy
Capacity for self-control	Random restlessness Impatience and impulsivity
Learned and social behavior	Diminution in or loss of initiative; power to make judgments, plan, and organize Increased social dependency
Ability to learn	Mental slowness and rigidity of thought Reduced learning capacity
Emotion	Irritability, silliness, lability of mood, apathy, and increased or diminished sexual drive

From Lezak,[5] with permission.

into self-help groups and become involved in the care and rehabilitation of the patient.

Lezak[5] studied 200 families who had a brain injured relative. She found that caregiving relatives felt trapped and isolated. They described themselves as often being subjected to violence and criticism by other relatives. In this situation, many spouses felt that they had a nonparticipating partner in their marriage. It was as if they were neither married nor single, and they felt frustrated in their sexual and affectional needs. Problems in the household led to children displaying divided loyalty to either parent. Table 16–1 categorizes the behavioral change brought about by severe head injury, described by Lezak.[5]

Oddy and Humphrey[6] studied 50 young adults 6 months after a severe (post-traumatic amnesia greater than 24 hours) closed head injury. Patients who suffered limb injury, matched for age and social class, formed a comparison group. A close relative completed a symptom checklist of 37 items relating to personality changes, somatic, sensory, cognitive, and psychiatric symptoms. Table 16–2 illustrates the symptoms in the patient most frequently reported by the relative, and shows that one third or more of the relatives describe memory difficulty, tiredness, impatience, and loss of temper.

Post-traumatic amnesia (PTA) and time of return to work correlated positively with the relatives' view of significant problems in the patient, but no significant association was demonstrated with the patients' sex or social class, nor was an outstanding compensation claim important in this respect. These results suggest that the social problems of head injury patients are secondary to personality change, itself a consequence of the injury. Six months after injury, there was no evidence to indicate serious disruption in marital relationships.

An Israeli study[7] compared wives of military brain injured patients with wives of paraplegics and staff members. Assessments were carried out 1 year after the injury. Head injury wives reported more selfish,

Table 16–2. HEAD INJURED PATIENTS' SYMPTOMS MOST FREQUENTLY REPORTED BY RELATIVES

Relatives (n = 48)	No. Relatives
Has trouble remembering things	21
Becomes tired very easily	18
Often impatient	17
Often loses temper	16
Is often irritable	15
Has difficulty with eyes	12
Sometimes bumps into things	11
Is often restless	10

From Oddy and Humphrey,[6] with permission.

childish, demanding, and dependent behavior in their husbands. They complained that their spouses took a smaller share in running the household, particularly in caring for the children. The result was a reduction in family leisure time and in time spent in contact with other relatives, with a consequent disruption in relationships. As in Oddy and Humphrey's study,[6] wives of the head injured patients reported a marked reduction in sexual activity.

McKinlay and coworkers[8] questioned relatives of men who had suffered severe blunt head injury in the year following trauma. The patients were consecutive referrals to a neurosurgical center, and all had suffered PTA greater than 48 hours. The relatives interviewed bore the major day-to-day responsibility for the care of the patient, and they commonly reported problems with the patient of a psychologic and emotional nature. Over two thirds of the relatives stated that the injured person was slow, tired, and irritable. Other significant problems mentioned were poor memory, impetuous behavior, tension and anxiety, bad temper, personality change, depressed mood, and headaches.

How do severely injured patients compare with minor injury patients as viewed by the relative? This has been assessed by listing the 10 most common complaints of the relatives of severe head injury patients and comparing the response made by the relatives of minor head injury patients to the same complaints.[9] There was a statistically significant difference in the level of reporting between the minor and severe head injury relatives in favor of the latter (p <0.001 in all cases). In addition, at least 30 percent of the relatives of severely injured patients reported each of the symptoms as a problem (Table 16–3).

What head injury patients' relatives report reflects their perception of events and may not be related to the severity of the injury in physical terms. Such subjective impressions are often based on poor information; for example, in an examination of 50 young patients with severe head injury together with their relatives, almost half of the relatives were dissatisfied with the quality of information given to them during the patients' hospitalization.[10] The response of 40 of the relatives is shown in Table 16–4, which also emphasizes the fact that, at this time of cri-

Table 16–3. MINOR AND SEVERE HEAD INJURY PATIENTS' SYMPTOMS REPORTED BY RELATIVES

Relatives' Complaint	Minor Head Injury % (n=41)	Severe Head Injury % (n=42)
Personality change	20	67
Change in work capacity	2	62
Bad tempered	10	50
Household routine upset	0	50
Depressed	22	50
Increased anger	12	45
Relative's health affected	0	40
Changeable mood	7	33
Avoids company	7	31
Childish behavior	7	31

*χ^2 for each complaint >5.9, p<0.01.
Adapted from Livingston, Brooks, and Bond.[9]

sis, relatives are not receptive to detailed information. In such circumstances, there is a clear need for simple and concise information to be packaged in such a way that it is understood by relatives. Obviously information will have to be given during the acute admission but this needs to be repeated and reinforced on several occasions, during ad-

Table 16–4. COMMENTS OF 40 RELATIVES OF HEAD INJURY PATIENTS ON INFORMATION DURING HOSPITALIZATION

Comments	No. Relatives
Did not get any information	1
Did not understand what doctor said	4
Believed doctors never tell the truth	3
Believed doctor was too busy	2
Believed doctor would not answer our questions	2
Was afraid and did not listen	1
Did not want to hear what doctor said	1
Received too little information, no further comments	4
Received good information	22

From Thomsen,[10] with permission.

mission, on discharge, and in the months that follow.

RELATIVES' BURDEN

Oddy and associates[11] studied closed head injury patients, aged between 16 and 39, who had a PTA greater than 24 hours. Fourteen married patients were interviewed together with their respective spouses. Forty single patients were interviewed with their relative; 30 mothers and 10 fathers. More than half the relatives 6 and 12 months after the injury reported that they were experiencing stress as a result of the head injury. Relatives related this stress to some aspect of the patient's current condition, including poorly controlled behavior, fear of epilepsy, and physical stress resulting from coping with physical disabilities. This work suggests that relatives appear to be able to adjust to tangible disabilities such as paraplegia or loss of a limb, but the emotional and psychologic consequences of brain damage are harder to accept.

In the study by McKinlay and colleagues,[8] relatives were asked to assess subjectively the burden imposed on them by the patient, using a seven-point rating scale. The reliability of this method was assessed by repeating 10 interviews with each rater. Personality and behavioral changes were most frequently reported as stressful, but there was no consistent relationship between relatives' burden and the severity of the injury as assessed by PTA.

Which features of personality change in the patients are most burdensome for relatives? Brooks and McKinlay[12] found that the association between patients' personality change and relatives' burden increased over time. At 6 months, poor control of temper, social withdrawal, loss of affection, lack of energy, cruelty, meanness, and unreasonableness were singled out as being associated with high burden in relatives. At 12 months, these features were still important in terms of the relatives' burden. As time elapsed the relatives showed a decreasing ability to accept, and cope with, these negative changes in the patient's behavior.

In two more recent studies from Glasgow[9, 13] male patients were recruited from a neurosurgical center, and a woman in the family was interviewed together with the patient, at home. A comparison group of minor head injury patients and their relatives were also assessed.

Burden on the relatives was assessed by means of the Perceived Burden Scale, which was devised for this study. The relatives of the severely injured patients, as might be expected, recorded significantly higher levels of perceived burden (p <0.001) compared with the relatives of the minor injury patients. This high self-rating of burden continued in the relatives of the severely injured throughout the year following injury.

Studies with follow-up over several years confirm that the deficits following head injury often persist for years with consequent burden on relatives. Brooks and associates[14] traced head injury patients' families 5 years after the injury and succeeded in reassessing 42 out of 50 patients—76 percent of the original sample. Dropouts were due to death, inability to be located, and, in one case, the discovery of premorbid epilepsy. Seventy-four percent of the relatives, compared with 60 percent at 1 year postinjury, reported continuing personality change in the patient. Sixty-four percent continued to report, in addition, slowness, memory impairment, irritability, and bad temper. The most marked increase was observed in threats of violence, said to be twice as common 5 years after the injury.

The distribution of burden changes from 1 to 5 years after the injury, with a preponderance of low to medium burden at 1 year and a preponderance of medium to high burden in the relatives at 5 years postinjury (Table 16–5). This increasing burden on relatives is associated with continuing and,

Table 16–5. NUMBER OF RELATIVES IN EACH SUBJECTIVE BURDEN CATEGORY AT 1 AND 5 YEARS

Subjective Burden		1 year		5 years	
Score	Description	N	%	N	%
1–2	"Low"	18	43	4	10
3–4	"Medium"	14	33	13	33
5–7	"High"	10	24	22	56
Total		42		39	

From Brooks et al,[14] with permission.

in some instances, worsening change in personality and behavioral outcome in the head injury patients.

In a 7-year follow-up,[15] the percentage of patients' relatives in the high burden group remained high at 47 percent. Eighty-five percent or more of the relatives are in the medium to high burden category and at least 46 percent are in the high burden category at any one time—thus, there was no significant change over time. In this study, the relatives' subjective burden seemed to be related to both the severity of the injury and the nature and magnitude of behavioral change in the patients.

A series of United Kingdom studies has found that relatives report a high burden in living with severe head injury victims. Relatives find emotional and behavioral changes in the patient most burdensome. Although relatives of severely injured patients report greater burden than relatives of those with minor head injury, there does not appear to be a simple relationship whereby burden on the relative increases with the severity of injury. This latter point would appear to confirm the importance of nonphysical patient factors in terms of relatives' burden, since these factors are in themselves not simply related to severity of the injury. In the studies which are to be described, burden on relatives is objectively assessed by measuring relatives' psychosocial adjustment.

PSYCHOLOGIC DISTRESS IN RELATIVES

Rosenbaum and Najenson[7] found greater disturbance in the wives of brain injured men than with the wives of paraplegic patients or staff members. The wives of the head injured soldiers recorded high levels of depression and irritability. The depression was said to be associated with a lack of positive reinforcement, as wives of the brain injured had fewer pleasurable activities, either at home or elsewhere. Sexual activity was reduced in the head injured couples but the authors felt that this was associated with interpersonal difficulties rather than a physical consequence of head injury.

Oddy and coworkers[11] administered the Wakefield Depression Inventory to relatives of severe brain injury victims. They found that at 1 month after the injury, 39 percent

of the relatives scored in the depression "caseness" range, and this was significantly greater than the scores obtained subsequently. At 6 months after the injury, 20 percent of the relatives scored in this range and at 12 months 23 percent, figures that are comparable to normal United Kingdom community samples.[16] Mood disturbance in the relative and severity of injury in the patient were not related, but there was a significant positive association between relatives' depression ratings and the relatives' perception of the patients' personality change. Interestingly there was a tendency toward parents of the head injured being more depressed than spouses but the number of spouses involved was small.

Two Glasgow studies[9, 13] have found significant anxiety in relatives. In these studies, psychologic distress was measured by means of the General Health Questionnaire (GHQ-60)[17] and the Leeds Scales for the assessment of anxiety and depression.[18] When relatives of severe head injury patients are compared with minor head injury patients, they differ significantly in terms of caseness on the GHQ, with the relatives of the severely injured being more disturbed. This greater disturbance appears to be due to greater levels of anxiety rather than depression (Table 16–6). As much as 40 percent of the relatives of the severely injured patients had anxiety case levels compared with 19 percent of the minor injury relatives. When the relatives of the severely injured patients are followed-up over 1 year, the GHQ and Leeds scores are consistent—that is, the high levels of psychologic distress continue whether in terms of severity of distress or percentage of cases at each time of sampling.

The GHQ 60 has four subscales, measuring somatic complaints, anxiety and insomnia, social dysfunction and severe depression. The relatives of severely injured patients report significantly more social dysfunction and anxiety/insomnia compared with minor injury patients' relatives at 3 months after injury.[19]

Wives' and mothers' scores on the GHQ 60 and Leeds scales were compared at 3 and 6, and 6 and 12 months.[13] No statistically significant differences were recorded but the numbers in each group were relatively small, in some instances being fewer than 20. Further studies are required with larger

Table 16–6. CASENESS IN RELATIVES

Variable	N	Cases	Noncases	Cutoff Score	χ^2	Probability
GHQ						
Mildly injured	37	4	33	>12	8.52	0.003
Severely injured	42	24	18			
Leeds Anxiety Scale						
Mildly injured	41	8	33	>7	5.14	0.02
Severely injured	42	19	23			
Leeds Depression Scale						
Mildly injured	41	3	38	>7	2.23	0.13
Severely injured	42	9	33			

From Livingston, Brooks, and Bond,[9] with permission.

numbers to assess whether there is a differential outcome dependent on relationship to the head injured.

There are significant positive correlations between the level of symptomatic complaints made by the patients and the relatives' psychologic distress.[13] On the rating instrument used, these complaints reflected high levels of personality and behavioral change as well as physical symptoms. Often, subjective complaints by the patients accounted for more than 20 percent of the variance in the relatives' GHQ 60 and Leeds anxiety responses, suggesting a link between the patients' current level of functioning and its impact on relatives.

Relatives of patients who suffer severe brain injury report high levels of psychologic distress, especially symptoms of anxiety. The anxiety appears to be related to the nonphysical consequences of trauma to the head, particularly the symptomatic complaints made by the patients. Again, no simple relationship between increasing severity of injury and increasing distress in the relatives has been demonstrated.

SOCIAL IMPACT OF HEAD INJURY ON RELATIVES

Oddy and colleagues[20] studied social recovery following head injury. They found no evidence of strain or increased friction in the family or marital relationships 6 months after the injury. Unlike the Israeli findings,[7] sexual functioning appears to have improved by this time. However, this survey was based on a consecutive sample of patients selected specifically for rehabilitation.

As such, they included a younger age group, and there was a skew toward upper socioeconomic groups.

In a subsequent study,[6] Oddy's group report increasing friction toward the end of 1 year in single head injury patients living with their parents, but at 2 years this also appears to have recovered. There was much less social disturbance within the families of married patients. Poor social functioning in the relatives was found to be related to personality change in the patients, possibly because highly disturbed patients curtailed social contact in the family home with friends and relatives and made it difficult for relatives to leave the patient on his or her own.

Weddell and coworkers[21] assessed severe brain injury patients and their families, who had been involved in rehabilitation. All patients were younger than 40 years old, presumably a factor in their selection for rehabilitation. Head injury families somewhat surprisingly appeared to enjoy closer involvement, perhaps because relatives compensated for the patients' limited social contacts by staying at home with them or possibly because they felt the need to supervise the patient. Since head injury is often associated with heavy alcohol taking, confinement to the house and thus reduced opportunity to obtain alcohol may have its advantages for some relatives.

Livingston and colleagues[9] used the Social Adjustment Scale in self report format (SAS-SR)[22] to assess social adjustment. Three months after injury there was no difference in global social functioning between the relatives of minor and severe head injury patients, nor was there any difference in the relatives' functioning at work, in social and leisure activities within the extended family, or with the nuclear family. There was, however, significantly poorer functioning in the marital role (p <0.04) and within the nuclear family (p <0.01). The results support the idea that functioning in roles within the family home was impaired 3 months after the injury.

There was deterioration in global social functioning at the 6-month assessment of the relatives of the severe injury patients, and this deterioration was still present at 12 months.[13] There was a trend for the mean role scores in work, social and leisure, extended family, marital, parental and nuclear family functioning, to be above those recorded by Weissman and coworkers[23] in their community survey of social adjustment. Social adjustment in terms of role performance thus appears to evolve more slowly than psychologic distress.

Although the literature on social impairment following head injury is conflicting, this may reflect the varying populations used. Studies that have used objective measures of social functioning point to slowly evolving role changes and diminished contacts outside the home. Relatives are placed in the position of caring for highly dependent people, often with little obvious physical incapacity but marked behavioral problems.

REHABILITATION OF FAMILIES WITH HEAD INJURY

Relatives under great stress, burdened by the care and management of head injury victms, may be unable to deal effectively with the day-to-day problems they encounter with their injured family member, or to make effective plans for the future. Often, decisions have to be made about rehabilitation, adaptation of the house or car, and the possibility of occupational retraining. Impending compensation claims often complicate the issue. It is important, therefore, to understand how psychosocial maladjustment within the families of head injured patients develops so that this knowledge may be incorporated into the planning of coordinated rehabilitation.

While rehabilitation centers for head injured patients are commonly found in the United States, there are very limited facilities in the United Kingdom. Such facilities that do exist in the United Kingdom tend to be oriented toward dealing with physical impairment; head injured patients with severe behavioral difficulties are referred for psychiatric management. Many victims of head injury with the poorest outcome may remain unsuitably placed in acute psychiatric wards, sometimes for up to 2½ years.[24]

Since the consensus in the literature indicates that a physical care/rehabilitation model is inappropriate and there is a need for family involvement in rehabilitation programs, another model of management involving both care and treatment has to be considered. One possible model is that of psychiatric rehabilitation which is concerned with addressing social, psychologic, and biologic deficits.[25] The process of rehabilitation involves identification, prevention, and minimization of these deficits. The organization of such treatment and care involves a multidisciplinary team approach and, most importantly, the treatment is problem centered. Individually tailored programs are worked out following an individual behavior analysis. Since the aim of psychiatric rehabilitation is maintenance within the community or restoration to the community, the family must be involved. Care and treatment is often organized on a day-attendance basis. Day attendance enables the practical work of rehabilitation to be carried out under supervision with staff encouragement in the day unit, and the techniques can later be applied in the family home. This avoids the problem of failure to generalize therapeutic work to the home following discharge from the inpatient rehabilitation program. Day care can provide an appropriate milieu to foster independence and encourage self-reliance. As well as providing treatment, such centers are often geared toward providing care of those left with long-term handicaps.

Severe head injury results in multiple handicaps with a variable time course of recovery. Relatives involved in the caregiving suffer significant psychiatric and social disturbance and there is a link between the relatives' disturbance and nature of the patients' symptoms. Head injury rehabilitation may, therefore, be organized on a similar basis to psychiatric rehabilitation. After assessment of patient and relatives by multidisciplinary teams, an individual program of care and treatment is outlined—in essence, a family management program.

Head injury rehabilitation teams draw on the skills of neurosurgeons and trauma surgeons, rehabilitation medicine specialists, psychiatrists, psychologists, nurses, physiotherapists, occupational therapists, and social workers. In countries where there is a highly developed system of primary care by family practitioners, close liaison between them and the rehabilitation team is often productive. Family practitioners are often well aware of the family background, and this includes a knowledge of how the family copes with stress, both individually and as a unit.

The two cases that follow are drawn from those seen by the author during his studies of head injury families.[26] They are described because they illustrate the interactive effect of head injury on the relatives and how a family assessment is important in head injury rehabilitation.

Case 1. A 30-year-old tire fitter suffered a severe head injury when he was struck by a car outside work. The incident occurred during the lunch break and he had no memory of the event. The post-traumatic amnesia lasted for 6 weeks. The first 2 weeks in the hospital were spent in a neurosurgical unit, but no operative procedure was carried out. After 6 more weeks in a district general hospital, the patient was discharged to his parents' care, although he had a home of his own.

A number of problems were evident upon discharge. The patient remained dysarthric and had a spastic gait. His personality changed, and he became sullen and moody with limited tolerance of frustration. He returned to his own house after 9 months because it was nearby and because his parents' ability to cope with him had been stretched to the utmost.

Two years after the injury on evaluation at home, speech and walking had improved but dysarthria was still evident and the patient required the use of a walking stick. He had no contact with his former friends and his social life consisted of infrequent outings with his parents.

On each home visitation, the patient's mother talked of her profound gratitude to doctors for her son's recovery. It was obvious that she had been drinking alcohol. She gave an impression of intense, suppressed anger. She denied there were any specific problems with her son's care but she al-

ways had difficulty indicating how much she was doing for him. She also indicated that her husband did not help in the management of their son.

Research assessments[9,13] showed high levels of anxiety but not of depression in this patient's mother. She reported little social activity. She was anxious to talk after an initial period of reticence. At the end of the last visit, she broke down in tears and confessed that she found the task she had to face more than she could bear.

Case 2. A 32-year-old skilled engineer fell from a high scaffold while at work in the shipyards. He denied any alcohol intake and alleged that the company had been negligent as they had failed to ensure that the scaffold planking was free of grease. He sustained a severe head injury resulting in a PTA of 8 weeks' duration. Neurosurgical evacuation of a hematoma followed, in the course of which a large area of infected skull bone was removed. The patient's wife frequently remarked about his appearance but indicated quite strongly that she did not wish the bony deficit to be replaced with an acrylic graft. Apart from this, there were no obvious physical handicaps but the patient consistently complained of fatigue.

The patient was apathetic at first, although this disappeared within 4 months. Cognitive impairment (slow thinking, poor ability to learn with consequent disorientation) was evident to his wife and confirmed by examination, but the patient denied any such difficulties. At interview he seemed a little facile and disinhibited. He insisted on driving the family car. During one visit to the home, the patient's wife indicated that the couple had given up sexual intercourse for 3 months. She stated that this was a sacrifice, meant as a thanksgiving offering to God for her husband's survival.

Clinically, this woman appeared tense and resentful, but although she expressed a willingness to complete questionnaires, asked very many questions about the purpose of the study and the confidentiality of the responses. Her early scores showed mildly elevated anxiety, which later increased. The clinical impression remained one of consistent tension. It was obvious that her resentment was meant for her husband but could not be directed toward him in his present predicament. Encouragement to ventilate these feelings met with strong denial. At the end of the assessment year, a claim for compensation was being pursued and it seemed unlikely that the patient would ever return to skilled work.

In Case 1, the patient has a variety of physical, social, and psychologic problems. The physical problems required physiotherapy in order to encourage graded remobilization and to advise about appropriate walking aids and the adaptation of a vehicle suitable for the patient's use. Since the pace of physical recovery is often more rapid than that of personality and behavioral deficits,[27] physiotherapy can provide a welcome boost to morale. There is a need to review progress regularly and to set further goals.

In this case, occupational therapists should provide craft and other task-oriented activity. The skill of the occupational therapist lies in providing tasks within the patient's ability that have relevance to either re-employment or day-to-day activities. Many of these tasks involve working in a group, in situations that allow for the development of social skills vital for the patient's functioning in the family and other social groups. In this setting, interpersonal interactions can be seen in vivo. Observing poor temper control and frustration and noting the flash-points and triggers thereof provides useful information to feed back to patients and their relatives, along with strategies for dealing with these problems. Occupational therapists will have access to various programs for industrial retraining and will be aware of the possibility of various forms of sheltered employment for the future.

The team psychologist's role in rehabilitation is to assess behavior and cognition, especially when these are either maladaptive or leading to impaired function. Feedback from the occupational therapist's group-oriented activities will obviously be helpful. In Case 1, frustration and temper outbursts were of particular concern to the family. An analysis of behavior has to consider both the antecedents and the consequences, as well as the behavior itself. Successful rehabilitation leads not only to the elimination of unwanted behavior, but also to learning new responses and strategies for coping.

The mother of the patient in Case 1 requires additional help herself. Counseling, education, and support are important, as well as an opportunity to learn more adaptive stress-reducing techniques. She needs to learn how to deal with her son's difficulties without resorting to alcohol. A first step should be encouragement to articulate her

feelings about her son and his behavior and to indicate what she considers to be the limits of her tolerance. In addition, a program of anxiety management, based on relaxation training techniques, should help in coping with her son's and her own difficulties. Much of this work with relatives is tackled by nurse therapists in the rehabilitation team.

Information is not satisfactorily conveyed to head injured patients' relatives.[10] If relatives' anxieties are to be allayed, they need clear and simple information about the likely outcome as well as the pace of recovery for different handicaps. This may be conveniently approached by a relatives' support and information group at the rehabilitation center, or by links with self-help support organizations such as Headway (in the United Kingdom) or the National Head Injury Foundation (in the United States).

Relatives' support groups are becoming more popular in many different aspects of family management. Beside providing support, these groups can inform, and an element of therapy can be incorporated in the group for the relative.[28] They can also teach the relatives techniques to facilitate management of the patients. Such techniques involve suggestions about coping with a behavioral problem or about how much to do for physically handicapped relatives. The mother in Case 1 would doubtless benefit from such an approach, particularly as she gave a strong impression of overinvolved caring. In addition, relatives' support groups can act as a focus for pressure groups to appeal for improved facilities or to engage in fund raising for research and resources.

The patient in Case 2 had difficulties mainly involving behavioral and psychologic handicaps. Although it was clear that repair of the patient's skull deficit would help him to reintegrate socially, his wife demonstrated marked anxiety about the procedure, possibly because she feared he might not survive the operation. Again, information and counseling should have a priority in this case for both patient and relative. An occupational therapist would play a considerable role in attempting to obtain industrial retraining and resettlement in a more suitable environment vital for this man's self-esteem and for his relationship with his wife.

Psychologists are increasingly focusing on structured programs to manage cognitive impairment following head injury. In Case 2, it seems likely that there were marital difficulties prior to the head injury. Some joint marital counseling of the couple, preferably at home, would be beneficial. Involvement of a social worker here could be of considerable help. As well as exploring possibly longstanding relationship difficulties, there is a need to focus on sexual functioning after severe head injury, dispelling any anxieties that this may lead to physical harm. The couple obviously needs encouragement to discuss its difficulties.

At present in the United Kingdom, many relatives of head injured patients receive minor tranquilizers[29] for anxiety, but simple behavioral and counseling treatments often may be just as effective (e.g., the patient in Case 2) and is less hazardous in the long run, particularly in view of recent concerns about the habit-forming potential of benzodiazepine drugs. Tranquilizers prescribed by the family practitioner or psychiatrist may, however, be beneficial in the short term until the rehabilitation program gets fully under way, particularly if the anxiety is at such a level that the relative's ability to cope is compromised.

One aspect of multidisciplinary rehabilitation programs that is not often emphasized is that they enable the provision of continuous assessment. This helps define the outcome for the head injured patient's family, an exercise often required if litigation is being pursued. Thus, a longitudinal view can be taken of the family, both from observation in the rehabilitation day unit and some observations in their home.

Cases 1 and 2 substantiate the view that a premorbid record of instability in the relative is likely to predispose him or her to breakdown following the stress of living with a person who has suffered severe head injury.[19] Such a record of instability would be obvious in the form of psychiatric consultation and hospitalization but it may simply take the form of difficulty in adjusting to stress, in which case the observations of family practitioners are helpful. Relatives' past illness experience, whether psychiatric or physical, seems to be highly predictive of their subsequent psychosocial function following the family member's head injury.[19] Thus, it is possible to predict to some extent those relatives who are most likely to have difficulty adjusting to living with serious illness and disability, and this emphasizes the need to begin rehabilitation as soon as possible in the hope of preventing secondary deficits appearing in patients and their relatives.

The link between past illness experience and current adjustment difficulty has been explored in the psychiatric literature. Following a large survey in the Camberwell district of London, Brown and coworkers[30] proposed a two-stage model of the causation of depression. In this work, early loss of a parent "sensitized" women, making them more vulnerable to depression in later life. The presence of current life stresses such as the lack of a confiding partner, not being involved in paid employment outside the home, and having young children at home acted as triggers in the development of depressive illness. It is possible that relatives of head injured patients were initially sensitized by previous illness experience themselves, and the trigger that leads to their psychosocial maladjustment is the stress of coping with daily symptoms in the patient.

It should be remembered that the burdens of severe head injury on the family are not intermittent or episodic. In such situations, friends or relatives, by offering to look after a patient for a period of time during the day or evening, may permit a much needed break for a relative. Some self-help groups will organize this for their member. A break from the burden of constant caring can be obtained by organizing a "holiday," or brief admission for the patient, a model of which is often provided by the geriatric and psychogeriatric services. The patient's disabilities will determine the most appropriate place for this admission, although if he or she is involved in a day rehabilitation program, it would be ideal if this care were offered by the rehabilitation unit, thus enabling the program to continue.

Rehabilitation professionals also play a role in indicating to the family the likely prognosis. Which deficits are likely to recover and which to persist? Is the patient likely to return to work, and if so, what sort of job is he or she likely to obtain? Will there be need for constant support by a relative? All these questions have to be considered carefully in assessing the level of a claim for compensation. The preparation of such cases often require many months of work, but detailed reports from members of the rehabilitation team do assist the court in determining the level of compensation. The final outcome in head injury is often only evident several years after the injury, and in many cases the outcome of the legal process is delayed even longer. Progress in rehabilitation can be aided by the early payment of an interim award, a practice that may in fact reduce the final payment if the outcome has been improved.

In conclusion, patients with severe head injury, by virtue of their dependence on close relatives, impose a stress on the family system. Some families may be unable to cope, resulting in psychosocial adjustment difficulties in the relatives. These family difficulties have to be tackled, as do the handicaps of the head injured patients themselves. Comprehensive head injury rehabilitation programs therefore view head injury as a family problem, requiring a team effort by families and therapists alike in order to permit as high a level of adaptation for the family as possible.

REFERENCES

1. Livingston, MG: Families who care. Br Med J 291:919, 1985.
2. Jennett, B and MacMillan, R: The epidemiology of head injury. Br Med J 1:101, 1981.
3. London, PS: Some observations on the course of events after severe injury of the head. Ann Roy Coll Engl 41:460, 1967.
4. Romano, MD: Family response to traumatic head injury. Scand J Rehabil Med 6:1, 1974.
5. Lezak, MD: Living with the characteriologically altered brain injured patient. J Clin Psychiatry 39:592, 1978.
6. Oddy, M and Humphrey, M: Social recovery during the year following severe head injury. J Neurol Neurosurg Psychiatry 43:798, 1980.
7. Rosenbaum, M and Najenson, T: Changes in life pattern and symptoms of low mood as reported by wives of severely brain injured soldiers. J Consult Clin Psychol 44:681, 1976.
8. McKinlay, WW, Brooks, DN, Bond, MR, et al: The short term outcome of severe blunt head injury as reported by relatives of the injured persons. J Neurol Neurosurg Psychiatry 44:527, 1981.
9. Livingston, MG, Brooks, DN and Bond, MR: Three months after severe head injury: psychiatric and social impact on relatives. J Neurolog Neurosurg Psychiatry 48:870, 1985.
10. Thomsen, IV: The patient with severe head injury and his family. Scand J Rehabil 6:180, 1974.
11. Oddy, M, Humphrey, M and Uttley, D: Stresses upon the relatives of head injured patients. Br J Psychiatry 133:507, 1978.
12. Brooks, DN and McKinlay, WW: Personality and behavioral changes after severe blunt head injury: a relative's view. J Neurol Neurosurg Psychiatry 46:336, 1983.
13. Livingston, MG, Brooks, DN and Bond, MR: Patient outcome in the year following severe head injury and relatives' psychiatric and social functioning. J Neurol Neurosurg Psychiatry 48:876, 1985.
14. Brooks, DN et al: The five year outcome of severe blunt head injury: a relative's view. J Neurol Neurosurg Psychiatry 49:764, 1986.
15. Brooks, DN et al: The effects of severe head injury upon patient and relative within seven years of injury. J Head Trauma Rehabil 2(3):1, 1987.
16. Goldberg, D, Kay, C and Thompson, L: Psychiatric morbidity in general practice and the community. Psychol Med 6:565, 1976.
17. Goldberg, D: The Manual of the General Health Questionnaire. NFER Publishing, Windsor, Berkshire, England, 1978, p 1.
18. Snaith, RP, Bridge, GW and Hamilton, M: The Leeds Scales for the self-assessment of anxiety and depression. Br J Psychiatry 128:156, 1976.
19. Livingston, MG: Head injury: The relatives' response. Brain Inj 1:8, 1987.
20. Oddy, M, Humphrey, M and Uttley, D: Subjective impairment and social recovery after closed head injury. J Neurol Psychiatry 48:611, 1978.
21. Weddell, R, Oddy, M and Jenkins, D: Social adjustment after rehabilitation: a two year follow up of patients with severe head injury. Psychol Med 10:257, 1980.
22. Weissman, MM and Bothwell, S: Assessment of social adjustment by patients' self-report. Arch Gen Psychiatry 33:1111, 1976.
23. Weissman, MM et al: Social adjustment by self-report in a community sample and in psychiatric outpatients. J Nerv Ment Dis 166:317, 1978.
24. Gloag, D: Rehabilitation after head injury. II. Behavioral and emotional problems, long term needs and the requirements for services. Br Med J 290:913, 1985.
25. Royal College of Psychiatrists: Psychiatric Rehabilitation in the 1980s. Report of the Working Party on Rehabilitation. The Social and Community Psychiatry Section. Greenways, London, 1980, p 1.
26. Livingston, MG: The outcome of severe head injury in men and its psychosocial impact on a close female relative. MD Thesis, Glasgow University, 1986, p 157.
27. Jennett, B et al: Disability after severe head injury: observations on the use of the Glasgow Outcome Scale. J Neurol Neurosurg Psychiatry 44:285, 1981.
28. Livingston, MG: Families and illness. Br J Hosp Med 7:51, 1987.
29. Livingston, MG: Assessment of need for co-ordinated approach in families with victims of head injury. Br Med J 293:742, 1986.
30. Brown, GW, Harris, TO, Copeland, JR: Depression and loss. Br J Psychiatry 129:125, 1976.

Chapter 17

Minor Head Injury

J. DOUGLAS MILLER, M.D., Ph.D.
PATRICIA A. JONES, Dip. Phys., M.Sc.

Minor head injuries comprise between 70 and 85 percent of all head injury admissions to the hospital. For many years this large group of patients was considered to have sustained a trivial brain injury and were expected to make full recovery. Patients who did not were frequently branded as malingerers or neurotics. In recent years the attention of clinical neuropsychologists has turned to these patients, revealing that a surprisingly high proportion suffer cognitive, memory, and other neuropsychologic deficits following minor head injury. Parallel studies of concussional head injury in the experimental laboratory have shown clearcut examples of axonal and other structural brain damage, even in circumstances in which only brief loss of consciousness had been produced by the experimental injury. This stands in contrast to studies of computerized tomography (CT) in patients with minor head injury, in which no abnormality is usually seen. More light has been shed on this area by the recent application of magnetic resonance scanning (MRI), in which abnormal areas in the brain may be observed in cases of minor head injury, even in patients in whom CT is normal. Considerable interest is now being developed in the definition of neuropsychologic and behavioral problems following minor head injury, and it is hoped that a detailed study of cases of minor head injury may reveal new information regarding the problems of patients with more severe injuries.

DEFINING MINOR HEAD INJURY

The simplest definition of minor head injury is based on the Glasgow Coma Scale (GCS), which defines minor head injury as patients who score 13, 14, or 15 on the Glasgow Coma Sum Score.[1] This definition implies that patients included in the category of minor head injury are those who have spontaneous eye opening or open their eyes to command, who obey commands in terms of motor function and speak in formed sentences, but who are either confused and disoriented or fully oriented. Of the patients who score the full 15 points on the Glasgow Coma Scale, there must have been a history of head injury and circumstances upon first evaluation at the hospital that led to the patient's admission. These might include evidence of skull fracture or a penetrating head wound. Thus, the definition of any population of patients with minor head injury must also take into account the guidelines that were used to govern which patients seen in the emergency room were admitted to the hospital and which were discharged.

In 1984, guidelines for initial management after head injury were published by a group of British neurosurgeons.[2] These guidelines are shown in Table 17–1; the key factors leading to hospitalization are the presence of confusion or any other depression of the level of consciousness at the time of examination, and clinical or radiologic evidence of a skull fracture. In these guidelines, brief amnesia following trauma, but with full recovery afterward, was not regarded by itself as sufficient indication for admission. Previously, a history or loss of consciousness or post-traumatic amnesia (PTA) of however short duration was often regarded as an indication for hospital admission. This change in guidelines for admission has meant a considerable reduction in the number of patients admitted without

**Table 17–1. GUIDELINES
FOR ADMISSION AFTER
HEAD INJURY**

1. Any depression of level of consciousness including confusion (GCS<15)
2. Signs of neurologic dysfunction
3. Evidence of skull fracture
4. Seizure, severe headache, recurrent vomiting
5. Assessment difficult—alcohol, drugs, age
6. Concomitant illness—diabetes, hemophilia, anticoagulants
7. Social concerns—young child, single elderly patient

Note: Brief loss of consciousness followed by full recovery is *not* an indication for admission. Patients who are discharged *must* have written instructions.

any evident increase in the complication rate in those patients allowed home without admission. In Edinburgh there were 1919 admissions for head injury in the year prior to the revision of the guidelines for admission. Following the introduction of the revised guidelines, annual head injury admissions fell successively to 1635, 1306, 1193, and 1158 cases. The reduction in head injury hospital admissions was entirely confined to minor head injuries.

Most patients admitted to the hospital with minor head injuries do not have any special features such as skull fracture, abnormal neurologic signs, cerebrospinal fluid (CSF) rhinorrhea, or multiple injuries. The problem is that along with this majority of patients there is an important minority who may be harboring a compound depressed skull fracture, a fracture of the base of skull with a cranionasal fistula, or other significant injuries.[3] The significance of these injuries is that they may be complicated by the development of infections in the craniospinal space—meningitis, or even an abscess, can cause further brain damage. The strategy for managing patients with minor head injury must include a system of diagnosis that will allow the clinician to identify in a cost-effective way the small number of patients with significant lesions in the brain or elsewhere from among the large number of patients who were hospitalized while slightly confused and who will go on to make an uncomplicated recovery, have a short hospital stay, and be free of residua thereafter.[4-6]

THE CONCEPT OF CONCUSSION

One of the continuing puzzles in head injury research is the pathophysiologic basis for the phenomenon of concussion, in which a patient becomes briefly unconscious after a blow to the head, recovers consciousness, and goes on to make an apparently full recovery. Loss of consciousness implies major interference with the functioning of the reticular activating system in the brainstem.[7] Other features of concussion that also suggest brainstem dysfunction include changes in blood pressure, heart rate, peripheral circulation, and respiration. Although most patients make an apparently full recovery, careful screening of the patients now reveals that as many as one third of them have post-traumatic symptoms and signs that may last for 3 months or longer and may prevent return to work or full activity for at least that period of time. Whereas some of these patients have a pre-injury background of neurotic problems and no detectable postinjury neurologic deficit, an equal number of patients have persistent signs of minor neurologic dysfunction if they are searched for assiduously. Examples are finger and hand incoordination or vestibular dysfunction shown on oculonystagmography.

Because minor injuries do not ordinarily result in death, there is virtually no supportive pathologic evidence to indicate the precise loci and nature of brain damage associated with the syndrome of concussion. Indeed, it is possible that the entire phenomenon may be based on dysfunction rather than on observable pathologic damage. Its rapidly reversible state suggests transient physiologic or biochemical dysfunction, possibly of neurotransmitter release or uptake, but in the absence of real proof this view is essentially speculative.

An approach to this problem has been to study animal models of concussive head injury of graded and repeatable severity. There are major drawbacks in comparing function and dysfunction in animal and human nervous systems. Differences in the relative proportions of fore and hind brain and in the relationships among the brain, the surrounding skull, and the dural infoldings greatly limit the analogy between "concussive" injury in an animal and the same phenomenon in a human.[8] It is, however, possible to define a stereotyped physiologic response to experimental concussive injury that has been common to all species studied so far, ranging from the mouse to the subhuman primate. This response consists of rapid but transient elevation of blood pressure; irregular respiration or even apnea, the duration of which is related to the severity of injury; and a decrease in electroencephalographic activity, the duration of which is also a function of the severity of injury.[9] Intracranial pressure is transiently elevated, the height and duration of the increase being loosely related to the severity of injury. Following these immediate changes there is dysfunction of the cerebrovascular system such that the normal regulatory responses of the cerebral vessels to changes in arterial carbon dioxide and oxygen tension and in blood pressure are impaired or abolished.[10, 11]

Studies involving the use of intravascular tracer substances have shown temporary impairment of blood brain barrier dysfunction in vessels close to the midline raphe of the brainstem. Intravascular horseradish peroxidase can be observed leaking from the vessels and being taken up by astrocytes in the vicinity. Electron microscopic studies clearly show that the transport of intravascular tracer through the capillary wall is by the medium of vesicular transport rather than due to opening of tight interendothelial cell junctions.[12] The leakage phenomenon is only temporary. If the injection of intravascular tracer is delayed more than 2 hours from the time of injury, the tracer remains within the vascular system.

Other subtle changes are seen following minor concussive brain injuries in the experimental subject.[13] Diffusely scattered swellings of axons in the cerebral white matter can be seen, somewhat similar to the retraction balls observed by pathologists in cases of severe closed head injury that survived for some weeks after the time of injury. In the past it was considered that such retraction balls represented extrusion of axoplasm from the torn end of a divided axon. Recent elegant electron microscopic studies have shown that, in some cases at least, the localized axonal swelling occurs without division of the axon and appears to be due to a localized failure of axoplasmic transport, causing axoplasm to build up behind the zone of transport failure. Later studies of white matter neuropathology following minor concussive head injury and using metal impregnation techniques have shown diffusely scattered areas of axonal degeneration. However, it is not yet clear whether there is a continuous link between the observation of segmental failure of axonal transport and subsequent axonal degeneration.

The experimental neuropathologist has, therefore, been able to demonstrate both transient and permanent abnormalities in the brain following minor concussive head injury of a severity that is normally followed by evidently full functional recovery and normal behavior of the experimental animal. It is likely that such transient disturbances can explain the phenomenon of concussion with its temporary coma and rapid return of full consciousness, and the scattered permanent features may explain the residual subtle disturbances of function following minor head injury that include impairment of rapid mental data processing or rapid finger movement. There is almost certainly a spectrum of structural damage that extends from minor head injury in a continuum to cases classified by the clinician as moderate and severe head injury. There remains, however, a wide discrepancy between the profound neurologic dysfunction and the histologically observable changes associated with concussion. Hayes and his colleagues[14] have recently proposed that activation of a cholinergic neural system located in the rostral pons may represent the functional basis for the transient unconsciousness and behavioral suppression associated with concussion.

In ranking the severity of minor concussional head injuries in the human and in trying to assess how much long-term dysfunction is to be expected, one of the most useful yardsticks is the duration of PTA, measurement of which is unavailable in the experimental animal. Post-traumatic amnesia is the length of time from the point of injury until return of continuous memory.[15] Its duration is usually at least three times that of the period of observed loss of consciousness. An injury that is followed by a PTA of less than 1 hour is considered mild; early return to work with no sequelae is anticipated. When PTA is between 1 and 24 hours, the injury should be considered moderate in severity. Post-traumatic problems of headache, dizziness, incoordination, and some persisting abnormal neurologic signs are more frequent among patients in this category. When PTA is between 1 day and 1 week in length, the injury should be considered severe and the family warned that post-traumatic sequelae, with some degree of permanent disability, are to be anticipated. When PTA lasts more than 7 days, the injury is considered very severe and a full return of neuropsychologic function would be the exception rather than the rule.

In testing for the return of memory and thus the end of the period of PTA, the Galveston Orientation and Amnesia Test (GOAT) is useful.[16] The test formalizes the questions that may be asked of a patient to determine the degree of orientation and uses a scoring system in which 100 is a perfect score and 75 indicates emergence from PTA. The significance of the GOAT is that formal neuropsychologic testing is not feasible until the GOAT score exceeds 75.

Although PTA is a useful yardstick, it is by no means infallible; one major problem is that the older that patients are and the more severe any preinjury brain dysfunction was, the longer will be the PTA associated with a given severity of injury. It is largely because the majority of head injuries are in healthy young adults whose preinjury neuropsychologic function is normal, that the PTA is of such value.

EPIDEMIOLOGY OF MINOR HEAD INJURY

In Edinburgh all adult head injuries occurring within the city and all major head injuries occurring in southeastern Scotland are admitted to a single head and spinal injury unit staffed by neurosurgeons and neuroanesthetists that forms part of the regional department of Clinical Neurosciences.[6, 17] This 20-bed head injury unit is located in the principal accident hospital for the region.

In 1981 a total of 1919 head injured patients were admitted to the head injury unit.[6] Of these, 1616 injuries (85 percent) were considered to be minor, with a low mortality of 0.4 percent. Nevertheless, about 20 percent of these patients with mi-

nor head injury had other significant injuries and 10 percent had skull fractures. In 1982, the revised guidelines for hospital admission following head injury were implemented. While the adoption of this policy increased the number of skull radiographs being performed, it almost certainly resulted in a pronounced decline in the number of patients with minor head injury that were admitted to the hospital. In 1983, a law was enacted in the United Kingdom making it compulsory to wear a seatbelt if traveling in the front seat of a car. This change in United Kingdom law also produced a reduction in certain types of head injury, most notably combined craniofacial injuries. In 1986 the prospective survey of head injury admissions to our unit was repeated, to assess the cumulative influence of the changes in admission policy and in the seatbelt law. The total number of head injury admissions had fallen from 1919 in 1981 (of which 1616 or 85 percent were minor head injuries) to 1008 in 1986, of which 702 (70 percent) were considered minor cases. When the 1981 and 1986 figures were compared, the numbers of severe and moderate head injuries had remained constant: the reduction in total head injury admissions was entirely due to the pronounced fall in minor head injury admissions (Table 17–2). This strongly suggests that the change in head injury admission criteria had been extremely effective. We have not noted any increase in unexpected head injury deaths in hospital or out of hospital since adopting this revised head injury admission policy.

In both series of head injuries the average age of patients with severe, moderate, and minor injury was between 35 and 40 years.

Table 17–2. HEAD INJURY ADMISSIONS IN 1981 AND 1986*

Category	1981	1986
Severe (GCS 8 or less)	93 (5%)	113 (11%)
Moderate (GCS 9–12)	210 (11%)	193 (19%)
Minor (GCS 13–15)	1616 (84%)	702 (70%)
Total	1919 (100%)	1008 (100%)

*Before and after introduction of admission guidelines.

Table 17–3. SEVERITY OF HEAD INJURY IN ELDERLY AND YOUNGER PATIENTS

Category	65 Years and Over	Under 65 Years
Severe	26 (6%)	79 (5%)
Moderate	46 (10%)	168 (11%)
Minor	377 (84%)	1324 (84%)
Total	449 (100%)	1571 (100%)
Male:female ratio	55:45	73:27

Although the largest groups of patients are in the age groups 11 to 20 years old and 21 to 30 years old, there are a substantial number of patients with head injury over 65 years old.[18] Unlike head injuries in younger patients, of which 75 percent are males, elderly women and men are equally likely to sustain head injuries (Table 17–3). Almost 40 percent of the minor head injury patients over age 65 also had concurrent medical disorders, often undiagnosed and untreated.[19] We concluded that in head injured patients over age 65, even with the most minor of head injuries, chest radiograph, electrocardiograph (ECG), complete blood count and film, blood sugar, blood urea, and serum electrolytes should be measured in all cases.

The most common cause of minor head injury is a domestic accident or fall, accounting for 40 percent of cases. The next most common cause is road traffic accidents, and in patients with minor injury— particularly the elderly—pedestrian acci-

Table 17–4. CAUSES OF MINOR HEAD INJURY IN ELDERLY AND IN YOUNGER PATIENTS

Cause of Injury	65 Years and Over (n = 377)	Under 65 Years (n = 1324)
Domestic/fall	77%	34%
RTA–vehicle occupant	5%	20%
RTA–pedestrian	12%	8%
Assault	4%	26%
Sport/work	0	12%

RTA = road traffic accident.

dents are by far the most common.[20] Assaults (20 percent) are the next most frequent cause with injuries at work or during sport accounting for 5 percent or less of minor head injuries (Table 17–4).

SKULL FRACTURES

In 1981 the overall incidence of skull fracture in patients admitted following head injury was 14 percent, whereas in 1986 this proportion had risen to 24 percent. This difference in the incidence of skull fracture is accounted for by the change in admission policy which favored discharge from the accident and emergency department without admission to hospital of patients who were alert and oriented and who did not have a skull fracture—even if such patients had been briefly unconscious after a minor head injury. The actual numbers of patients with skull fractures were similar in the two 1-year cohorts, 272 in 1981 and 246 in 1986. The incidence of skull fracture was highest in patients with severe head injury, 53 percent and 47 percent in 1981 and 1986, respectively; in moderate head injury the incidence was 28 percent and 36 percent, respectively, while in patients with minor head injury the incidence of skull fracture was 8 percent and 14 percent, respectively, for 1981 and 1986. This applied only to linear skull fractures, the position with depressed skull fracture being quite different; most patients with depressed skull fracture had suffered a minor head injury as defined on the Glasgow Coma Scale.[21] In 1981, 28 of 39 patients with depressed skull fracture (72 percent) had sustained a minor head injury, while in 1986 the equivalent figures were 16 of 22 patients (73 percent).

Intracranial hematomas are common in patients with severe head injury (30 to 50 percent), less common in moderate head injury (5 to 10 percent), and rare in minor head injury (less than 1 percent). It is, however, of equal importance to detect the hematoma in all cases, so that avoidable brain damage can be averted. There is an important association between the presence of skull fracture of any type and the presence of an intracranial hematoma.[17, 22] This association is not apparent in patients with severe head injury, because intracranial hematoma is so common in all categories of severely

**Table 17–5. SKULL FRACTURE VERSUS
INTRACRANIAL HEMATOMA**

Category of Injury	Hematoma	No Hematoma	Total
Severe			
Skull fracture	27 (49%)	28	55
No fracture	15 (39%)	23	38
$\chi^2 = 0.84$; NS	42 (45%)	51	93
Moderate			
Skull fracture	15 (30%)	48	63
No fracture	4 (3%)	143	147
$\chi^2 = 23.83$; p<0.001	19 (9%)	191	210
Minor			
Skull fracture	6 (4%)	148	154
No fracture	4 (0.3%)	1458	1462
$\chi^2 = 29.73$; p<0.001	10 (0.6%)	1606	1616

NS = not significant.

head injured patients. However, in patients with moderate and minor head injury the presence of a skull fracture significantly increases the risk of intracranial hematoma being present. Thus, in 1981 4 percent of patients with minor head injury who had a skull fracture had an intracranial hematoma, whereas only 0.3 percent of patients with minor head injury who had no skull fracture had an intracranial hematoma. In 1986 the equivalent percentages were 11 percent of patients with skull fractures and only 1.4 percent of patients without skull fracture (Table 17–5).

Alcohol is a common confounding factor in the assessment of patients with head injury, particularly minor head injury. More than one third of patients admitted to the head injury unit in 1981 had consumed alcohol shortly before the head injury; for minor head injuries, the proportion overall was 37 percent. In 1986, the figures were very similar, in that 39 percent of the 702 patients with minor head injury had consumed alcohol, often in large quantities, shortly before the head injury. Males are two to four times more likely than females to have consumed alcohol prior to head injury.

MULTIPLE INJURIES

A considerable proportion of all patients with head injury, whatever the severity, have injuries elsewhere in the body of sufficient severity to warrant intervention by other specialists. These injuries may significantly influence the need for, and the form of, rehabilitation measures. In 1981, 55 percent of the 93 severely head injured patients and 26 percent of the 210 moderately head injured patients had multiple injuries, whereas 372 (23 percent) of the 1616 patients with minor head injury had multiple injuries. In 1986 the proportions of patients with multiple injury were even higher, at 65 percent of patients with severe head injury, 44 percent of patients with moderate head injury, and 41 percent of those with minor head injury. Thus, the prognosis and rehabilitation needs of a person with a minor head injury may be heavily influenced by the presence of other accompanying injuries. The most common associated injuries are to the face and facial skeleton, followed by limb injuries, injuries to the trunk, and spinal injuries.

CT SCANNING

When CT scanning first became available for patients with head injury, its immediate impact and benefit was in the rapid diagnosis of intracranial hematomas requiring urgent surgical decompression, mostly in patients with severe head injury. With increasing experience and progressively widening application of CT scanning in head injury, it was soon recognized that sequential CT studies in severely head injured patients would provide an index of prognosis. CT scanning of selected patients with moderate

Table 17–6. CT SCANS AND EXTRADURAL HEMATOMAS (EDH) TREATED IN 1981 AND 1986

Category of Injury	1981					1986				
	CT (%)	EDH Found (op)	G/M	S/V	D	CT (%)	EDH Found (op)	G/M	S/V	D
			Outcome					*Outcome*		
Severe	72 (77%)	10 (10)	4	4	2	99 (88%)	7 (7)	4	2	1
Moderate	57 (27%)	5 (3)	3	1	1	112 (58%)	6 (6)	6	0	0
Minor	52 (3%)	2 (1)	2	0	0	115 (16%)	8 (5)	7	0	1*
Total	181 (10%)	17 (14)	9 (53%)	5 (29%)	3 (18%)	326 (32%)	21 (18)	17 (81%)	2 (9%)	2 (9%)

*Posterior fossa hematoma; patient GCS 15 on admission.
Op = operated.
G = good recovery.
S = severe disability.
M = moderate disability.
V = vegetative.
D = dead.

and minor head injuries would often reveal parenchymal lesions that explained prolonged confusion or focal neurologic abnormalities in these patients.

In 1981 more than three quarters of the 93 severely head injured patients admitted to our unit had at least one CT scan, but only 8 percent of moderately head injured patients and 3 percent of those with minor head injuries were submitted to CT scanning, and this was usually because of subsequent neurologic deterioration. By 1986 the proportion of patients in all of these categories subjected to CT scanning had risen significantly, to 88 percent of severely head injured patients, 58 percent of moderately head injured patients, and 16 percent of those with minor head injuries. It has been our experience and that of others that the increase in the numbers of patients with minor head injury subjected to CT scanning has increased the proportion of extradural hematomas detected in patients still in a good neurologic state (Table 17–6). A number of asymptomatic intracranial hematomas have also been detected—that is, intracranial hematomas unassociated with neurologic deterioration.

Magnetic resonance imaging, even more recently available, has already shown lesions in patients with head injury in whom CT scan has been entirely normal.[23] There appears to be a better correlation between subtle neuropsychologic deficit and abnormalities on MRI than between the neuropsychologic evaluation and the results of CT.

MINOR HEAD INJURIES IN THE ELDERLY

The majority of patients admitted to hospital after head injuries are young and male, and the characteristics of these patients tend to predominate in most published reviews of head injury. Patients over 65 years old do, however, constitute a considerable proportion of all head injured patients and present some particular problems. Patients over 65 years old constituted 15 percent of the total number of 1919 head injury admissions in 1981 and 16 percent of the 1008 admissions in 1986. These proportions are the same if only minor head injuries are considered. The major difference between elderly patients with head injury and younger patients is that in the elderly population the same number of women and men are admitted. In southeastern Scotland alcohol is just as great a problem in elderly head injured patients as in younger patients. Moreover, in the elderly, concomitant medical disorders and social problems related to capacity to cope when living alone tend to feature much more prominently than in head injuries in younger patients. Six weeks after a minor head injury, more than 40 percent of elderly patients were significantly less mobile and one in six of those who had lived in their own home prior to injury were unable to return.[20]

MANAGEMENT AND OUTCOME IN PATIENTS WITH MINOR HEAD INJURY

The first stage in management of these patients is an assessment of the risk of intracranial hematoma or other severe complications. The other part of the assessment relates to the presence of concomitant medical disorders or domestic circumstances, including the presence of dementia, which might make the observation period following head injury impossible in the patient's own home. Patients admitted to hospital are observed for signs of a depressed level of consciousness and/or the development of abnormal neurologic signs, signs of intracranial infection, or the development of any concomitant medical problems such as cardiac arrhythmia, respiratory disturbance, or metabolic disorder. In our practice, patients with minor head injury who require admission, according to the accident and emergency department, will have a full neurologic examination. Then they will begin to undergo sequential neurologic nursing observation, including scoring on the Glasgow Coma Scale (GCS), pupil size and response to light, and comparison of motor power on the left and right sides of the body. If the GCS has not returned to a score of 15 after 24 hours, or if there are persisting abnormal neurologic signs, we arrange for CT scanning. This is done earlier, soon after admission, if these signs occur in the presence of a skull fracture. This is because the presence of a skull fracture raises severalfold the chance of there being an intracranial hematoma. If there are persisting mental or medical problems in elderly patients, a geriatric medical consultation is requested and a simple battery of medical investigations is arranged, including chest radiograph and ECG, hemoglobin and blood count, urea and electrolytes, and blood and urinary sugar and protein levels. The majority of patients with minor head injury make a rapid recovery and can soon be discharged from the hospital. In 1981, 74 percent of patients with minor head injury admitted to our unit were discharged within 1 day, and a further

20 percent returned home within a week of the time of injury; 5 percent remained hospitalized for periods ranging from 1 week to 1 month, and 1 percent were in the hospital for more than 1 month. In 1986, following the change in admission policy for patients with minor head injuries, there was a considerable reduction in the proportion of these patients who were admitted for periods of 24 hours or less, from 74 percent down to 16 percent. Admission for periods of 2 to 7 days was the practice in 76 percent of the patients with minor head injuries who were admitted, while for patients hospitalized between 1 week and 1 month the figure was 6 percent, and for more than 1 month 1 percent. In both of these cohorts of patients, admission periods of 1 month or longer were nearly always because of the presence of pre-existing dementia and difficulties with placement of the patient.

The duration of hospital stay provides only an incomplete picture of the degree of recovery from a minor head injury. In 1981 Rimel and her colleagues[1] reported that one third of patients with minor head injuries had still not been able to return to their previous level of work or student activity 3 months after the injury. In patients with moderate head injury (GCS 9 to 12) the proportion of patients not back at their former level of activity at 3 months was over 60 percent.[24] In the Edinburgh studies 3 percent of patients with minor head injury were still considered to be severely disabled 1 month after the injury [1981 study[6]] while in 1986 2 percent of patients with minor head injury were considered to be severely disabled at 1 month (unpublished study).

In some cases, disability persisting 1 month or more after a minor head injury is related to concomitant injuries elsewhere in the body, or to pre-existing medical or psychobehavioral problems. However, in most cases, particularly in young patients, the cause of the disability is related to the head injury itself and often can be associated with a demonstrable structural or functional disorder of the brain resulting from head injury.[25] There appears to be a spectrum of post-traumatic disorders ranging from deficits clearly visible in virtually all severely head injured patients to a relatively low rate of persisting obvious deficit in patients with minor head injury. Nevertheless, it is true that the more assiduously neurologic or psychologic abnormalities are sought, the more frequently they are found in head injured patients of all grades of severity.[26] The main complaints of those who have sustained minor head injury are headache and dizziness, as well as neurologic problems such as diplopia, tinnitus and deafness, and loss of balance and stability.[27, 28] Psychologic problems include memory loss, particularly for recent events, and slowing down of the capacity to verbally process information or to make a motor response.[29–36] Impaired or inappropriate emotional responses and psychiatric disturbance may also follow minor head injury.[37, 38] In patients with minor head injury more persisting symptoms tend to be aggregated under the broad heading of postconcussional syndrome.

Postconcussional Syndrome

This term appears to be a label for a large number of diverse symptoms that include headache, dizziness or feelings of light headedness and instability, tinnitus, deafness, irritability and difficulty of controlling anger or sadness, loss of sexual interest, difficulty with sleeping, ease of tiring, impairment of memory, short attention span, and episodes of depression and of uncontrolled rage.[39] The mix of such symptoms varies from patient to patient as does the relative severity of the various elements of this disorder (Table 17–7).

Over the years opinions concerning the basis of the postconcussional syndrome have ranged between two extremes. In one view these patients are malingering, simulating a disorder for reasons of personal gain associated with litigation following the accident that caused the head injury.[40, 41] In the other view every one of the symptoms is organic in origin, related to minor but persisting disorders. Vasomotor control malfunction is responsible for headaches and other paroxysmal disturbances; auditory-vestibular dysfunction accounts for tinnitus and dizziness; and disorders of the medial temporal structures and brainstem connections cause difficulties with sleep pattern, memory, attention, and concentration.[42–44]

Taylor and Bell[45] demonstrated abnormalities of cerebral blood flow velocity in a number of survivors of minor head injuries and strongly advanced the organic theory as the basis for the postconcussional syndrome. Henry Miller,[40] on the other hand, was an eloquent proposer of the behavioral theory. Perhaps the most reasonable compromise has been that proposed by Cartlidge and Shaw,[46] who examined a large number of patients with postconcussional syndrome. They performed detailed tests of brainstem function such as oculonystagmography and at the same time took a careful history of any preinjury behavioral abnormality, such as frequent visits to the doctor with diagnoses of a nonorganic nature.[46]

In essence, Cartlidge and Shaw were able to divide patients with postconcussional syndrome into two equally sized groups. The first was a predominantly organic group in whom the symptoms had begun soon after injury and persisted for many months. In these patients there were subtle neurologic changes indicative of persisting dysfunction many weeks after the injury. In virtually all of these cases the symptoms had subsided more or less completely within 1 year after the injury. In the second group of patients objective signs of neurologic dysfunction

Table 17–7. SYMPTOMS AFTER MILD HEAD INJURY
(GCS 13–15)

Symptom	Discharge (n = 847)	3 Months (n = 542)	6 Months (n = 485)	12 Months (n = 301)
Headache	46%	41%	30%	29%
Dizziness	14%	25%	14%	13%
Amnesia	13%	23%	17%	21%
Weakness	10%	15%	8%	8%
Diplopia	5%	9%	4%	6%
Tinnitus	2%	13%	9%	10%
Deafness	2%	11%	9%	7%

From Alves et al.,[27] with permission.

were usually lacking. There was a strong history of frequent minor illnesses and visits to the family doctor prior to the head injury. The postconcussional symptoms tended to begin only after an interval and frequently persisted for periods beyond 1 year from the time of injury. In these cases it was believed that the postconcussional syndrome was part of a broader syndrome of illness behavior that the patient had adopted as a response to the injury and to the events thereafter, which frequently included impending litigation.

This division may be an oversimplification of the problem, however. Many patients who have persisting symptoms following a minor head injury are puzzled and frightened by the symptoms, even fearful that they may be going mad because they have been told by medical advisors that the injury was trivial and full recovery is to be expected. A sympathetic explanation to such patients may reduce the subsequent incidence of postconcussional symptoms or their impact on the patient's lifestyle.[47, 48]

DISCHARGE AND FOLLOW-UP

Prior to discharge a full neurological examination should be carried out, including tests of balance and gait. The patient should be rechecked for any other undetected injuries—for example, a fracture of the odontoid process of the axis or ligamentous instability of the spine or limb joints. If patients have a fracture of the skull base it is good practice to repeat the skull radiograph with a brow-up lateral view prior to discharge in case there is an accumulating aerocele, and to obtain flexion and extension views of the cervical spine if the patient has any persisting complaint referable to the neck.

The social and domestic circumstances of the patient should be established before discharge to home, to family members, or to an institution, to ensure that the patient, particularly the elderly, will be able to cope satisfactorily. The patient and a relative or close friend must be given easy and rapid means of re-establishing contact with the hospital.

Follow-up, ideally at a head injury clinic, should occur within 2 weeks of discharge, to be repeated at 6 weeks and again only if indicated. At the follow-up visit, the duration of PTA can be established, providing a retrospective index of the severity of the brain disturbance that followed the injury. Any symptoms suggestive of development of a chronic subdural hematoma should be asked about, as well as symptoms suggesting development of postconcussional syndrome. In examining the patient, olfactory sensation should be tested. Anosmia follows more than 5 percent of head injuries, mainly those involving frontal or occipital impact.[49] Finally, an assessment of the patient's functional or disability status should be made.[50–52]

It is recognized that these recommended practices are all in some way a counsel of perfection, but if they were widely adopted and the patient with a minor head injury had easy access to sympathetic and informed advice and supervision, much anxiety and morbidity might be avoided and other problems considerably reduced.

This approach to the sequelae of minor head injury is more likely to be successful than drug therapy. However, antidepressants have been proposed for certain persistant and appropriate postconcussional symptoms.[35] More often, symptomatic drug treatment is applied on an entirely empirical basis, patients often receiving combinations of analgesics, tranquilizers, anxiolytics, and sedatives at night. Frequently, however, this treatment only adds to the patient's problems. As a corollary to the cholinergic hypothesis of brain dysfunction following minor or moderate head injury, Hayes and his associates[14] have proposed that anticholinergic agents, started as soon as possible after injury, may mitigate or prevent some of the unwanted sequelae of injury. Experimental evidence is cited in support of this proposal but the outcome of clinical trials is awaited.

CONCLUSION

Minor head injury poses a very slight threat to life, and most patients remain in the hospital only for a day or two. Nevertheless, a third or more of them suffer prolonged post-traumatic sequelae and many have measureable neuropsychologic deficits. Few of these patients receive the benefit of advice and treatment from rehabilitation teams. It is likely that much benefit could be obtained if more of them had access to such advice and help.

REFERENCES

1. Rimel, RW et al: Disability caused by minor head injury. Neurosurgery 9:221, 1981.
2. Jennet, B et al: Guidelines for initial management after head injury in adults. Br Med J 288:983, 1984.
3. Dacey, RG et al: Neurosurgical complications after apparently minor head injuries. J Neurosurg 65:203, 1986.
4. Kalsbeek, WD et al: The National Head and Spinal Cord Injury Survey: Major findings. J Neurosurg 53 (Suppl):S19, 1980.
5. Mendelow, AD et al: Admission after mild head injury: benefits and costs. Br Med J 285:1530, 1982.
6. Miller, JD and Jones, PA: The work of a regional head injury service. Lancet 1:1141, 1985.
7. Symonds, C: Concussion and its sequelae. Lancet 1:1, 1962.
8. Denny-Brown, D and Russell, WR: Experimental cerebral concussion. Brain 64:93, 1941.
9. Millen, JE, Glauser, FL and Zimmerman, M: Physiological effects of controlled concussive brain tumour. J Appl Physiol 49:856, 1980.
10. Lewelt, W, Jenkins, LW and Miller, JD: Autoregulation of cerebral blood flow after experimental fluid percussion injury of the brain. J Neurosurg 53:500, 1980.
11. Lewelt, W, Jenkins, LW and Miller, JD: Effects of experimental fluid percussion injury of the brain on cerebrovascular reactivity to hypoxia and hypercapnia. J Neurosurg 56:332, 1982.
12. Povlishock, JT et al: Vascular permeability alterations to horseradish peroxidase in experimental brain injury. Brain Res 153:223, 1978.
13. Povlishock, JT et al: Axonal change in minor head injury. J Neuropathol Exp Neurol 43:225, 1983.
14. Hayes, RL et al: Metabolic and neurophysiologic sequelae of brain injury. A Cholinergic hypothesis. J Cent Nerv Syst Trauma 3(2):163, 1986.
15. Russell, WR and Smith, A: Post-traumatic amnesia in closed head injury. Arch Neurol 5:16, 1961.
16. Levin, HS, O'Donnell, VM and Grossman, RG: The Galveston orientation and amnesia test: A practical scale to assess cognition after head injury. J Nerv Ment Dis 167:675, 1979.
17. Miller, JD: Minor, moderate, and severe head injury. Neurosurg Rev 9:135, 1986.
18. Pentland, B et al: Head injury in the elderly. Age and Aging 15:193, 1986.
19. Roy, CW, Pentland, B and Miller, JD: The causes and consequences of minor head injury in the elderly. Injury 17:220, 1986.
20. Wilson, JA et al: The functional effects of head injury in the elderly. Brain Injury 1:183, 1987.
21. Miller, JD and Jennett, B: Complications of depressed skull fractures. Lancet 2:991, 1968.
22. Mendelow, AD et al: Risks of intracranial haematoma in head injured adults. Br Med J 287:1173, 1983.
23. Levin, HS et al: Magnetic resonance imaging and computerised tomography in relation to the neurobehavioral sequelae of mild and moderate head injuries. J Neurosurg 66:706, 1987.
24. Rimel, RW et al: Moderate head injury: completing the clinical spectrum of brain trauma. Neurosurgery 11:344, 1982.
25. Levin, HS, Benton, AL and Grossman, RG. Neurobehavioural Consequences of Closed Head Injury. Oxford University Press, 1982.
26. Levin, HS et al: Neurobehavioural outcome following minor head injury—a three center study. J Neurosurg 66:234, 1987.
27. Alves, WM et al: Understanding post traumatic symptoms after minor head injury. J Head Trauma Rehabil 1:1, 1986.
28. Colohan, ART et al: Neurologic and neurosurgical implications of mild head injury. J Head Trauma Rehabil 1:13, 1986.
29. McLean, A et al: Psychological functioning at 1 month after head injury. Neurosurgery 14:393, 1984.
30. Gronwall, D and Wrightson, P: Delayed recovery of intellectual function after minor head injury. Lancet 2:605, 1974.
31. Gronwall, D and Wrightson, P: Memory and information processing capacity after closed head injury. J Neurol Neurosurg Psychiatry 44:889, 1981.
32. McMillan, TM and Glucksman, EE: The neuropsychology of moderate head injury. J Neurol Neurosurg Psychiatry 50:393, 1987.
33. MacFlynn, G et al: Measurement of reaction time following minor head injury. J Neurol Neurosurg Psychiatry 47:1326, 1984.
34. Rutherford, WH, Merrett, JD and McDonald, JR: Sequelae of concussion caused by minor head injuries. Lancet 1:104, 1977.
35. Rutherford, WH, Merrett, JR and McDonald, JR: Symptoms at one year following concussion from minor head injuries. Injury 10:225, 1979.
36. Barth, JT et al: Neuropsychological sequelae of minor head injury. Neurosurgery 13:529, 1983.
37. Dikmen, S and Reitan, RM: Emotional sequelae of head injury. Ann Neurol 2:492, 1977.
38. Lishman, WA: The psychiatric sequelae of head injury—a review. Psychol Med 3:304, 1973.
39. Cook, JB: The post concussional syndrome and factors influencing recovery after minor head injury admitted to hospital. Scand J Rehabil Med 4:27, 1972.
40. Miller, H: Accident neurosis. Br Med J 1:919, 992, 1961.
41. Miller, H and Cartlidge, N: Simulation and malingering after injuries to the brain and spinal cord. Lancet 1:580, 1972.
42. Taylor, AR: Post-concussional sequelae. Br Med J 3:67, 1967.
43. Rowe, MJ and Carlson, C: Brain stem auditory evoked potentials in post concussion dizziness. Arch Neurol 37:679, 1980.
44. Bergmasco, BP et al: Brain stem auditory evoked potentials in post concussional syndrome. Int J Neurol Sci 4:281, 1982.
45. Taylor, AR and Bell, TK: Slowing of cerebral circulation after concussional head injury. Lancet 2:178, 1966.
46. Cartlidge, NEF and Shaw, DA: Head Injury. WB Saunders, London, 1981.
47. Relander, M, Troup, H and Bjorkesten, G: Controlled trial of treatment for cerebral concussion. Br Med J 4:777, 1972.

48. Bremner, DN, Gillingham, FJ. Patterns of convalescence after minor head injury. J Roy Coll Surg Edinburgh 19:94, 1974.

49. Miller, JD: Head injury. In Miller, JD (ed): Northfield's Surgery of the Central Nervous System. Blackwell Scientific Publications, Edinburgh and Oxford, 1987, p 795.

50. Mahoney, F and Barthel, DW: Functional assessment: the Barthel index. MD State Med J 14:61, 1965.

51. Livingston, MG and Livingstone, HM: The Glasgow assessment schedule. Clinical and research assessment of head injury outcome. Int Rehabil Med 7:145, 1985.

52. Affleck, JW et al: Rehabilitation status: A measure of medico-social dysfunction. Lancet 1:230, 1988.

Section III
Conclusion

MICHAEL R. BOND, M.D., Ph.D.

This section deals with both minor and major head injuries, the greater part of the contents being concerned with the latter. Nevertheless, it should be remembered that patients who sustain relatively trivial injuries account for up to 85 percent of all head injury hospital admissions and of these 15 to 20 percent are elderly. Also, multiple injuries in association with minor head injury are more common than might be thought, with 20 to 40 percent of patients being involved. Despite the apparent mildness of injury to the head, structural brain damage does occur in a significant proportion of patients, accounting for some of the hitherto unexplained cognitive and behavioral changes following minor injuries.

The consequences of all brain injuries may be grouped into those that are physical, cognitive, and emotional and behavioral, and the resultant secondary effects that take place within the family system.

In order to provide the reader with an understanding of the scientific basis of recovery of functions within the nervous system, the author of the first chapter in this section discusses a range of possible mechanisms by which this process may occur at the cellular level, though the exact intrinsic mechanisms involved are not fully understood. Similarly, the way in which variations in recovery at a cellular level and responses to environmental influences occur is uncertain. Nevertheless, there are implications for pharmacologic, physical, and psychologic therapies that might influence the processes described. In fact, the problem of epilepsy described in Chapter 7 underlines not only the relationship of this problem to the nature and extent of injury but also provides a useful model for examining the influence of various drugs on this particular malfunction of the central nervous system. Other neurologic deficits vary from the highly specific effects on cranial nerves, among which the first and third are most often damaged, to abnormalities of peripheral nerves and such problems as changes in cerebrospinal fluid (CSF) production and circulation. Often cranial nerves do not recover from injury and rehabilitation has to focus on devising compensatory or substitution strategies to overcome patients' difficulties. Peripheral nerve injuries do recover, however, though not completely in some cases. Regarding CSF circulation, the late complication of post-traumatic hydrocephalus is amenable to surgical treatment.

Medical and orthopedic complications are commonly associated with head injury. They should be detected early and usually can be dealt with quite effectively. However, sometimes there are difficulties in making diagnoses in patients who are unconscious or in states of altered consciousness, and the chief aid to detection here is awareness of the possibilities and vigilance on the part of the clinician. The later physical complications of hypertonicity and movement disorders form well-defined syndromes, which every clinician working in rehabilitation should recognize. They vary widely both in type and in the extent to which spontaneous recovery occurs. The clinician should be aware of the wide range of pharmacologic, nonsurgical, and surgical techniques available for their relief or amelioration, and these issues are discussed extensively in Chapter 10.

Disorders of communication involving

speech and a wide range of cognitive functions represent a major handicap, which frequently slows the process of recovery. Communication is a vital skill needed by patients in a range of rehabilitative processes and the therapist should remember that attention must be paid to environmental factors and that account must be taken of emotional lability, if present. Cognitive deficits, such as disturbances of memory, interfere with communication and so with rehabilitation.

The range of cognitive deficits following severe brain injury is well understood and has been extremely well documented over the years, as described in Chapter 12. One of the main points made by the author is that considerable variation exists in terms of recovery and eventual optimal functioning between different aspects of cognition. Moreover, the point is made that cognitive performance on tests in the laboratory does not necessarily match problem-solving behavior in everyday life. Cognitive functions may be influenced by a variety of factors including the injured person's degree of motivation and mood. For example, depression is not uncommon among brain injured patients and may influence cognitive performance negatively to a profound extent.

Turning to other aspects of the mental consequences of severe brain injury, Chapter 13 outlines issues arising from studies of behavioral disorders, which are of particular significance because the various forms provide some of the most difficult problems to be handled by both clinicians and family members. In fact, of all the deficits that may occur, behavioral problems provoke the greatest stress among families. Until recently, little attempt had been made to place emotional and behavioral disturbances in the context of a formal diagnostic framework. However, this can be achieved by using the criteria for organic mental disorders as defined in the revised version of the third edition of the Diagnostic and Statistical Manual of Mental Disorders of the American Psychiatric Association (DSM-III-R). Small additions have been made to the classification in order to accommodate all the major forms of post-traumatic behavioral and emotional disorders, and it is hoped that clinicians will use this system to ensure greater accuracy in allocating patients to appropriate diagnostic categories.

Disturbance of sexual life for patients following head injury is an important subject. Chapter 15 makes it clear that these disturbances may be primary—that is, related to endocrine abnormalities or damage to the autonomic nervous system—or that they may be secondary to emotional and personality change. The management of the injured person is a very sensitive matter in which attention must be paid to the patient's level of sexual development, his or her civil status, and the feelings and attitudes of partner or spouse. Expertise in this area is developing, and the authors of the chapter describe the blend of physical, pharmacologic, and psychologic techniques that may be required on the basis of a team approach to deal with the complexities of this difficult issue.

Chapter 16 reveals how great a burden is imposed upon the caretakers of the severely brain injured person. In fact, about one third of those caring for the severely injured show evidence of a psychiatric disorder, usually anxiety or depression, during the first postinjury year. Long-term studies in Scotland and Denmark show that levels of stress are maintained year after year among many relatives and that the chief cause lies in the behavioral problems of the brain injured person and the high levels of dependency shown by many. A whole range of methods of relief should be available for relatives, but for many, little support is accessible. The development of the National Head Injury Foundation in the United States, Headway in Britain, and various self-help groups in other countries within the past decade represents a response to this need, which clinicians should seek to support fully.

Chapter 17, dealing with minor head injuries, is new to the book. The problems posed by patients having minor injuries are different in nature, as well as in degree, from those of the severely injured, and they require different management. One of the needs is for counseling at an early stage if neurotic reactions to the relatively trivial physical and cognitive effects of the injury are to be prevented. For example, a significant proportion of young patients with minor head injuries do not return to work as quickly as might be expected, though extensive testing of cognitive deficits that do occur reveals that most have disappeared within a month of injury. This links with other findings that show that the early development of headache, dizziness, and irritability, sometimes known as the post-traumatic syndrome, may well disappear quite quickly. When such symptoms arise at a later stage in recovery and after any neurologic and psychologic signs of damage have cleared, it can be understood that a purely psychologic reaction has occurred to which will be added increasingly elements of abnormal sickness behavior lasting, perhaps, for many months.

To conclude, Section III underlines the range of physical, mental, and behavioral/social problems that occur after head injuries of varying severity. The main tasks for those involved in rehabilitation are two: first, they should be alert to all the possible consequences of brain injury and methods for managing them, and second, they should endeavor to determine which of the methods of rehabilitation they use are most effective—preferably by using appropriate scientifically designed studies.

SECTION IV

SPECIALIZED METHODS OF ASSESSMENT

J. Douglas Miller, M.D., Ph.D., Editor

Chapter 18

Physiatric Assessment for Rehabilitation

D. NATHAN COPE, M.D.

Traumatic brain injury (TBI) is a major disorder in terms of incidence, disability, and cost. It also is a condition that every rehabilitation physician can expect to see often during his or her practice. The physiatrist needs to have a basic understanding of the significant factors involved in recovery from and treatment of TBI. The physiatric assessment is usually the initial point at which a traumatically brain injured patient begins interacting with the rehabilitation system. The physiatrist has the responsibility to develop and oversee all of the varied needs of the brain injured patient. The results of the physiatric evaluation should logically lead to proper decisions regarding development of this comprehensive treatment.

Few areas of rehabilitation medicine present as much difficulty in assessment as the brain injured patient. The TBI patient is often unable to fully cooperate with the assessment process. Successive TBI patients will present in such widely differing states and with such varying syndromes that the practitioner with marginal experience in TBI may feel significant confusion, uncertainty, and frustration when evaluating these patients. It may be felt that early assessment in particular is less important since the severity and course of the TBI patient, and hence the ultimate specific needs for rehabilitation, will usually declare themselves with time anyway. However, reluctance to assess the status and treatment needs of the acutely injured TBI patient at an early stage may lead to delay or denial of appropriate treatment with demonstrated morbidity.[1]

It is the intention in this chapter to provide a general conceptual framework for assessment by which the physiatrist may place the multiple problems of the TBI patient in perspective, and which will assist in the development of an overall treatment approach.

ROLE OF THE PHYSIATRIST IN EVALUATION

The physiatrist plays a central role in the rehabilitation assessment of the TBI patient, acting as a bridge of knowledge across those acute medical and surgical concerns that are properly the initial focus of care after severe brain trauma to the later physical, behavioral, and social problems that may follow severe head injury. It is possible to differentiate those conditions that preclude initiation of comprehensive rehabilitation from those that may be adequately managed medically in a non–intensive care rehabilitation environment. Without necessarily being expert in all areas of the rehabilitation care of the TBI patient (for example, the neuropsychologic or the vocational), the physiatrist nevertheless should have an extremely broad grasp of the potential of each rehabilitation specialty to contribute to the overall treatment program and recovery of the patient. At the conclusion of the assessment the physiatrist should also be able to formulate and initiate a general plan and timeframe for appropriate rehabilitation interventions by this wide range of disciplines which will lead to optimum comprehensive care and outcome. The physiatrist also plays a major role in the decision algorithm regarding acceptance or nonacceptance into an acute rehabilitation program, the most common destination for the severely injured surviving patient. Finally, the physiatrist usually is the rehabilitation specialist who is called to the treatment scene soonest after injury, and therefore can prevent delays in initiating treatment and the complications such delays may create.

PURPOSE OF THE EVALUATION

The information gained from the evaluation should be sufficient to allow decisions regarding the individual and specific needs and treatments for each patient. These should be based on as accurate a prediction as possible of the outcome of the patient's illness. While performing each evaluation it is most effective to keep in mind the realm of feasible treatment alternatives. The large number of specific problems that each TBI patient presents to the clinician, and their complexity, makes it impractical to obtain a definitive assessment of each during the initial examination. The physiatrist will direct most attention to relevant problems. These issues will vary from case to case and even in the same patient at different stages in the recovery process. For example, an evaluation performed in the surgical intensive care unit upon a newly injured and semiresponsive patient will focus upon joint, skin, and bladder management; initial family contact; and whether or not the patient is ready for a move to a higher level of care. Exact characterization of motor control or neuropsychologic deficits is not usually feasible or crucial at this stage. On the other hand, for the patient first seen some years after injury, focus needs to be on neuropsychologic, social, and vocational function; mobility issues are likely to be less important and will not change.

Although these examples seem self-evident, one of the major problems the inexperienced physician tends to encounter in evaluating the TBI patient is that of being overwhelmed by the multiplicity of problems that are present and by the lack of specificity of many of the deficits. By addressing these problems in an unstructured

manner the clinician risks attending only to those with which he or she is most comfortable, or which are simply the most self-evident, or those which the patient identifies as most troublesome. Each of these approaches will fail to identify problems that ought to be addressed.

Acquiring sufficient experience with the TBI patient is the best means of obtaining skill in differentiating these priorities. The course of recovery and the variety of syndromes after TBI are still too unpredictable for any straightforward formula. Nevertheless, this chapter attempts to provide some sense of direction to this process.

COURSE OF RECOVERY

One of the most characteristic features of TBI is the importance of the passage of time in the recovery process. It cannot be emphasized too strongly that one should always consider the length of time since injury in making an assessment of the TBI patient. This feature of TBI contrasts most sharply, for example, with the assessment of spinal cord injury where accurate predictions of physiologic recovery are possible in most cases within a few weeks of injury.

This progressive recovery has led investigators to consider whether there might be some principles involved in recovery which could be mathematically described, allowing the development of "recovery curves."[2] If such lawful relationships could be found and described by means of tables or formulas, then not only would the problem of prediction of recovery be greatly advanced, but also the groundwork for properly matching groups of TBI patients to compare various treatment regimens would be more feasible.[3] Although a number of attempts have been made to construct such recovery curves, no clinically satisfactory mathematical or tabular system has yet appeared. It has been proposed that we do not have sufficient data regarding the natural history of various TBI syndromes to develop such curves. Certain early indexes such as measurement of neurologic status (especially with the use of the Glasgow Coma Scale[4] and radiographic examination (CT scan),[5,6] have been shown to have some significance as predictors of long-term outcome. No measure, however, has demonstrated a sufficiently strong correlation with the degree of disability to be clinically useful to identify cohorts of TBI patients for planning various treatment needs. Batteries of measures have been proposed as possible means of accurately predicting outcome, but no such battery is clinically available at present. In any event we must accept early uncertainty about the functional outcome of any particular TBI patient.

Acknowledging the variations inherent in this process of recovery, one can still differentiate groups of patients on the basis of certain clinical features. Most obvious in this regard is the duration of coma, or of post-traumatic amnesia (PTA) for the less severely injured patient. Clinical experience and multiple studies have proven that the patient who recovers consciousness within days following injury has a much better outcome than the patient who remains in coma for weeks or months. Many other clinical features can be correlated with outcome. These are discussed elsewhere in this text and the physiatrist should be familiar with them to aid in clinical assessment. Even if a mathematical curve cannot be precisely constructed, it is helpful to use clinical data to conceptualize such a curve (Fig. 18–1). Every patient function (F), be it level of arousal, motor recovery, speech and language capability, activities of daily living, social skills, or some other, can generally be expected to follow an asymptotic pattern of recovery. Important features of such recovery are that from an original preinjury level

of 100 percent ability, at the point of injury the particular function drops to unmeasurable levels (or 0 percent). Following a variable length of time first indications of return can be discerned with varying rates or slopes of recovery. With the passage of time recovery gradually slows and approaches an asymptote where no discernible practical further recovery occurs, leaving a fixed deficit (D).

For differing patients, varying rates of recovery of equivalent functions may be seen. Certain relationships usually apply to these curves. The longer the delay before the apparent reappearance of a function, the slower the rate of recovery. The slower the rate of recovery, the larger the final fixed deficit. The clinical ability to estimate such curves and the ultimate level of deficit can be improved by taking multiple measurements of the same function over time.

To apply these concepts to the assessment process, it is clear that every measurement of deficit or functional loss is dependent on the time after injury at which the measurement is obtained. For example, the significance of a particular deficit in attention or motor ability depends on whether it is observed in the first moments or in the days, weeks, or months following head trauma. The same qualification applies to other deficits that may be seen after TBI. The ultimate level of recovery of function may be most accurately assessed after the speed or slope of the recovery is assessed. In practice this means that the initial assess-

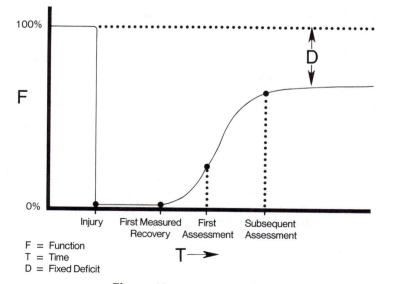

Figure 18–1. Recovery curve.

ment of the patient may be more directed to establish accurate baselines of function against which later change may be contrasted. It is usually futile to try to make a long-term prognosis for the TBI patient at first observation.

Varying types of function characteristically seem to recover at differing rates. In general, the basic arousal functions recover earlier and more quickly, the gross motor behaviors less quickly, and the more complex social abilities most slowly.[7] In practice there are four clinical intervals following TBI in which the physiatrist assesses a patient: in the emergency or neurosurgical setting; in the acute rehabilitation period; in the subacute rehabilitation period; and in the very late, "chronic" period. Discussion of the assessment will address each of these periods separately, although issues germane to each interval may apply to another in individual cases.

Emergent or Neurosurgical Phase

The physiatrist is often the first member of the rehabilitation team to be called to the bedside of a head injured patient. This often occurs in the surgical intensive care unit shortly after the time of injury. At times there is some hesitation by neurosurgeons to obtain such rehabilitation consultation before the patient is "ready for rehabilitation." Since a number of patients either recover too quickly and fully to require traditional rehabilitation or never recover sufficiently to indicate a need for the traditional comprehensive rehabilitation care, this approach has some logic. However, this early period is the optimum time for such an evaluation. The benefit of such early assessment is twofold. First, earlier preventive measures that maintain physiologic status are begun; complications are avoided. It is better to begin a positioning program immediately to prevent later development of decubiti. Similar points are applicable to joint maintenance, nutritional support, protection from aspiration through avoidance of ill-advised feeding programs, initiating bowel and bladder management, and so on. These concerns ought to be a component of the acute care team interventions and may have already been addressed before the

physiatric assessment. Unfortunately, this is not always the case, and it is only with the long-term perspective upon recovery which the physiatrist brings that these problems receive adequate attention.

Second, the physiatrist brings to the scene skills that are of benefit to the patient: proper positioning, ranging, and if necessary, casting and orthoses are often started by the physiatrist. The diagnosis of unsuspected peripheral nerve injuries is facilitated in this setting by careful physical examination and electrodiagnostic procedures. Evaluation of the spastic patient for nerve or motor-point blocks should also be considered.

Ideally, early assessment of the TBI patient by the physiatrist should not be separated from treatment. For the severely brain injured patient and his or her family, the emergency and acute medical setting is often the beginning of a long process of emotional anguish, grieving, education, and adaptation. In the emergency period families frequently and actively seek and acquire information regarding the nature and significance of the injury. From all they observe, learn, and experience, they quickly develop attitudes with which to deal with this emotional "crisis." A great deal of evidence indicates that under such intense emotional distress, patients (or in the case of TBI, families) rapidly develop psychologic defenses or coping mechanisms. Often, these defenses prove to be obstacles to the latter treatment and progress of the patient.[8] Various problems may develop. For example, magical, unrealistic expectations of recovery may arise often from casual statements by intensive care unit (ICU) staff about the potential for rehabilitation to restore lost abilities. Conversely, negative staff attitudes toward the extent of possible recovery may, when proved wrong, lead to a hostile, adversarial attitude toward medical personnel in general, resulting in later problems for the rehabilitation team regarding family cooperation and trust. What is clearly appreciated about these family emotional responses is that they evolve quite rapidly—in most cases within a few weeks of the onset of the injury—and once evolved they are, if maladaptive, characteristically extremely difficult to modify.

These processes are explained by crisis theory from the field of psychiatry. Crisis theory involves several important laws of human behavior. Individuals have characteristic coping mechanisms. When faced with a period of extreme psychologic stress, the "crisis," they respond with various strategies to solve the problem or relieve the distress. Serious illness frequently constitutes such a crisis. The coping mechanisms may be either adaptive or maladaptive in nature. That is, although a particular mechanism may relieve distress, it may do so in two ways: first, in a manner that strengthens the individual or social unit and that has long-term adaptive value; or second, a mechanism that sacrifices long-term adaptiveness for short-term relief of symptoms. Examples of the first, or adaptive, coping mechanisms include seeking specific information about the illness, allowing it to be placed in perspective, and to permit realistic planning for future needs. It may be seeking support, either from professional sources or from friends and extended family. It includes beginning to understand cognitively and emotionally and to accept the implications of the illness event; it also includes beginning to grieve for the lost or injured family member. Developing specific technical skills to assist in patient care is another example.

Examples of maladaptive coping mechanisms include such obvious ones as excessive denial (insisting that the preinjury situation is reattainable); magical thinking that innovative, unproved, or "mystical" treatments will accomplish what standard treatment cannot; and avoidance, through simply absenting from the hospital and bedside, or perhaps through misuse of alcohol or medications. The inappropriate anger and hostility that families may display toward the health care team is often a maladaptive projection of anger about the injury itself.

Since these adaptive or maladaptive coping mechanisms routinely develop within a few weeks and since they rapidly become integral and hardened behaviors, it is essential to avoid delay in their treatment. It is better to prevent such maladaptive psychologic behaviors from developing than to have to treat them after they have emerged and been adopted by the distraught family. A principal reason for early assessment, therefore, is to allow this immediate evaluation and intervention with the family.

The rehabilitation of the brain injured patient is as much a social as a medical process. The major mistake made in planning a rehabilitation program for these patients is to consider the matter in terms of the patient's problems alone. A major determinant of success in rehabilitation is in the social support systems—in their level of strength and sophistication. Patients for whom there is no support, or for whom such support is inadequate or inappropriate, fare significantly worse regardless of the degree or type of direct rehabilitation treatment.

The implications of this fact for the physiatrist who is planning a program for the newly injured patient is that treatment solely aimed at direct physical care is only half a program. An assessment of the family (or social support system) and an active treatment program *for it* should be made at the first opportunity. Therefore, the physiatrist seeing the TBI patient in the ICU or on the surgical wards must also assess and make initial contact with the family. Two errors should be avoided. The first is to assume the family treatment issues can be postponed until a more convenient time or until more definitive information about the status and specific treatment plans are available. The second is delegation of the approach to the family to another member of the rehabilitation team.

The psychologic crisis begins for the family at the moment of the injury. One of the primary tasks of an early assessment of the brain injury patient and his family is to obtain information about how crisis resolution is proceeding. Is the family reasonably informed about the injury and its implications? If not, are there signs that they have been given inappropriate or incorrect information? Perhaps the family has been distorting what has been told them. If a maladaptive coping mechanism is identified, immediate intervention is indicated. This usually entails counseling and educating the family, and may involve the physiatrist alone, or frequently also the psychology and social service staff. It is the responsibility of the physiatrist, however, to assess the need for intervention and see that it is initiated immediately.

Another frequent tendency is to delegate this family interaction to other members of the rehabilitation team such as the social worker, the rehabilitation nurse, discharge planner, or psychologist. While a great deal of the counseling and education is usually performed by these other team members, it cannot all be done in this manner. This is particularly true in the early phases of care when families regard the issue in mainly medical terms. Only "the physician" carries the credibility to convince family members initially of the severity of the injury and the limitations of curative medical or surgical approaches. Later, the counseling role of the physician may become significantly less, but it cannot be abrogated in this first phase of care.

A further related point bears mention. In almost all cases, the information given the family is bad news. Beyond the fact of survival, all the professional estimates of future recovery will be far short of family hopes. There will be a great deal of resistance to accepting such information, and it is usually necessary to "earn" sufficient credibility with the family to make the transmission of such bitter information acceptable. The primary requirement in accomplishing this, after basic technical competence, is to give time to the family. By listening to the family, sharing their fears, concerns, and memories, the physiatrist is establishing a basic level of trust and caring that will allow the later effective transmittal of information and advice. The most perceptive and accurate recommendations will be rejected when given by the physiatrist who spends only a few moments with the patient and even less with the family. Unfortunately, there is no shortcut in this area. Any time spent with the family in the acute situation will be amply repaid in the longer term.

Acute Phase

In the acute phase of recovery, the assessment goals are similar to those in the emergent phase, but the information to be gained by the evaluation is usually substantially greater. As more time has passed since injury (normally a number of weeks or months), there are more "points" on the recovery curve (Fig. 18–1) of that particular patient to be used in establishing prognosis. At least three points can usually be ascertained. First is the point at which injury occurred. The second is the point at which recovery of functions was first observed to occur (e.g., the time after injury when consciousness, speech, motor control, ability to follow commands, or urinary continence first returns). It may be necessary to scrutinize the medical records, particularly nursing and therapy notes, and to interview medical staff and family to ascertain this information. Finally, the third point is established as the current level of function. In addition, the obscuring effects of associated medical and surgical conditions have usually passed, making current function a more accurate reflection of underlying central nervous system deficit than in the emergent period.

It should be possible at this juncture to estimate the approximate final functional outcome of the individual patient and to plan a course of treatment that will move toward these goals. This treatment may involve admission to an acute hospital-based rehabilitation program, but may also include referral to long-term coma management programs, skilled nursing facility–based rehabilitation programs, day programs, or home care.

The success of family adaptation and understanding of the head injury and recovery process should now be evident. Maladaptive coping processes, as well as secondary morbidity such as depression or financial difficulties, should also be clearer. There is an equal need to provide sufficient time for the family in this postinjury phase, but the requirements are somewhat different. By this time families tend to be more knowledgeable regarding head injury and the physician should expect probing questions that require accurate technical knowledge and awareness of current TBI treatment alternatives.

Subacute Phase

At some point between 6 and 18 months after injury, the medical condition of the TBI patient has usually been definitively treated. The patient has usually had some exposure to a rehabilitation process, although the occasional patient will have had none. The approximate final level of disability is usually self-evident, particularly those disabilities that are closely related to specific afferent or efferent neurologic activity. Specific sensory, motor, and balance deficits have reached close to maximal levels of recovery. The practical question in this situation is whether the functional expression of the overall neurologic recovery is factitiously diminished due to inadequate prior treatment (e.g., if disuse atrophy has produced generalized weakness, if sensory isolation has reduced coordination or cognitive function, or if contracture has produced sufficient inefficiency or pain to interfere with the maximum potential use of the limb). In these situations of secondary disability, specifically focused rehabilitation intervention may produce substantial functional gains. At the extreme, if no rehabilitation has been previously provided, a totally misleading picture of central nervous system deficit may be produced. A trial of comprehensive therapies for some weeks may be necessary to resolve this question. If an active comprehensive rehabilitation program has been ongoing, the issue is to assess recent progress within that program and to determine the appropriateness and need for further treatment.

Chronic Phase

A case can be made for the lifelong rehabilitation follow-up of the significantly head injured patient. After optimum function has been attained by active rehabilitation, late functional loss can occur if a supportive environment to maintain function is not present.[9] This may manifest itself as physical disability or as loss of more complex functions such as educational or vocational involvement and social isolation.

The overall stress level and psychologic health of the family unit should be assessed. The stresses on the family with a head injured member increase rather than decrease with the passage of years.[10, 11] Intervention to preserve the integrity of the family may be crucial.

The TBI patient is at risk for late medical and surgical complications that may first present as an insidious or overt deterioration of function.[12] Most important in this regard are late development of seizure disorders, hydrocephalus, intracranial mass lesions (e.g., chronic subdural hematoma), or infection.[13] A more general risk is of any medical condition that goes unnoted due to the patient's ability to communicate his or her health status. Patients also tend to accumulate medication regimens with risk of re-

sultant secondary toxicity, particularly organic brain syndromes.

Assessment in this period must therefore concentrate upon maintenance of function. Any deterioration indicates a need for evaluation, first to rule out significant medical or surgical problems and second to alert to any breakdown in the environment and supports necessary to maintain function.

HISTORY AND NATURE OF INJURY

Although specific features of TBI are discussed elsewhere in this text, a brief discussion of the most significant elements to be included in an assessment is given. Differentiation between diffuse and focal injuries is often helpful in assessing the likelihood of significant recovery, particularly in those localized functions such as language, vision, pyramidal tract control, and the like. Although diffuse brain injury due to high-energy deceleration may be the clear initiator of injury, a large majority of patients with such injury suffer additional secondary brain injury from hypoxia, increased intracranial pressure, or both. Records indicating need for respiratory resuscitation, a dilating pupil or other lateralizing sign, and ICU records of intracranial pressure can, for example, give evidence regarding these issues. Following craniotomy, inquiry must be made regarding need for protective headgear due to skull defects or for cranioplasty. History of persistent drainage of CSF from ears or nasopharynx, or other evidence of fracture through sinuses or base of the skull should alert to the risk for late CNS infection.

Information regarding prior acute treatment is necessary for those conditions that require further attention. Of particular concern are seizures, fractures, feeding tubes, cranial defects, ventricular shunts, and infections.

It is usually necessary to obtain a review of systems from family and those involved in the patient's prior health care. Similar considerations apply to history of premorbid conditions. Specific inquiry should be made regarding drug or alcohol abuse, learning disability, and attention deficit disorder prior to the injury; it is known that all three are strong risk factors for acquiring TBI. Ad-

5

ditionally, in the United States, the pre-existence of "developmental disabilities" entitles the patient to extensive medical and educational coverage, which might not otherwise be available. Psychiatric conditions such as schizophrenia or bipolar affective (manic-depressive) disease should be ascertained, so that subsequent behavioral disorder, if it occurs, may be properly understood.

Finally, a clear sense of the patient's highest level of preinjury functioning needs to be obtained. It is evident that no rehabilitation program can improve a patient beyond this premorbid level, yet inadvertently unrealistic goals are surprisingly often set because of neglect of this simple principle.

The social environment must be defined. Not only the family weaknesses and strengths but also financial and legal aspects need clarification. Is there a financial limit to the amount of treatment feasible for the patient? Is the family financially well enough situated to allow a member (parent or spouse) to cease employment and manage a home program?

A history of current behavior is important. This also should be obtained from a variety of independent sources, including family and medical personnel. It is necessary to ask specifically about those behavior deficits that are known to occur with high frequency after TBI, which nevertheless are often not spontaneously reported. Notorious in this regard are deficits in short-term memory, contrasted with adequate longterm recall. Certain "frontal lobe" deficits such as social inappropriateness and lack of initiation or perseveration may also only be revealed by direct inquiry. Lack of social judgment or sensitivity may also need eliciting. More positive symptomatology, such as social intrusiveness, irritability, and aggression are usually mentioned spontaneously, but if not, inquiry should be made.

Judgment in areas of safety, financial management, driving, and plans for future activities should all be assessed for appropriateness. Sexual behavior is usually affected as a consequence of diminished social sensitivity and impulse control. At times, a true hypersexuality occurs and may require specific evaluation, but loss of libido is most common. Suicidal feelings, intent, and behavior, although usually not predominant, need to be assessed.

At the highest level, an assessment of the success of return to a viable social adjustment is important. Even for those TBI patients who make good physical and cognitive recovery, a pervasive subtle loss of higher social perception often leads to social isolation, behavioral deterioration, and maladaptations such as alcohol or drug abuse.

An outline of the salient elements of the history is presented in Table 18–1.

Table 18–1. History

Nature of injury
Evidence of secondary brain injury
Skull defect
Dural tears or leaks
Treatment
  Surgery
  Cranial defect
  Shunts
  Infection
Review of systems
  Often necessary to get from family and medical staff
Premorbid conditions
  Drug abuse or alcoholism
  Learning disability or attention deficit disorder
  Psychiatric conditions
    Suicidal
    Psychotic
Highest level of premorbid functioning
Social situation
  Family—a source of support, either spouse or other family member should be identified
  Financial
  Legal
Current behavior and function
  Need to obtain from family and staff as well as patient
  1. Deficits
    Memory (especially short-term)
    Attention
    Frontal: initiation, perseveration
    Lack of insight
    Denial
  2. Positive symptoms
    Aggression
    Intrusiveness
  3. Judgment
    Safety
    Money
    Plans for future/problem solving
Sexuality
Suicidal ideation/behavior
Social
  Isolation
  Inappropriate

COMPLICATIONS

A variety of other medical problems are associated with severe TBI. These have been surveyed and reported by others,[14] and are detailed in Chapter 9. However, certain specific problems bear particular emphasis. Spinal cord injury is a frequent concomitant of TBI. Unfortunately in the comatose patient it may not be appreciated at the time of injury. Discovery may come weeks after the injury, yet certain spinal injuries such as atlantoaxial subluxations can be associated with sudden death. A good rule is to obtain a radiograph of the spine in every high-energy brain injured patient. Seizure disorders are usually self-evident; however, post-ictal or interictal confusion and mental impairment may factitiously reduce function if the epileptic nature of the disorder is not appreciated. Conversely, in a patient receiving anticonvulsants, impairment of cognition routinely occurs; withdrawal of medication may elicit much higher functional capability. As a more general aspect, the TBI patient is exquisitely sensitive to the effects of all CNS active drugs, and similar considerations apply.

Hydrocephalus may occur at any time following TBI. Its onset may be particularly deceptive when it occurs late after the injury, and a high level of suspicion of any functional deterioration must be maintained.

Infection, malnutrition, or any other physiologic stress including fatigue and sensory deprivation will alter the picture of the TBI patient and make accurate assessment of underlying capacities difficult. To the extent possible, all such modifying influences should be corrected before a definitive assessment is made. Patients who appear to be in vegetative state may become responsive when septicemia or catabolism is corrected.

Finally, environmentally induced etiologies for behavior problems should be considered after elimination of medical causes. Aggression, even severe assaultiveness, may be a reaction to situation-specific frustration or discomfort; these circumstances should be defined and corrected.

PHYSICAL EXAMINATION

Certain aspects of the physical examination bear mention. The time of day at which the examination is performed is critical, as easy fatiguability and excessive sleepiness are well known in the head injured. It may be optimal to perform the examination early after patient rising (although this is not always best), or to perform the examination at differing times of day to assess this influence. If a patient has been transported a long distance to the examination site it is usual to see a decrement in ability due to fatigue. The position of the patient is significant. Certain reflexes and posturings will be accentuated by certain body positions, and the supine position generally produces a less satisfactory level of alertness and behavior than the upright. Always try to examine the patient in part in an upright posture, even if that involves supported sitting or placement in a wheelchair. Multiple examinations are generally necessary to obtain an accurate representation of capacity. It should be appreciated that recent surgery or even general anesthesia will produce longer-lasting deficits in the injured patients' behavior than in that of the non–brain injured.

An extensive mental status examination is essential. This examination should concentrate upon neurobehavioral syndromes rather than more traditional psychiatric concerns. Excellent manuals are available as guides.[15]

The motor picture in relation to tone, spasticity, abnormal reflexes, and coordination evolves over a number of months. As a rule, no definitive decision, particularly regarding surgical releases or tendon transfers, should be made before 18 months after injury.

NEUROPHYSIOLOGIC STUDIES

Neurophysiologic studies such as the electroencephalogram (EEG) and cortical evoked potentials (EPs) have a limited role in the general rehabilitation assessment of the TBI patient. EEGs are useful in the diagnosis of specific seizure activity and type. However, a normal EEG does not rule out a seizure process. EEGs are indicated with questions of true brain death, diagnosis of particular seizure type, and in certain medicolegal situations (e.g., to provide evidence of an organic condition in mild TBI). Cortical evoked potentials may be useful in co-matose patients in predicting outcome. In addition they may be useful if questions of specific sensory loss are germane, for example, hearing or vision.[16] The EPs are also useful in medicolegal situations, to provide evidence supporting a clinical diagnosis of organic brain damage.

RESULT OF ASSESSMENT

The assessment should culminate in an appropriate decision in regard to treatment; the physiatrist needs to connect the assessment result to decisions about treatment. The decision is not simply whether or not to admit to an acute rehabilitation facility. In general a decision to observe, admit, treat, or refer should be made. The responsibility is with the rehabilitation physician to ensure that the TBI patient is referred to the appropriate type of treatment or treating facility, and that appropriate follow-up is done, even if acute inpatient care is not indicated. The extent of this network of programs to which referral may be made has been described;[17] it includes non–hospital-based acute rehabilitation facilities, residential and transitional programs, day programs, specialized educational programs, lifetime care facilities, and behavioral management programs.

Observation may be chosen to allow more urgent medical or surgical issues to resolve or in some cases to allow the course of recovery to become more clear. For example, a patient in a coma will be observed for a number of weeks to determine whether return of consciousness will occur, allowing admission to an intensive rehabilitation program, or whether the persistent

vegetative state will develop, in which case the appropriate referral is to a specialized skilled nursing facility or coma management program. Even if observation is the first chosen course of action, all maintenance care and family interventions need initiation immediately.

Those patients who will require a comprehensive, hospital-based, inpatient rehabilitation program usually declare themselves within a short time of injury although extended delay in recovery from coma is not unknown.[18] A rule of thumb that will select perhaps 80 to 90 percent of the appropriate candidates for this level program is to include all patients who are in a coma more than a week but less than 4 to 6 months. Although these guidelines are approximate and should not be adhered to rigidly, they will include the majority of patients who have sufficient neurologic recovery to benefit from intensive rehabilitation treatment (with increased function and quality of life) and will exclude those who have only such minor deficits so as to not require the extensive medical, nursing, and laboratory support of these inpatient rehabilitation programs. For those patients who have less than 1 week of coma, a majority will probably not require extensive inpatient rehabilitation care. However, it is appreciated that long-lasting cognitive and behavioral deficits will be present in these patients. Therefore, appropriate follow-up in clinic and referral to psychologic, educational, and vocational programs as appropriate are indicated. A thorough and accurate assessment should permit the physiatrist to choose the appropriate program or intervention at the proper time for each patient. This will ensure an optimum outcome and facilitate the proper utilization of scarce treatment and financial resources.

REFERENCES

1. Cope, DN and Hall, K: Head injury rehabilitation: Benefit of early intervention. Arch Phys Med Rehabil 63:433, 1982.
2. Hiorns, RW and Newcombe, F: Recovery curves: Uses and limitations. Int Rehabil Med 1:173, 1979.
3. Baddely, A, Meade, T and Newcombe, F: Design problems in research on rehabilitation after brain damage. Int Rehabil Med 2:138, 1980.
4. Teasdale, G and Jennett, B: Assessment of coma and impaired consciousness. Lancet 2:81, 1974.
5. Rao, N et al: Computerized tomography head scans as predictors of rehabilitation outcome. Arch Phys Med Rehabil 65:18, 1984.
6. Timming, R, Orrison, WW and Mikula, JA: Computerized tomography and rehabilitation outcomes after severe head trauma. Arch Phys Med Rehabil 63:154, 1982.
7. Mackworth, N, Mackworth, J and Cope, DN: Towards an interpretation of head injury recovery trends. In: Severe Head Trauma: A Comprehensive

Medical Approach. A report to the National Institute for Handicapped Research, Washington, DC, Project 13-P-59156/9, pp VII:1–VII:65, 1982.

8. Romano, MD: Family response to traumatic head injury. Scand J Rehabil Med 6:1, 1974.

9. Rusk, HA, Block, JM and Lowman, EW: Rehabilitation following traumatic brain damage: immediate and long term follow-up in 127 cases. Med Clin North Am 53:677, 1969.

10. Bond, MR, Brooks, DN and McKinlay, W: Burdens imposed on the relatives of those with severe brain damage due to injury. Acta Neurochir [Suppl] (Wien) 28:124, 1979.

11. Rosenbaum, M and Najenson, T: Changes in life patterns and symptoms of low mood as reported by wives of severely brain-injured soldiers. J Consult Clin Psychol 44:881, 1979.

12. Jennett, B and Teasdale, G: Management of Head Injuries. FA Davis, Philadelphia, 1981.

13. Cope, DN, Date, ES and Mar, EY: Serial computerized tomographic evaluations in traumatic head injury. Arch Phys Med Rehabil 69:483, 1988.

14. Kalisky, Z et al: Medical problems encountered during rehabilitation of patients with head injury. Arch Phys Med Rehabil 66:25, 1985.

15. Strub, RL and Black, WF: The Mental Status Examination in Neurology, ed 2. FA Davis, Philadelphia, 1985.

16. Rappaport, M et al: Evoked brain potentials and disability in brain-damaged patients. Arch Phys Med Rehabil 58:333, 1977.

17. Cope, DN: Traumatic closed head injury: Status of rehabilitation treatment. Sem Neurol 5(3):212, 1985.

18. Tanheco, J and Kaplan, PE: Physical and surgical rehabilitation of patient after 6-year coma. Arch Phys Med Rehabil 63:36, 1982.

Chapter 19

Physical Therapy Assessment

PAMELA W. DUNCAN, M.A., P.T.

The motor deficits following head trauma are variable and complex. The purpose of the physical therapy assessment is to identify the causes of movement dysfunction, develop an appropriate treatment program, and establish realistic short- and long-term goals. A thorough assessment of the head trauma patient includes a general assessment of cognitive, perceptual, and behavioral features; communication abilities; and a detailed assessment of sensorimotor function. The sensorimotor determinants of motor performance are range of motion and biomechanical alignment, sensation, muscle tone, strength, synergistic organization, balance, and adaptability. The head trauma patient may have any combination of deficits that cause motor control problems. Once the patient's motor control problems have been identified, the therapist must analyze all the factors that affect motor control and finally generate hypotheses about the relative contribution of the altered functions to the patient's motor deficits.

In view of the variability in extent and type of deficits following head trauma, assessment of the sensorimotor system should be seen as a continuum. In the comatose patient the therapist should first observe the patient without intervention; note the resting postures; evaluate spontaneous movements; assess the patient's responses to tactile, auditory, and visual stimulation; and finally, record range of motion and resistance to passive movements. As the patient's arousal level improves, more specific assessments of the sensorimotor determinants can be undertaken.

COGNITION/BEHAVIOR

Cognition is defined as "all processes by which sensory information is transformed, reduced, elaborated, stored and used."[1] Good cognition is crucial for motor learning or relearning and for performance of purposeful motor tasks. Most cognitive functions are observed by a physical therapist while detailed assessment and interpretation is performed by psychologists, speech pathologists, and occupational therapists. The cognitive functions that should be recognized by the therapist are (1) level of consciousness and alertness, (2) orientation, (3) short- and long-term memory, (4) attention span, (5) level of agitation and anxiety, (6) ability to problem-solve, and (7) ability to organize and sequence movements. The Rancho Los Amigos cognitive scale is a good tool to document cognitive function (Table 19–1).

PERCEPTION

Perception is the "dynamic process of receiving (perceiving) the environment through sensory impulses and translating these impulses into meaning based on a previously developed view of the environment."[2] Our motor behavior is determined by how we perceive our environment. Perceptual deficits in head trauma patients lead to misinterpretation of the environment and inappropriate movement performances. For example, if the patient has a distorted perception of vertical, his or her balance will

Table 19–1. RANCHO LOS AMIGOS COGNITIVE SCALE

I. No Response:. Unresponsive to any stimulus.

II. Generalized Response: Limited, inconsistent, nonpurposeful responses, often to pain only.

III. Localized Response: Purposeful responses; may follow simple commands; may focus on presented object.

IV. Confused, Agitated: Heightened state of activity; confusion, disorientation; aggressive behavior; unable to do self-care; unaware of present events; agitation appears related to internal confusion.

V. Confused, Inappropriate: Nonagitated; appears alert; responds to commands; distractable; does not concentrate on task; agitated responses to external stimuli; verbally inappropriate; does not learn new information.

VI. Confused, Appropriate: Good directed behavior, needs cueing; can relearn old skills as activities of daily living (ADLs); serious memory problems; some awareness of self and others.

VII. Automatic, Appropriate: Appears appropriate, oriented; frequently robot-like in daily routine; minimal or absent confusion; shallow recall; increased awareness of self, interaction in environment; lacks insight into condition; decreased judgment and problem solving; lacks realistic planning for future.

VIII. Purposeful, Appropriate: Alert, oriented; recalls and integrates past events; learns new activities and can continue without supervision; independent in home and living skills; capable of driving; defects in stress tolerance, judgment, abstract reasoning persist; many function at reduced levels in society.

Prepared by Professional Staff Association, Rancho Los Amigos Hospital, Inc., Downey, California.

be precarious and motor responses to postural displacements will be inappropriate. Perception is a complex function to test and is usually evaluated by psychologists or occupational therapists; however, prior to analyzing movement deficits and establishing a program, the physical therapist must have an understanding of some key perceptual functions; visual orientation, right/left orientation, depth perception, verticality, body schema, neglect, and the presence of apraxias.

SENSORIMOTOR DETERMINANTS

Range of Motion

The prolonged immobilization, movement dysfunction, and abnormal tone associated with head trauma may produce contractures and loss of range of motion. Compromised range of motion limits the functional range for movement, alters the normal muscle length–tension relationship, as well as impairing normal biomechanical alignment. All these factors contribute to excessive effort in movement, faulty postures, and gait deviations.

In order to evaluate the true status of joint motion, range of motion should be evaluated with slow passive movements to minimize the influence of abnormal tone. Standard goniometric readings should be recorded for all major joints.

When assessing joint motion, joint play should also be evaluated. "Joint play movements are those accessory movements that can be produced passively at a joint, but cannot be isolated actively."[3] For example, during shoulder flexion, the head of the humerus must glide down to prevent jamming of the head against the acromion process. Without this accessory movement, the motions of flexion and abduction are limited and often become painful.

Biomechanical Alignment

The patient's alignment over his or her base of support will influence the effort required to stay upright and will modify the muscle tone, as well as determining which movement synergies are appropriate for mobility and stability. Poor biomechanical alignment can therefore contribute to poor motor control. Because of the frequent occurrence of musculoskeletal injuries in head trauma, a careful analysis of postural alignment may explain some of the observed motor control deficits.

Sensation

Sensation plays an important role in motor learning for feedback on performance and encoding new equilibrium points for other programs. Sensation is especially important for production of appropriate muscle force, complex multijoint movements, and coordination of agonist and antagonist timing. In the low-level patient with limited responsiveness, sensory functions may be grossly evaluated by observing the patient's response to sensory stimulation. For example, does the patient look or move in response to touch? When the patient can follow simple commands, tactile sense, joint position sense, sharp/dull discrimination, and stereognosis should be evaluated with traditional methods. Vision and visual fields also should be grossly checked. Therapists should review all ophthalamic reports. Distorted vision (i.e., blurred, double vision) will compromise balance and may alter the selection of movement strategies.

Strength

The inability to produce an appropriate voluntary contraction and alterations in motor unit recruitment and timing are common problems observed in patients with head trauma. Yet many clinicians have assumed that in upper motor neuron lesions limited strength is not a primary motor deficit, but rather secondary to abnormal tone. The primary motor cortex plays a major role in regulating recruitment and frequency of motor neuron firing for muscle force production; therefore, paresis is an expected consequence when the cortex or the descending motor tracts are disrupted. The presence of antagonistic coactivation and impaired reciprocal inhibition contribute to the paresis but are not always a primary factor in limiting force production.

The assessment of strength in head trauma patients should include the capability to isolate and generate a muscle force against gravity in the prime movers. The scoring system devised by the Medical Research Council[4] can be used to document function in key muscle groups. In addition, the patient's ability to produce force throughout the range of motion, at different speeds, and for several repetitions is a necessary part of the assessment.

Isokinetic testing in some select patients who are able to follow instructions and who are able to flex and extend against gravity may be used to provide information about the process of force production, power, and fatiguability.[5] The following measures can be documented by such testing: (1) peak torque, (2) time to peak torque, (3) limb excursion, (4) velocity-torque relationships, (5) time between reciprocal movements, (6) ability to attain and sustain a submaximal torque, and (7) ability to repeatedly produce force.

Muscle Tone

Abnormal muscle tone is a classic motor deficit in head trauma. It is usually evaluated by subjectively rating the patient's resistance to passive movement. The tone abnormality may be very severe in decerebrate rigidity or may be mild and elicited in only fast movements. Tone fluctuates. It is frequently influenced by position in space, anxiety, and infection. Because tone is such a salient feature of head trauma, we have assumed that it is the cause of many of our motor dysfunctions, yet abnormal tone is a symptom of upper motor neuron damage and does not necessarily cause all other movement deficits.[6]

The increased resistance to passive movement is often called "spasticity." When the patient moves actively, resistance may be noted in the antagonist and this is also called spasticity, yet the "spasticity" observed in passive movement may not be the same as that observed in active movement. As therapists we are often successful in reducing the hypertonicity in response to passive movement, yet when the patient attempts to move volitionally, his "spasticity" increases. This may be explained by the fact that the restraint to passive movement is due to a different pathophysiology than restraint to active movement. For example, the restraint to passive movement may be due to a hyperactive stretch reflex, and restraint to active movement is due to abnormal regulation of the neuron pool. This abnormal regulation causes prolonged recruitment of motor units and delays cessation of antagonistic contractions at the end of the movement.[7] Disorders of reciprocal inhibition also contribute to increase restraints during active movement.[8]

When evaluating and treating patients, it is important to closely analyze "spastic" behaviors and hypothesize about the potential cause. Otherwise, inappropriate treatment techniques may be selected. For example, resistance to passive movement that is due to the hyperactive stretch reflex may respond well to drug therapy, physical modalities, slow stretch, and rotation; but if the problem is abnormal programming of the motor neuron pool for reciprocal movement, the patient's active movements will not necessarily be improved by the previously mentioned treatment.

The pendulum drop test provides an objective measure of passive restraint in certain muscle groups.[9] The Cybex II isokinetic dynamometer, which incorporates an electrogoniometer and recorder, can be used to perform a pendulum drop test. For example, to test the knee extensor muscles:

1. The patient is positioned in a sitting or supine position on the Cybex table.
2. The patient is stabilized to the table with thigh, pelvis, and trunk straps.
3. The dynamometer input shaft is positioned laterally over the knee's axis of rotaton and the shin pad of the dynamometer arm is strapped just proximal to the malleoli.
4. The stylus of the position angle is adjusted.
5. The speed of the isokinetic dynamometer is adjusted to 300 degrees per second.

6. The patient is instructed to relax completely.
7. The lower leg is then raised up by the examiner until the knee is fully extended.
8. Paper speed is set at 25 mm per second.
9. The patient is reminded to relax the leg, which is then dropped by the examiner.
10. Steps 6 through 9 are performed five more times (the first three trials are to ensure the patient is relaxed, and the last two trials are recorded).

In normal subjects, the recordings obtained in sequential drops are not significantly different. The normal extremity falls through the available range of motion without constraint and usually demonstrates from 5 to 6 oscillations (Fig. 19–1). Patients with spasticity often fail to reach 90 degrees of flexion on the first oscillation and may actualy experience a reversal in direction of movement. In addition, they have fewer oscillations (Fig. 19–2).

The restraint in the antagonist that occurs during active voluntary movements may be assessed clinically by comparing torque produced during voluntary reciprocal movement to torque produced during unidirectional movement. For example, a patient whose primary movement problem is prolonged activation of the quadriceps will produce minimal knee flexor torque during reciprocal movement (extension/flexion) but will be able to produce significantly more

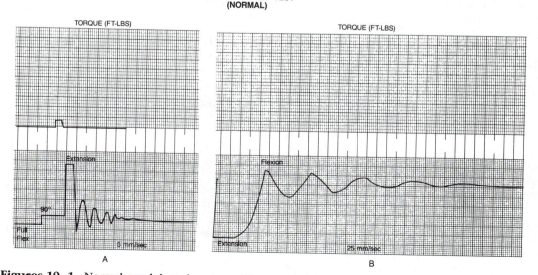

Figures 19–1. Normal pendulum drop test. *A,* Paper speed at 5 mm/sec. *B,* Paper speed at 25 mm/sec.

PENDULUM DROP TEST
(SPASTICITY)

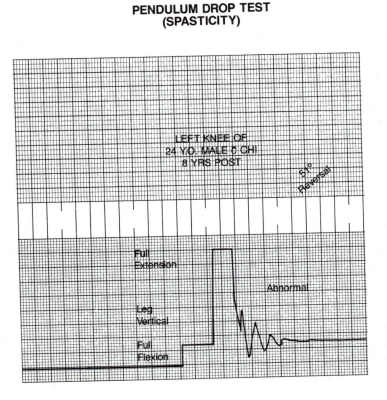

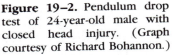

Figure 19–2. Pendulum drop test of 24-year-old male with closed head injury. (Graph courtesy of Richard Bohannon.)

knee flexion torque when flexing the knee only. This problem will become worse as velocity of exercise increases.

Synergistic Organization

All movements consist of functionally related patterns of muscle contractions (synergies), which have fixed spatial-temporal relationships. These synergies simplify the control of movement for the central nervous system.[10] The normal CNS has an uncanny ability to predict exactly which muscles should work and the exquisite timing of these contractions. For example, if a standing person voluntarily lifts his or her arm, muscular activity in the trunk and contralateral lower extremity precedes the muscle activity in the upper extremity.[11] This sequence of muscle activity provides the postural support for the movements. Normal movements require an interweaving of synergies to provide postural control and many options for movement.

In head trauma patients the synergistic organization of movement may be disturbed in many ways. In severe damage, the patient's movement may be limited to primitive reflexes (asymmetrical tonic neck, symmetrical tonic neck, tonic labyrinthine reflexes, and positive support). Milani-Comparetti theorizes that these primitive reflexes are primary motor programs that are modified and expanded upon in development.[12] In CNS damage the abnormality is not due to acquisition of abnormal reflexes but to loss of a variety of movement patterns. Often the head trauma patient's movements are limited to stereotyped patterns of flexion (flexion, abduction, external rotation) and extension (extension, adduction, internal rotation). These gross movement patterns in the lower extremity may be sufficient for a functional, yet abnormal, gait. In the upper extremity, however, if the patient's movements are limited to gross patterns of flexion and extension, the movements are not functional. The loss of selective motor control should be viewed as a disorder of voluntary movement that is due to the malfunction of the upper motor neuron centers which participate in the programming and execution of movement, rather than a result of "spasticity."

In other cases of disorganization of syner-

Table 19–2. ANALYSIS OF ALL THE FACTORS THAT COULD CONTRIBUTE TO A MOTOR DEFICIT

I. Observe motor deficit

II. Assesses factors that could cause the motor deficit

Inability to develop an upper extremity protective extension reaction
1. Cognitive—The patient is not alert or oriented enough to respond.
2. Perception—The patient's perception of vertical is distorted.
3. Range of motion—The patient has insufficient shoulder abduction, elbow extension, wrist extension, and hand opening.
4. Sensory—The patient has impaired sensory integration (vision, vestibular, somatosensory) to provide feedback about displacement.
5. Weakness—The patient has paralysis and unable to abduct, and extend upper extremity.
6. Tone—The patient has excessive and prolonged muscle activity in flexors.
7. Synergistic organization–The patient's movement patterns are limited by primitive movement patterns (i.e., asymmetrical tonic reflex, tonic labyrinthine reflexes, and so on) or restricted to gross patterns of flexion and extension. The patient has difficulty in timing of muscle activity, which causes ataxia and tremors.

III. Evaluate (decide which of the factors are contributing to motor deficit)
IV. Select intervention strategies
V. Treat

gistic organization, the patient may have a variety of movement pattern available, but the timing of the muscular contractions are abnormal during posture and movement. These timing deficits produce the symptoms of ataxia and tremor and are present when there is damage to the cerebellum or basal ganglia.

Balance

Balance is a complex function that requires sensory inputs (vision, somatosensory, and vestibular), motor programs (postural synergies), and neuromuscular function (muscle contractions, range of motion, and biomechanical alignment). Without exquisite balance control, movement will not be purposeful and coordinated. Therefore, careful analysis is crucial for treatment planning and success. Many head trauma patients have balance impairments, which should be carefully evaluated. This evaluation should not only include a rating of balance in different positions but should also analyze the factors that are contributing to poor postural control. Many of the factors previously evaluated (i.e, range of motion, biomechanical alignment, strength, synergies) will provide useful information for diagnosing the cause of balance deficits. However, more detailed assessment should be included. For example, the ability to balance under different sensory conditions, eyes open–eyes closed, with impaired somatosensory input, and during visual conflict should be included. (See Shumway-Cook and Horak[13] for more detailed description of these balance assessment techniques.) In addition to evaluating static balance, the patient's balance during self-initiated movements and during postural perturbations should also be analyzed.

Adaptability

Adaptability is the flexibility in the CNS that allows it to program and execute movement patterns under a variety of conditions and environments. The ability to vary speed, force, and amplitude of movements and to move in different environments should be assessed.

CONCLUSION

In view of the complexity and variability in motor control deficits in patients with head trauma, there is no one form of assess-ment that is appropriate for all patients. The appendix is an outline of assessment strate-gies. Assessment should be viewed as a dy-namic process in which the determinants of motor control are evaluated. The most im-portant evaluation that can be performed on head trauma patients is a proper clinical evaluation to determine which of the mani-festations of CNS damage are contributing to the disability (Table 19–2). By an appro-priate analysis of the missing components of motor control, treatment programs can be appropriately and realistically developed.

REFERENCES

1. Adamovich, BB: Cognitive assessment and rehabili-tation of closed head injured patients. Paper pre-sented at Postgraduate course on Rehabilitation of the Brain Injured Adult. Williamsburg, VA, June 6–8, 1985.
2. Bouska, MJ, Kauffman, NA and Marcus, SE: Disor-ders of the visual perceptual system. In Umphed, D (ed): Neurological Rehabilitation. CV Mosby, St Louis, 1985, p 552.
3. Kessler, RM and Hertling, D: Management of Common Musculoskeletal Disorders. Philadelphia, Harper and Row, 1983, p 22.
4. Medical Research Council: Aids to the examination of the peripheral nervous system. Her Majesty's Stationery Office, London, 1976.
5. Watkins, M, Harris, BA and Kozlowshi, BA: Isoki-netic testing in patients with hemiparesis: A pilot study. Phys Ther 64:183, 1984.
6. Burke, D: Stretch reflex activity in the spastic pa-tient. EEG (Suppl 36):172, 1982.
7. Sahrmann, SA and Norton, BJ: The relationship of voluntary movement spasticity in the upper motor neuron syndrome. Ann Neurol 2:460, 1977.
8. Miller, S and Hammond, GR: Neural control of arm movement in patients following stroke. In Van Hof, MW and Mohn, G (eds): Functional Recovery from Brain Damage. Elsevier–New Holland, Amsterdam, 1981, p 259.
9. Bohannon, RW and Larkin, PW: Cybex II isokinetic dynamometer for the documentation of spasticity. Phys Ther 65:46, 1985.
10. Bernstein, N: The Co-ordination and Regulation of Movements. Pergamon Press, Oxford, 1967.
11. Paltser, Y and Elner, AM: Preparatory and compen-satory period during voluntary movement in pa-tients with involvement of the brain of different localization. Biofizika 1:142, 1967.
12. Milani-Comparetti, A: Pattern analysis of normal and abnormal development: the fetus, the newborn and the child. In Slaton, D (ed): Development of Movement in Infancy. University of North Carolina, Chapel Hill, 1980.
13. Shumway-Cook, A and Horak, FB: Assessing the in-fluence of sensory interaction on balance: Sugges-tion from the field. Phys Ther 66:1548, 1986.
14. Fregly, AR and Graybiel, A: An ataxia test battery not requiring rails. Aerospace Med 39:277, 1982.
15. Graybiel, A and Fregly, AR: A new quantitative ataxia test battery. Acta Otolaryngol Stockholm 61:292, 1966.
16. Wolfson, LI et al: Stressing the postural response: A qualitative method for testing balance. J Am Ger Soc 34:845, 1986.

Appendix: Assessment Strategies for Head Trauma Patients

I. Cognition

☐ Is patient arousable to sound (e.g., ring a bell) or to his or her "name"? If not, can you elicit a rooting or sucking reflex in response to facial stimulation?

☐ Is patient alert? Can he or she track objects with visual or auditory stimulation?

☐ Does patient follow directions (one-two-three step commands)?

☐ Is patient oriented to person, place, and time? Is patient able to recognize family and friends?

☐ Is the patient able to selectively attend or is he or she easily distracted?

☐ Does the level of alertness fluctuate?

☐ Does patient demonstrate any memory deficits (short-term, intermediate, long-term)?

☐ Is the patient a verbal or nonverbal communicator?

☐ Can the patient organize and sequence tasks?

☐ Does the patient display the ability to problem-solve?

II. Emotional

Is the patient

☐ Confused, agitated
☐ Irritable
☐ Labile
☐ Apathetic
☐ Impulsive
☐ Depressed
☐ Unmotivated
☐ Denying disability
☐ Persevering
☐ Egocentric

III. Perceptual

Does the patient have

☐ Perception of body in space
☐ The ability to discriminate figure ground
☐ Correct body schema
☐ Neglect
☐ Right/left orientation
☐ Apraxias

IV. Range of Motion

A. In order to evaluate the true status of joint motion, range-of-motion testing should be performed slowly and passively. If range of motion is within normal limits, the available range should be recorded.

B. If range of motion is not within normal limits, joint play should be assessed by passively gliding the joint surface and rate mobility according to following scale:

0 = Ankylosed
1 = Moderate hypomobility
2 = Mild hypomobility
3 = Normal
4 = Mild hypermobility
5 = Moderate hypermobility
6 = Severe hypermobility

V. Biomechanical Alignment

While the patient sits or stands (if patient is able to assume these positions) analyze postural alignment of head, shoulders, pelvis, knees, and feet and evaluate symmetry in weight bearing.

VI. Strength

A. *Force:* Evaluate key muscle groups:
Lower extremity: Hip flexors, extensors, and abductors; knee extensors and flexors; ankle dorsiflexors
Upper extremity: Scapular protractors; shoulder flexors and abductors; elbow extensors and flexors; and wrist extensors
Trunk: Flexors and extensors

Scoring for strength: Medical Research Council Muscle Grading[4]
0 = No movement or contraction whatsoever
1 = A palpable contraction, but no movement observed
2 = Movement seen at the appropriate joint with gravity eliminated
3 = Able to move the joint against gravity
4 = Able to move the joint against resistance, but less than normal side
5 = Fully normal strength

B. *Isokinetic Testing*
For more advanced patients, this tool provides information about the process of force production, power, and fatiguability. The following measures can be documented:

1. Time to generate peak torque
2. Peak torque
3. Time peak torque is held
4. Time between reciprocal movements
5. Limb excursion
6. Maximum speed at which torque can be generated
7. The ability to attain and sustain a given submaximal torque isometrically

VI. Muscle Tone

A. Note increased resistance to quick stretch in the upper extremities (UE) and lower extremities (LE) (UE: pectoralis major, biceps, triceps, wrist flexors, finger flexors; LE: hip flexors and extensors, adductors, quadriceps, hamstrings, gastrocnemius)

Scoring:

0 = Flaccid

1 = Minimal to moderate hypotonia

2 = Normal tone

3 = Moderate resistance to stretch

4 = Severe resistance to stretch

B. For more advanced patients a drop test on the Cybex dynamometer (described in the chapter text) with speed at 300 degrees will give more quantitative information about muscle tone.

C. What alters the patient's muscle tone?
Position _____, Effort _____, Fatigue _____, Emotional Stress _____, Temperature _____

VII. Active Restraint to Movement

A. Ask the patient to slowly and then quickly reciprocally flex and extend the elbow and knee.

B. Ask the patient to move unidirectionally (i.e., flex the knee only). Then compare the force produced and range of motion accomplished during unidirectional movement with that produced during reciprocal movement (i.e., extension of knee, then flexion).

Scoring:

0 = Patient is unable to reverse direction of movement

1 = Impaired—patient is able to reverse, but reversal is slow and jerky

2 = Normal—quick reversal of direction of movement

VIII. Synergistic Organization

A. *Volitional Movement*

Observe patient's volitional movements in supine, sitting, and standing and make the following qualitative assessments of the available motor patterns of extremities and trunk.

☐ No available movement

☐ Movements are performed only in stereotypical flexion and extension synergies

☐ There is an ability to combine components of the stereotypical synergies

☐ Movements are selective without synergy dependence

☐ Movements are influenced by primitive reflexes (asymmetrical tonic neck, tonic labyrinthine, positive support) or associated reactions

☐ Movements are ataxic

☐ There is a resting or intentional tremor

☐ Movements are of normal speed and coordination

IX. Functional Movement Patterns

Assess the spontaneous automatic use of extremities, head, neck, and trunk during functional activities of rolling, supine to sit, sit to stand, and stand.

Scoring for functional tasks:

0 = No spontaneous use of limbs, head, neck, and trunk

1 = Delayed, weak, or inefficient* use of limb, neck, and head

___

*Efficiency: as determined by sense of effort, associated movements, and minimization of energy expenditure during movement.

2 = Quick, efficient, spontaneous use of limb, head, neck, and trunk

X. Balance Activities
A. *Static Balance*

	Eyes Open	Eyes Closed
1. Sitting		
2. Standing		
3. Unilateral Stance on Right Leg		
4. Unilateral Stance on Left Leg		

Scoring for static positions
0 = Cannot maintain balance for more than 5 seconds without support
1 = Can maintain balance 5–59 seconds or with significant postural sway
2 = Can maintain balance for more than 60 seconds, little postural sway

Scoring for unilateral stance
0 = Cannot maintain balance longer than 1–2 seconds
1 = Stands balanced for 4–9 seconds
2 = Stands balanced for more than 10 seconds

B. *Sensory—Organization Test;*[13] *Modified Fregly Scoring*[14, 15]

1. Standing, normal stance on floor, eyes   Standing barefoot, feet in normal   Score: Max 150 Trial 1 _____

open (Fig. 19–3)   alignment, stand   2 _____
                            for 30 seconds   3 _____
                            with eyes open   4 _____
                                                             5 _____

                                                    Score: Max 150

2. Standing, normal   Standing barefoot,   Trial 1 _____
   stance on floor, eyes feet in normal   2 _____
   closed (Figure 19–4)   alignment, stand   3 _____
                          for 30 seconds   4 _____
                          with eyes closed   5 _____

                                                    Score: Max 150

3. Standing on floor,   Eyes open, wearing   Trial 1 _____
   wearing visual dome   visual dome, feet in   2 _____
   (Fig. 19–5)   normal alignment,   3 _____
                          stand for 30   4 _____
                          seconds   5 _____

                                                    Score: Max 150

4. Standing, normal   Standing on foam sur-   Trial 1 _____
   stance eyes open on a face, feet in normal   2 _____
   foam surface (Fig.   alignment, stand   3 _____
   19–6)   for 30 seconds   4 _____
                          with eyes open   5 _____

                                                    Score: Max 150

5. Standing on a foam   Standing on foam sur-   Trial 1 _____
   surface, eyes closed   face, eyes closed,   2 _____
   (Fig. 19–7)   feet normal align-   3 _____
                          ment, stand for 30   4 _____
                          seconds   5 _____

                                                    Score: Max 150

6. Standing on foam sur- Standing on foam sur-   Trial 1 _____
   face wearing visual   face, eyes open,   2 _____
   dome (Fig. 19–8)   wearing visual   3 _____
                          dome, feet in nor-   4 _____
                          mal alignment for   5 _____
                          30 seconds (stand
                          for 30 seconds)   TOTAL SCORE: _____

Scoring: Each subject is given a maximum of five trials to maintain balance under each sensory condition. Failure to maintain balance is defined as dropping one or both arms or the displacement of the foot before the 30-second period is completed. The number of seconds stood prior to failure is recorded. Using a modified Fregly scoring system, a maximum score of 900 (5 trials times 30 seconds times 6 conditions is possible over the six sensory conditions).

C. *Dynamic Balance—during self-initiated movements*

Diagonal reach to left   Diagonal reach to right

1. Sitting (Fig. 19–9)

☐ Head righting
☐ Trunk righting
☐ Postural reactions in opposite upper extremity
☐ Postural reactions in both lower extremities
☐ Resumes vertical

2. Standing (Fig. 19–10)

☐ Head righting
☐ Trunk righting
☐ Weight shift
☐ Postural reactions in extremities
☐ Resumes vertical

Scoring for self-initiated movements and small perturbations:
0 = No postural adaptation and weight shift or significant delay in response
1 = Inefficient, weak postural adaptation and weight shift, or mild delay in response
2 = Efficient, quick postural adaptations, and appropriate weight shift

D. *Dynamic Balance—in response to perturbations*

A simple and quick assessment of postural response, the Postural Stress Test has been developed by Wolfson and colleagues.[16] A pulley and weight system is used to deliver a destabilizing force at the waist level of each subject. (Fig. 19–11) (see the original article for construction information). During this test each subject stands with arms at sides, feet 6 to 12 inches apart, and with back toward the pulley system. Each of three specified weights (1½, 3, and 4½ percent of body weight, with a maximum of 10 pounds) is used to produce a destabilizing force. Subjects are informed that their balance will be disturbed and that their goal is to maintain their balance during the test. The motor response that the subjects used to recover the balance after each perturbation are videotaped. Scores are based on the 9-point scale described by Wolfson and colleagues[16] (Fig. 19–12).

Postural Stress Test[16]

1. Number of trials with effective balance
   0 _____
   1 _____
   2 _____
   3 _____

2. Balance Strategy Score
   Trial 1 _____
   Trial 2 _____
   Trial 3 _____

TOTAL _____

XI. Adaptability of Motor Patterns

If the patient has volitional and spontaneous movement patterns, qualitatively assess motor patterns as the speed, force, amplitude, postural base, and sensory conditions are altered.

For example, if the patient is ambulatory you may assess adaptability of gait pattern by altering:

☐ Speed: slow, fast
☐ Sensory conditions
☐ Pattern requirement: toe walking, heel walking
☐ Balance on balance beam
☐ Accuracy: follow specified steps suggested
☐ Environment (crowded, obstacles, different floor surfaces)

Scoring for adaptability:
0 = Unable to perform or significant deterioration in motor pattern
1 = Minimal or moderate deterioration in motor pattern
2 = Performs motor pattern with good selectivity, speed, and adaptability

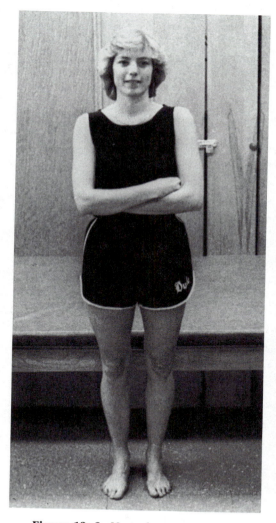

Figure 19–3. Normal stance, eyes open.

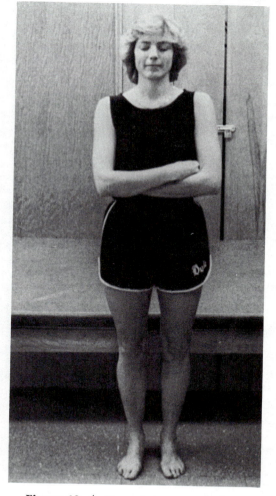

Figure 19–4. Normal stance, eyes closed.

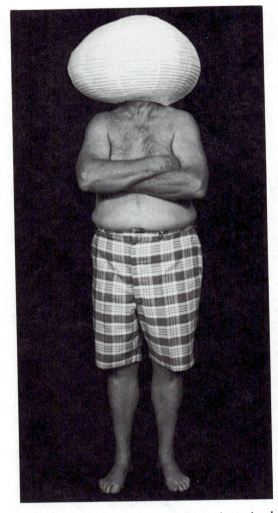

Figure 19–5. Normal stance, wearing visual dome.

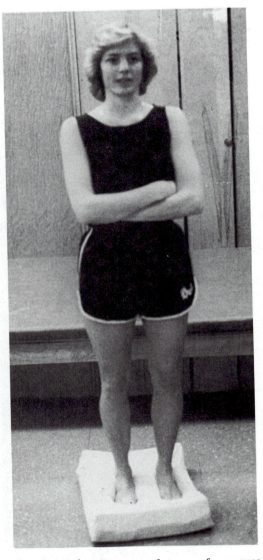

Figure 19–6. Stance on foam surface, eyes open.

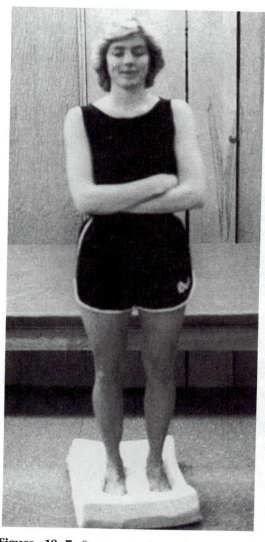

Figure 19–7. Stance on foam surface, eyes closed.

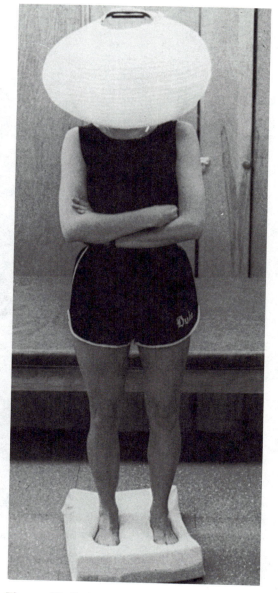

Figure 19–8. Stance on foam surface, wearing visual dome.

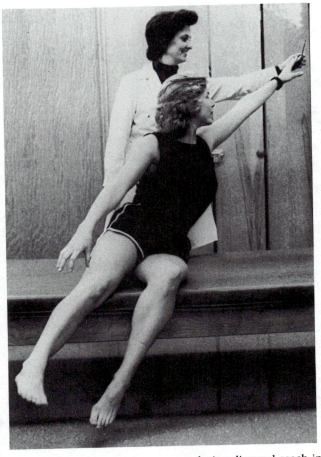

Figure 19–9. Normal postural responses during diagonal reach in sitting.

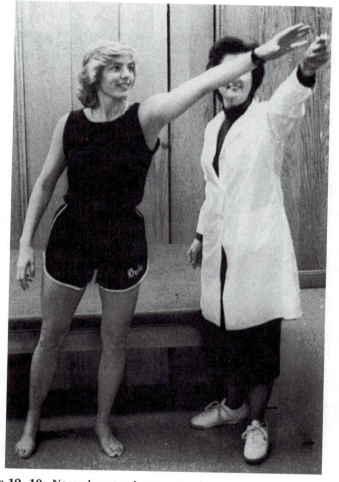

Figure 19–10. Normal postural responses during diagonal reach in standing.

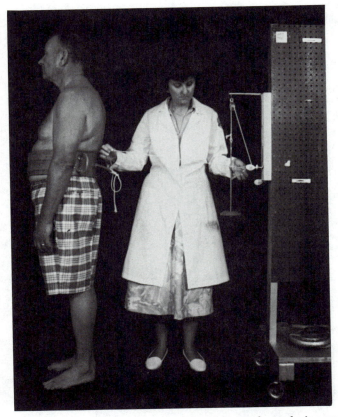

Figure 19–11. Pulley weight system to deliver destabilizing force during postural stress test.

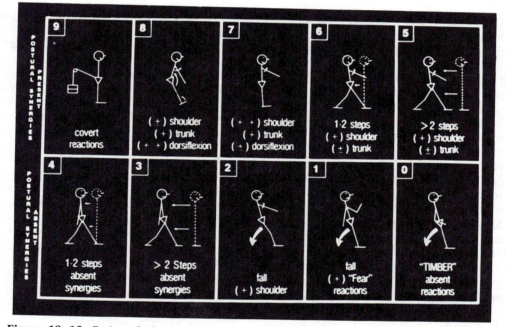

Figure 19–12. Rating of adaptive balance strategies. (From Wolfsen et al.[16] with permission.)

Chapter 20

Occupational Therapy Evaluation

BARBARA ZOLTAN, M.A., O.T.R.

The occupational therapist treating head trauma patients is presented with a complex, challenging patient population. Head trauma, by virtue of its diffuse nature, results in a broad constellation of residual problems with no patients presenting the same clinical picture. The therapist therefore must rely on a diverse repertoire of theoretical constructs, observation, evaluation, and treatment techniques as guides in developing individualized, quality treatment programs. No matter what specific techniques are used, the ultimate goal of treatment is increased function.

This chapter is solely devoted to occupational therapy evaluation techniques. (For additional information on occupational therapy treatment of head injury, the reader is referred to Chapters 24 and 25 and references 1 through 3.) Although no two head injury patients are exactly alike, guidelines and rationale for evaluation and treatment do exist. For purposes of evaluation and treatment, for instance, the patient may fall into two general categories—low-level and high-level. The first- or lower-level patient has been termed "primary"[1] or "semicomatose," as well as being described by response level (i.e., generalized response, localized response, and so on).[4]

No matter what terminology is used, the low-level patient will exhibit decreased level of awareness, as well as severe motor, language, cognitive, perceptual, visual, behavioral, and/or functional deficits. The patient at this level would be appropriate for a "coma/progressive rehabilitation program."[5]

When the patient is able to interact actively with his or her environment, even though perhaps inconsistently or inappropriately, the patient progresses to a more advanced clinical level requiring different evaluation and treatment techniques. The patient at this level may have visual, perceptual, motor, cognitive, or behavioral deficits; however, these deficits are not sufficient to render the patient completely functionally dependent.

Occupational therapy evaluation techniques and procedures will differ depending on the patient's level of functioning. The previously described general categories of patients provide a framework for occupational therapy evaluation needs. It behooves the therapist, however, to always remain cognizant that the head trauma patient falls into and progresses on a continuum. The patient may display any number or degree of deficits in a variety of combinations.

The remainder of this chapter describes the techniques of occupational therapy evaluation for both levels of head trauma patients just described. The general evaluation categories described will include visual, perceptual motor, motor, sensorimotor, oral motor, mobility, functional cognitive, and functional. Specific areas within each category are also discussed.

LOWER-LEVEL PATIENT

Motor Picture

Evaluation of the patient's motor picture includes the following: postural reflexes, head and total body control, muscle tone, coordination, active movement, and joint range of motion.

Postural Reflexes

The presence of abnormal postural reflexes is probable. Observed reflexes can include decerebrate or decorticate rigidity (or a combination of or fluctuating between both),[6] positive supporting, asymmetrical tonic neck reflex, symmetrical tonic neck reflex, tonic labyrinthine reflex, extensor thrust, decreased equilibrium, righting and protective reactions, and/or associated reactions. The occupational therapist evaluates the level of integration of these and other reflexes through structured observations and formal reflex testing.[8] Poor integration of primitive reflexes will result in decreased rotational movements, decreased trunk segmentation, postural insecurity, and decreased isolated movement.[9] Table 20–1 outlines observation of the presenting problem, the reflex responsible for the observed problem and the potential functional implications related to the reflex.[1]

Head/Total Body Control

Abnormal reflexes and tone, as well as muscle weakness, will affect head control. In addition, brainstem damage prevents the necessary stimulation to the carotid sinus to regulate tone in antigravity muscles. Trunk control or musculature will be altered by these same underlying deficits. The evaluation of head, neck, and trunk control should be carried out in a number of positions throughout the day. Assessment is done through direct observation during static and dynamic activities as well as through therapist feeling of changes in tone with positional change, static positioning, and testing for righting or equilibrium reactions. The

Table 20–1. ABNORMAL POSTURAL REFLEX MECHANISM

Observation	Reflex	Functional Implication
Severe plantar flexion, clawing of toes, inversion of ankle	Positive supporting reaction—extensor tone predominates	Cannot bear weight without facilitating extensor pattern; poor balance reactions with rigid limb, small base of support for foot
Neglect of one side and head off to right or left	ATNR—increased extensor tone on jaw (preferred) side and increased flexor tone on skull (neglected) Rule out visual-perceptual deficits	Prevents reach, grasp, and midline activity, imbalance of muscle tone, decreasing selective movement, mostly in upper extremities
Severe flexor spasticity of upper extremities, severe extensor tone of lower extremities	STNR—flexed head increases flexor tone of upper extremities and extensor tone of lower extremities and vice versa	Will affect coordination, reciprocal movements, total body function; can develop contractures; decreased ability to bear weight on upper extremities in transfers
Severe extensor spasticity and adduction of lower extremities when supine in bed	TLR—extensor tone predominates in supine and flexor tone in prone (depends on position of head in space)	Cannot roll over (i.e., bend leg to roll or bring shoulder forward to roll), decreased mobility, sitting, and transfers; cannot bear weight on lower extremities
Increased spasticity in arm while ambulating	Associated reactions—increased spasticity in some part of the body produced by forceful activity of another part	Functional activities, such as writing, and dressing and other purposeful movements of normal hand can increase flexor spasticity of affected hand

Adapted from Zoltan and Rykman,[1] with permission.

therapist should also remember that the patient's level of awareness will have a direct effect on his head and trunk control.

Range of Motion

Loss of range of motion at one or more joints is common in the head trauma patient. The brain's failure to inhibit abnormal postural reflexes and the patient's increased tone can result in joint contractures and deformities. The comatose patient who is immobilized for an extended period often develops heterotopic ossification and calcification. It is therefore crucial for the occupational therapist to assess range of motion in detail through goniometry measurements. The therapist must become aware of and control for potential loss of range of motion as soon after the onset of injury as possible.

Muscle Tone

Normal muscle tone, or the resistance a muscle presents to stretch, is a continuous state of mild muscle contraction.[10] Abnormally high or low muscle tone will result in impaired functional abilities and general joint and mobility problems.

Disorders of muscle tone that the head injury patient may exhibit are flaccidity, spasticity, and/or rigidity. The patient may be flaccid at one joint and rigid at another. The occupational therapist must also remember that the patient's muscle tone pattern is constantly fluctuating and therefore requires ongoing evaluation.

The occupational therapist can evaluate muscle tone through passive movement or quick stretching of muscles,[11] and/or through patient observation and handling before, during, and after a given treatment procedure.

When using the passive movement method, spasticity will be characterized by a portion of free range of movement, a strong muscle contraction, followed by free movement with continued stretch.[11]

Rigidity—simultaneous contractions of agonist and antagonist muscles—is characterized by increased resistance to passive stretch throughout the entire range of motion.[12]

An additional method of tone evaluation

is through repeated observation and feeling of changes in tone throughout transitional movements or dynamic activities.[7, 13] The therapist observes and feels postural changes, compensation patterns, and abnormal movement patterns before, during, and after an activity. This method of tone evaluation is becoming popular with today's therapists.

No matter what method of evaluation the occupational therapist employs, it is crucial to indicate what specific type of tone problem the patient displays, as the underlying mechanisms and proposed treatment will differ depending on the specific problem. (For additional information on muscle tone evaluation, the reader is referred to references 1, 2, 3, 7, and 13.)

Sensorimotor Picture

The sensorimotor evaluation of the semicomatose patient identifies what sensory input or modality elicits a patient response or reaction. This evaluation establishes whether the patient is able to respond to his or her environment on even the most basic level. Tactile, olfactory, gustatory, auditory, visual, and kinesthetic senses are all evaluated. General guidelines for evaluation are provided by Zoltan and Rykman[1] as follows*:

Pain
Evaluate for reponse to pinprick on upper and lower extremities and face. Is the response generalized or localized? Assess whether the response is away from, toward, delayed, or absent.

Deep Pain
Pinch the patient on the leg, arm, or neck and note response (same as for pain), or put pressure on fingernail with a hard object like a pen.

Oral Area
Refer to testing of oral reflexes (Table 20–2). If patient is prone to seizures, placing ice on lips can set off seizures.

Olfactory
See if the patient can be aroused with noxious odors. Watch out for rebound phe-

---

*Reproduced with permission from C.V. Mosby Co., St. Louis, Missouri.

Table 20–2. ORAL REFLEXES

Area Evaluated	Age	Function	Stimulus	Response
Face	Birth to life	Appropriate level of sensitivity allows for touch awareness. Motor component allows for food handling and expression	Pressure to perioral area and temples. Functional muscle test	Appropriate toleration of pressure; isolate muscle function coordination evaluation
Tongue	Birth 4–6 mo 10–12 mo	Tongue elevation. Lateralization. Tip elevation; moves and locates food in mouth; directs food back in mouth to be swallowed	Feeding cortical command; manually palpate with index finger or rubber seizure stick	Elevation; lateralization, tip elevation, rapid lateralization
Soft palate	Birth to life	Elevation; allows food to escape nasal cavity	Light touch on lateral portion of soft palate	Soft palate elevation
Rooting	Birth to 3–5 mo	Assists in locating food source	Touch on corner of lip or cheek	Rooting reflex can cause possible impedance of normal or motor function; head turned toward stimulus, open mouth, and tongue slightly protracted. Sustained reflexive
Bite	Nonreflexive after 3–5 mo	Allows introduction of food and leads to chewing	Padded tongue blade or rubber seizure stick on patient's tongue, gum, and tooth surfaces	Sucking with buccinator and orbicularis oris compressing; subsequent swallow
Sucking and swallowing	Birth to 3–5 mo	Initial intake of food; sucking followed by swallowing	Nipple; straws of various diameters	Swallowing
Swallowing	Birth to life	Food intake of solids and fluids; nutrition	Stretch digastric and geniohyoid muscles; depress spoon or tongue blade half way back on tongue, introduce eyedropper full of fluid	
Coughing	Birth to life	Prevents aspiration	Observe for voluntary or spontaneous coughing	Coughing
Gag	Birth to life	Prevents aspiration, triggers swallowing mechanism	Apply pressure on posterior third of tongue	Simultaneous head and jaw extension with rhythmical protrusion of tongue and contraction of pharynx

From Zoltan and Rykman,[1] with permission.

nomena. Noxious stimuli will have an arousing effect, whereas pleasant odors will have a calming effect. Various smells may be used to arouse the patient before a treatment session.

Gustatory

Investigate response to taste. This can be used as a stimulation technique or for working on the oral feeding mechanisms. For example, sour tastes help with lip pursing, which in turn helps with sucking. This area is mentioned because the patient may need to be aroused to adequately assess level of awareness.

Auditory

Use a bell, jingle keys, clap hands, or simply talk to see of the patient responds to sound. Note if the patient turns the head or eyes toward the sound, or if there is merely a startle response. Note if response is generalized, localized, delayed, or absent. Abnormal postural reflex mechanisms may prevent the patient from responding. Positioning should be optimal.

Tactile

Note if there is any response to touch, rubbing, vibration, or different textures. Response could be the same as for auditory stimulation. Fine tactile discrimination cannot be assessed with the patient with head injury at the lower level, but responses can be observed to combine with observations of other responses to derive a clinical picture.

For all areas of sensorimotor evaluation, note whether the patient's response is positive, negative, or neutral. Also note whether the response is delayed, generalized, localized, and/or purposeful. (For additional information on sensorimotor evaluation, the reader is referred to reference 9.)

Active Movement

Related to the patient's tone, joint mobility, reflex mechanisms, and strength is the degree and quality of active movement. The head injury patient with poorly integrated reflexes and tone deficits will display limited isolated active movements. It is likely that movements will be synergistic in nature. The key then for the occupational therapist is to evaluate not only the presence of active movement but also the quality of this movement.

The patient's active movement is evaluated in all positions and planes of movement and observed on an automatic, or subcortical level as well as a cortical level. Each joint is analyzed separately as the patient may have active isolated control at one joint and synergistic movement at another. The degree of stability and mobility around the joint is analyzed with and without intervention. In addition, how the present degree of active movement affects and relates to functional activities is assessed. The following documentation examples are provided to illustrate the key components of an active movement evaluation. All cases evaluate upper extremity movement with each patient displaying a different level of recovery.

SAMPLE SELECTIVE MOVEMENT EVALUATIONS

Example 1

RUE: Sitting—Exhibits severe increased tone in shoulder girdle, with abnormal movement patterns consisting of scapular retraction, shoulder elevation and abduction, and elbow flexion. Patient compensates for decreased proximal control with trunk elongation on the right. Distal hand function is partially selective, with only gross release present. Patient unable to use right hand functionally.

Goals: 1. Mobilize trunk and shoulder girdle in preparation for minimal assist rolling.

2. Distal grasp and prehension tabletop activities with proximal stabilization and inhibition.

Example 2

LUE: Sitting—Full selective movement proximally. Moderately increased flexor tone in wrist and fingers which limits hand function to level of a gross assist to dominant right hand.

Goal: Decrease flexor tone of wrist and fingers sufficient for patient to increase left hand use to effective function assist in bilateral activities (i.e., washing dishes, opening/closing containers, and so on)

Example 3:

RUE: Sitting—Severe hypotonus in shoulder girdle, minimum increased flexor tone in elbow, wrist, and fingers. Patient able to effect and put to functional use all grasp and prehension patterns. Fine motor manipulation skills are performed with decreased speed and accuracy. In gravity eliminated plane patient able to use hand as a functional assist, i.e., bend over to put sock and shoe on.

Goals: 1. Proximal stabilization with distal fine motor manipulation activities.

2. Monitor positioning needs of shoulder.

Coordination

As the lower-level patient begins to initiate movement, problems with gross or fine motor coordination may become evident. The patient's incoordination may be caused by primitive reflexes or abnormal tone as previously described. In addition, a primary cause of incoordination in the head trauma patient is ataxia.

Ataxia is characterized by errors in direction and rate of movement. The patient may display disturbances in posture and balance, gait, speech, eye movement, and extremity movement as a result of ataxia. The patient may also display dysmetria (difficulty with limb placement during voluntary motion) or dysdiadokinesia (decreased ability for rapid alternating movements) and/or movement decomposition (segmental movements rather than in one smooth pattern).[3]

The evaluation of coordination with the lower-level patient is restricted to clinical observation rather than formal standardized testing. The occupational therapist observes for coordination deficits in all positions and transitional movements and in all planes of movement, before, during, and after therapeutic intervention. If the patient reaches a level at which beginning activities of daily living (ADL) are appropriate, coordination is evaluated during these tasks. For the higher-level patient, standardized evaluations may be used.

GROSS VISUAL SKILLS

Basic oculomotor skills should be evaluated with the patient in the sitting position with the head upright. If required, provide positioning equipment to help the patient maintain head control. The areas to assess in the lower-level patient are attentiveness, tracking (ocular pursuits), and visual field deficits or neglect.

Attentiveness—Note if the patient focuses on bright objects, pictures, or people.

Note not only what the patient attends to, but for how long.

Tracking—Note if the patient can follow a moving bright object. Evaluate all planes of movement (up/down, side to side, diagonal and rotatory). Note completeness and quality of eye movement (i.e., nystagmus, jerkiness, and/or delayed response).

Visual Fields/Neglect—Although the integrity of the patient's fields or the presence of visual neglect cannot be specifically evaluated in the low-level patient, the therapist should observe any differences in response between body sides.

Oral Bulbar Status

Any or all oral reflexes may be impaired as a result of head trauma. These deficits will result in impaired or no ability to eat, drink, or speak. The clinical evaluation of oral reflexes is presented in Table 20–2. In addition to these reflexes, the therapist should evaluate jaw stability, facial sensitivity, and breathing.

The occupational therapist must have a clear understanding of the normal anatomy and functional phases of swallowing as well as the effects of different-level food consistencies on the patient's oral bulbar status. (For additional information on these and other areas related to oral bulbar evaluation, the reader is referred to references 1, 9, and 14.)

In addition to the occupational therapist's clinical evaluation, videofluoroscopy may be of considerable value.[14, 15] Videofluoroscopy is basically a modified barium swallow that can reveal mobility problems in the oral cavity and pharynx.[14] Any head injury patient who "... is aspirating, whose swallowing disorder is of pharyngeal origin, or who has a pharyngeal component, should be referred for a videofluoroscopic study."[14]

Level of Awareness

The low-level head injury patient's level of awareness will affect all other categories of functioning. Fluctuations in active movement, head control, or the ability to participate in functional tasks are often related to concurrent fluctuations in level of awareness.

The low-level patient's level of awareness is assessed through structured clinical observation throughout the day with input from nursing and any additional team members. The assessment should include levels in both structured and unstructured environments in all positions (i.e., in wheelchair, bed). The patient's level of awareness may change significantly just by going from a lying to a sitting position. As noted in the sensorimotor evaluation portion of this chapter, evaluate changes in awareness as a result of sensory stimulation from specific sensory modalities. Also note changes in awareness when family members are present. Often, the patient's parents or spouse can elicit an increased level of awareness when the therapist cannot. If this is the case, utilize family members in the evaluation and treatment process to best maximize the patient's potential. Keeping a daily log or diary filled by all team and family members is an excellent way of establishing baseline performance as well as measuring patient progress.

ADVANCED/HIGHER-LEVEL PATIENT

Motor Skills

POSTURAL REFLEXES

Although the integration of postural reflexes in the advanced patient is significantly better than in the low-level patient, more subtle deficits may be present. Most commonly existing deficits include associated reactions and residual changes in tone from the influence of tonic neck reflex (TNR), asymmetrical tonic neck reflex (ATNR), and tonic labyrinthine reflex (TLR). In addition, righting and equilibrium reactions are often delayed or functionally ineffective.

For the higher-level patient, formal reflex testing is not usually indicated. Balance and equilibrium reactions, associated reactions and any changes in tone related to primitive reflexes should be tested and observed during functional transfers, bed mobility, total body function activities, and ADL.

HEAD/TOTAL BODY CONTROL

Head control of the advanced-level patient is usually good. Total body function,

on the other hand, may be affected for basic ADL such as dressing and for higher level bending, reaching, or carrying activities. The occupational therapist assesses the patient's deficits through structured clinical observation of relevant functional and mobility tasks, and/or a formalized physical capacity evaluation.

RANGE OF MOTION

Some residual range of motion loss may be present even in higher-level patients. As with the lower-level patient, goniometric measurements are indicated. if contractures are encountered, the presence of soft tissue calcification or bony deformity must be identified by radiographic procedures.

MUSCLE TONE

Most of the problems with muscle tone that occur in the lower-level patient may also be found in the higher-level patient, although to a lesser degree. For instance, the higher-level patient may display mild or no hypertonicity in performing basic hygiene or dressing, while showing increased tone for walking, reaching, or community tasks. Tone in the high-level patient may also be assessed through the passive stretch method or through patient observation and feeling during mobility and functional tasks. The main difference between the evaluation of tone for the two patient levels lies in the activities in which the patient can participate.

ACTIVE MOVEMENT

General principles and techniques related to the active movement evaluation of the low-level patient hold true for the high-level patient as well. Usually the major additional component of the high-level patient's evaluation is the hand function evaluation. The therapist evaluates whether the patient has isolated control of gross grasp/release, lateral pinch, palmar prehension, and fingertip prehension.[1] The Carroll Upper Extremity Function Test can be a helpful tool in the hand function evaluation of this level patient.[16] The therapist should compare the patient's hand function both with and without provision of proximal stability. As the patient progresses, the hand function evaluation should include measures of object manipulation skills and fine finger dexterity.

COORDINATION

Coordination deficits, as outlined for the lower-level patient, may also be present to a lesser degree in the high-level patient. Structured clinical observation of incoordination as previously described is indicated. In addition, the high-level patient can be given more formal standardized tests. For upper extremity/hand coordination—for instance, the Jebsen Hand Function Test,[17] Purdue Pegboard,[18] or Minnesota Rate of Manipulation[19]—may be indicated.

MOBILITY

The areas of mobility evaluation for the high-level patient can include wheelchair mobility, bed mobility, and functional transfers. Wheelchair management and mobility includes the evaluation of skills such as locking of brakes, removal of footrests, and wheelchair propulsion both within the hospital and in the community. The bed mobility evaluation should include the assessment of skills such as rolling, scooting, and supine/sitting bed edge and vice versa. The transfer evaluation should include bed/chair to tub, toilet, furniture, and car transfers. Included in the transfer assessment is the identification of required durable medical equipment for successful task completion. For all areas of the mobility evaluation, the therapist must note how visual, perceptual, cognitive, and physical deficits affect performance.

SENSORY MOTOR

More formalized sensory testing can be administered with the higher level patient. Areas that should be tested include tactile discrimination (sharp/dull), light touch, stereognosis, temperature sense, proprioception, and kinesthesia. Impaired sensation can affect the patient's safety for ADL, such as in the kitchen, or with bathing or hygiene. Impaired proprioception and/or kinesthetic sense can affect the patient's body image or motor planning in any task. (For specific sensory testing procedures, the reader is referred to the references.[1, 2, 9.]

Gross Visual Skills

The occupational therapist should evaluate visual attentiveness, ocular pursuits, visual neglect, and visual fields. In addition, saccadic eye movements can be evaluated with the high-level patient. More formal testing of visual skills is possible with the high-level patient. In addition to gross visual skills deficits, the head injury patient may have double vision, blurred vision, decreased convergence, and nystagmus. If the patient appears to have difficulty in any of these areas, the therapist should recommend a complete eye examination. The patient's visual status will affect all other testing and therefore should be given prior to perceptual motor and cognitive evaluations. (For specific testing procedures for visual skills testing, the reader is referred to references 20 through 22.)

Perceptual Motor Evaluation

The perceptual motor evaluation should consist of testing for apraxia (all levels and types), body scheme disorders, form size and depth perception, part-whole integration, figure-ground perception, and position in space. Detailed information about these deficits is presented in Chapter 24. (For additional detailed information pertaining to the occupational therapist evaluation of these deficits, see references 20 and 21.)

Functional Cognitive Evaluation

The head injury patient may exhibit deficits in the following cognitive areas: attention, orientation, memory, initiation, planning, problem-solving, insight, mental flexibility, abstraction, calculation, and higher intellectual functions. Several disciplines may be involved in cognitive evaluation. The neuropsychologist, for instance, may administer psychometric testing. The clinical psychologist may use qualitative projective testing. The role of the occupational therapist in cognitive evaluation pertains to cognitive deficits as they relate to the patient's functional status.

The occupational therapist's main tool for functional cognitive evaluation is structured clinical observation and activity analysis. The following is an example of clinical observation/activity analysis for the cognitive skill of initiation.

Evaluation of Initiation[20]*

TEST NO. 1: CLINICAL OBSERVATION AND ACTIVITY ANALYSIS

General Guidelines for Evaluation

1. Observe the patient in a number of settings.
2. Consider the amount of structure and cueing required for initiation of activity by the patient.
3. Establish functional baseline measures. Consider the frequency and severity of the problem as it relates to function. Select relevant functional areas or tasks as the basis for evaluation and reassessment.

SPECIFIC AREAS AND QUESTIONS TO CONSIDER AND EVALUATE

1. Are there any associated behavioral problems, such as flat or blunted affect? Behavioral outbursts? Disinhibition?
2. Is the patient's behavior generally passive? Does the patient respond passively to questions or suggestions?
3. What does the patient do during the day? Does someone have to organize activities for him or her?
4. What, if any, activities can the patient self-initiate without cueing or structure?
5. What cueing method or sensory modality appears to be the most effective? For example, do tactile or kinesthetic cues work better than visual or auditory cues?
6. Is the patient aware that he or she has an initiation problem? Does the patient accept the problem when it is pointed out?
7. Is an associated attentional or memory problem affecting initiation abilities? To improve validity, rule out decreased attention, processing, language, apraxia, and psychologically based (versus organic) depression as causes of poor performance.

Such structured analysis can be used by the occupational therapist for all cognitive skills. (For additional information on cognitive evaluation, the reader is referred to references 20, 23, and 24.)

ACTIVITIES OF DAILY LIVING EVALUATION

As soon as the patient initiates active movement and can interact purposefully with the environment, the patient's hygiene, feeding, and dressing skills can be evaluated. A complete kitchen and homemaking evaluation should also be initiated when appropriate. The therapist evaluates how the patient's motor, perceptual, visual, and/or cognitive deficits affect functional independence. For instance, if the patient cannot put on a shirt, is it due to apraxia, visual neglect, or perhaps distractibility? The degree and type of physical assist and verbal cueing required for task completion must be noted. As the patient progresses, the therapist should initiate community skills, driving, and prevocational evaluations.

Community Skills

The community skills evaluation should range from the lowest level (e.g., the assessment of basic money handling skills) to the highest level (e.g., grocery or department store shopping and budgeting tasks). The evaluation should take place initially within the hospital and progress to graded levels of community settings. The amount and type of physical and verbal assistance required is noted, incorporating the patient's physical, visual, perceptual, and cognitive abilities.

Prevocational

When comprehensive disability and physical capacity evaluations have been completed and the patient has plateaued in functional independence, the prevocational evaluation may be initiated with the higher-level patient. The therapist can use standardized tools such as the Tower,[25] Microtower, or Valpar[26] system, as well as job simulation tasks whenever possible. Work site evaluations should also be initiated and relevant information elicited from the patient's employer or supervisor.

---

*Reproduced with permission from Slack, Inc., Thorofare, NJ.

Driver Evaluation

In many facilities, it is the conjoint role of the occupational therapist and the adaptive driving instructor to share an active involvement in the head injury patient's driving evaluation. The evaluation begins in the hospital with a complete disability assessment including skills that relate specifically to driving. For example, the patient's depth perception would be evaluated with a road sign test, and figure-ground ability may be tested with a driving scene.

In addition to the disability evaluation, the therapist must perform a comprehensive medical history including medications, seizures, and the like. Information on premorbid driving habits and records should also be obtained.

If deemed appropriate, after the in-hospital evaluation, the patient should be taken for a road test. The influence of physical, visual-perceptual, and cognitive abilities on the patient's ability to drive safely and effectively are assessed. The need for adaptive driving steering devices is also identified.

SUMMARY

The preceding information is provided as an overview and basic rationale for occupational therapy evaluation techniques. Subsequent to the clinical evaluation, the therapist establishes an individualized treatment program with the final goal of optimal function. As previously mentioned, the head injury patient presents a diverse clinical picture requiring a specialized evaluation and treatment approach. With this in mind, the reader is encouraged to seek out additional resources to refine knowledge and skill level.

REFERENCES

1. Zoltan B, and Rykman, D: Head injury in adults. In Lorraine Pedrette (ed): Occupational Therapy: Practice Skills for Physical Dysfunction, ed 2. CV Mosby, St Louis, 1985.
2. Trombley, KA and Scott, AD: Occupational Therapy for Physical Dysfunction, ed 2. Williams and Wilkins, Baltimore, 1983.
3. Umphred, D: Neurological Rehabilitation. CV Mosby, St Louis, 1985.
4. Rancho levels of Cognitive Functioning. The Professional Staff Association of Rancho Los Amigos Hospital, Downey, Ca, 1979.
5. Program Title for Meadowbrook Neurologic Care Center, 340 Northlake Drive, San Jose, CA 95117.
6. Bricolo, A et al: Decerebrate rigidity in acute head injury. J Neurosurg 47:680, 1977.
7. Bobath, B: Adult Hemiplegia: Evaluation and Treatment, ed 2. William Heinemann, Medical Books Ltd, London, 1978.
8. Fiorentino, M: Reflex Testing, Methods for Evaluating CNS Development, ed 2. Charles C Thomas, Springfield, IL, 1973.
9. Farber, S: Neurorehabilitation: A Multisensory Approach. WB Saunders, Philadelphia, PA, 1982.
10. Pedretti, L: Evaluation of muscle tone and coordination. In L. Pedretti (Ed): Practice Skills for Physical Dysfunction. CV Mosby, St Louis, 1985.
11. Trombley, KA and Scott, AD: Evaluation of motor control. In Occupational Therapy for Physical Dysfunction, ed 2. Williams and Wilkins, Baltimore, 1983.
12. De Myer, W: Technique of the Neurologic Examination: A Programmed Text, ed 2. McGraw Hill, New York, 1974.
13. Davies, P: Steps to Follow. Springer-Verlag, Berlin, 1985.
14. Logemann, JL: Evaluation and Treatment of Swallowing Disorders. College Hill Press, San Diego, Ca, 1983.
15. Linden, P and Siebens, AA: Dysphagia: Predicting laryngeal penetration. Arch Phys Med Rehabil 64(6):98, 1983.
16. Carroll, D: A quantitative test of upper extremity function. J Chron Dis 18:479, 1965.
17. Jebsen, RH et al: An objective and standardized test of hand function. Arch Phys Med Rehabil 50:311, 1969.
18. Purdue Pegboard: Examiner's Manual, Chicago, Science Research Associates, Inc, 1968.
19. Minnesota Rate of Manipulation Tests: Examiner's Manual. Circle Pines, MN, American Guidance Service, Inc, 1969.
20. Zoltan, B, Siev, E and Freishtat, B: Perceptual and Cognitive Dysfunction In the Adult Stroke Patient, Rev Ed. Slack, Inc, Thorofare, NJ, 1986.
21. Zoltan, B et al: Perceptual Motor Evaluation for Head Injured and Other Neurologically Impaired Adults, Santa Clara County, CA, 1984.
22. Lieberman, S, Cohen, AH and Rubin, J: NYSOA K-D test. J Am Optom Assoc 54(7):631, 1983.
23. Lezak, MD: Neuropsychological Assessment. Oxford University Press, New York, 1976.
24. Wilson, BA and Moffat, N (eds): Clinical Management of Memory Problems, Aspen Systems Corp, Rockville, MD, 1984.
25. Tower System: Evaluator's Manual. I.C.D. Rehabilitation and Research Center, New York, 1967.
26. Valpar Component Work Samples Series, Valpar Corp, Tucson, AZ, 1974–1977.

Chapter 21

Speech and Language Assessment

MICHAEL E. GROHER, Ph.D.

THE RATIONALE

Success in the assessment of speech and language deficits following traumatic head injury depends on the clinician's recognition that *speech* and *language* by themselves are only parts of the communication process; speech refers to the motor aspects of production, while language is the sum of its phonologic, syntactic, and semantic constituents. An individual may be able to articulate perfectly three consecutive sentences that do not violate semantic or syntactic rules yet be unable to communicate with the listener. Conversely, the person may not demonstrate any audible speech or linguistic form yet be able to communicate successfully with the listener by deliberate gesture, an eyeblink, a facial expression, or a body movement. The process of communication spans these extremes. In a broad sense, success in communication is a reflection of how well one relates to the environment in solving problems. In the human, articulated speech and language often are the most usual vehicles used in this relationship, even in so-called tasks of nonlinguistic problem-solving. Experiences with this environment are coded in memory for future use. Expressions of this experience surface through language as sentences that, in the normal brain, connect logically to formulate thoughts for use in solving the daily challenges the environment presents. Individuals with traumatic brain injury often fail to communicate effectively with the environment, and the speech and language assessment of head injured patients needs to delineate those factors that are responsible for such failure.

This approach to evaluation is tied closely with the need to understand the components of speech and language as part of the patient's total cognitive structure. A measure of the patient's cognitive skills, of which speech and language are only a part, should be highly correlated with the ability to be a successful communicator, regardless of the mode of expression. In this context, it becomes important to gather data that will describe not only the patient's motor speech and linguistic skills, but also his or her ability to respond and relate to the environment. Adopting the philosophic approach of measuring the patient's *communication effectiveness* (the ability to solve problems presented by the environment), rather than just speech and language, will allow the clinician to describe more accurately the wide range of potential disability seen in this patient population. This group ranges from totally uncommunicative patients who respond inconsistently to familiar sounds to patients with well-articulated speech and seemingly normal linguistic skills who find it difficult to hold a job because they are unable to follow instructions or communicate effectively with their coworkers.

The extensive range of functional disability forces the examiner to be familiar with a wide variety of measures and approaches to evaluation that can be applied at bedside, in the clinic, or in the patient's home or workplace. At bedside, the clinician must focus on aspects of cognition that are prerequisite to successful linguistic performance. Those aspects include attention to and discrimination among visual and tactile inputs, assignment of meaning to these inputs, memory of these stimuli, and any attempts to react to these stimuli. In the clinic, the clinician will need concurrent documentation of how the patient's cognitive deficits, particularly attentional, memory, and perceptual disability, will affect emerging linguistic skills. In the patient's home or workplace the clinician must have the tools to measure the patient's ability to use linguistic skills to solve daily problems. Each stage of recovery will dictate the use of different approaches to measurement if one is interested in documenting the patient's communicative capacities. Clearly, the typical standardized aphasia language battery will be insensitive to documentation of the patient with severe injury who responds consistently only to his or her name; nor will it be useful in explaining why the patient cannot solve thinking problems utilizing language skills that are judged to be syntactically and semantically sound.

Because of the variability in severity of communication disabilities and in the amount and rate of recovery seen in this population, the examiner needs to have an assessment protocol and tools that allow for maximum amounts of flexibility. Measures must be chosen with the goal of describing as accurately as possible the patient's communicative effectiveness at any particular time during recovery. Comparisons of change in performance over time in head injury patients are most meaningful when the comparison focuses on change in the individual's own test performance rather than on the performance in comparison to another group of traumatically injured patients. The volatility of change seen in this population makes documentation of individual change a more utilitarian measure. The assessment protocol not only should describe the patient's communication deficits and their severity, but also should be biased toward discovering what particular pattern of conditions in the environment facilitate the patient's communication with that environment. Documentation of these conditions will provide the data for treatment. The inseparable relationship between the cognitive requisites for effective communication and the language needed to accomplish it often dictates the types of measures needed and how one interprets those measures. As Hagen[1] has pointed out, in the assessment of patients with traumatic head injury, there is a distinct need to discover the type and level of nonlinguistic cognitive dysfunction in order to adequately interpret the linguistic disturbance. If one is to provide a comprehensive assessment of the communicative intent and strategies of the traumatically injured, the evaluation, regardless of severity of involvement should be flexible enough to document linguistic competencies while manipulating cognitive demands such as speed of processing and/or dependence on memory. Hagen[1] correctly asserts that an understanding of a patient's linguistic potentials is achieved best if the assessment of communication focuses on eight processes of cognition:

1. Attentional abilities including alertness, awareness, attention span, and selective attention
2. Discrimination of touch, sight, and sound
3. Temporal ordering
4. Retention span, including immediate, recent, and remote memory
5. Categorization
6. Association and integration
7. Analysis and synthesis
8. The ability to maintain sequential, goal-directed behavior

The information (nonlinguistic and linguistic) that can be gathered from both standardized and nonstandardized measures that sample each one of these cognitive processes should provide the examiner with a description of how well the patient can communicate with a changing environment, which in turn will provide an index of his or her communication efficiency. It is this reciprocal interaction between linguistic and nonlinguistic skills that best describes the problems of the traumatically injured.[1]

Because of the variability in the cognitive and linguistic severity levels and recovery rates, and because this potentially can demand a wide range of clinical observations and psychometric tests, the assessment of the patient's communication effectiveness will be most useful if the data are interpreted with the combined efforts of the speech/language pathologist, neuropsychologist, and the attending medical staff.

THE BEDSIDE EVALUATION

Evaluation of the patient's communicative effectiveness in the acute stage of injury not only can provide important prognostic information,[2] but also can facilitate the patient's medical management and recovery. If the treatment team is aware of the patient's communicative strengths, medical care is facilitated because the patient can more easily cooperate with requests, and through proper input structure may be able to communicate basic needs. These strengths also can be reinforced in a coordinated effort by approaching the patient in a similar manner. For instance, if the patient responds best to gesture and short auditory input from the left visual field, then this fact should be communicated to staff and family. In time, the treatment for the patient's communication deficits may be that he or she reponds in a similar manner to stimuli presented from the right. The benefits from the knowledge of how best to communicate with the patient, therefore, can serve as the treatment the patient will receive while bedridden.

The information that is gathered at bedside will be dictated by the patient's ability to cooperate. The choice of assessment tool also is dependent on the patient's level of alertness and/or willingness to cooperate and length of attention span. Data will be gathered from repeated observations of the patient's responses to sensory input, attempts at motor initiation, and scores on psychometric batteries from both formal and nonformal evaluations of communication.

THE SENSORY/MOTOR END ORGAN

Evaluation of the acutely ill patient must begin with a basic assessment of the integrity of the end organ sensory and motor mechanisms needed for the comprehension and motor expression of language. This includes evaluation of hearing, vision, and limbs (for expressive gesture), together with attention to the cooperative processes of articulation, phonation, and respiration needed for intelligible speech production. What can be accomplished in this assessment and the reliability of data gathered will depend on the patient's ability to cooperate. However, even for patients who are unwilling or unable to cooperate, inferences about end organ integrity can be made.

Audiometric screening of hearing can be accomplished at bedside without the patient's total cooperation. Observations of the patient's eyes or facial expressions when sound is introduced can provide a gross measure of attention to noise at known sound pressure levels. Cessation of agitated movement when sound is introduced also can serve as an indicator of cochlear integrity. If needed, and if the patient's behavior is not too erratic, evoked potentials to sound can be elicited in a quiet environment, thus providing an objective measure of hearing. The patient's ability to localize sound from hand clapping or bell ringing, by turning the head or by the cessation of movement, is a gross measure of hearing. Comparison of responses from the patients right and left should be made.

Whether or not the patient has the motoric ability to gesture as a mode of communication can be assessed by observations of volitional and nonvolitional limb movement. Attention should be given to coordination and planned intention and in what circumstances movement is most regular and purposeful.

Integrity of the visual system is measured by systematic observations of the patient's reaction to light, threat, and ability to track moving objects. Retinal abnormality is assessed by ophthalmologic inspection. Reaction to familiar faces and objects also can provide basic information about visual integrity.

Objective measures of respiratory capacities needed to effect phonation are difficult to obtain. However, patients who are receiving respiratory supports, or those with high cervical lesions with vital capacities less than 2 liters may not be able to be heard because of poor respiratory support for speech. Those who are tracheotomized will have the further complication of an open airway. Nonvolitional, irregular respiratory patterns also may confound the use of adequate vocal volume needed for attempts at volitional speech. Phonatory capacity can be assessed by documentation of vocalizations made in unresponsive states to noxious or theatening stimuli. Severely reduced respiratory capacities may preclude phonatory assessment even if the vocal folds are intact. Tracheostomy prevents adequate evaluation of the patient's ability to coordinate respiration with phonation unless the patient can cooperate to occlude the tube and attempt to phonate. Long-term intubation may be suggestive of phonatory incompetence; however, visual inspection of glottic and subglottic structure can be accomplished at bedside to rule out any secondary traumatic effects such as granuloma or paralysis. Inferences of end organ strength can be made by observations of the support structure needed, such as the tongue, facial muscles, velum, and oropharynx. Inability to manage secretions and/or extensive atrophy of structure is suggestive of severe weakness that would compromise speech production.

INFORMAL COMMUNICATION MEASURES

Informal measures of communication made at bedside are attempts to establish the nature of the cognitive deficits as they affect communication. They should be done after peripheral motor and sensory systems have been assessed because pathology in end organs will affect the approach to the evaluation of the cortical integrity and, if not explored fully, will contaminate test interpretation.

Because of characteristically short attention spans and fluctuating levels of consciousness, informal measures must be designed to gather a maximum amount of information in a short period of time. Most often, their design will not only sample linguistic skills directly but also focus on cognitive prerequisites for language. As language recovers, direct formalized assessment batteries can be used.

Inherent to the design of informal measures is that they have the flexibility to sample a wide variety of behaviors, detailing the circumstances of the patients best communicative performance. The test should be easy to administer, using few props and/or testing booklets. Ease of administration is important in establishing the reliability of the measure, since multiple samples of performance must be done by different examiners in an effort to determine a level of communication competence and to document recovery. Because of fluctuation of performance, multiple measures done frequently will provide the most reliable data

base upon which statements of recovery and prognosis can be made.

Informal assessment should begin by careful observation of the patient's physiologic status, formulating assumptions about cognitive/linguistic function that might assist in guiding more detailed evaluation or in forming an immediate diagnostic impression. In this circumstance, evidence for localizable deficits should be sought. For instance, observation of unilateral hemiplegia would help localize pathology to the right or left brain. Assumptions regarding the possibility of more linguistic disorders (left brain) versus the presence of perceptual disturbance (right brain) would follow. The presence of restraints suggests confusion and diffuse pathology, and perhaps an inability to cooperate with direct assessment. Disorders of posture manifested as neglect or denial can be suggestive of the best side to approach in assessment if inputs are to be appreciated. Differentiation between the communicative disorders associated with the vegetative state, locked-in syndrome, akinetic mutism, and mutism (see Chapter 11 for descriptions) can be made through observations of posture and the evaluation of basic language and the peripheral speech mechanism.

In uncooperative or severely impaired patients, data relative to communication prerequisites must be gathered systemically and recorded by each member of the health care team. Because each member may be gathering data, the system should be simple and kept at the bedside. Recording should focus on any environmental stimulus event such as light, touch, sound, language, or a familiar face, and the patient's response. Daily recordings (Table 21–1) are then analyzed for consistencies in pattern of response. Emerging patterns are used to document change in communicative awareness and to reinforce desired patterns for treatment. Selected behaviors such as "vocalizes to familiar faces" can be assigned numerical values after a week's gathering of data: 0 = not observed; 1 = present less than 50 percent of the time; 2 = present more than 50 percent of the time; 3 = consistently present. The nursing notes should document any signs of the patient's ability to cooperate with nursing care as an informal measure of cognition. It is particularly important to document this over time, as patients who are

Table 21–1. SAMPLE STIMULUS/RESPONSE RECORDING SHEET OF COMMUNICATIVE BEHAVIORS*

	Day 1	
	Stimulus	*Response*
AM	Hand clap, left ear	Note
	Dish fell on floor	Startled
	Turned patient	Nonintelligible vocalization
PM	Called patient's name	Opened eyes
	Flashlight at head of bed in patient's face	Tracked visually for 5 seconds
	Familiar visitor	Attempted to vocalize
	Unfamiliar visitor	Smiled
	Suctioned	Vocalized, nonintelligible
Night	Received medication	Spit, said "no"
	Changed dressing	None
	Changed dressing	Resisted, pushed hand away
	Held patient's hand	Squeezed hand in return

*Data should be kept on a 24-hour basis. Patterns of response are analyzed every week, or more often if necessary.

improving respond positively to the structure that routine nursing care provides.

Even though informal measures are not standardized, they should attempt to adhere to more structure than random recordings, especially as cognition improves. Assessment of basic arousal mechanisms should be followed by evaluation of selective attention or the ability to sustain attention to an outside stimulus. Documentation of the capability to attend is an important measure of cognitive reorganization. Responses to external stimuli should be divided into *differentiated* and *nondifferentiated*.[1] Differentiated responses are considered to indicate an improvement in cognitive function. As distinguished from undifferentiated responses, they represent the patient's ability to inhibit responses to stimuli after the stimulus is withdrawn. Documentation of the patient's ability to initiate a response without an external stimulus is an important barometer of change, an indication of the patient's cognitive attempt to relate, rather than merely react, to the environment. As the patient begins to respond to stimuli selectively and initiate responses, the appropriateness of these responses must be judged and will serve as a measure of change.

Informal measures that seek to provide information beyond the basic arousal and discriminative level will sample a broader range of communicative capacities and generally will be hierarchically arranged in levels of abstraction. For instance, matching tasks involving common objects will precede categorization of the same objects, while matching two similar words will precede matching a word to an object. Tests that sample sequential skills should proceed from repetitive finger-tapping, to pointing to objects in order, to sequencing cards that tell a story. In patients with established verbal skills, confrontation naming and memory skills should be assessed. Use of a verbal fluency task that requires the patient to name in 60 seconds animals in a given category (i.e., farm animals) or words that begin with a specific letter is a most useful measure because it requires the cognitive manipulation of categorization within a linguistic (naming) context. Such a measure has been demonstrated to be a reliable predictor of recovery at 3 months in survivors of head injury.[3] Investigations of memory should be divided into immediate, recent, and remote; immediate memory recall is commonly tested at bedside with digit repetition, recent memory is tapped by asking the patient to enumerate the items eaten for breakfast, and remote memory is a confirmation of items from the patient's biographic past.

As cognition improves, the patient's ability to sustain attention will allow for attempts at administering more formalized screening tools. Suggested measures that sample linguistic skills as they pertain to

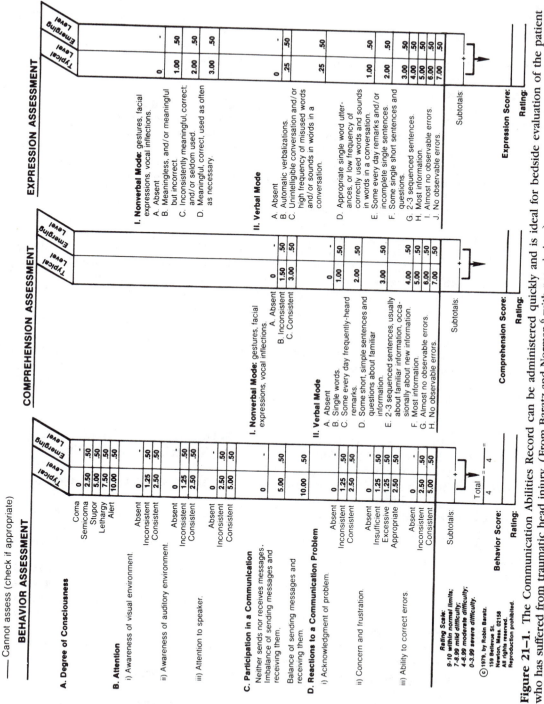

Figure 21–1. The Communication Abilities Record can be administered quickly and is ideal for bedside evaluation of the patient who has suffered from traumatic head injury. (From Baratz and Norman,[6] with permission.)

levels of cognition are the *Bedside Evaluation Screening Test* (BEST),[4] the *Aphasia Language Performance Scales* (ALPS),[5] and the *Communication Abilities Record.*[6]

The BEST is a screening test of language designed to assess communicative competencies at bedside in eight categories: conversation, expression, naming objects, describing objects, repeating sentences, pointing to objects, pointing to picture parts, and reading. Individual subtest scores and a total overall score is used for comparison to normative data on two groups of aphasics. Scores are used to rate impairment in seven categories ranging from mild to no deficit, to moderate/severe, to profound. In addition to the patient's linguisitc performance, the examiner is asked to rate various cognitive abilities such as orientation, appropriateness, pragmatics, error recognition, and speed of response. Individual subtests are designed to assess four graded levels of performance with easier tasks requiring less information or having additional cues. For instance, in "pointing to objects," the patient receives the maximum score for correctly pointing to the "thin straight nail," but is given the minimum number of points for "show me a nail." As the examiner progresses through each subtest, the patient's level of performance can be quickly established, minimizing frustration and fatigue. For most patients, the BEST can be completed in 10 to 15 minutes. This feature is particularly useful in assessing the traumatically injured because the streamlined administration assists in providing the patient with the positive reinforcement necessary to sustain attention during a bedside evaluation.

The ALPS was constructed to be used at bedside, eliciting information about communication through natural interaction between the examiner and the patient. Each linguistic category (listening, talking, reading, writing) has 10 subtest items arranged in increasing levels of complexity. The examiner is encouraged by approach and with repetition and cueing to elicit the patient's best response. Scoring is simple, and the examination is easily repeatable on a daily basis. Reliability and validity measures involving comparison to longer, more standardized measures have been reported.

Developed as a measure to quickly assess and chart cognition and language in patients

in acute care settings, the *Communication Abilities Record* rates the patient's behavior, comprehension, and expression. Ratings are obtained from descriptions of the patient's actual behaviors, rather than from elicited behavior. For instance, in the verbal mode of the expression section, response scores based on the presence of specific behaviors such as "has automatic verbalizations," "demonstrates some single short sentences and questions," and "can produce two or three sequenced sentences." The behavior section asks the examiner to rate performance in four areas that provide useful information as measures of prelinguistic competencies: consciousness, attention, participation in communication (messages sent and received), and reactions to a communication problem (acknowledgment, frustration, error recognition). Decision making in scoring is facilitated by the fact that patients can receive credit if the required behavior has just begun to emerge, yet has not fully manifested itself according to the test's criteria for that particular level. Patients are rated in each test category on a weighted 10-point scale, with 9 to 10 representing normal scores, 7 to 8.99 indicating minor impairment, 4 to 6.99 moderate difficulty, and 0 to 3.99 severe involvement (Fig. 21–1).

FORMAL ASSESSMENT OF COMMUNICATION

Standardized Measures

Test batteries used in the assessment of communication skills of aphasic adults frequently are administered in the evaluation of the linguistic competencies of the traumatically head injured patient. Batteries that are used most often include the *Minnesota Test for Differential Diagnosis of Aphasia* (MTDDA),[7] the *Boston Diagnostic Aphasia Examination* (BDAE),[8] the *Porch Index of Communicative Ability* (PICA),[9] the *Western Aphasia Battery* (WAB),[10] and the *Communicative Activities of Daily Living* (CADL).[11]

These test measures require patient cooperation while sitting in upright positions for prolonged periods of time (at least 1 hour) to obtain maximum validity. Therefore, attempts to use these measures will be most rewarding after orientation improves (predictive of increased patient cooperation)[1] and after verbal skills emerge (frequently between 1 and 6 months).[12] The value of standardized measures lies in their recognized ability to describe systematically linguistic deficits. While each test provides normative data for score comparison, most are standardized according to patients with linguistic deficits secondary to vascular rather than traumatic causative factors (see Chapter 11 for a discussion of differences in language deficits between traumatic and vascular etiologies). These batteries are limited in their sensitivity in measuring patients with severe cognitive/linguistic deficits and in their failure to adequately describe residual communication problems, especially more than 6 months after injury. As linguistic skills improve, patients frequently do well on all standardized linguistic tests except for the most difficult subtests, reducing the tests' sensitivity as diagnostic tools. Hagen[1] feels that when recovering patients reach level 7 (automatic-appropriate) on the Rancho Los Amigos Cognitive Scale, the global disturbance of language has remitted sufficiently to enable patients to do well with the categorical aspects of language that are measured by standardized aphasia batteries. Residual communication deficits in recovering patients manifest themselves more in pragmatic and problem-solving aspects of language than in tasks that specifically assess phonologic, syntactic, and semantic processes. Standardized aphasia batteries now in use sample these latter processes only and are, therefore, insensitive to the documentation of residual communication disturbance. Hagen[1] found that as patients improve they do well in the controlled testing situation imposed by standardized aphasia batteries; however, conversational and linguistic problem-solving skills remain impaired, and aphasia batteries typically do not measure or analyze these skills. Sarno,[13] however, points out that while functional communication skills may appear intact, the use of standardized measures often reveals deficits that are undetected in casual conversation.

The most comprehensive test battery, the *MTDDA* provides a broad sampling of linguistic behaviors. Because of its length, dividing the test into shorter sections is most useful with the traumatically injured and can be accomplished easily because of its design. Particularly useful are the subtests evaluating reading, writing, mathematics, and phonemic discrimination. The *PICA* can be administered in 1 hour, and its simple design and scoring system make it particularly suitable to this population. Because each patient response can be scored from 1 to 16, the PICA is able to describe not only the accuracy of the patient's response but also the quality of the response which often reflects the interplay between cognition and language. Analysis of patterns of response can reflect how the patient solves a linguistic problem. For instance, patients whose performance is characterized by the score of 10 (suggestive of an accurate response with self-corrective behavior to achieve the response) may display such behavior because they momentarily lose concentration or have associative difficulty but are able to persevere toward the correct answer. Patients who achieve many scores of 8 or 9 are capable of responding correctly, but need additional task information to do so. Patients with a predominance of scores in the 11 and 12 range have difficulty processing all of the elements of a stimulus, suggestive of associative or integrative disorders. Patients who make many errors at the beginning of each subtest often evidence difficulty in shifting topics, whereas those with correct responses in the middle but not at the end of subtests may have attentional or concentration difficulty. A description of the patient's processing skills, then, is accomplished effectively with the PICA scoring system. Use of this scoring system with any other aphasia battery or test of cognition is appropriate and desirable. Used eclectically, subtests II and III (associative gestural tasks) and the subtests of naming, sentence completion, and graphic skills are most useful. Although standardized primarily on patients with vascular disease, the PICA does provide norms on patients with bilateral disease, making its use with the traumatically injured more valuable than other aphasia batteries.

The *Boston Diagnostic Aphasia Examination* is a comprehensive battery most useful in documenting focal brain disorders. Subtests that yield the greatest predictive and descriptive information with this population include the auditory and reading comprehension subtests, repetition tasks, the parietal lobe battery, and an analysis of the patient's response both verbally and graphically to the "cookie theft" picture.

Similar in design to the Boston Diagnostic Aphasia Examination, the *WAB* not only provides an aphasia quotient (AQ) but also provides a performance quotient (PQ). In combination, apropos to this population, the AQ and PQ provide a cognitive quotient (CQ) indicative of whole brain performance. Using the test's fluency rating and information content scaling provide useful data. The test's strength is its ability to identify both focal and diffuse disease.

In an attempt to avoid some of the unnatural communicative situations inherent in standardized aphasia batteries, the *CADL* was designed to test more functional communication skills, using a series of subtests that recreate actual communicative situations such as ordering, phoning, and asking for and receiving directions. It provides a broad index of how well a patient can solve some everyday problems utilizing any available cognitive and/or linguistic skills.

Other standardized language measures that evaluate the anomic and subtle auditory comprehension deficits characteristic to this population include the *Boston Naming Test*[14] and the *Revised Token Test*.[15] The *Revised Token Test* also is valuable when administered as an oral expressive, rather than as a comprehension task. In this form it has been described and used as *The Reporter's Test*.[16]

Test Administration and Interpretation

With this population one often has difficulty administering standardized measures because of poor patient cooperation due to distractibility and poor concentration. Completion of any single battery is rare in one sitting, and most are not adaptable to bedside use. Repeated administration of aphasia batteries with the traumatically injured reveals that some subtests from each battery not only provide a broad description of linguistic competence, but allow, through the novelty of the subtest design, for maximum patient cooperation and attention. These subtests were enumerated in the previous section on standardized measures. The eclectic approach to evaluation invalidates normative comparisons, but fulfills the main requirement in assessment by providing a broad description of communication efficiency. As mentioned previously, normative comparisons of traumatically injured patients to scores obtained by aphasics with vascular insufficiency is probably invalid.

Strict adherence to administrative procedure should be attempted, but frequently is impossible if the examiner seeks to determine those conditions that facilitate the patient's communication effectiveness. Modifications in testing procedure that will achieve this goal include liberal use of visual and auditory cues, alone and in combination; repetition of, and/or demonstration of subtest instructions, freely moving from one subtest to another because of patient-generated conditions even if it is not completed; employing short and long testing sessions to study the effects of time modifications (e.g., presenting the same subtest at 5- or 30-minute intervals); and presenting subtests with and without time constraints as a measure of task efficiency.

Diagnostically, comparisons between patient scores achieved with and without testing modifications are useful in determining the exact points at which communication fails. Similarly, comparisons between informal and formal test battery scores will provide the most accurate assessment of functional communicative capacities. For instance, it is not uncommon for patients who demonstrate adequate verbal skills in conversation to be unable to verbalize effectively when confronted with a structural task such as "Tell me what you do with a pen." These differences can assist in documenting inconsistencies in patient performance on similar tasks but with different cognitive demands. As the patient recovers such differences may become more subtle, but measures sensitive to describing changes in linguistic skills as cognitive demands increase or decrease need to be employed.

The PICA scoring system is particularly useful in providing a method of scoring patient behaviors, allowing the clinician to evaluate variations in a pattern of patient response errors under similar task conditions. A similar approach in analysis has been suggested by Hagen[1] and is summarized in Table 21–2.

**Table 21–2. VARIATIONS IN PATTERN OF ERRORS WITHIN
SIMILAR TASK CONDITIONS**

A. Random and fluctuating errors across time—suggests attention span and/or selective attention problems

B. Errors that occur on the first several stimuli of tasks but not later in the task, across test tasks—suggests attentional/selective attention impairments

C. Errors that consistently occur during the last several stimuli of tasks but not earlier—suggests attentional, selective attention, or retention span fatigue

D. Clustering of errors at relatively similar time intervals during a task—suggests problems with amount and duration of stimuli, and gives insight into what would be optimal for a given patient relative to these parameters during treatment

E. Errors decrease relative to certain types of cues: auditory, visual, visuomotor, contextual, breaking up stimulus into its parts, providing whole idea, and so on—suggests problems with categorization, association, and/or analysis/synthesis

F. Errors increase/decrease with rate, amount, and duration of stimuli—affects all cognitive abilities

G. Errors increase in relation to complexity—suggests impaired memory abilities, including retention span and/or weakened categorization, association, and analysis/synthesis problems

H. Responds appropriately to parts of stimulus but not whole, or vice versa—suggests associative, integrative, analysis/synthesis impairment

I. Poor carryover of responses to previous tasks to succeeding ones—suggests cognitive shift problems

MEASURES OF LANGUAGE AS A PROBLEM-SOLVING TOOL

As patients recover, the examiner needs to be aware that many specific linguistic incompetencies will improve, giving way to communication deficits emerging in tasks that involve language as a problem-solving tool. A different set of assessment measures must be employed if the evaluation is to describe these residual deficits. The patient may be a functional communicator, in situations not requiring cognitive demands on the linguistic system such as informal conversation, but skills may deteriorate under conditions of stress, which usually represents a departure from premorbid performance. Testing emphasis should shift from a singular analysis of linguistic performance to include measures that manipulate the cognitive supports for linguistic competence. Most tests will involve aspects of memory, analysis of parts of information, judgment, reasoning, sequencing, and synthesis—all of which may be assessed through linguistic and nonlinguistic input and output channels. The measures selected should be able to evaluate the patient's communicative effectiveness by measuring the changes in linguistic performance as cognitive demands increase.

Currently there is no single test battery that encompasses measurement of linguistic skills in relation to their use in solving problems. Most often the examiner must assemble a group of subtests from recognized test measures, and from subtests that are informally designed and may be particular to a single examiner. Scoring strategies will not necessarily parallel those recommended by the test, since entire testing instruments are given infrequently. However, it is helpful to choose tests that report means and standard deviations for each subtest such as those provided by the Wechsler Memory Scale.[17] Emphasis in scoring should be focused on an analysis of the patient's efficiency in solving problems linguistically, providing an understanding of which processes fail to respond normally. Care must be taken to select and interpret measures that do not unfairly exceed expected premorbid levels of cognitive function.

The examiner will need to focus the evaluation of communication effectiveness away from the specific components of linguistic elements toward an analysis of pragmatic rules and behaviors involved in communication exchanges. Pragmatic analyses explore communicative intentions and interactions: Was the message sent so as to be correctly received? What output modalities were used? What was the extent of emotional involvement? How much redundancy, pause time, facial expression, and body language were used? How much time did it take to send the message?

The Language Sample

The elicitation and analysis of a language sample is the most important diagnostic tool in the evaluation of traumatically injured patients who have developed conversational skills that appear normal on clinical assessment screenings.

The sample should contain data for both verbal and graphic output (on identical tasks for comparative analyses) elicited consecutively in the following circumstances:

1. Automatic conversation
2. Picture description
3. Explanation of similarities and differences
4. Problem solving (conclusions)
5. Sequencing
6. Inferences
7. Environmental conversation

Five to 10 minutes of output in each category provides enough data for analysis. Verbal output should be taperecorded for future study.

Automatic conversation should be elicited from the patient on a topic familiar to or interesting to the patient. Questions about the patient's family or prior occupation would be appropriate.

A *picture description* task requires more specific use of language than automatic conversation. Pictures should be selected that might be known to interest the patient. The examiner's goal should be to elicit specific information.

Explanation of similarities and differences requires direct analysis of information and reformulation into specific explanations. Questions ranging from concrete items such as "How are a pear and an apple alike?" to more abstract questions such as "How are a pen and a pencil different?" can be used. Of use in this examination are the items presented in workbook form by Tomlin.[18]

Graphic and verbal problem solving is tested by presenting patients with familiar problems such as "What would you do if your pipes were leaking?" in an effort to evaluate their skills in drawing conclusions about familiar situations. With some patients

it is appropriate to begin this subtest with more concrete items that assess verbal closure skills, such as "You clean the floor with a *(mop)*." The verbal problem-solving treatment tasks described by Huisingh and co-workers[19] also can be used as diagnostic tools.

Sequential language tasks can be divided into three parts: story retelling, sentence construction, and the patient's ability to sequence a common activity without cues. Story retelling requires the examiner to read a story that is three paragraphs in length (length can be varied dependent on the patient). The patient is asked to retell the story in the correct order. Sentence construction (such as having the patient construct two different sentences with the same word) is a useful measure of divergent thinking.[20] After completing this portion, the patient is asked to explain the sequence involved in changing a tire, baking a cake, or getting ready for a date.

The patient's response to information of paragraph length (either self-read or read to the patient) involves analyzing and being able to make a prediction or *inference* based on that information. The computer software designed by Volin and Groher[21] is suitable for both diagnosis and treatment of linguistic inferential processes.

Assessment of *environmental conversation* is best elicited if the clinician creates a role-playing model, presenting the patient with real-life situations such as ordering food, opening a check account, buying stamps, using the phone book, requesting directions, or buying clothes. The clinician typically plays the role of the clerk, and must continue the conversation by asking the patient appropriate questions. Giving the patient one or two prearranged "problems," such as anticipating a wrong size or not having enough money when buying a pair of pants, helps guide the activity and ensures elicitation of an adequate sample. If the patient is employed, an evaluation of communicative needs in the work environment through role playing can be accomplished if the examiner has prior knowledge of the patient's place of employment.

Other Measures

The majority of verbal tasks also require elements of auditory comprehension as they relate to linguistic problem solving. Subtle auditory deficits can be evaluated further with the *Revised Token Test.*[15]

Specific evaluation of reading skills in five categories particularly useful in the evaluation of the traumatically brain injured (inference, assumption recognition, deduction, interpretation, and evaluation of arguments) has been designed by Watson and Glaser.[22] The test can be modified to assess auditory processing skills in the same categories. Designed primarily for patients with aphasia, the *Reading Comprehension Battery for Aphasics*[23] is a useful tool for detailing on what levels the processes involved in reading may be disordered. The patient's ability to comprehend humor and ambiguity, often impaired in the traumatically injured, can be evaluated using subtests from the *Clinical Management of Right Hemisphere Dysfunction.*[24]

The clinician may find it useful to compare the information obtained from linguistic problem-solving tests with the information obtained from nonlinguistic problem-solving tests. These tests usually are visually biased; however, they can be used as effective predictors of linguistic problem-solving ability in patients whose verbal skills have been decompensated but whose perceptual abilities remain intact. Nonlinguistic problem-solving tasks chosen will parallel those used in direct linguistic analysis. These include the Visual Sequencing and Visual Closure subtests of the *Illinois Test of Psycholinguistic Abilities;*[25] the *Test of Nonverbal Intelligence,*[26] (provides means and standard deviations with percentile rankings); the similarities, block design, object assembly, and picture arrangement subtests of the *Wechsler Adult Intelligence Scale;*[27] and the *Nonverbal Test of Cognitive Skills,*[28] a test that relies on visual memory and requires the patient to make manual manipulations.

Test Interpretation

It is important that the elicited language sample and other tests of cognition that sample communication effectiveness receive an analysis relative to the pragmatic aspects of the interaction between patient and examiner such as the one suggested by Hutchinson and Jensen.[29]

Their analysis is completed by examining three aspects of communicative exchange. Part one includes a total numerical count of utterances, the number of speaking turns taken during the exchange, and the number of utterances per turn. Analysis of the speech act, defined as the speaker's intent exclusive of syntax, is the second part. Analysis in this section includes tabulation of representatives (assertions), directives (requests), expressives (how one feels), and commissives (commitments the speaker makes to a future course of action). Part three is a tabulation of the number of topics initiated, utterances on the same topic, the number of times the patient continues on the topic initiated by the clinician, and the number of utterances not related to the topic. This final section can be expanded to include a numerical count of the number of utterances that are inappropriate, irrelevant, confabulatory, fragmented, out of sequence, circumlocutory, or tangential and concrete as suggested by Hagen.[1] Although some of the tabulations in these categories often overlap, making strict separation difficult, operational definitions can be applied so that demarcation is easier. The goal of pragmatic analysis is description of the patient's ability to use language in solving problems. There are no normative data upon which to make comparisons; therefore, comparisons must be individualized. The *Clinical Management of Right Hemisphere Dysfunction*[24] test protocol provides guidelines for rating pragmatic communication skills that includes a simple and effective rating scale of nonverbal communication, conversational skills, use of linguistic context, and narrative organization (Table 21–3). The battery also includes a format for scoring the patient's graphic skills (Table 21–4). This scoring format is a good example of how an examiner can operationally define parameters and assign a scoring system that is useful in the description of communicative behavior.

As the patient attempts to use his or her linguistic and nonlinguistic communicative skills in problem solving, the clinician must develop a system for analyzing not only the response but also how the patient came to that response. This will include an analysis of the strategies or nonstrategies the patient uses in the attempt to use language to meet self-generated communicative needs or to

Table 21–3. A PROPOSED GUIDELINE FOR ASSISTANCE IN RATING PRAGMATIC COMMUNICATION SKILLS

A. Nonverbal Communication

	1	2	3	4	5
Intonation	Flat or stereotyped		Limited or inappropriate		Appropriate
Facial expression	None		Limited or inappropriate		Appropriate
Eye contact	Cannot establish or maintain eye contact		Needs cues to establish or maintain eye contact		Appropriate
Gestures and proxemics	Inappropriate or does not use		Inconsistent appropriate use		Appropriate

B. Conversational Skills

	1	2	3	4	5
Conversational initiation	Inappropriate or does not initiate		Inconsistent appropriate initiation		Appropriate
Turn-taking	Does not obey signals		Inconsistently responsive to signals		Adequate
Verbosity	Over 50% of responses are verbose or tangential		25% to 50% of responses are verbose or tangential		Appropriate response length

C. Use of Linguistic Context

	1	2	3	4	5
Topic maintenance	Maintains topic less than 25% of the time		Maintains topic 50% of the time		Maintains topic
Presupposition	Presupposes too much and/or too little 50%		Presupposes too much and/or too little 25% to 50%		Appropriate
Referencing skills	Inappropriate referencing		Inconsistent appropriate		Appropriate

D. Organization of a Narrative

	1	2	3	4	5
Organization	Disorganized		Some organization but lacks a unifying theme		Adequate
Completeness	More than 50% of details are missing and/or inaccurate		25% to 50% of details are missing or inaccurate		Adequate

From Burns et al,[24] with permission.

Table 21–4. A PROPOSED FORMAT FOR SCORING A PATIENT'S GRAPHIC OUTPUT

	1	2	3	4	5
Visuospatial disorganization (superimposed letters and lines and lines progressing on a diagonal)	Always present (100%)		Present part of the time (50%)		Adequate
Left-sided neglect (writing begins to right of appropriate left-hand margin)	Always		Part of the time or center placement		Not present
Omissions of letters	30 or more omissions		15 omissions		Less than 3 omissions
Omission of strokes (e.g., unclosed *a's* and *o's*, *i's* undotted, *t's* uncrossed, and so on)	100 or more omissions		50 omissions		Less than 10 omissions
Perseveration of strokes and/or letters	30 or more		Less than 15		Less than 3
Ambiguous sentences	50% or more of sentences unclear		25% or more of sentences unclear		One or less unclear sentence
Run-on sentences	Always present (100%)		Present part of the time (50%)		Not present
Incomplete sentences	Always present (100%)		Present part of the time (50%)		Not present
Grammatical errors	(10)		(5)		One or none
Phonetically based spelling errors	80% or more		40%		Correct
Visually based spelling errors	80% or more		40%		Correct

Total _____

From Burns et al,[24] with permission.

respond to clinician probes. Such a system has been proposed by Hagen,[1] who feels that an analysis of the pattern of problem solving is, perhaps, more important than the correct answer. Tabulation of patient behaviors in the following categories has been suggested:[1] immediate solution recognition, study of the task before attempting a solution, taking an organized and systematic approach, solving the problem with impulsive trial-and-error strategies, developing alternate strategies that are appropriate, overattending to detail, needing prompts to start, benefiting from assistance, and transferring assistance appropriately to the next task. Additional behaviors to tabulate include needing constant prompts to continue working, giving up easily when the solution is not clear, and attempting to change the rules the task demands in an effort to solve a dilemma. Other psychologic components such as anger, frustration, apathy, disinhibition, and depression also should be coded as part of the analysis.

CONCLUSION

The assessment of speech and language skills in adults with traumatic head injury should be guided toward obtaining a broad description of the patient's communicative effectiveness (how well the patient relates to the environment through linguistic channels), rather than solely focusing on phonology, syntax, and semantics. A description of communication effectiveness will be closely tied to the patient's cognitive competence. Thus, the examiner must screen cognition and interpret linguistic test results, aware of fluctuation in and increased demand on communicative exchanges as tasks require more attention, vigilance, memory, and problem solving.

Because the traumatically injured widely vary in communicative performance and because recovery rates are unpredictable, the clinician must be prepared to assess patients at all severity levels, adapting measures to fit individual needs. Different stages of involvement require different administration and interpretive technique as the patient progresses from prelinguistic, to emerging language, linguistic, language as a problem-solving tool, to prevocational and vocational stages of recovery.

In the acute stages of dysfunction, the bedside assessment will measure the patient's ability to relate to the environment. Responses to gross environmental stimuli such as noise, light, and touch form the basis of the evaluation. As the patient recovers, the evaluation should focus on linguistic competencies using formal measures of language. With further recovery, the evaluation should focus on how effectively the patient can use linguistic skills in solving problems that require language. The measures needed to perform this evaluation often consist of a collection of subtests designed to explore the interplay between language performance and cognitive demands.

Interpretation of test results should be guided toward an analysis of behavioral patterns that influence communication effectiveness. Systems of scoring linguistic competencies should be simple enough to be easily replicated so as to respond to and describe the relationship between the patient's changing cognition as it affects linguistic performance. Analysis of communicative pragmatics and the patient's ability to use language to solve problems imposed by the environment should be the focus of the assessment as the patient recovers.

REFERENCES

1. Hagen, C: Language disorders in head trauma. In Holland, A: Language Disorders in Adults. College-Hill Press, San Diego, 1983.
2. Teasdale, G and Jennett, F: Assessment of coma and impaired consciousness. Lancet 2:81, 1974.
3. Brooks, DN et al: Cognitive sequelae of severe head injury in relation to the Glascow Outcome Scale. J Neurol Neurosurg Psychiatry 49:549, 1986.
4. West, J and Sands, E: Bedside Evaluation Screening Test. Aspen Systems Corporation, Rockville, MD, 1986.
5. Keenan, JS and Brassell EG: Aphasia Language Performance Scales. Pinnacle Press, Murfreesboro, TN, 1975.
6. Baratz, R and Norman, S: Communication Abilities Record. Newton, MA, 1979.
7. Schuell, H: Minnesota Test for the Differential Diagnosis of Aphasia. University of Minnesota Press, Minneapolis, 1972.
8. Goodglass, H and Kaplan, E: The Assessment of Aphasia and Related Disorders. Lea and Febiger, Philadelphia, 1983.
9. Porch, BE: Porch Index of Communicative Ability. Consulting Psychologist Press, Palo Alto, CA, 1981.
10. Kertesz, A: The Western Aphasia Battery. Grune and Stratton, New York, 1982.
11. Holland, AL: Communicative Abilities in Daily Living: A Test of Functional Communication for Aphasic Adults. University Park Press, Baltimore, 1980.
12. Levin, H: Aphasia in closed head injury. In Sarno, MT: Acquired Aphasia. Academic Press, New York, 1981.
13. Sarno, MT, Buonaguro, A and Levita, E: Characteristics of verbal impairment in closed head injured patients. Arch Phys Med Rehabil 67:400, 1986.
14. Kaplan, E, Goodglass, H and Weintraub, S: Boston Naming Test. Lea and Febiger, Philadelphia, 1983.
15. McNeil, MR and Prescott, TE: Revised Token Test. University Park Press, Baltimore, 1978.
16. DeRenzi, E and Ferrari, C: The Reporter's Test: a test sensitive to detect expressive disturbances in aphasics. Cortex 14:279, 1978.
17. Wechsler, D and Stone, CP: Wechsler Memory Scale. The Psychological Corp, New York, 1945.
18. Tomlin, KJ: Workbook for Adult Language and Cognition, Workbook 3, Reasoning. Lingui Systems, Moline, IL, 1984.
19. Huisingh, R et al: Situational Language, A Pragmatic Approach to Problem Solving. Lingui Systems, Moline, IL, 1984.
20. Adamovich, B, Henderson, J and Auerbach, S: Cognitive Rehabilitation of Head Injured Adults. College-Hill Press, San Diego, 1985.
21. Volin, R and Groher, M: Language Stimulation Software #7, Inferences. Aspen Systems Corp, 1986.
22. Watson, R and Glaser, S: Critical Thinking Appraisal. The Psychological Corp, San Antonio, TX, 1980.
23. LaPointe, L and Horner, J: Reading Comprehension Battery for Aphasia. CC Publications, Tigard, OR, 1979.
24. Burns, MS, Halper, AS and Mogil, SI: Clinical Management of Right Hemisphere Dysfunction. Aspen Systems Corp, Rockville, MD, 1985.

25. Kirk, SA, McCarthy, JJ and Kirk, WD: Illinois Test of Psycholinguistic Abilities. University of Illinois Press, Urbana, 1968.

26. Brown, L, Sherbenon, RJ, and Dollar, SJ: Test of Nonverbal Intelligence: A Language-Free Measure of Cognitive Ability. Pro-Ed, Austin, TX, 1982.

27. Wechsler, D: Wechsler Adult Intelligence Scale. The Psychological Corp, New York, 1955.

28. John, GO and Boyd, HF. Nonverbal Test of Cognitive Skills. Charles E Merrill Publishing, Columbus, OH, 1981.

29. Hutchinson, JM and Jensen, M: Evaluation of discourse in communication. In Obler, LK and Albert, M: Language and Communication in the Elderly. DC Heath, Lexington, MA, 1980.

Chapter 22

Neuropsychological Assessment

WILLIAM J. LYNCH, Ph.D.

DEFINITION AND BACKGROUND

Neuropsychological assessment involves the evaluation of cerebral functions through the administration of standardized tests or procedures. There are similarities between neuropsychological and neurologic examinations, but the two procedures differ both in detail and in breadth of focus. The neuropsychological evaluation typically involves the administration of a number of tests or procedures that seek to determine the integrity of the patient's higher cortical functions. There is no real attempt to evaluate the central nervous system (CNS) below the level of the cerebral cortex, although some neuropsychologists do try to assess cerebellar functions as well. The neurologist attends to cortical as well as to subcortical, brainstem, spinal, and peripheral components of the CNS. While being more comprehensive in scope, the neurologic examination is less detailed than the neuropsychological evaluation in its assessment of cognitive and perceptual-motor abilities dependent upon the cerebral cortex.

Another distinction between the two lies in the information sought by each. The neuropsychological evaluation provides information relevant to the diagnosis and prognosis of a brain disorder, but it can also define areas of strength and weakness that can be helpful in designing a treatment program. The neurologic examination is intended to identify pathology of the CNS as a basis for medical treatment, not to serve as a comprehensive assessment of patients' cognitive impairments and prognosis for their improvement.

Neuropsychological evaluations can provide a comprehensive baseline for pre-treatment and post-treatment (including drug therapy or surgery) comparisons. Most stroke or head injury rehabilitation programs employ such serial testing in order to document change. This is not to say that the neurologic examination cannot provide valuable information in this regard, but that its strength lies in its ability to detect neuropathology at all levels and not in documenting complex cognitive deficits.

The original efforts of Halstead,[1] Luria,[2] and Reitan[3] stemmed from a desire to organize and standardize — at least to some extent — the procedures employed by individual clinicians involved in the assessment of brain impaired individuals. Golden and colleagues[4] have extended this effort considerably with their reorganizing and restructuring of Luria's original neuropsychological investigation.[5] The following section will examine each of these approaches, as well as a more recent development known as the "Process Approach," which owes its origins to Luria but which has long been championed by Milberg and others.[6]

DESCRIPTION OF THE PROMINENT TEST BATTERIES OR APPROACHES

Halstead-Reitan Battery

Halstead[1] gathered a number of procedures that he felt would be sensitive to frontal lobe dysfunction. These procedures emphasized problem solving, attention, vigi-

310

lance, abstraction, motor speed, and incidental memory. Each measure had to be shown to discriminate consistently between controls and patients with frontal lobe pathology. Halstead's espousal of a formal test battery and his establishment of cut-off scores to evaluate individual patient's performances were among his principal contributions to the field of clinical neuropsychology. He used cut-off scores to develop his concept of an "impairment index" (wherein each impaired score among the 10 scores obtained in his original battery counts as 0.1) as a measure of overall level of performance.

Reitan elaborated on and in some ways extended Halstead's groundwork by adding several measures to the battery, and as a result, it is now known as the "Halstead-Reitan Battery."[7] Reitan included measures of psychometric intelligence (Wechsler Intelligence Scale for Children[8] or Wechsler Adult Intelligence Scale[9] [WAIS]); academic achievement (Wide Range Achievement Test [WRAT] by Jastak and Jastak[10]); a standardized cortical sensory evaluation (the Sensory-Perceptual Examination); a measure of hand-grip strength; a measure of visual-motor searching, sequencing, and set switching (the Trail Making Test); and a measure of nondominant finger-tapping speed (Halstead measured only dominant finger tapping). Reitan also eliminated two of Halstead's original measures (Time-Sense and Critical Flicker Frequency) because of their inferior ability to discriminate between normal and lesioned patients. The resulting set of tests, along with a brief description of each, is provided in Table 22–1.

Reitan[11] suggests four methods of inference in the interpretation of neuropsychological test data:

1. **Level of Performance:** How well the patient performed relative to some cut-off score. The impairment index reflects level of performance.

2. **Patterns of Performance:** An analysis of differences in scores within the battery as they reflect strengths, weaknesses, and variability in performance. As an example, a patient may perform well on verbally oriented measures, while nonverbal skills may reflect significant deficit.

3. **Specific Behavioral Deficits or Pathognomonic Signs:** Are there any signs that are found only in pathological conditions? While not encountered in all patients, these deficits are felt to confirm the presence of a neurological disorder. Examples of pathognomonic signs are hemiparesis, visual field defects, and aphasia.

4. **Comparison of Performance of the Two Sides of the Body:** An analysis of the performance of the right and left sides of the body on motor and sensory tests. For example, patients with strongly lateralized cerebral lesions will have consistent motor and/or sensory impairment on the contralateral side of the body.

Luria's Neuropsychological Investigation

Although Luria's work had been well publicized over the years since World War II, it was not until Christensen[12] published her translation and compilation of his assessment methods that his investigative technique became widely understood. Because Luria's approach to assessment and treatment was highly intuitive and improvisational, it was difficult for many clinicians trained in the structured battery approach (Halstead-Reitan) to comprehend its fine points. Luria's approach is based upon his theory of functional systems, which considered complex psychological processes to be the result of an interaction of a number of brain regions involved in arousal, sensory analysis, and motor output. He correctly pointed out that acts such as writing, reading, or naming must be considered multidetermined. An inability to perform such activities does not imply a specific lesion site; rather, it implicates any one of the components of the *system* that mediates that ability. Thus, an inability to read aloud could stem from a failure in visual, receptive language, or expressive speech abilities (or a combination of these). A related presumption is that any function that does *not* include a given system will be unaffected by damage to that system.

Luria's neuropsychological investigation (LNI) is composed of 11 principal segments, each having two or more subsections. These segments and subsections are listed in Table 22–2.

Scoring the LNI is impressionistic, although a three-point system (none, slight,

Table 22–1. HALSTEAD-REITAN BATTERY (AGES 15 AND OLDER)

Test Name	Brief Description	What Test Measures
Halstead's Original Tests		
1. Category Test	208 slides divided into 7 subtests; patient must discern an abstract principle by which each is organized via trial and error with immediate feedback provided by a bell (correct) or buzzer (incorrect). Score is number of errors.	Attention, visual problem solving, ability to generate and test various hypotheses, ability to attend to and make constructive use of feedback, ability to generalize from familiar to new yet similar situations.
2. Tactual Performance Test (TPT)	Modified Seguin-Goddard Formboard is employed. Patient is blindfolded; empty board in upright position is placed in front of patient along with the 10 wooden blocks. Patient must replace all the blocks as fast as possible using first the dominant, then the nondominant hand, and then using both hands together on three consecutive trials. Time limit varies from 10–15 min per trial. After this, board is removed, patient's blindfold is removed, and he must then draw the board and block shapes from memory. Scoring consists of total time, and number of block shapes recalled and located.	Motor problem solving, transfer of training from one trial to the next, tactile-motor-spatial integration, spatial and tactile memories, incidental learning.
3. Seashore Rhythm Test	30 pairs of tone patterns are presented via tape recording. Patient must indicate "same" or "different." Score may be given as a rank or as an error total.	Attention, concentration, nonverbal auditory discrimination and memory.
4. Speech Perception Test	60 nonsense words are presented via tape recording. Response form has 4 choices for each word. Patient underlines choice. Score is number of errors.	Attention, concentration, verbal auditory discrimination, high-frequency sound discrimination.
5. Finger Tapping Test	Using a mechanical counter affixed to a $9 \times 9.5''$ board, patient taps as rapidly as possible for 10 seconds. Preferred and nonpreferred hands are used alternately until 5 trials per hand are obtained. Score is mean taps over 5 trials. The preferred hand counts in impairment index.	Motor speed, with a small proprioceptive component. Also the ability to sustain a regular tapping rhythm, thus basal ganglia or cerebellar disease may hinder performance.
Additional Measures		
6. Grip Strength	Using a hand dynamometer calibrated in kilograms, patient squeezes with preferred and nonpreferred hands in alternating sequence. Score is given as mean kilograms of pressure for 2 or more trials for right and left hands.	Strength of the upper extremities.

Table 22–1. *(Continued)*

Test Name	Brief Description	What Test Measures
7. Trail Making Test	Using pen or pencil, patient must rapidly connect 25 circles scattered on $8.5 \times 11''$ paper. Part A consists of numbers 1–25; Part B contains numbers 1–13 and letters A–L, and patient must *alternate* the order (e.g. 1-A-2-B-3-C, and so on). Score is given in terms of seconds required for each part, as well as the number of errors made. (Reitan has used a "credit score" based on seconds.)	Visuomotor speed, scanning, searching, dealing with alphabetic or numeric information, visual sequencing, and set-switching ability.
8. Aphasia Screening	32 items dealing with aspects of language as well as other abilities such as right-left orientation and copying designs. Scoring is not quantitative; items are scored as right or wrong with no summary score. The emphasis is on noting "pathognomonic signs" of pathology (see further on).	Communicative abilities, including verbal, graphic, and gestural; lateral orientation; spatial organization; and drawing praxis.
9. Sensory-Perceptual	Cortical sensory abilities are evaluated by a series of tasks, including double simultaneous stimulation, tactile shape recognition, and visual field testing by confrontation. Scoring consists of recording errors on either side of the body. Visual field problems are recorded.	Cortical sensory functions; assesses the presence of sensory neglect or "extinction" phenomena; visual fields and stereognosis.

or severe) of rating disturbances is provided on the test forms. A sheet containing five diagrams depicting the brain in various aspects is included, so that the clinician can indicate the specific site of a lesion.

There are three main stages in the investigation. The first consists of the administration of numerous brief tests evaluating the status of the principal systems ("analyzers" in Luria's terminology) that mediate primary visual, auditory, kinesthetic, and motor functions. The second stage deals with more specific tests suggested by the patient's performance during the first stage. According to Christensen, testing at this stage is "strictly individualized." The emphasis here is on qualitative rather than quantitative observations. Stimuli may be presented at varying rates, for example, in order to evaluate the critical factors at work in the failure to perform a task. The third and final stage

consists of the formulation of a conclusion based on the information obtained. The clinician must identify the etiology of the deficit and the ways in which it intrudes upon the patient's cognitive and perceptual-motor activity. The detailed analysis of the results will lead to an identification of one or more "syndromes" of "symptom complexes," which will ultimately point the way to the locus of the lesion.

While the LNI is not commonly administered in its entirety as a screening device in traumatic head injury programs, many clinicians in the United States make use of Luria's approaches and procedures in analyzing a patient's pattern of strengths and weaknesses in treatment planning. Luria's approach provides the clinician with a central organizing scheme for evaluating and understanding the impact of a brain lesion on a patient's abilities.

Table 22–2. PRINCIPAL SEGMENTS AND SUBSECTIONS OF LURIA'S NEUROPSYCHOLOGICAL INVESTIGATION

Segment	Subsections
1. Preliminary conversation	a. State of patient's consciousness
	b. Principal complaints
2. Motor functions	a. Functions of the hands
	b. Functions of the mouth (oral praxis)
3. Acousticomotor organization	a. Perception and reproduction of pitch
	b. Perception and reproduction of rhythm
4. Higher cutaneous and kinesthetic functions	a. Cutaneous sensation
	b. Muscle and joint sensation
5. Higher visual functions	a. Visual perception
	b. Spatial orientation
	c. Intellectual operations in space
6. Impressive speech	a. Phonemic hearing
	b. Word comprehension
	c. Understanding simple sentences
	d. Understanding logicalalal grammatical structures
7. Expressive speech	a. Articulation of speech sounds
	b. Repetition of speech sounds
	c. Naming
	d. Narrative speech and fluency
8. Writing and reading	a. Phonetic analysis of words
	b. Writing
	c. Reading
9. Arithmetic skill	a. Comprehension of number structures
	b. Arithmetic operations
10. Mnestic processes (Memory)	a. Learning
	b. Retention and retrieval
	c. Discursive intellectual activity

From Christensen,[12] with permission.

Luria-Nebraska Neuropsychological Battery

The Luria-Nebraska Neuropsychological Battery (LNNB) is a standardized version of the LNI developed by Golden and colleagues.[13] In its current form,[14] the LNNB consists of 11 clinical and 5 summary scales, along with 8 localization and 28 factor scales. The LNNB differs from the LNI in that it provides both for formal scoring of each item (on a 0-1-2 or a 0-2 ordinal scale) as well as for a conversion of the obtained raw scores to standard (T) scores, which are then plotted on various profiles for later analysis. The LNNB also provides age and education adjustments when plotting a patient's T scores. The profile elevation and impairment scales[15] are among the most recent additions to the original 14 scales, and represent an effort to develop more valid in-

terpretive rules for analyzing LNNB profiles. Table 22–3 summarizes the clinical and summary scales of the LNNB (form I).

The LNNB is available in forms I and II, the latter of which includes a new scale, C12 (Intermediate Memory) that supplements the C10 scale. C12 makes use of longer delays on recall tasks. While the LNNB has gained wide acceptance in the United States, there have been some expressions of caution regarding organization of the items,[16] as well as independence of the scales.[17]

Additional Techniques

A number of additional assessment techniques are not part of the standard batteries just described. Memory and language assessment are inadequately represented in these

Table 22–3. CLINICAL AND SUMMARY SCALES OF THE LURIA-NEBRASKA NEUROPSYCHOLOGICAL BATTERY

Scale Name	Number of Items	What the Scale Evaluates
C1 (Motor functions):	51	Basic and complex motor functions (including fingers, hands, tongue, mouth; drawing)
C2 (Rhythm)	12	Rhythm and pitch perception and production
C3 (Tactile functions)	22	Kinesthetic, proprioceptive sense; tactile recognition of symbols and objects
C4 (Visual functions)	14	Visual object naming, discrimination, spatial perception (clock, map, forms)
C5 (Receptive speech)	33	Discrimination and comprehension of elementary, speech sounds, words, phrases, sentences
C6 (Expressive speech)	42	Ability to express simple speech sounds, words, phrases, sentences, stories. Responsive and spontaneous speech
C7 (Writing)	13	Spelling, copying, writing to dictation, spontaneous writing
C8 (Reading)	13	Simple and complex reading skills
C9 (Arithmetic)	22	Math knowledge and skills
C10 (Memory)	13	Recall of words (lists, sentences, stories), rhythms, gestures
C11 (Intellectual Processes)	34	Intellectual functions, including abstract thinking, math problem solving, categorizing, vocabulary
S1 (Pathognomonic)	34	Items that best discriminate normal and brain-damaged subjects, reflecting overall level of deficit
S2 (Left Hemisphere)	21	Items dealing with left hemisphere functions (motor, sensory)
S3 (Right Hemisphere)	21	Items dealing with right hemisphere functions (motor, sensory)
S4 (Profile Elevation)	28	Items most highly correlated with the average T score of the summary scales[15]
S5 (Impairment)	22	Items most highly correlated with number of scales above a critical level[15]

batteries, and for this reason it is common to employ one or more specialized tests in addition to the standard ones.

Language Functions

In most clinical settings, speech pathologists are called upon to perform detailed assessments of a patient's language functions. The most frequently employed comprehensive assessment tools are the following:

1. *Boston Diagnostic Aphasia Examination* (BDAE)[18] evaluates the principal components of language in order to determine qualitative and quantitative features of the patient's communicative system. Impaired patients are classified into categories such as Broca's, Wernicke's, conduction, or global aphasia. Performances are scored on an ordinal rating scale, and are then transformed to a Z-score profile for ready reference.

2. *Minnesota Test for the Differential Diagnosis of Aphasia* (MTDDA)[19] is a detailed procedure that attempts to methodically determine the precise problem of language by systematically examining each principal aspect of speaking, comprehending, and writing. Scoring is "pass-fail" in nature.

3. *Porch Index of Communicative Ability* (PICA)[20] is a procedure consisting of 18 subtests divided among graphic (6), verbal (4), and gestural (8) response requirements. The PICA is unique in that it employs a 16-point multidimensional scoring system that translates behavior into a numeric value. The PICA, unlike the BDAE or Minnesota tests, is not designed to diagnose aphasia or label a person's communicative

problem but to quantify the person's communication competence in a variety of situations. The PICA is particularly useful in initial assessment, treatment planning, and outcome measurement.

In addition to these comprehensive procedures, there are some useful brief measures that deal with specific language disturbances. The *Token Test*[21] measures verbal comprehension by requiring the patient to follow a series of simple and complex spoken commands (e.g., "Touch the red square" or "If there is a black square, pick up the blue circle"). The test materials consist of 10 variously shaped and colored plastic tokens. Because of the minimal output requirements, the Token Test is considered a relatively pure measure of verbal comprehension. The *Neurosensory Center Comprehensive Examination for Aphasia*[22] evaluates language (expression and comprehension), repetition, reading, and writing. Norms are available for aphasics, right-hemisphere damaged patients, and normal subjects.

Holland[23] published the *Communicative Activities of Daily Living* (CADL), which was designed to assess practical, "real-life" communication skills such as filling out forms, reading product labels, understanding common signs, and expressing emotional states. The CADL is one of the few language assessment tools that directly evaluates how a patient actually *uses* language skills in daily life. Language assessment is further discussed in Chapter 21.

Memory Functions

Memory assessment in rehabilitation typically focuses on recall of verbal or visuospatial information. The most popular memory test in the United States has been the Wechsler Memory Scale (WMS).[24] The WMS consists of eight subtests measuring the following abilities: personal/current information, orientation, mental control (sequencing), story recall, digit recall, memory for designs, and paired-associate learning. Raw scores for each subtest are added, and the total is converted to an age-weighted sum by referring to a table provided in the manual. The age-weighted sum is then transformed to a memory quotient, which is similar to a deviation intelligence quotient (IQ) (mean of 100 ± 15). In recent years, age norms for each subtest, as well as for immediate and delayed presentation formats of stories and designs, have been published.[25-27] A long-awaited revision of the WMS, the Wechsler Memory Scale-Revised or WMS-R, is now available. The WMS-R contains many improvements including both immediate and delayed presentations for several of the subtests.

Visual memory is often evaluated with measures such as the Revised Benton Visual Retention Test (RBVRT).[28] The RBVRT consists of 10 designs, most consisting of two central figures and one smaller peripheral figure. Scoring is simple and is graded according to the gravity of the error made. A helpful feature of the RBVRT is the availability of three parallel forms.

Some recent additions to the memory testing field are the Randt Memory Test (RMT)[29] and the Denman Neuropsychology Memory Scale (DNMS).[30] The RMT consists of the following seven "modules":

1. General information
2. Five items
3. Repeating numbers
4. Paired words
5. Short story
6. Picture recognition
7. Incidental learning

Modules 2, 4, 5, and 6 are repeated 24 hours after the primary test administration. In an effort to enhance patient compliance, these repeated measures may be administered either in person or by telephone. Norms for the RMT are derived from 300 normal subjects (divided among seven 10-year age intervals) and a clinical group of 80 patients. One of the strong points of the RMT is its apparently low correlation with psychometric intelligence. In an unpublished study[31] comparing the WMS and the RMT with the WAIS-R, it has been reported that the RMT, while correlating substantially ($r = 0.74$) with the WMS, correlates less than the WMS with the WAIS-R ($r = 0.40$ versus $r = 0.66$). The basic RMT requires 20 to 25 minutes to administer (plus the 24-hour follow-up), and is available in a standard and a computer-administered and -scored version.

The DNMS is a more comprehensive memory assessment tool that requires about

1 hour to administer. It is similar to the WMS-R in that it yields verbal, nonverbal and full-scale memory quotients. The subtests of the DNMS include the following:

Verbal	Nonverbal
Immediate recall of story	Immediate recall of figure
Paired associate learning	Musical tones and melodies
Memory for digits	Memory for human faces
Remote verbal information	Remote nonverbal information
Delayed paired associates	Delayed recall of a figure
Delayed recall of a story	

Norms for the DNMS are provided for ages 10 through 69, with a total normative sample of 246. Raw scores for each subtest are converted to age-weighted scaled scores, much as is done with the WMS-R. The item content of the DNMS is in some ways unique among the typical memory measures in use today. For example, its inclusion of a *nonverbal* remote information subtest requires the patient to recall the appearance or shape of commonly experienced objects such as the Eiffel Tower or a "No Smoking" sign. The figure employed on the DNMS is the Rey-Osterrieth Complex Figure[32] used by many neuropsychologists.

Several additional memory measures have been found to be useful both as assessment tools and as techniques for monitoring cognitive change during rehabilitation. Perhaps the most notable of these is the Paced Auditory Serial Addition Task (PASAT).[33] The PASAT requires the patient to attend to a lengthy series of digits presented at a predetermined pace. Starting with the second digit, the patient must report the sum of the current and preceding digit. The PASAT has been shown to be a reliable measure of cognitive progress following traumatic head injury.[34]

Levin and colleagues[35] have introduced the Galveston Orientation and Amnesia Test (GOAT) as a method for quantifying the presence and duration of post-traumatic amnesia (PTA). These investigators define PTA as the time from return to consciousness to the return of immediate memory following a head injury*. The GOAT is useful in documenting recovery of amnesia and disorientation, and a number of validation studies are presented by the authors. Mack[36] presents an excellent critical review of these and other memory assessment techniques in head injury.

Neuropsychological Assessment in Rehabilitation Settings

Neuropsychological assessment can be useful from the standpoints of diagnosis and of treatment. The following sections will highlight the applications of neuropsychological assessment in rehabilitation settings.

BASELINE DETERMINATIONS

Neuropsychological assessment is helpful in determining the patient's initial status with regard to cognitive and perceptual-motor abilities. By comparing the patient's performance with that of an appropriate normative group, the clinician can establish a comprehensive baseline for future comparison. Progress in general, as well as in specific areas, can be documented by comparing periodic evaluations with baseline data.

IDENTIFICATION OF STRENGTHS AND WEAKNESSES

Aside from determining levels of performance, neuropsychological assessment is useful in specifying areas of strength and weakness in rehabilitation patients. Due to the recent advances in neurodiagnostic techniques (e.g., computed tomography, magnetic resonance imaging, or positron emission tomography), there is little need for the neuropsychologist to attempt to localize brain lesions. What neuropsychological assessment can provide is a method for identifying a patient's assets or strengths versus liabilities or weaknesses. Such information is crucial in the development of a

---

*The classical definition of PTA is that interval from the onset of injury to the return of continuous day-to-day memory.

problem list and treatment plan. The rehabilitation team needs to know not only what the patient is currently able and unable to do, but what he or she may be expected to achieve after treatment. Comprehensive assessment can define competence in such areas as memory, intelligence, academic achievement, perceptuomotor skills, activities of daily living (ADL), and personality.

One manner in which information relating to relative strengths and weaknesses can be displayed is the T-score profile. The patient's raw test data are transformed to a series of standard scores having a mean of 50 and a standard deviation of ± 10. Such profiles permit the clinician, patient, and family to view all performances according to a common reference point without having

to constantly recall normal and abnormal ranges for raw scores. Table 22–4 illustrates a portion of the computer-generated T-score profile developed by the author at the Brain Injury Rehabilitation Unit (BIRU) at the Palo Alto, California, Veterans Administration Medical Center.

T scores falling in the 10 to 39 range are considered below average and thus, liabilities or weaknesses. Scores in the 40 to 60 range are considered average, with those above 60 deemed superior. T scores in the latter ranges may be considered relative strengths for the patient.

It must be emphasized that the determination of deficits should not rely solely on neuropsychological test scores. Although important, these scores often do not accu-

Table 22–4. SAMPLE OF BIRU T-SCORE PROFILE PRINTOUT*

BRAIN INJURY REHABILITATION UNIT VA MEDICAL CENTER–PALO ALTO, CA, T-SCORE LISTING

Patient: Sample T-Score Profile
Examiner: Lynch

Date Tested: 4/15/87
Handedness: R

Measure	Raw	T Score	
Verbal Weighted Score:	45	46	
Performance Weighted Score:	32	38	
V-P Difference:	13	26	
Wechsler Memory Scale (MQ):	97	48	
Mini-Mental State	18	20	
Trail Making Test–Part A:	150	0	
Trail Making Test–Part B:	345	0	
Basic Aphasia Examination:			
Overall average:	13.4	44	Average
Verbal:	12	33	Borderline
Graphic:	12.7	44	Average
Gestural:	14.11	47	Average
Motor Tests:			
Grip/Dominant:	45	49	
Grip/Non-dominant:	35	43	
Grip/Difference:	10	36	
Finger Tapping/Dominant:	34	40	
Finger Tapping/Non-dominant:	24	41	
Finger Tapping/Difference:	10	30	
Foot Tapping/Dominant:	34	47	
Foot Tapping/Non-dominant:	33	48	
Purdue Pegboard/Dominant:	11	31	
Purdue Pegboard/Non-dominant	7	28	
Purdue Pegboard/Both:	4	28	
Purdue Pegboard/Total:	22	28	

Deficit Index = 0.34
Average T Score = 34
Level of Impairment is: Marked

*The norms used are based upon normal adults and thus should not be applied to any other groups or age ranges.

rately represent what a patient actually does in the "real world." For example, test scores do not address the issues of whether a behavior is carried out completely or consistently.

In addition to standard neuropsychological assessment techniques, many clinicians will want to employ some structured measure of ADLs. The author has adapted and modified a measure entitled the Rating of Patient's Independence, or ROPI.[37] The ROPI consists of 18 separate task areas, organized into the three general clusters of self-care, socialization, and communication. The task areas of the ROPI are listed below:

Cluster	Tasks
Self-care	Dressing, grooming, toilet activities, ambulation, eating
Socialization	Health awareness, memory, scheduling, interpersonal activities, transportation, occupation/avocation, personal business, housing
Communication	Speech, understanding, reading, writing, gestural

Scoring is multidimensional, ranging from 1 (cannot do task) to 15 (does task normally, as before the injury). Average independence levels are calculated for each task as well as for each cluster. Finally, an overall average is derived by averaging all tasks. The reader is referred to a recent chapter by Lynch[38] for a more detailed description of the ROPI scoring system and profile. In addition to the ROPI, there are a number of recently published measures of independence that may be of use in head injury assessment. The Scales of Independent Behavior[39] and the Vineland Adaptive Behavior Scales[40] are two of the more prominent examples of widely distributed measures with national norms. There has been a recent effort to develop a nationally standard functional assessment tool for data gathering and research purposes. This measure — the Functional Independence Measure, or FIM — is described in detail elsewhere.[41]

Once enough data have been gathered to permit an accurate depiction of the patient's assets and liabilities, it is helpful to employ a standard problem list as a means of organizing the treatment effort. Examples drawn from one such standard list developed expressly for head injury rehabilitation are provided in Table 22–5.

PRESCRIPTIONS FOR TREATMENT

Once problems have been identified, the next step in the treatment process involves deciding upon specific treatment strategies. This is accomplished by selecting treatment tasks that either retrain impaired skills or that provide alternate methods for accomplishing a task. By analyzing the pattern of performance on neuropsychological tests, the clinician can identify abilities that appear to be maintained, impaired, or (at least temporarily) "lost." It is important to identify retained abilities, as these must often be exploited in treatment of more impaired skills.

In determining treatment, it is helpful to first assess the patient's status with regard to basic cognitive and sensory-motor processes such as arousal, alertness, attention, concentration, and motor skill. More complex abilities such as memory, mathematical computation, and abstract reasoning depend upon these fundamental processes. Thus, neuropsychological assessment that deals with reaction time, mental status, simple memory, and simple motor performance is regarded to be of primary importance in determining treatment approaches.

Qualitative aspects of test performance

Table 22–5. ITEMS FROM THE STANDARD PROBLEM LIST DEVELOPED BY LYNCH AND MAUSS-CLUM[42]

1. Memory difficulty: general or specific
   a. Auditory
   b. Visual
   c. Spatial
2. Impaired language processing: general or specific
   a. Reading comprehension
   b. Word recognition
   c. Auditory comprehension
   d. Writing
   e. Word finding
   f. Fluency
   g. Spelling
3. Math difficulty

are also crucial in inferring strengths and weaknesses in head injured patients. Careful observation of the patient under various conditions (e.g., quiet versus noisy) and on a variety of test procedures will provide useful information pertaining to the patient's typical problem-solving strategies, recognition of and response to failure, capacity for abstract reasoning, and persistence at demanding tasks. Such information is used to determine not only *what* treatments are to be employed, but also *how* and *when* they are to be instituted into the patient's treatment program.

The reader is referred to the work of Conboy and others,[43] Diller and Gordon,[44] Craine,[45] Luria and colleagues,[46] and Prigatano and others[47] for a more thorough presentation of the role of neuropsychological assessment in the development of treatment prescriptions.

Prediction and Determination of Outcome

Neuropsychological assessment can provide useful data for the prediction and for the determination of outcome after head injury. Most of the predictors in the literature relate to neurosurgical or neurological variables such as length of coma, motor response patterns, or pupillary reactions,[48] and other factors such as age and duration of post-traumatic amnesia (PTA) that appear to be significant.

One of the most widely used measures of post-head injury status is the Glasgow Coma Scale (GCS).[49] The GCS consists of a 15-point scale measuring responses such as eye opening, best motor response, and verbal response. Bond[50] states that while 90 percent of patients with GCS scores of 8 or less are in a coma, none of those having scores of 9 or more are comatose. It has been reported, for example, that when the GCS score is 11 or more during the first 24 hours after coma, 87 percent of head injured patients will attain a level of "moderate disability" or "good recovery" on the Glasgow Outcome Scale (GOS).[51] The GOS consists of four levels of outcome for surviving patients: vegetative, severely disabled, moderately disabled, and good recovery.[52] A brief description of each of the GOS levels is given at the bottom of this page.[53]

Many outcome measures focus upon the patient's quality of life following head injury. Jennett[54] suggests that the following factors be considered in determining quality of life:

1. Activities of daily living
2. Mobility/life organization
3. Social relationships
4. Work (level)
5. Present satisfaction
6. Future prospects

Such a comprehensive approach to assessing quality of life is essential in determining the impact of head injury on patients who are involved in lawsuits. When testifying in court, the neuropsychologist must be mindful of all of these factors in his or her effort to describe the effect of a head injury on an individual.

Rappaport and others[55] at the Santa Clara Valley Medical Center in San Jose, Califor-

Level	Descriptor
Vegetative state	Absence of function of the cerebral cortex; patient shows no significant response to the environment. Patients who can follow a command or say a single word are rated "severe," rather than "vegetative."
Severe disability	Patient is conscious but requires assistance in ADLs every day. Degree of dependency may vary from total to partial. Jennett uses the term "conscious but dependent" to describe this group.
Moderate disability	Jennett refers to this group as "independent but disabled." Due to mental and/or physical deficit, patient can no longer perform at previous level of work or social activity. Patient may be able to work as long as deficits do not affect work activity.
Good recovery	Despite minor mental and/or physical deficits, patient is deemed *able* to return to work and other social functions, even if such has not yet occurred.

nia, developed the Disability Rating Scale (DRS), consisting of 8 categories of disability. Each category is assigned a numerical value according to a set of standard scoring criteria. The scoring categories include (1) arousability, awareness, and responsibility; (2) cognitive ability for self-care activities; (3) dependence on others; and (4) psychosocial adaptability. The DRS uses some elements of the GCS, and has been found to be both a reliable and useful scale for quantifying disability level both on admission and at discharge.

It has been reported that GOAT scores are predictive of recovery from mild head injury.[56] In a sample of 50 patients who recovered from mild head injury, 42 (84 percent) had GOAT scores of 81 or more. The authors also reported that no patients who had PTA (as defined by a GOAT score of 75 or less) longer than 1 month had a long-term good recovery.

Roberts[57] described a detailed system for predicting long-term outcome after head injury. He stated that the three crucial variables in determining prediction of outcome are (1) the *degree of neurologic dysfunction* during the acute stage, (2) the *rate* at which recovery from neurophysical disability takes place, and (3) the patient's *age* at the time of injury.

Porch and colleagues[58] reported that in stroke patients, communicative status at various points in time can be predicted with some accuracy by a combination of test data (from the PICA) and the patient's age. The authors conclude that accuracy improves when predictions of outcome are made beyond the first month after onset, and when the prediction spans a relatively short period of time (i.e., from the first to the 12th month).

Klonoff and others[59] investigated predictors and indicators of quality of life in 71 closed head injury patients from 2 to 4 years after injury. They found that the combination of the predictor variable, initial Glasgow Coma Scale score, and the indicator variables of motor functioning, memory and constructional ability were most strongly related to patients' reports of quality of life. According to reports by relatives (using a standard scale of adjustment), severity of head injury and motor disability related strongly to quality of life.

In summary, measures of outcome should be both comprehensive and operationally defined. The trend in the field of head injury rehabilitation is toward measures that are based on ADL or similar functional behaviors, while the use of purely psychometric measures is receiving declining support.

Organization and Presentation of Neuropsychological Data

The usefulness of neuropsychological test data is dependent to a great extent on the manner in which the information is organized and presented. Halstead-Reitan test data were originally presented in the form of a set of raw scores arranged on a summary sheet. Aside from being difficult to interpret by those unfamiliar with the distribution of scores for each test, the raw score summary sheet failed to take into account age and educational influences on certain test performances (especially memory and perceptual-motor tasks). A reasonable solution to this problem was to employ standard scores that would in effect place all scores on a common scale relative to the mean performance of a relevant normative sample.

In addition to individual T scores, two other level of performance summary scores may be obtained. The deficit index (DI), first described by Knights and Watson,[60] involves the calculation of the percentage of T scores that fall at or below 30. A DI of 0.2 or greater is considered significant. The average T score is simply the mean of all T scores obtained.[61] At the BIRU, we have combined these two measures by using a decision tree. Figure 22–1 illustrates the decision model used to determine general level of performance.

It should be emphasized that, although useful, level of performance is only one of several ways to interpret neuropsychological test data. The following case will illustrate how neuropsychological tests can be helpful in determining the deficits sustained by a head injured patient.

Case 1. The patient was a 30-year-old married male with a high school education when he sustained a closed head injury after losing control of his four-wheel drive vehicle. A CT scan revealed a right temporoparietal contusion, left temporoparietal subdural hematoma, and subarachnoid

CRITERIA FOR EVALUATING NEUROPSYCHOLOGIC PROFILES

I. DATA REQUIRED:

A. DEFICIT INDEX (DI): The percentage of T-scores falling at or below 30 .

B. AVERAGE T-SCORE (AT): The average or mean of all T-scores obtained.

II. DECISION TREE:

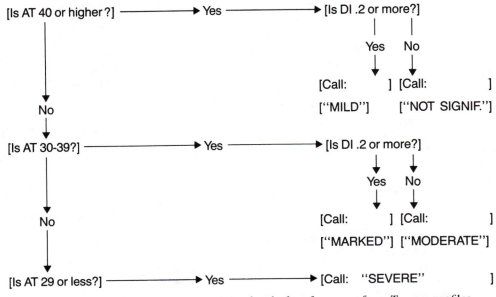

Figure 22–1. Decision model for determining level of performance from T-score profiles.

hemorrhage. Admission blood alcohol level was 0.33 g percent. Eye movements were roving and disconjugate; corneal reflexes were intact; oculocephalic reflexes were absent. Both upper extremities responded to pain, but the lower extremities did not. He was unconscious for several days, and by the third week in the hospital he began to look around and follow simple commands. Post-traumatic amnesia was estimated to have lasted for 8 weeks.

He was transferred from the initial acute care hospital to a rehabilitation facility after 5 weeks. He then underwent occupational, speech, and physical therapies over a period of 23 weeks. At that point, he was admitted to the Palo Alto Veterans Administration Brain Injury Rehabilitation Unit (BIRU) for outpatient cognitive rehabilitation.

On admission, he was evaluated by a battery of neuropsychologic tests (Table 22–6). The results indicated defective general psychometric intelligence, with a verbal IQ of 73, and a performance IQ of 62. His best performance on the WAIS-R was on the measure of simple attention, while he performed poorly on measures of visuomotor coordination; new learning, visual sequenc-

ing, perceptual organization, practical knowledge, and fund of general information. The WRAT-R indicated significant impairment of simple word recognition, while arithmetic and spelling were somewhat less depressed.

On the Wechsler Memory Scale (WMS), the patient obtained a memory quotient of 53, reflecting defective general immediate memory functioning. Mental status assessment using the Mini-Mental State (MMS) yielded a raw score of 15, which is in the impaired range (normal score is 27 to 30).

The neuropsychologic measures were in the severely impaired range with regard to level of performance. Halstead's impairment index would have been 1.0, indicating that all constituent measures were in the impaired range.

Motor measures indicated normal and symmetrical manual grip strength and finger tapping, while foot tapping was significantly slower on the right side. Fine motor dexterity was bilaterally slow, with the left hand performing 33 percent slower than the right. On the tactual performance test (TPT), the patient performed very poorly with either hand alone, as well as with both hands together, although the right hand was

Table 22–6. RAW SCORES ON BASELINE NEUROPSYCHOLOGICAL MEASURES FOR CASE 1

Trail Making (sec):
Part A: Disc. at 300 sec
Part B: Not attempted

Grip Strength (kg):
R = 52
L = 45

Purdue Pegboard (30 sec):
R = 9   L = 6
B = 4   T = 19

Wide-Range Achievement Test:
Reading: <46 (Standard Score)
Spelling: 71
Arithmetic: 68
Average T Score: 24
Deficit Index: 0.68 (Severe)

WAIS-R:
Verbal IQ   = 73
Performance IQ = 62
Full Scale IQ   = 66
Subtests:

Verbal: Performance:
INF   = 3   PCO = 5
DSP   = 8   PAR   = 4
VOC   = 6   BLD   = 4
ARI   = 5   OBJ   = 3
COM = 4   DSY   = 1
SIM   = 5

Wechsler Memory Scale:

Memory Quotient = 53
Basic Aphasia Exam (Rating/Impairment):
Overall Average = 8.56 (Marked)
          Verbal = 9.6 (Marked)
       Graphic = 6.9 (Marked)
       Gestural = 9.2 (Marked)

Category Test: 119
Tactual Performance Test:
    Right: 10.00 (min/block)
    Left: 2.85
    Both: 5.00 Memory: 2
    Total: 4.48 Local: 0
Finger Tapping (10 sec):
R = 47
L = 46
Foot Tapping (10 sec):
R = 26
L = 30

Mini-Mental State:

Raw Score = 15

---

worse than the left. Recall of the shapes and their locations was poor, indicating impaired incidental learning and spatial memory.

Aphasia screening assessment revealed marked communicative impairment on all modalities: verbal, graphic, and gestural. His typical responses required repetition and clarification of instructions. Nonverbal abstract reasoning, inductive problem solving, and set-shifting were severely impaired.

On the ROPI (Table 22–7), he was significantly impaired on all of the principal domains (self-care, socialization, and communication). His overall score was characteristic of individuals who are generally in need of direct assistance or supervision in ADL.

After 20 months of treatment the patient's outcome scores on these same measures indicated substantial improvement in a number of areas. Table 22–8 summarizes his performances at discharge. On the WAIS-R, he evidenced a slight increase in general psychometric intelligence, due in large part to an 11-point increase in the performance IQ. The patient showed considerable change on the WRAT-R reading subtest, improving from a standard score of below 46 to 86.

Performance on the WMS improved by 17 points, although it remained in the borderline range. A relatively greater increase was noted on the Mini-Mental State, which was normal (raw score = 27) at discharge. The measures of general level of performance also reflected improvement. His ATS increased by 10 points, while his deficit index decreased by 39 percent.

Motor testing indicated a slight improvement in strength and fine manual dexterity, especially with the left hand. The TPT was performed much more efficiently with regard to time, although the patient's ability to recall the proper locations remained impaired.

Aphasia testing improved from a level of marked communicative deficit on admission to a level of moderate on all modalities. The Halstead Category Test result indicated impairment at discharge, although the number of errors declined slightly from 119 to 94.

On the ROPI, the patient improved by an

Table 22–7. BASELINE AND OUTCOME DATA ON RATING OF PATIENT'S INDEPENDENCE (ROPI) FOR CASE 1*

Measure	Baseline	Outcome (20 mo)
Overall average	8.56	12.36
Self-care	9.6	12.8
Socialization	6.9	10.6
Communication	9.2	13.7

*ROPI scores range from 1 (cannot do task) to 15 (does task normally).

**Table 22–8. RAW SCORES ON FINAL NEUROPSYCHOLOGICAL
MEASURES FOR CASE 1**

Trail Making (sec):
Part A: 70
Part B: 257

Grip Strength (kg):
R = 61
L = 50

Purdue Pegboard (30 sec):
R = 11   L = 10
B = 8   T = 29

Wide-Range Acheivement Test:
Reading: 86 (Stand. Score)
Spelling: 84
Arithmetic: 76
Average T Score: 34
Deficit Index 0.29 (Marked)

WAIS-R:
Verbal IQ   = 79
Performance IQ = 73
Full Scale IQ   = 73

Subtests:

Verbal:		Performance:	
INF	= 5	PCO	= 6
DSP	= 8	PAR	= 6
VOC	= 8	BLD	= 5
ARI	= 6	OBJ	= 8
COM	= 7	DSY	= 3
SIM	= 6		

Wechsler Memory Scale:
Memory Quotient = 70
Basic Aphasia Exam (Rating/Impairment):
Overall Average = 12.36 (Moderate)
Verbal = 12.8 (Moderate)
Graphic = 10.6 (Moderate)
Gestural = 13.7 (Moderate)

Category Test: 94
Tactual Performance Test:
  Right: 2.5 (min/block)
  Left: 3.3
  Both: 1.6 Memory: 5
  Total: 2.3 Local: 0
Finger Tapping (10 sec):
R = 44
L = 37
Foot Tapping (10 sec):
R = 29
L = 27

Mini-Mental State:
Raw Score = 27

---

average of about 4 rating points on each of the summary scales. In fact, when he left the BIRU, he was able to drive a pickup truck and could attend classes for the disabled at a nearby community college. His writing and verbal communication skills were noticeably improved, although they continued to be impaired. This assessment not only enabled us to document some of the improvements in cognitive function that had occurred during the patient's 20 months of treatment, but also assisted us in developing appropriate postdischarge educational and vocational plans.

SUMMARY

While constituting only a component of the total process of evaluation, neuropsychological assessment plays a critical role in the quantitative and qualitative assessment of a patient's cognitive strengths and weaknesses. Each of the approaches detailed in this chapter (Halstead-Reitan, Luria, and Luria-Nebraska) has particular strong points as well as important shortcomings. None is sufficiently comprehensive to preclude the need to employ additional specialized assessment procedures in order to properly define the patient's cognitive status. When correctly employed and interpreted, neuropsychological test data can be a highly effective way of identifying problems and of measuring both progress and outcome in treatment programs. The clinician should attempt to evaluate these three major approaches in terms of their ability to provide timely, comprehensible, practical, and reliable information concerning patients' present and predicted neuropsychological status. It bears emphasizing that neuropsychological assessment in head trauma rehabilitation must transcend the relatively simple function of detecting and localizing cerebral dysfunction. Assessment is most useful to the treatment team if the test data are related to problems in self-care, socialization, or communication.

REFERENCES

1. Halstead, W: Brain and Intelligence: A Quantitative Study of the Frontal Lobes. University of Chicago Press, Chicago, 1947.
2. Luria, A: Higher Cortical Functions in Man. Basic Science Books, New York, 1966.
3. Reitan, R: An investigation of the validity of Halstead's measures of biological intelligence. Arch Neurol Psychiatry 73:28, 1955.
4. Golden, C, Hammeke, T and Purisch, A: Diagnostic validity of a neuropsychological battery derived

from Luria's neuropsychological tests. J Consult Clin Psychol 46:1258, 1978.

5. Golden, C, Purisch, A and Hammeke, T: Luria-Nebraska Neuropsychological Battery: Forms I and II (manual). Western Psychological Services, Los Angeles, 1985.

6. Milberg, W, Hebben, N and Kaplan, E: The Boston process approach to neuropsychological assessment. In Grant, I and Adams, K (eds): Neuropsychological Assessment of Neuropsychiatric Disorders. Oxford University Press, New York, 1986, p 65.

7. Reitan, R and Wolfson, D: The Halstead-Reitan Test Battery: Theory and Clinical Interpretation. Neuropsychology Press, Tucson, 1985, p 16.

8. Wechsler, D: Wechsler Intelligence Scale for Children. Psychological Corporation, New York, 1949.

9. Wechsler, D: Wechsler Adult Intelligence Scale. Psychological Corporation, New York, 1955.

10. Jastak, J and Jastak, S: The Wide Range Achievement Test, ed 3. Jastak Associates, Wilmington, 1978.

11. Reitan, R: A research program on the psychological effects of brain lesions in human beings. In Ellis, N (ed): International Review of Research in Mental Retardation. Academic Press, New York, 1966, p 153.

12. Christensen, A-L: Luria's Neuropsychological Investigation (text), ed 1. Spectrum Publications, New York, 1975.

13. Golden, C, Purisch, A and Hammeke, T: Luria-Nebraska Neuropsychological Battery: Manual. Western Psychological Services, Los Angeles, 1980.

14. Golden, C, Purisch, A and Hammeke, T: Luria-Nebraska Neuropsychological Battery: Forms I and II. Western Psychological Services, Los Angeles, 1985.

15. Sawicki, R and Golden, C: The profile elevation scale and the impairment scale: two new summary scales for the Luria-Nebraska Neuropsychological Battery. Int J Neurosci 23:81, 1984.

16. Delis, D and Kaplan, E: Hazards of a standardized neuropsychological test with low content validity: comment on the Luria-Nebraska Neuropsychological Battery. J Consult Clin Psychol 51:396, 1983.

17. Crosson, B and Warren, R: Use of the Luria-Nebraska Neuropsychological Battery in aphasia: a conceptual critique. J Consult Clin Psychol 50:22, 1982.

18. Goodglass, H and Kaplan, E: The Assessment of Aphasia and Related Disorders. Lea and Febiger, Philadelphia, 1972.

19. Schuell, H: The Minnesota Test for the Differential Diagnosis of Aphasia. University of Minnesota Press, Minneapolis, 1965.

20. Porch, B: The Porch Index of Communicative Ability. Vol. 2: Administration, Scoring and Interpretation, ed 3. Consulting Psychologists Press, Palo Alto, 1981.

21. DeRenzi, E and Vignolo, L: The Token Test: a sensitive test to detect disturbances in aphasics. Brain 85:665, 1962.

22. Spreen, O and Benton, A: Neurosensory Center Comprehensive Examination for Aphasia. Neuropsychology Laboratory, Victoria, BC, 1969.

23. Holland, A: Communicative Abilities in Daily Living. University Park Press, Baltimore, 1980.

24. Wechsler, D and Stone, C: A standardized memory scale for clinical use. J Psychol 19:87, 1945.

25. Osborne, D and Davis, L: Standard scores for Wechsler Memory Scale subtests. J Clin Psychol 34:115, 1978.

26. Russell, E: A multiple scoring method for the assessment of complex memory functions. J Consult Clin Psychol 43:800, 1975.

27. Ivison, D: The Wechsler Memory Scale: preliminary findings toward an Australian standardization. Austral Psychol 12:303, 1977

28. Benton, A: Revised Visual Retention Test, ed 4. Psychological Corp, New York, 1974.

29. Randt, C, Brown, E and Osborne, D: A memory test for longitudinal measurement of mild to moderate deficits. Clin Neuropsychol 2:184, 1980.

30. Denman, S: Denman Neuropsychology Memory Scale Manual. Sidney Denman, Charleston, SC, 1984.

31. Wright, D and Brown, E: Memory versus intelligence in the Randt Memory Test and the Wechsler Memory Scale. Veterans Administration Medical Center, New York City (undated, unpublished manuscript).

32. Osterrieth, P: Le test de copie d'une figure complexe. Arch Psychol 30:206, 1944.

33. Gronwall, D: Paced auditory serial addition task: A measure of recovery from concussion. Percept Mot Skills 44:367, 1977.

34. Gronwall, D: Rehabilitation programs for patients with mild head injury: components, problems, and evaluation. J Head Trauma Rehabil 1:53, 1986.

35. Levin, H, O'Donnell, V and Grossman, R: The Galveston orientation and amnesia test: a practical scale to assess cognition after head injury. J Nerv Ment Dis 167:675, 1979.

36. Mack, J: Clinical assessment of disorders of attention and memory. J Head Trauma Rehabil 1(3):22, 1986.

37. Porch, B and Collins, M: The rating of patient's independence. (unpublished document), 1974.

38. Lynch, W: Neuropsychological rehabilitation: description of an established program. In Caplan, B (ed): Rehabilitation Psychology Desk Reference. Aspen Systems Corp, Rockville, MD, 1987.

39. Bruininks, R et al: Scales of Independent Behavior. DLM Teaching Resources, Allen, TX, 1985.

40. Sparrow, S, Balla, D and Cicchetti, D: Vineland Adaptive Behavior Scales. American Guidance Service, Circle Pines, MN, 1984.

41. Granger, C et al: Advances in functional assessment for medical rehabilitation. Topics Geriat Rehabil 1:59, 1986.

42. Lynch, W and Mauss-Clum, N: Brain injury rehabilitation: Standard problem lists. Arch Phys Med Rehabil 62:223, 1981.

43. Conboy, T, Barth, J and Boll, T: Treatment and rehabilitation of mild and moderate head trauma. Rehabil Psychol 31:203, 1986.

44. Diller, L and Gordon, W: Rehabilitation in clinical neuropsychology. In Filskov, S and Boll, T (eds): Handbook of Clinical Neuropsychology. John Wiley & Sons, New York, 1981, p 702.

45. Craine, J: Principles of cognitive rehabilitation. In Trexler, L (ed): Cognitive Rehabilitation: Conceptualization and Intervention. Plenum Press, New York, 1982, p 83.

46. Luria, A, et al: Restoration of higher cortical function following brain damage. In Vinken, P and Bruyn, G (eds): Handbook of Clinical Neurology, Vol 3. North Holland, Amsterdam, 1969, p 368.

47. Prigatano, G et al: Neuropsychological Rehabilitation After Brain Injury. Johns Hopkins University Press, Baltimore, 1986.

48. Jennett, B: Management of Head Injuries. FA Davis, Philadelphia, 1981, p 317.

49. Teasdale, G and Jennett, B: Assessment of coma and impaired consciousness: a practical scale. Lancet 2:81, 1974.

50. Bond, M: Standardized methods of assessing and predicting outcome. In Rosenthal, M et al (eds): Rehabilitation of the Head-Injured Adult. FA Davis, Philadelphia, 1983, p 102.

51. Jennett, B, Teasdale, G and Braakman, R: Prognosis in a series of patients with severe head injury. Neurosurgery 4:283, 1979.

52. Jennett, B and Bond, M: Assessment of outcome after severe brain damage: a practical scale. Lancet 1:480, 1975.

53. Jennett, B: The measurement of outcome. In Brooks, N (ed): Closed Head Injury. Oxford Medical Publications, Oxford, 1984, p 37.

54. Jennett, B: The measurement of outcome. In Brooks, N (ed): Closed Head Injury. Oxford Medical Publications, Oxford, 1984, p 42.

55. Rappaport, M et al: Disability rating scale for severe head trauma patients. Arch Phys Med Rehabil 63:118, 1982.

56. Levin, H, O'Donnell, V and Grossman, R: The Galveston Orientation and Amnesia Test: a practical scale to assess cognition after head injury. J Nerv Ment Dis 167:675, 1979.

57. Roberts, A: Severe Accidental Head Injury. Macmillan, New York, 1979.

58. Porch, B et al: Statistical prediction of change in aphasia. J Speech Hear Res 23:312, 1980.

59. Klonoff, P, Costa, L and Snow, W: Predictors and indicators of quality of life in patients with closed head injury. J Clin Exp Neuropsychol 8:469, 1986.

60. Knights, R and Watson, P: The use of computerized test profiles in neuropsychological assessment. J Learn Disabil 1:696, 1968.

61. Kiernan, R and Matthews, C: Impairment index versus T-score averaging in neuropsychological assessment. J Consult Clin Psychol 44:951, 1976.

Section IV
Conclusion

J. DOUGLAS MILLER, M.D., Ph.D.

In the assessment of the head injured patient the neurologic examination has to be adapted to cope at one end of the spectrum, with the elicitation of minor neurologic dysfunction and subtle indications of disability, while at the other extreme the comatose patient is unable to cooperate at all with the examiner and special techniques are involved in eliciting evidence of neurologic function or dysfunction. In many ways the challenge for the specialized evaluations carried out by the physiatrist; physical, occupational, and speech therapist; and the clinical psychologist is even greater. In the management of head injury early assessment is desirable, often at a stage when the patient is inaccessible to verbal command and at a later stage when the assessment needs to be more detailed, difficulties for the assessor arise because the patient may be dysphasic, may have a short attention span, may have inappropriate or antisocial behavior, and often has impaired short-term memory. Considerable patience, skill, and understanding is required in building up the accurate picture of the patient's disabilities that is so essential to the planning of a suitable treatment regimen.

Until relatively recently the assessment of the head injured patient at the bedside or in the outpatient clinic was made more difficult by a lack of understanding of the pathophysiology of head injury. Partly as a result of wartime experience much attention was focused on focal brain injury, particularly by the clinical psychologist, and over-rigid differentiations between diffuse and focal injury were made. It is now recognized that even the patient who has a missile wound of the head will have some element of diffuse brain dysfunction and damage of both primary and secondary types, as well as the more obvious focal brain lesion. The patient who has suffered a head injury of blunt acceleration/deceleration type will certainly have a large amount of diffuse brain injury, often of axonal type scattered in the white matter, but such patients also have elements of focal brain injury, particularly at the frontal and temporal poles. Therefore, assessments must provide an approach to the global assessment of brain function; many of the late problems suffered by head injury patients reflect these diffuse forms of dysfunction.

In this section on specialized methods of assessment some overlap has been inevitable. No apology is made for this because it is a realistic description of the day-to-day experience of the authors. For making assessments standardization would be ideal. This has been exemplified by the widespread international use of the Glasgow Coma Scale for the neurologic assessment, particularly of the severely head injured patient. Such standardization becomes much more difficult to achieve in these more specialized methods of assessment because of the difficulty that some patients have in completing all the tests or completing them all at one time, or in the use of tests that simply do not cover all of the problems experienced by the patient. There is, however, widespread recognition of the immense value of standardization of head injury assessment.

A common theme in these assessment methods is the growing realization that the challenge is to be able to assess function in head injured patients in real life situations. There is appreciation of the importance of functional impairment owing not to primary inability to perform a task, but to undue proneness to distraction from the task because of irritability, bad temper, short-term memory loss, or short attention span. All who work with head injured patients recognize these problems and the heartening message for the future is that many workers are steadily progressing toward the development of a battery of tests that will accurately define and describe the day-to-day problems of the head injured survivor.

SECTION V

TREATMENT APPROACHES

Mitchell Rosenthal, Ph.D., Editor

Chapter 23

Strategies for Improving Motor Performance

MARY ANNE RINEHART, M.S., P.T.

NATURE OF THE PROBLEM

Motor impairment is one sequela of head trauma. The nature or extent of residual motor impairment has been correlated by various authors to outcome scales.[1-4] A large percentage of head trauma survivors is likely to have some degree of motor impairment. Although residual physical or motor impairment does not appear to have as high a frequency as cognitive impairment,[3, 5] it is not always possible to distinctly separate motor and cognitive performance. Scales that measure motor and cognitive function may not always take into consideration that these variables can be dependent upon each other. For example, apraxia resulting in reduced motor performance is dependent on the loss of the cognitive function of ideomotor planning. Therefore, motor and cognitive functional losses in the head trauma patient merit equal consideration and attention.

The principal problem in the treatment of motor deficits is lack of known effectiveness of one treatment regimen versus another. Treatment of head trauma in general is relatively new in the field of medicine. In the realm of treatment for motor dysfunction, increased effort at measuring treatment effectiveness is essential and feasible.

One problem in determining the extent of motor deificits and the effectiveness of treatment is the lack of qualitative assessment scales. Measurements of motor performance are often broad categorical items such as ambulation or self-care. Within these generalized functions are many components covering a broad spectrum of motor activities. Quality of movement has been addressed in only a couple of studies,[6, 7] yet it is the quality of movement that distinguishes the effectiveness of treatment and refinement of independent performance of tasks.[8]

Strategies to improve motor performance discussed in this chapter are intended to provide concepts for treatment planning. Strategy has been defined as the overall approach or plan for obtaining a specific goal.[9] Prior to selecting specific treatment plans one needs to consider why and how motor performance can be improved.

EFFICACY OF TREATMENT

In order to determine why or how treatment of motor deficits can be effective, sensorimotor oganization must be considered. When considering the motor system, one needs to remain aware that the sensory system is an integral part of motor function. The nervous system programs motor output, which is continuously dependent on sensory feedback for the correct execution of the movement.[10] In head trauma the impairment of sensory feedback produces numerous problems in motor performance. Treatment directed at affecting the sensorimotor system could result in improved motor performance. Although musculoskeletal problems such as fractures or heterotopic ossification may impair motor performance

331

(without a direct relationship to sensory receptors) they do not constitute the majority of motor problems.

Improvement in motor performance may be the result of spontaneous recovery or plasticity of the central nervous system (CNS).[11, 12] Spontaneous recovery may be evident as the person emerges from a coma. The motor system is essentially intact and loss of performance is due to the coma. Edema of the brain may resolve, which usually occurs within a couple weeks posttrauma, and motor performance could dramatically improve.[13] For the majority of patients seen for rehabilitation, spontaneous recovery is a minimal factor in improvement.

Plasticity of the CNS does exist and may be the most efficacious reason that sensorimotor improvement can occur following brain trauma. The CNS was once thought to be incapable of change or plasticity after its development. Evidence of plasticity includes at least two mechanisms: collateral sprouting and unmasking. In collateral sprouting, intact axons establish synaptic connections in areas where degenerated axons have occurred.[11] Neural reorganization or unmasking is a process in which neural structures and pathways not formerly used for a given function, are developed to provide improved motor performance.[12]

Some of the factors that influence plasticity are environment,[14] complexity of stimulation,[15] repetition of tasks,[16] and motivation.[17] An enriched environment, one in which a variety of controlled stimuli is provided, has been shown to encourage dendritic growth.[14] Other studies have demonstrated that complex stimuli and repeated practice are needed to augment plasticity.[15, 16] Motivating the patient to perform a task is essential for any training effect to occur.[17] Likewise, Black and colleagues demonstrated that a delay in implementing therapy in monkeys with cortical lesions resulted in less improvement of function.[18] At 6 months following the lesion, monkeys with a delay in therapy had 67 percent return of previous function, while those receiving immediate therapy had 82 percent return. Plasticity can be affected by treatment that is instrumental in providing the necessary environment, complexity and repetition of tasks, and motivation to perform motor activities.

Beginning treatment as soon as possible following the trauma is another consideration in the efficacy of treatment. Early treatment intervention for head trauma has been shown to reduce the total length of hospitalization.[7] The sooner rehabilitation was initiated after the acute hospital phase, the less time was needed before the patient could be discharged from an inpatient environment. This phenomenon indicates that earlier intervention prevents complications which might retard progress in motor performance and, therefore, treatment goals can be achieved sooner. Physical complications such as joint contractures are preventable even in the comatose patient. Unfortunately, if proper attention during the acute phase is not given to treatment that prevents contractures, the ultimate motor performance goals require increased effort and timelines to achieve.

Because acute trauma triage is aimed at life-threatening functions, management of extremity fractures or wounds is frequently delayed. Also the treatment of the fractures may be less than ideal if the physician believes coma is permanent or death is certain. Consultation between therapists and orthopedic physicians could reduce the secondary skeletal complications that prevent the maximum level of motor performance possible following the coma. The orthopedist seldom sees the patient after the period of coma and is not aware of how the surgical or fixation techniques affect the long-term outcome.

Ideally, treatment should be aimed at restoring lost function, and consideration must be given to compensatory movement patterns—particularly during the early phase of the treatment program. The early introduction of compensatory movement patterns is likely to prevent the restoration of more normal movement patterns. Pressures on the therapist from the patient or family and hospital expectations to decrease the length of stay often result in teaching compensatory movements with or without assistive devices. Perhaps more attention should be given to discussing alternatives and their rationale with patients or families to achieve more qualitative goals. Obviously social and economic factors do play a role in the patient's goals and should be considered in all aspects of treatment planning.

Related to the efficacy of treatment is

knowing when to stop treatment. When it is evident that an individual has achieved a certain goal, we should discontinue the current treatment program, or implement a new treatment plan in accordance with another goal. If our goal is not achieved and various treatment approaches have been tried, we often have a difficult time accepting the fact that the patient is at a plateau. The CNS is capable of change but not always at the pace we would like. As therapists we can avoid frustration for ourselves and patients if we can learn to recognize a plateau and deal with it pragmatically. Putting a patient on an exercise program at home for several months and then reassessing the patient for further improvement in motor performance is an acceptable alternative. It is beneficial not only to recognize a plateau but also to appreciate when treatment should be reinstituted months or years post-trauma. Reassessment at intervals enables the therapist to observe changes, both losses or improvements, in motor performance and establish a new treatment plan as indicated.

TREATMENT CONSIDERATIONS

There are at least four principles that should be incorporated into treatment plans to improve motor performance. One or more of these principles will be used in any treatment process.

One of the principles in treating motor dysfunction is *the need to facilitate movement*. Generally, we want to facilitate normal patterns of movement, but with the comatose patients our purpose may be to facilitate any movement while at the same time not causing excessive repetition of abnormal movement patterns. For example, scraping the sole of a comatose patient may elicit a flexor withdrawal pattern of that lower extremity. The flexor withdrawal reflex is a primitive reflex pattern in an adult, but this movement pattern may be elicited occasionally if achieving good joint flexion is difficult due to severe extensor posturing. Many treatment techniques exist to facilitate normal movement patterns (such as altering the position of the neck or body, applying resistance to certain body parts, guiding the part through the correct pat-

tern, providing biofeedback, applying tactile input, and so forth).

A second principle for treatment is *the need to inhibit undesirable characteristics of movement patterns*. For example, lesions of the basal ganglia or cerebellum and their pathways can unmask tremors, ataxia, or other losses of timing and sequencing of movement that cause excessive movement. Techniques to dampen unwanted movement include visual and kinesthetic cues, resistance to body parts, and controlled timing of the movement. Effectiveness of treatment for such movement disorders seems to be less than that provided for other motor dysfunctions. Perhaps we have yet to find more plausible treatment methods or possibly the neural plasticity capabilities are less for the basal ganglia and cerebellum.

Another principle of treatment is that *muscle strength and endurance must be sufficient to achieve normal movement*. Damage to the motor cortex and its association areas results in the loss of upper motoneurons and subsequently muscle strength. Additionally, muscle atrophy does occur in patients with upper motor neuron lesions.[19] Since head trauma patients are likely to be in a coma and immobilized in bed for a period of time, muscle atrophy can occur with resultant loss of strength. Sahrmann and Norton have shown that spasticity is not the only factor in the paucity of movement in persons with upper motor neuron lesions.[20] Rather the lack of a sufficient number of functioning motoneurons to perform the desired movement is the major contributing factor to lack of movement. Endurance should also be considered in motor performance. In patients following a coma or in those that seldom move unless facilitated, there can easily be a decrease in endurance. Therefore, sustained inactivity results in decreased motor performance.

The last principle is that *motor learning occurs best under certain circumstances*. The head trauma patient may relearn functional motor skills in much the same manner as the skills were originally learned. There are three general stages for learning a motor skill: understanding the task, establishing sensory and motor associations, and integrating the movement patterns at an automatic level.[21] Numerous circumstances affect the stages of motor learning, including learning set, attention, motivation, past experience, and type of stimulus.[22] Obviously, the ideal circumstances are not always present for motor learning treatment, but must be strived for to achieve the desired goal. For example, the patient may not be able to attend to the task, so the first step in the motor learning process would be to develop an increased attention span before the next step of the task is undertaken. Analysis of the motor control problem can enable the therapist through treatment to assist the patient in learning the desired skill.

TREATMENT PLANNING

Determining a treatment plan for head trauma patients poses some unique problems compared with that for other rehabilitation diagnoses. For example, relatively predictable neurologic sensory and motor patterns of recovery are known for spinal cord injury or stroke patients. Long-term functional goals can be fairly confidently set and then a treatment plan can be established which correlates with the evaluation findings and the goal. A comatose head trauma patient requires a treatment plan based on the evaluation findings but with restricted short-term goals. The limited goal may be to prevent loss of joint range of motion. As the patient becomes more alert and changes in motor control can be observed and assessed the treatment plan is modified and more measurable functional goals are established. Likewise, if several weeks pass with no improvement in alertness or motor control, plans should be made to put the patient on an infrequent treatment program and to periodically assess for improvement or deterioration. Teaching other medical personnel or the family how to provide essential treatment may also be a necessary cost-effective method of treating unresponsive patients.

Other factors to consider in treatment planning for improving motor performance are behavior and cognition. Although behavioral and cognitive problems can exist in patients with other rehabilitation diagnoses, both generally do not occur at the degree of severity as in head trauma patients. A major emphasis in treatment plans needs to be on behavioral and cognitive dysfunction. If these problems are not considered, the therapist and quite possibly the patient will become highly frustrated with the lack of progress in any one direction. For example, the treatment plan for a patient with a motor control problem of a dominating extensor synergy of the lower extremity when standing could include:

1. Kneeling to achieve good hip control without the influence of simultaneous knee and ankle extension
2. Standing with the ankle in dorsiflexion to decrease plantar pressure influences and facilitate reciprocal inhibition of plantar-flexor muscles
3. Resistive exercises to the hip flexor, abductor, and external rotator muscles to encourage a balance of muscle control influences

All of these activities would make a sensible treatment approach for the motor control problem but are doomed for failure if the patient's behavior or cognitive problems preclude such motor performance. If the patient becomes agitated when kneeling, treatment 1 will be ineffective. If the patient's attention span is too short to remain standing on the heel, then treatment 2 is inappropriate. Finally, if verbal requests to hold against resistance cannot be comprehended, then treatment 3 is not feasible. The altered treatment plan may be a totally different one or a modification of the previously described ones which incorporates the behavioral and cognitive problems. Such plans might include, for example, resistance (without verbal instructions) to hip and ankle flexion while the patient is rolling; kneeling may be tolerated if the patient is distracted during the activity. (See Chapters 12 and 13 for in-depth information on behavioral and cognitive problems.) All rehabilitation team members must have at least a general knowledge of physical and mental dysfunction, since one affects the other. Particular emphasis must be directed by the physical therapist toward treatment planning that consideres the cognitive and behavioral problems in the treatment program for motor performance.

A second major concern in treatment of motor problems is secondary complications. Fractures of the skull and facial bones, vertebrae, and extremities affect the treatment plan. Skull fractures or other problems that require removal of part of the skull pose no significant problem for therapeutic exercises. The use of a helmet is necessary for protection of the brain, but all physical activities can still be done. Facial bone fractures usually do not interfere with treatment except that mandibular fractures curtail oral-motor activities. The coincidence of spinal cord injury and head injury is fairly common.[23] Spinal cord damage may not be recognized initially when the patient is unable to communicate and sensorimotor function is disrupted cortically as well. Ultimately symptoms may be manifested such as flaccid lower extremities, Brown-Sequard sensorimotor pattern, and movement of upper extremities with little or no movement of lower extremities.

Fractures of the extremities affect treatment plans during the period of immobilization (see Chapter 9). Frequently, standard methods of surgery and/or immobilization are not feasible. Surgery may need to be delayed as a result of acute respiratory distress or unstable vital signs. Immobilization with traction may not be practical for a patient with increased agitation or if it increases the chances of pressure areas or further bony distortion. The therapist may be able to determine the most feasible type of immobilization, given the patient's physical constraints.

Brachial plexus injuries occur frequently with head trauma, particularly when resulting from motorcycle accidents. Brachial plexus injury is suspect in the presence of a clavicular fracture or a dislocated shoulder. The injury may not be obvious in a comatose or flaccid hemiplegic patient.

Hydrocephalus is another complication to which the therapist should be attuned. A decrease in motor performance would be a strong indicator of increased hydrocephalic pressure, which may also be accompanied by increased lethargy. A malfunctioning shunt or the need for a shunt can readily be determined by the physician when the observed symptoms are reported.

A significant number of head injury patients receive prophylactic medications to prevent or control seizures. Increased lethargy or decreased performance may be indicative of toxicity to the medications. Therapists may also be the first to note petit mal seizures since activities or communication are momentarily interrupted. These seizures should be readily distinguishable from motor impersistence and loss of attention.

Heterotopic ossification is another complication that can occur with head trauma (see Chapter 9). Of particular interest to physical or occupational therapists are the painful joints and loss of joint range of motion. The ability to prevent a decrease in joint range of motion is compounded if the patient has difficulty understanding the problem. Activities that encourage the patient to stretch his or her own joints are often necessary for the person who cannot accept manual stretching by the therapist. Positioning to achieve a prolonged stretch may also be effective. The painful stage of this procedure usually only lasts several weeks; it is during this period that treatment priorities must focus on maintaining joint range of motion. Even after the pain and inflammation around the joint subside the bone formation continues, so one cannot abandon treatment. However, with a decrease in pain it is usually easier to design a treatment program that includes other needs while incorporating maximum movement of the traumatized joint.

TREATMENT APPROACHES

The treatment approaches for comatose head trauma patients have a different emphasis than those for patients no longer in coma. For purposes of this discussion the treatment approaches for the comatose patient are considered first. Recognizing that there is no precise demarcation between coma and postcoma regarding motor performance, treatment approaches for both phases may overlap.

Coma

Plum and Posner defined coma as a state in which psychological and motor responses to stimulation are either completely lost (deep coma) or reduced to only rudimentary reflex motor responses (moderately deep coma).[24] Strategies for improving motor performance for patients in a coma are directed toward altering abnormal motor responses and facilitating appropriate responses. Treatment emphasis includes sensory stimulation, preserving joint range of motion, and positioning. Additional therapeutic techniques may be necessary, depending on the specific problem; for example, chest physical therapy for residual pneumonia or immobilization devices for orthopedic complications such as joint sprains or dislocations.

Sensory Stimulation

Sensory stimulation in the comatose patient is used for arousal and to elicit appropriate patterns of movement. In this context, sensory stimulation is considered as methods to primarily tap the five basic senses. In the comatose patient multiple avenues of stimulation may provide a summation of stimuli sufficient to affect the reticular activating system for arousal. Furthermore, it is initially difficult to determine which sensory modalities are functioning, although auditory and visual evoked potentials provide some information for these two modalities. Using sensory stimuli can give an empirical means of assessing the patient's responses and quantifying those responses. Taste can be stimulated by solutions of the basic taste modalities: sweet, sour, salty, and bitter. A cotton swab can be dipped in the solution and then applied to the outside of the gums or teeth. It is not necessary to touch the appropriate taste receptors of the tongue with the solutions as the saliva will reach the responsive areas. The cotton swab must be applied externally to the teeth or gums in cases of jaw fractures or strong bite response. Responses to this form of stimuli are no response, protective or avoidance response, and good oral motor response which includes no excessive grimacing or bruxism.

Scents may be used to stimulate olfactory reception but do not appear to be a very powerful form of sensory stimulation in the comatose patient. Patients with a tracheostomy will not benefit from odors since they do not breathe through their nose and are unlikely to capture the scent.

The auditory system is stimulated by radio, television, and the human voice. One should approach comatose or semicomatose patients as if they can hear and comprehend what is being said. Explaining to the person what treatment is being done in a simple and concise manner may prevent startle reactions or agitation.

Visual stimulation may be evoked at the bedside by pictures and mobiles. The treatment area can augment visual input by using posters, mirrors, multicolored beach balls, and pinwheels to encourage spontaneous eye movement and fixation.

Tactile stimulation is employed in turning the person in bed, bathing, and dressing. Therapeutic tactile techniques for the low-level patient should concentrate on neck, facial, and oral areas. Head and neck control is one of the first areas needed to achieve an upright position. Tapping and stroking neck musculature can facilitate those muscles opposed by the asymmetrical tonic neck reflex (ATNR), while pressure may inhibit the muscles influencing the ATNR. Facial and oral responses to tactile stimulation are important for eating and speech. Treatment may include inhibition of avoidance to tactile stimulation around the face and mouth, and facilitation for sucking, chewing, swallowing, and breath control. An oral hygiene stick can be used to provide gentle tactile stimulation to the lips, gums, and tongue. To facilitate mouth closure, light pressure with the finger above the upper lip can be used, and for a clenched jaw, pressure to the temporomandibular joint and masseter muscles can provide relaxation of the lower jaw.

The family can readily be involved in providing sensory stimulation which in turn gives the family a feeling of value through participation. Family involvement in treating the comatose or semicomatose patient is beneficial for two reasons. First, it gives the family opportunity and responsibility for assessing real changes to treatment in the patient. Second, when family members are involved in care and treatment they are less apt to complain to or become frustrated with medical staff when improvement is not occurring, as they are already aware of it.

Precautions should be taken in applying sensory stimulation, since the patient may have adverse responses. Sensory bombardment may lead to increased reflex responses or avoidance reactions which will not lead to the desired motor outcomes. For example, icing around the mouth or to other body areas may evoke a desirable response or it may produce a strong primitive reflex response such as the snout reflex or ATNR. In this case, the sensory modality would be contraindicated. Sensory stimulation that produces adverse responses can only be justified if it also elicits other more beneficial responses. Awareness of the patient's responses determines the appropriate therapeutic sensory modality to use and when to cease using it, based on desired responses.

Positioning

Positioning is part of the treatment program for comatose or semicomatose patients. One of the benefits of positioning is good joint alignment, which will ultimately affect motor performance. Positioning in the bed and wheelchair can diminish undesirable postures. Cerebral edema usually subsides within 2 weeks after trauma; therefore, if other medical complications are not present, the patient can be positioned prone and sitting.

Patients often have a combination of primitive tonic neck and labyrinthine reflexes. For patients with strong extensor influences to the joints when in the supine position, sitting can achieve prolonged flexion of lower extremity joints and decrease the possibility of equinus deformities. If strong flexion responses are present in the lower extremities, standing on a tilt table can provide a prolonged stretch and inhibition to the flexor muscles and likewise prevent hip and knee flexion contractures. Positioning that prevents joint contractures is a more cost-effective treatment method than is serial casting and should be tried as the first treatment method. Also, a good bed or sitting positioning program reduces the potential for joint contractures more effectively than does passive range of motion by itself. Positioning inhibits undesirable tonic reflex influences and provides prolonged muscle stretch, which passive range of motion does not accomplish. Sitting or standing for comatose patients is important for physiologic benefits and also provides proprioceptive stimulation and visual feedback through increased alertness.

Frequently, washcloths are placed in the hands of comatose patients who have strong finger flexor spasticity to prevent skin breakdown due to sweating of the palm and the fingernails pressing into the skin. A wooden dowel or cone placed in the palm for grasping is more likely to inhibit the increased flexor tone by firm pressure to the flexor muscles.

Range of Motion

Joint range of motion needs to be preserved or restored at any stage of recovery but can be a greater problem during the comatose stage when active movement is zero to minimal. As previously mentioned sensory stimulation techniques and positioning are treatment methods to preserve joint range of motion. Passive range of motion is also necessary to various joints since bathing, positioning, and the like do not provide full range to each joint. Shoulder and hip rotation, hip abduction, finger abduction, and forearm supination are all examples in which passive range of motion is the most effective treatment method. Neck and trunk flexibility must not be overlooked, which can easily happen when the abnormal postures of the extremities are so much more apparent.

Accessory motions of the joint must also be considered and treated as needed. For example, if the shoulder remains protracted and internally rotated the anterior capsule of the shoulder joint is likely to become tight. For a tight anterior capsule the treatment would be to push the head of the humerus posteriorly. If this accessory motion is not available, passive range of motion into shoulder flexion and external rotation will jam the head of the humerus against the acromioclavicular joint. Accessory motions can readily be lost in any immobilized joint and become even more important to evaluate and treat for joints immobilized due to fractures.

Serial casting is another method of treating joint range of motion problems in both coma and postcoma phases. An important consideration in casting for head trauma patients is their cognitive status. Many patients cannot tolerate having more than one joint casted at the same time. The process of casting takes time and the discomfort or annoyance produced by a cast must be considered when selecting the joint or joints to be casted. If the person is confused, easily agitated, or has poor short-term memory, casting one joint at a time is more likely to be successful. (For further information on casting techniques, see Booth and coworkers.[25])

Postcoma

Once the person is no longer in a comatose state, physical restoration is accomplished by emphasizing other treatment approaches. Analysis of the factors contributing to abnormal postures and movement or the lack of movement must be done to effectively design a treatment plan. Although various authors have expressed different theories and treatment techniques for neuromuscular disorders, there is no one technique that can be described as the only choice for the treatment of head trauma patients.[26–30]

Fay believed that patterns of movement are developmentally achieved.[26] Movement of the extremities begins with homolateral patterns progressing to homologous and finally to crossed diagonal patterns. Doman and Delcato developed treatment techniques based on taking a person through the patterns of movement espoused by Fay.[31] The patterns of movement are repeated until the person achieves success at one developmental level and then progresses toward the next level.

Brunnstrom developed a system of classifying and treating patients with hemiplegia based on observations of their recovery patterns.[27] One of Brunnstrom's theories is that during early recovery stages the basic synergy patterns of the extremities should be facilitated since they are an integral phase of recovery. Ultimately facilitation of movement patterns which deviate from the basic synergies are encouraged.

Kabat and Knott found that stretch and resistance to muscles while going through specific functional patterns of movement caused irradiation to the muscles involved and thus stronger muscle contractions.[28] Kabat's treatment techniques have been termed proprioceptive neuromuscular facilitation (PNF). Facilitation techniques of PNF may also be used at different points in the movement pattern to inhibit the antagonist or facilitate the agonist.[32]

The treatment techniques advocated by Rood are based on principles of developmental motor patterns to achieve stability or mobility and that sensory stimuli facilitate or inhibit the motoric responses.[29]

Bobath treatment techniques were developed for people with cerebral palsy and hemiplegia and are now commonly called neurodevelopmental techniques.[30] Essentially this technique is concerned with the inhibition of abnormal patterns of movement while facilitating normal patterns. This is accomplished by guiding the person through movement patterns approximating those found in normal development.

Harris also defined treatment techniques for persons with cerebral palsy.[33] He used the term "inapproprioception" to refer to athetoid movements in cerebral palsy (i.e., the proprioceptive system is providing poor feedback to the CNS regarding posture and movement). Abnormal postures lead to faulty feedback of body awareness and to shortened resting tension of the muscle. His concept is that hypertonic agonist muscles must be slowly stretched and then weak antagonist muscles facilitated and strengthened.

All of these techniques rely on facilitation techniques and the majority emphasize following developmental patterns. The developmental patterns of movement described by Fay, Rood, and Bobath are not the same nor are they all-inclusive for each phase of development. Since there has been no determination made that recovery patterns of adults with head trauma follow a developmental sequence or the patterns of stroke patients, caution needs to be exercised in extrapolating treatment theories and techniques to the head trauma population. Obviously certain patterns of movement are necessary to perform a given activity and these patterns may be achieved through activities such as crawling or coming to sitting. The rationale for these activities may be to facilitate motor control for scapular stability and upper extremity extension and not to achieve a developmental milestone. The rationale for most of the previously mentioned treatment techniques is based on common neurophysiologic principles. Some of the principles are reciprocal inhibition,[34] facilitation and inhibition of motoneurons by cutaneous stimuli,[35] and stimuli to a stretched muscle are excitatory to that muscle, depending on the position of the body.[36] A combination of treatment principles and techniques is essential in treating patients with head trauma, since variations in dysfunction exist within and between individuals. Treatment techniques selected should consider the physical, cognitive, and behavioral deficits exhibited by that person. Because these factors can change during the continuum of rehabilitation, various techniques may be selected at different points in time. In sum, there is no one best technique to activate motor performance under all circumstances.

Hypertonicity Treatment

Treatment techniques for the person with spasticity or hypertonicity are also dependent upon careful analysis of the symptoms. As stated by Duncan (Chapter 19), motor control is influenced by hypertonicity, which is a fluctuating phenomenon. Therefore, a patient may exhibit spasticity in the biceps muscle when sitting but not when prone, or the degree of spasticity may vary between morning and afternoon. Merely to determine that a person has spasticity in a given muscle does not provide enough information on which to base selection of treatment techniques. Passive and active movement during different body positions provides more complete information for treatment planning. Prolonged stretch by positioning or casting, cryotherapy to the hypertonic muscle, and facilitation of the antagonist muscle are methods of reducing the sensitivity of stretch receptors. Treatment to alter hypertonicity is essential to preserve joint range of motion and to reduce exaggerated motor responses.

The therapist should be careful about deciding that the loss of movement is only due to spasticity. As previously noted, Sahrmann and Harris have found that lack of movement can be due to muscle weakness and not just hypertonicity.[20, 33] For example, if the biceps muscle displays increased resistance to passive stretch and active movement only occurs in mid-range, one could conclude that spasticity of the muscle prevents the full range of active movement. The most likely reason active elbow flexion cannot be initiated from the neutral position is muscle weakness. In this example, to strengthen the biceps muscle the use of facilitation techniques, and not the inhibitory techniques, would be emphasized.

Peripheral nerve blocks by an injection of phenol or other anesthetic agents can denervate nerve fibers in the area of the injection and alter hypertonicity.[37, 38] The physical therapist may identify the potential benefits of a phenol block for a certain patient and present this information to the physician. Indications for a peripheral nerve block may include hypertonicity which interferes with function or joint integrity. For example, ambulatory function will be limited when the stretch receptors of the knee extensor muscles are so sensitive that standing causes an excessive overflow of activity to other lower extremity muscles. When other treatment measures do not alleviate this problem or surgical techniques are being considered, a phenol block may be of benefit. The physician will selectively inject the motor point of the offending knee extensor muscle. This may then reduce the overflow stimulus to the other muscles and allow functional ambulation to occur.

A successful or unsuccessful peripheral nerve block can provide information upon which to base a surgical decision. Peripheral nerve blocks with phenol are usually temporary but may allow for a functional movement pattern to be established prior to nerve regeneration (see also Chapter 10).[37]

Oral Motor Treatment

At Rancho Cognitive Level III and above, oral motor problems may be emerging and treatment can be emphasized for those deficits. Treatment for oral and dysphagia motor problems should also consider head and neck posture. The head and neck must be in good alignment for an adequate airway and functional jaw movements and swallowing. When the patient is in bed pillows should be removed if they are causing excessive neck flexion. When the patient is upright neck support may be needed to maintain the head in good alignment. Head and neck posture can be improved by many treatment techniques, such as rolling, proning on elbows, tapping neck extensor muscles, touch to the posterior head, and joint approximation through compression to the top of the head.

Abnormal oral behaviors including bruxism, clenched jaw, and drooling are influenced by tactile stimulation and improvement in other oral movements. Tactile stimulation to the face and oral areas needs to be assessed and treated if hyperesthetic or hypoesthetic responses occur. Facial expressions are often lacking in head injury patients but this is not commonly due to paralysis from the facial nerve. Affect and the associated facial expressions are a cerebral function and the loss of such is due to lack of sensory integration and function of other neuronal structures. If little or no reaction occurs with tactile stimulation to the face, gums, or tongue, then teatment should include such stimulation. If excessive grimacing or biting occurs with tactile stimulation, then treatment should be to reduce these exaggerated responses. This can be accomplished by tactile stimulation to the face, lips, and gums using firm and slow repetitions with a washcloth, cotton swab, or oral hygiene stick. As responses to tactile stimulation become more normal, jaw clenching and other exaggerated facial and oral reactions will decrease.

Motor performance of the tongue is important for movement of food inside the mouth, swallowing, and speech phonemes. If the patient is unable to follow verbal requests, tongue movements can be observed during spontaneous activities such as licking the lips and swallowing and in response to tactile stimulation. Touch to the tongue with a tongueblade or bite stick, if the bite is questionable, should produce avoidance or protective reactions. Normally the tongue will move away from the stimulus or try to remove it. If there is no movement, treatment consists of pressure to the sides and dorsum of the tongue using the tongueblade to encourage movement. When the patient can follow verbal requests, tongue movements (lateral, elevation, protrusion, and retraction) can be evaluated and strengthened by resistance against a tongue blade or manually. Functional movements can then be assessed to determine if the tongue can remove food between the teeth and cheek, retract during swallowing, and produce phonemes rapidly enough to provide quality of speech.

The soft palate elevates during swallowing and certain vocal sounds to close the nasopharyngeal cavity. If the soft palate is not functioning properly, speech has a nasal sound and food may enter the nasal passage.

Function of the soft palate can be assessed as it elevates and adducts reflexively with stimulation or with the sound "ah." If muscle weakness is present, activities involving sucking and blowing can strengthen motor control. Blowing can be done with matches or soap bubbles, which is a good spontaneous activity for low-level patients.

Posterior pharyngeal wall muscle activity is essential for swallowing. Function of these muscles is assessed by the gag reflex, which is stimulated by pressure on the posterior third of the tongue using a tongueblade. Impairment of the gag reflex in adults with a head trauma is usually seen in a hypoactive response.[39] Treatment consists of pressure to the posterior tongue or stroking the posterior pharyngeal wall with a tongueblade for a hypoactive gag reflex. A hyperactive gag reflex can be desensitized by firmly and slowly moving the tongueblade backward on the tongue.

Dysphagia occurs when one or more oral motor control problem exists. When tongue and soft palate movements and the gag reflex are funtioning, swallowing can be observed for timeliness and coordination. Feeding training can begin when oral motor components are functioning adequately and a functional cough is present. Problems may continue after eating has been initiated due to fatigue, decreased attention span, impaired taste, and the effects of drugs such as phenobarbital on salivation.

Motor Control Treatment

At Rancho Cognitive Levels III and above, motor control of the trunk and extremities becomes more relevant in treatment planning. Initially, treatment emphasis is to encourage spontaneous movement by inhibition of undesirable postures and facilitation of normal movement. The following activities are a sample of some treatment methods to achieve spontaneous movement and functional motor performance in the low-level patient:

Prone

Position	Patient prone on elbows with a foam wedge under the chest, or without wedge if position can be maintained	Purpose	Decrease extensor tone found in the supine position Facilitate shoulder flexion and abduction

	Facilitate neck control
	Facilitate shoulder girdle stability
	Stretch to and decrease tone in hip flexor muscles
	Allow spontaneous knee flexion and extension
Activities	Weight-shift side to side on elbows to inhibit shoulder extension/adduction posture, facilitate shoulder girdle musculature, and preparation for prone-to-supine rolling pattern
	Neck control by tapping or vibration to neck extensor muscles, looking at objects such as pictures at different locations and heights

Crawling

Position	Patient in crawling position over a bolster, or without bolster if the position can be maintained
Purpose	Decrease upper extremity postures of shoulder extension/adduction/internal rotation, elbow and wrist flexion
	Facilitate shoulder flexion/abduction, elbow and wrist extension
	Facilitate shoulder girdle and pelvic stability
	Facilitate protective and equilibrium reactions
Activities	Weight-shift side to side onto upper extremities, lower extremities, or both, to decrease elbow and wrist flexor muscle tone and facilitate elbow and wrist extensor muscles and shoulder girdle and pelvic stability
	Rolling the bolster forward and backward to facilitate spontaneous weight bearing, protective and equilibrium reactions
	Neck control as described under "Prone"

Kneeling

Position	Patient kneeling against a bolster, or without support if the position can be maintained
Purpose	Facilitate head and trunk control
	Inhibit total flexor or extensor pattern of lower extremities, facilitate hip extension with knee flexion
	Facilitate shoulder flexion/abduction in a more stressful environment

	Facilitate protective and equilibrium reactions
Activities	Weight-shift from side to side to facilitate hip stability and equilibrium reactions
	Tapping to facilitate back and hip extensor and hip abductor muscles
	Upper extremity movement with objects placed on top of the bolster to encourage balance while using upper extremities

Sitting

Position	Patient sitting on a mat with the feet on the floor or wooden block if the feet do not reach the floor; when sitting posture is fair to good add sitting on an air filled cushion
Purpose	Facilitate head and trunk control
	Inhibit total flexor or extensor pattern of lower extremities
	Facilitate protective and equilibrium reactions
	Facilitate upper extremity extension through support
Activities	Tapping of head and back extensor muscles or side of trunk to achieve upright and vertical head and trunk control
	Trunk movements forward, backward, to the sides, and rotation at first with upper extremity assistance to improve protective and equilibrium reactions, functional ability to come from sidelying to sitting, and so forth
	Weight-bearing on upper extremities at the side and behind the trunk to encourage upper extremity extensor patterns for functional purposes
	Alternately lifting the leg, extending the knee, and tapping the feet to facilitate reciprocal movements and timing of muscle activity in preparation for wheelchair transfers and ambulation
	Catching or kicking a ball and participating in similar activities while maintaining upright posture to improve balance and coordination of extremities
	Sitting on an air-filled cushion and maintaining balance while the cushion is tipped in various directions to spontaneously encourage protective and equilibrium reactions

Standing

Position	Patient standing with support (such as a standing frame) or without support if the position can be maintained	vation of desired muscles, for example, gastrocnemius-soleus muscle (relaxation) or peroneal muscle (activation)
Purpose	Facilitate protective and equilibrium reactions	Pelvic protraction and retraction while weight-shifting to facilitate pelvic rotation necessary for gait
	Facilitate head, trunk, and lower extremity control in preparation for gait	Trunk rotation without moving the lower extremities to facilitate spontaneous rotatory components for upright functional activities while decreasing the robot appearance due to lack of trunk rotation
Activities	Standing in a standing frame to achieve trunk control and facilitate weight-bearing on lower extremities; particularly necessary if one lower extremity has fractures or severe contractures	Balance board with weight-shifts side to side and also forward and backward with one leg in front of the other to increase rapid knee flexion and extension and equilibrium reactions necessary for gait
	Weight-shift on lower extremities side to side, forward and backward, or in PNF patterns to facilitate joint stability through approximation	
	Biofeedback during weight shifts to encourage relaxation or acti-	

Biofeedback Treatment

Electromyographic (EMG) biofeedback has been demonstrated to facilitate motor training in the stroke population, and the same success could be expected with the head trauma population.[40] EMG biofeedback is effective in muscle re-education to bring in the desired muscle response or to relax an undesired response. With this type of feedback the patient must have the visual or auditory ability and attention span to enable successful training. Other types of biofeedback devices are also useful in achieving a desired motor response.[41, 42] Auditory signal devices have been used on helmets or headbands to encourage good head control and on the trunk to help maintain upright sitting posture. For patients with a limited attention span, poor body image, or other body perceptual problems biofeedback devices can be an effective source of motor control training since they do not require a high degree of cortical effort by the patient. These devices also augment treatment since they can be worn for many of the hours the patient is not in physical therapy. The purpose of the devices can be easily understood by other ancillary staff and patient families so that these people can help monitor the response for successful results.

Functional Electrical Stimulation Treatment

Functional or neuromuscular electrical stimulation (FES) may also be a treatment resource to improve muscle activity.[43] The indications for its use are to improve muscle strength, facilitate joint range of motion, and control spasticity. The head trauma patient should be able to tolerate the electrical stimulation without increased agitation or FES is not appropriate. Patients may not be good candidates if their memory or attention span is too short and they are moving against the stimulus or do not leave the electrodes or stimulator alone.

Surgical Treatment

Surgical procedures may be indicated to correct joint deformities or muscle imbalance.[44] The physical therapist should be part of the decision-making process to determine when surgery is indicated and how the outcome of the procedure could affect the patient. Tendon releases to correct contractures will leave the person with decreased strength, which must be considered if functional use of the extremity will be sacrificed. Additionally, the therapist must use conservative measures of passive joint stretching, serial casting, and positioning prior to a surgical tendon release. If other soft tissue limitations of the joint are present, such as a tight capsule or ligaments, the tendon release will not accomplish the maximum results anticipated.

Surgical procedures to correct muscle imbalance, including tendon transfers or split anterior tibial tendon transfer, merit therapist input as to the feasibility of the surgery. The physical therapist should have a strong knowledge of the patient's functional abilities under varying circumstances which may not be readily observed by the surgeon. If hypertonicity varies with different postures the surgical transfer may unmask further problems. Strength of the muscles to be transferred needs to considered as well as functional ability to use the extremity following the transfer. The results of hand muscle transfers may not be practical if elbow and shoulder motor control are not sufficient for the surgical procedure to result in a functional outcome.

Following surgical tendon releases or transfer the therapist must be very actively involved in the postoperative care to achieve effective results.[44] Tendon releases require aggressive joint range of motion and positioning, and tendon transfers must be followed by muscle re-education and gentle active-assistive exercises.

Ambulation Treatment

Ambulation can be emphasized when trunk and lower extremity weight-bearing stability are performed without undue increases in abnormal postures. If balance reactions are not good, the stress of ambulation is likely to cause excessive increases in postural tone in an effort to maintain upright stability. The muscle control needed for lower extremity mobility during a step becomes too difficult to achieve when such hypertonicity impedes or prevents movement.

An area physical therapists may forget in their eagerness to have the patient ambulate is associated reactions. These reactions are particularly brought on by stressful activities and by situations that tax physical or emotional capacities. Ambulation may be too stressful for a person with a head injury and diminished physical capacities. One commonly seen associated reaction during ambulation is a pronounced increase in upper extremity posturing. Physical therapists should be cognizant of the total body during ambulation in order to determine if the patient is ready for this activity. If strong associated reactions are produced during ambulation, then treatment to reduce these reactions is necessary prior to initiating ambulatory activities. Poor equilibrium reactions, lower extremity weakness, or poor timing of muscle contractions are some of the dysfunctions that could make ambulation so stressful that strong associated reactions are produced. In this case treatment emphasis should not be on ambulation but on improving equilibrium reactions, lower extremity strength, or joint movement in smooth synergistic patterns in supine, sitting, and standing positions. When these functions have improved sufficiently, ambulation can then be initiated with the expectation that minimal or no associated reactions would occur. Assistive equipment may also be beneficial in decreasing associated reactions during ambulation. For example, a dynamic upper extremity sling can keep the extremity in good alignment during gait. A walker with small wheels on the front could reduce stress of ambulation for the patient with poor trunk control or equilibrium reactions. One must also be aware that ambulation with crutches or a cane requires good coordination and equilibrium reactions; therefore, many head trauma patients will continue to use a walker for a longer time to ensure safety and to decrease frustration caused by poor coordination.

Normally, ambulation is a subconscious activity, which is the goal with the head trauma patient. Continuous verbal reminders to the patient during gait are usually not appropriate. Head trauma patients may have a low frustration tolerance, poor short-term memory, and may be distractible. Behavior problems may be exacerbated by verbal reiteration during gait. For the most part physical therapists should be using touch or resistance to guide the trunk or lower extremities through the desired pattern during the gait cycle. Biofeedback devices can also lead to an improved gait pattern. For example, a buzzer that goes off when the heel is on the floor provides positive feedback to the patient that the movement was correct. This feedback is instantaneous and probably more accurate than the therapist's verbal feedback. The use of a video monitor may also be beneficial. Patients enjoy seeing themselves on the screen and show a premorbid characteristic of showing their best side for the camera. Patients observing themselves on the screen often spontaneously correct poor posture or achieve the desired performance level.

Orthotic devices may be necessary to allow safe and efficient ambulation. A Swedish knee cage can help prevent genu recurvatum during the stance phase of gait. If ankle dorsiflexion range of motion is adequate and yet the knee hyperextends during weight bearing, the likely cause is excessive gastrocnemius-soleus muscle activity. Gait training with the knee cage may provide the necessary feedback to prevent a habit from occurring. Plastic or double metal upright ankle-foot orthoses should be considered during gait if other treatment methods are not effective in producing a good gait pattern, sensory impairment is significant, or ankle instability is present. A longitudinal metatarsal arch support may correct pronation of the foot during stance. Minimal build-up of the shoe sole on the medial or lateral border may correct eversion or inversion of the foot, respectively.

Advanced ambulatory activities may be an essential part of the treatment program. Activities including jumping, hopping, running, and maneuvering through an obstacle course may improve the patient's lifestyle. Progress in advanced ambulatory activities will lead to increased ambulatory speed and coordination, as well as allow the individual to participate in recreational or vocational activities requiring such agility and performance.

Ataxia Treatment

Ataxia is a movement disorder resulting from disturbances of the cerebellum.[45] Muscle activity during ballistic movements demonstrates impairment in appropriate timing.

Dysmetric movements show prolonged activity of the agonist, causing too much movement, or of the antagonist, causing an abrupt stop or reversal of movement.[45] Rapid alternating movements show prolonged muscle activity in the antagonist delaying the timing of agonist activity. Therefore, ballistic movements may result in dysmetria or dysdiadochokinesia when there is a failure of muscle activity to start or stop at the appropriate time. Appearance of such movements during phasic movement is commonly called ataxia.

Treatment for ataxia should emphasize facilitation or inhibition of the agonist or antagonist muscles depending on which one is primarily contributing to the disorder. For example, during elbow flexion and extension prolonged firing of the biceps muscle will not allow the triceps muscle to move the elbow into extension. Inhibiting biceps muscle activity using a biofeedback apparatus could be a treatment source to improve timely motor control. Frenkel's exercises are another type of treatment to achieve improved timing of muscle activity (see Chapter 19).[46] Motor learning could be achieved with repetition of these exercises to produce coordinated movements. Weighted resistance is another type of treatment used for dysmetria. I have had minimal success with this type of treatment and believe that the additional proprioceptive feedback is not helpful in altering motor control when proprioception is intact. In fact, additional resistance may increase the prolonged firing of the muscle, if that is the problem. Weighted resistance would be more effective for motor control problems due to kinesthetic impairment, which the person with ataxia may or may not have.

Dizziness or Vertigo Treatment

Dizziness or vertigo are other symptoms head trauma patients may experience. Keim defined dizziness as a spatial disorientation characterized by a floating or light-headed feeling that is not due to a disturbance of any specific structure but rather due to generalized metabolic, emotional, or CNS disorders.[47] Vertigo is a spatial disorientation characterized by a feeling of turning or having objects rotate about oneself. It is caused by a disruption of the vestibular system. Impairment of balance is one of the most significant symptoms of vertigo disorders.[48]

Balance is the adjustment in posture of the neck, trunk, and extremity musculature in relation to the center of gravity and the position of the supporting surface.[49] Balance is a dynamic process that involves sensory and motor integration and reaction. Impaired sensory structures—including visual, proprioceptive, and vestibular—can lead to altered motoric balance synergies. For example, balance may be no problem when only the visual and proprioceptive systems are functioning, but when walking in the dark, vision is impaired and balance can be a problem. Each of the three sensory systems should be assessed while occluding the other systems, to provide information about which systems are functioning and to what extent. Also when one or more systems are not functioning compensatory posture patterns may occur in order to maintain or achieve balance.[50] The compensatory patterns may lead to neck or back pain, headaches, and generalized deconditioning. Depending on which system or systems are impaired the therapist can select the most plausible treatment. Drugs such as Valium and Transderm V patch are used to suppress the vestibular system. Physical therapy should include training in static and dynamic balance activities to alter problems of vertigo.[50] Possibly the exercises presented by Keim can be adapted for the head trauma patient who experiences vertigo (see Appendix to this chapter).[47]

SUMMARY

Treatment for motor performance problems in persons with head trauma is a challenging process due to the multiplicity of problems presented. The range of problems varies from no functional motor response to a minor loss of fine motor control. Due to the broad spectrum of clinical problems that can be presented, the therapist is stimulated to treat the complex needs of each patient. In addition to treating the complexity of motor performance problems identified, the deficits in cognition, communication, and behavior must be incorporated into the treatment process. The effectiveness of treatment programs for sensorimotor deficits are largely dependent on the interaction with the patient's cognitive, communication, and behavioral abilities. Modification of treatment plans can be a daily necessity depending, for example, on the patient's attention span, level of awareness, agitation, or comprehension.

A treatment program to improve motor performance requires consideration of at least four factors: facilitation of movement, inhibition of undesirable characteristics of movement patterns, muscle strength, and motor learning circumstances. One or more of these factors are addressed in any treatment process. General suggestions to facilitate and inhibit movement patterns, improve muscle strength, and provide an environment for motor learning were discussed. In the context of one chapter it is not possible to provide detailed treatment suggestions for each problem that could be encountered. Rather strategies were described for treatment planning related to various motor control deficits. Because the diffuse nature of head injuries precludes specific treatment techniques applicable to all circumstances, the therapist must select appropriate individualized treatment procedures.

Advances in treatment of motor performance problems during the last 10 years have been primarily due to a better understanding of neurophysiology. The concept of CNS plasticity has helped focus the basis for treatment. Goals and treatment plans are directed toward restoring normal movement patterns and not just compensatory patterns, since the probability of creating functional neuronal pathways does exist. We are also cognizant that loss of movement due to an upper motor lesion is not primarily due to spasticity. Therefore, attention to treating alterations in motor unit recruitment and timing are being emphasized and not just the inhibition of spasticity. Recognition that spasticity is not the primary cause for lack of movement and observations of surgical outcomes for persons with cerebral palsy have decreased the quest for tendon releases and muscle transfers. We are better able to determine how the surgical intervention will affect the motor performance of the entire individual and not just one joint. Our knowledge and skills in the use of biofeedback and FES devices has also expanded. As more quantitative measures of effectiveness are developed, treatment procedures for motor performance deficits will continue to become more refined.

Case Study. Karen, a 17-year-old female, sustained a traumatic head injury following an automobile accident. Upon admission to an acute care hospital she was severely comatose, had a fracture of the right mandible and left second rib, and had multiple contusions. Seven weeks after injury she was transferred to a rehabilitation center, still comatose, and with a nasogastric tube, tracheostomy tube, and Foley catheter inserted. Briefly stated, her sensory assessment revealed flexion and extension of the right elbow to pinprick to either upper extremity, and no response to pinprick to the lower extremities, as well as a protective blink but no visual tracking and bilateral nystagmus. Oral motor responses included a moderate bite reaction and hyperactive gag reflex. Motor control demonstrated random movements of the right upper extremity and minimal head control when sitting or being rolled from side to side. Muscle tone was moderately increased in the extensor muscles of the elbows and lower extremities, and mildly increased in both wrist and finger flexor muscles. Joint range of motion was normal except that dorsiflexion was −20 degrees bilaterally, and right ankle eversion was limited to neutral.

The initial treatment plan consisted of (1) increasing sitting endurance in a standard wheelchair with adaptive positioning devices including lateral trunk supports, head support, and lapboard; (2) gentle touch and pressure to the face to decrease the bite reaction; (3) tilt table for prolonged stretch to the heelcords; (4) motor activities including rolling, crawling position over a bolster, and short sitting. These latter activities were performed to influence vestibular disturbances, inhibit abnormal postures, and facilitate normal motor control of the neck and extremities.

One month later Karen started responding to some verbal requests, the tracheostomy tube was removed, and she followed objects with her eyes. Her bite reaction was now mild, tongue control was poor, and she could inconsistently chew and swallow ice chips slowly. Karen could roll to the left, supine to prone, and return with minimal assistance; sit with arms extended for support at 30-second intervals; and stand with feet flat on the tilt table. She was also using her right upper extremity to push away objects but seldom showed any movements of the left upper extremity or either lower extremity.

Two months after admission the nasogastric tube was removed. Left facial weakness was now apparent, bite reaction was gone, gag reflex was good, and the soft palate was hypoactive but she could blow out a match after several attempts. She was actively moving all joints of the right upper extremity and had some active movement of the left wrist and lower extremities. At this time resting tremor of the head and dysmetria of the right upper extremity became evident. Head control was now fair; she was rolling with standby assistance, achieving the crawling position with minimal assistance, coming to sitting with moderate assistance, and sitting with arm support for 2 minutes. Wheelchair transfers still required maximum assistance. Standing was now done in a standing frame with minimal assistance to maintain the trunk upright. Karen was shaking her head "yes" or "no" to questions but not speaking. Treatment emphasis continued to be on functional motor performance.

Four months after admission (6 months postinjury) Karen was at Rancho Cognitive Level V. She comprehended short messages, spoke three- to four-word phrases, and had dysarthria. Oral motor control showed the soft palate was good, tongue had good strength except that elevation of the tip was poor, and rapid tongue movements were not possible. Motor control of the right extremities was good and fair for the left sided extremities. The left upper extremity showed a predominant associated reaction of flexion during stressful activities. Karen was independent in sitting and needed minimal assistance for all wheelchair transfer activities. She was able to stand for a few seconds without assistance. Ambulation was added to the treatment program, done mostly in the pool where she could perform reciprocal movements easier and where negative associated reactions were absent. Outside the pool ambulation required standby assistance using a walker with front wheels, and a temporary left ankle-foot orthosis (AFO).

Six months after admission (8 months postinjury) Karen was discharged to her home in another community, where she would continue to receive outpatient therapies. At the time of discharge she was at Rancho Cognitive Level VII. She was speaking in sentences, her memory was good, and her safety judgment was fair. Sensory modalities were intact, mild dysmetria was present in the right extremities, and rapid alternating movements were moderately impaired in all extremities. All extremities had essentially good strength and control except the left shoulder and scapular muscles, which were fair. Hypertonicity was mild in the left lower extremity extensor muscles and upper extremity flexor muscles. Left ankle dorsiflexion was limited to neutral. Karen required standby assistance to do wheelchair transfers and ambulate

with a walker, and minimal assistance to get up and down from the floor and for stairs with a rail. Ambulation was very slow, taking 10 minutes to go 35 feet. Karen was still making progress in motor performance at the time of her discharge from inpatient status.

REFERENCES

1. Jennett, B, Bond, M and Brooks, N: Disability after severe head injury: Observations on the use of the Glasgow Outcome Scale. J Neurol Neurosurg Psychiatry 44:285, 1981.
2. Najenson, T et al: Rehabilitation after severe head injury. Scand J Rehabil Med 6:5, 1974.
3. Heiden, JS et al: Severe head injury: clinical assessment and outcome. Phys Ther 63:1946, 1983.
4. Becker, DP et al: The outcome from severe head injury with early diagnosis and intensive management. J Neurosurg 47:491, 1977.
5. Bond, MR: Assessment of the psychological outcome. In Ciba Foundation Symposium 34: Outcome of Severe Damage to the Central Nervous System. Elsevier Science Publications, New York, 1975, p 141.
6. Sweeney, JK and Smutok, MA: Vietnam head injury study. Phys Ther 63:2018, 1983.
7. Head Injury Rehabilitation Project: Final Report. Santa Clara Valley Medical Center, Project 13-P-5915619, National Institute for Handicapped Research, Washington, DC, 1982.
8. Talmage, EW and Collins, GA: Physical abilities after head injury. Phys Ther 63:2010, 1983.
9. Rothstein, J and Echternach, JL: Hypothesis-oriented algorithm for clinicians. Phys Ther 66:1388, 1986.
10. Brooks, VB: The Neural Basis of Motor Control. Oxford University Press, New York, 1986, p 5.
11. Wall, PD: Signs of plasticity and reconnection in spinal cord damage. In Ciba Foundation Symposium 34: Outcome of Severe Damage to the Central Nervous System. Elsevier Science Publications, New York, 1975, p 35.
12. Bach-y-Rita, P: Central nervous system lesions: sprouting and unmasking in rehabilitation. Arch Phys Med Rehabil 62:413, 1981.
13. Raichle, M, DeVivo, D and Hanaway, J: Disorders of cerebral circulation. In Eliasson, S, Prensky, A and Hardin, W (eds): Neurological Pathophysiology. Oxford University Press, New York, 1978, p 278.
14. Walsh, RN and Greenough, WT: Environments as Therapy for Brain Dysfunction. Plenum Press, New York, 1976.
15. Rosenzweig, MR: Animal models for effects of brain lesions and for rehabilitation. In Bach-y-Rita, P (ed): Recovery of Function: Theoretical Considerations for Brain Injury Rehabilitation. University Park Press, Baltimore, 1980, p 127.
16. Moore, J: Neuroanatomical considerations relating to recovery of function following brain lesions. In Bach-y-Rita, P (ed): Recovery of Function: Theoretical Considerations for Brain Injury Rehabilitation. University Park Press, Baltimore, 1980, p 9.
17. Glees, P: Functional reorganization following hem-

is[ph]erectomy in man and after small experimental lesions in primates. In Bach-y-Rita, P (ed): Recovery of Function: Theoretical Considerations for Brain Injury Rehabilitation. University Park Press, Baltimore, 1980, p 106.
18. Black, P, Markowitz, RS and Cianci, SN: Recovery of motor function after lesions in motor cortex of monkey. In Bach-y-Rita, P (ed): Recovery of Function: Theoretical Considerations for Brain Injury Rehabilitation. University Park Press, Baltimore, 1980, p 65.
19. Edstrom, LL, Grimby, L and Hannerz, J: Correlation between recruitment order of motor units and muscle atrophy pattern in upper motorneuron lesion. Experientia 29:560, 1973.
20. Sahrmann, SA and Norton, BJ: The relationship of voluntary movement to spasticity in the upper motor neuron syndrome. Ann Neurol 2:460, 1977.
21. Arnett, J: Acquisition of skill. Br Med Bull 27:266, 1971.
22. Bach-y-Rita, P: Brain Mechanisms in Sensory Substitution. Academic Press, New York, 1972, p 74.
23. Wilmot, CB et al: Occult head injury: its incidence in spinal cord injury. Arch Phys Med Rehabil 66:227, 1985.
24. Plum, F and Posner, J: Diagnosis of Stupor and Coma. FA Davis, Philadelphia, 1972.
25. Booth, BJ, Doyle, M and Montgomery, J: Serial casting for the management of spasticity in the head-injured adult. Phys Ther 63:1960, 1983.
26. Fay, T: The origin of human movements. Am J Psychol 111:644, 1955.
27. Brunnstrom, S: Movement in Hemiplegia. Harper and Row, New York, 1970, p 1.
28. Kabat, H and Knott, M: Proprioceptive facilitation technics for treatment of paralysis. Phys Ther Review 33:53, 1953.
29. Stockmeyer, SA: An interpretation of the approach of Rood to the treatment of neuromuscular dysfunction. Am J Phys Med 47:900, 1967.
30. Bobath, B: Adult Hemiplegia: Evaluation and Treatment. William Heinemann Medical Books, London, 1974, p 1.
31. Doman, RJ et al: Children with severe brain injuries, neurological organization in terms of mobility. JAMA 174:257, 1960.
32. Knott, M and Voss, DE: Proprioceptive Neuromuscular Facilitation. Harper and Row, New York, 1968, p 3.
33. Harris, FA: Muscle stretch receptor by hypersensitization in spasticity. Am J Phys Med Rehabil 57:16, 1978.
34. Sherrington, CS: Integrative Action of the Nervous System. University Press, Cambridge, 1974.
35. Hagbarth, KE: Excitatory and inhibitory skin areas

for flexor and extensor motoneurons. Acta Physiol Scand 26:1, 1952.

36. Magnus, R: Haltung. In Payton, O, Hirt, S and Newton, R: Neurophysiologic Approaches to Therapeutic Exercise. FA Davis, Philadelphia, 1977, p 63.

37. Felsenthal, G: Pharmacology of phenol in peripheral nerve blocks: A review. Arch Phys Med Rehabil 55:13, 1974.

38. Dimitrijevic, MR and Nathan, PW: Studies of spasticity in man. 90:1, 1967.

39. Winstein, CJ: Neurogenic dysphagia: Frequency, progression, and outcome in adults following head injury. Phys Ther 63:1992, 1983.

40. Wolf, SL: Electromyographic biofeedback applications to stroke patients. Phys Ther 63:1448, 1983.

41. Bjork, L and Wetzel, A: A positional biofeedback device for sitting balance. Phys Ther 63:1460, 1983.

42. Hallum, A: Subject-induced reinforcement of head lifting in the prone position. Phys Ther 64:1390, 1984.

43. Benton, LA et al: Functional Electrical Stimulation: A Practical Clinical Guide, ed 2. Professional Staff Association of Rancho Los Amigos Hospital, Downey, CA, 1981.

44. Garland, DE and Keenan, MA: Orthopedic strategies in the management of the adult head-injured patient. Phys Ther 63:2004, 1983.

45. Hallet, M: Physiology and pathophysiology of voluntary movement. Curr Neurol 2:351, 1979.

46. Weber, LM and Verbanets, J: Assessing balance performance in moderate brain injury. Top Acute Care Trauma Rehabil 1:84, 1986.

47. Keim, RJ: Dysequilibrium and the Vestibular System. Presented at Combined Sections Meeting APTA, Nashville, TN, 1983.

48. Black, FO: Vestibular causes of vertigo. Geriatrics 30:123, 1975.

49. Roberts, TDM: Neurophysiology of Postural Mechanisms. Plenum Press, New York, 1967, p 201.

50. Tangeman, PT and Wheeler, J: Inner ear concussion syndrome: Vestibular implications and physical therapy treatment. Top Acute Care Trauma Rehabil 1:72, 1986.

Appendix: Vestibular Exercises

GOALS

1. To develop proprioceptive and visual mechanisms to compensate for a disturbance in labyrinthine function
2. To improve muscle coordination in general
3. To practice balancing under everyday conditions with special attention to developing the use of the eyes, and muscle and joint sense
4. To train movement of the eyes independent of the head
5. To loosen the muscles of the neck and shoulder to overcome the protective muscular spasm and tendency to move "in one piece"
6. To practice head movements that *cause* dizziness and thus gradually overcome the disability
7. To become accustomed to moving about naturally in daylight and in the dark
8. To encourage the restoration of self-confidence and easy spontaneous movement

EXERCISE PROGRAM

1. **Eye Exercises:** Exercises are to be carried out for 15 to 30 minutes twice a day (while seated or in bed); at first slowly, then quickly
    a. Up and down (20 times)
    b. Side to side (20 times)
    c. Diagonal movements (20 times)
    d. Focusing on finger moving from 3 feet to 1 foot away from face (20 times)
2. **Head Exercises:** Exercises are to be done at first slowly with eyes open in primary position, then quickly; later with eyes closed (20 times each)
    a. Bending forward and backward
    b. Turning from side to side
    c. Tilting from side to side
    d. Diagonal movements
3. Coordinated movements of both the eyes and the head in the same direction as in 2
4. Shoulder shrugging and circling (20 times each)
5. While seated, bend forward and pick up objects from the ground (20 times)
6. **Standing Exercises:** Perform each 20 times
    a. Repeat exercise 1
    b. Change from sitting to standing position with the eyes open and shut
    c. Throw ball from hand to hand (above eye level)

    d. Throw ball from hand to hand under knee

    e. Change from sitting to standing, and turn around in-between

  7. **Full Activity:** Perform each 10 times

    a. Walk across the room with eyes open and then closed

    b. Walk up and down a slope with the eyes open and then closed

    c. Walk up and down steps with eyes open and then closed

    d. Sit up and lying down in bed

    e. Stand up and sit down in a chair

    f. Recover balance when pushed in each direction

    g. Throw and catch a ball

    h. Any game involving stooping or stretching and aiming, such as bowling and shuffleboard

Chapter 24

Remediation of Visual-Perceptual and Perceptual-Motor Deficits

BARBARA ZOLTAN, M.A., O.T.R.

Our ability to deal effectively with our environment is manifested in part by an ability to accurately perceive ourselves as well as the people and objects that surround us. The internalization of basic perceptual skills accomplished by the normal adult allows effective interaction with the environment without conscious thought to the perceptual process.

Perception, as the end product of the perceptual process, can be considered the individual's awareness of experiences and objects within the environment. This awareness is developed through the registration and integration of physical sensations from all sensory modes (i.e., touch, smell, taste, sight, and hearing) and mental processes. Just as the experiences of an individual are ongoing, so is the perceptual processing that accompanies these experiences. The significance of intact perceptual skills becomes apparent when one encounters the individual who lacks these skills. The head injured adult is a prime example of an individual whose perceptual skills have been severely disrupted. The head injured patient can display a breakdown in the perceptual process at any stage involving any or all of the senses. The following information pertains to one aspect of perceptual dysfunction, i.e., visual-perceptual dysfunction.

Visual-perceptual dysfunction is one of the most common devastating residual impairments of head injury. Recovery from visual-perceptual and perceptual-motor deficits takes longer than physical recovery, and research has established a correlation between the presence of perceptual deficits and functional outcome.[1–3] In a 4-year study of approximately 60 head injury patients, a significant correlation ($p < 0.01$) was noted among level of independence in community skills and praxis, ocular pursuits, visual attentiveness, position in space, body scheme, figure-ground perception, and form perception.[1] Baum and Hall, in a study of 37 head injury patients, demonstrated a significant relationship ($p < 0.01$) between constructional praxis and dressing.[2] Finally, Sivak and colleagues established that cognitive perceptual tests were good predictors of driving performance in brain damaged adults.[3] Given the close relationship between visual perception and function, the therapist treating the head injury patient must have a clear understanding and specialized skills pertaining to perceptual evaluation and treatment. The more refined the therapist's skill level, the more effective the treatment and ultimate outcome.

The following chapter describes specific visual, praxis, and visual-perceptual deficits; the inter-relationships among vision, perception, and cognition; general approaches of treatment; and clinical application of treatment through case studies. In addition,

Table 24–1. VISUAL DEFICITS COMMON TO THE BRAIN DAMAGED PATIENT

Deficit	Underlying Mechanism	Clinical Manifestation/ Resulting Deficit	Treatment
Double vision	Decreased extraocular control preventing both eyes from seeing the same object simultaneously; for example, third nerve palsy (one eye will deviate)	In severe cases the brain will suppress one image and focus with one eye; in borderline cases (and with fatigue) the patient will actually see double	Eye patching (alternate eye patched at least once every 1 to 2 days)
Decreased convergence	Convergence-accommodation reflex: contraction of medial rectus muscles, lens thickening by ciliary muscles, narrowing of pupils	Double vision or blurred vision for close fields; decreased depth perception	Patient drills for convergence (i.e., object brought in toward patient's nose on which he must focus)
Blurred vision	Impaired innervation of the focusing muscles	Vision blurred for both close fields and for distance	Prescription lenses; not always correctable
Nystagmus	Brainstem damage (especially vestibular system); cerebellar damage	Abnormal oscillations of the eyes resulting in blurred vision (decreased visual acuity)	Surgery, sensory integration therapy (developed originally for use with learning-disabled children but is being applied to the brain damaged adult)
Visual field loss	Right or left temporal or parietal lobe; optic nerve, radiations or chiasmal lesion	A variety of field deficits depending on location of lesion; these can include scotomas, hemianopsias, and quadrantanopsias	Train the patient to compensate for the loss through effective visual scanning
Decreased oculomotor skills:			
1. Ocular pursuits	Lesion in either hemisphere with or without brainstem damage	Difficulty or inability to track in any or all of the following planes, depending on location of damage: horizontal, oblique, vertical, or rotatory	Transfer of training approach; functional; computers and videogames; sensory motor approach
2. Saccadic eye movements	Frontal cortex (area 8)	Difficulty or inability in quick localization; difficulty in reading	Transfer of training; sensory motor approach; computers and videogames

From Zoltan et al.,[9] pp 104–105, with permission.

guidelines for choosing the correct approach or combination of approaches are provided.

VISUAL SKILLS DEFICITS

Visual skills deficits related to head injury can include double vision, decreased convergence or accommodation, blurred vision, nystagmus, visual field loss, and decreased oculomotor skills (i.e., pursuits or saccades). Any of these deficits will result in ineffective processing of visual input, which can result in perceptual disorders. Specific visual deficits, the underlying mechanism related to each deficit, clinical manifestation, and treatment ideas are summarized in Table 24–1.

Treatment for visual skills deficits, in addition to a transfer of training, functional, and sensory integrative approach, can include specific vision therapy and, when necessary, extraocular surgery.

Vision training involves the use of lenses and prisms which change the value and quality of light gradients entering the eye.[4] Optometric visual therapy can include "... anaglyph activities, various stereoscopes, tachistoscopes, cheiroscopes, saccadic fixators, rotators, prism readers, perimeters, and many other remedial tools."[4]

It is important to note that work with lenses, prisms, and additional visual retraining tools requires specialized knowledge. Optometric visual retraining should be done directly by or under the supervision of the neuro-ophthalmologist, or optometrist. It is crucial, however, that the therapist discuss and understand how the patient's visual deficits affect overall function. The optometrist and therapist together can design a treatment program that is within the visual capabilities of the patient and/or assist in the patient's visual processing.[4]

In addition to those deficits summarized in Table 24–1, the head injured patient may have related deficits in visual attention and visual neglect. Visual attention deficits are primarily the result of frontal lobe damage[5] and can be treated with a sensory integrative, transfer of training, and/or functional approach.

Visual neglect may be present in addition to or in the absence of a visual field cut, and may be associated with a spatial or body neglect. Associated lesion sites for neglect are the frontal lobe[6] and right or left occipital parietal and parietal damage.[7,8] Any of the approaches described later in this chapter may be effectively used to treat visual neglect.

APRAXIA

Apraxia is often a residual deficit of head injury. It is the inability to perform purposeful movements even though there is no loss of coordination, motor function, or sensation. There are several types of apraxia including constructional, ideomotor, ideational, and dressing apraxia. In addition, apraxia can be categorized by the body parts affected (i.e., buccofacial, unilateral limb, bilateral limb, and/or total body apraxia). Classes of actions may be further delineated as transitive (gestures or actions demonstrating the use of a missing object), conventional (gestures representative of culturally specific ideas), natural (nonculturally specific ideas), and/or nonrepresentative (actions conveying no message).[10] Patients may also have more difficulty with motor planning with tasks performed away from the body versus toward the body, or have difficulty in certain planes of movement. Two or more types of apraxia are usually seen in a patient. All of these factors and categories of apraxia deficits are evaluated and subsequently incorporated into the treatment planning process.

Treatment of apraxia is often frustrating for both the therapist and the patient. No matter what type of apraxia is evident, understanding underlying mechanisms as well as pinpointing the point of breakdown of a particular action or task is crucial.[11] For example, identifying that a patient is unable to put his shirt on is insufficient evaluation. Does the patient recognize the shirt? Can he orient the shirt to his body? Can he manipulate and position it effectively? These and other questions or observations pertaining to the subskills required of particular tasks provide meaningful data for treatment strategies. Similar task analysis for other problem areas related to motor planning deficits is likely to identify key deficits that generalize to many functional areas. For instance, closer examination or analysis may reveal that the patient consistently has difficulty with object manipulation in certain planes of movement no matter what the task.

Several treatment approaches can be used effectively with the apraxic patient if applied appropriately. For example, the transfer of training approach has been found to be effective in treating constructional apraxia. This same approach, however, would be less effective for patients with ideomotor apraxia who have difficulty wheeling their wheelchair. For these patients, a more functionally oriented approach combined with a sensory motor approach is appropriate. Generally, a combi-

nation of approaches is effective, as illustrated in the treatment of dressing apraxia. Obviously a functional approach is indicated for the dressing apraxic patient. Less obvious perhaps is the effective use of a neurodevelopmental and tactile-based treatment combined with the repetitive functional approach. For example, bilateral upper extremity weight-bearing tasks prior to having the patient put on an overhead T-shirt is effective in reorienting the patient to his or her body scheme. This reorientation provides a basis for the patient to understand and interpret how the body relates to and is

Table 24.2 TYPES OF APRAXIA COMMON TO HEAD INJURY PATIENTS

Deficit	Underlying Mechanism Lesion Site	Clinical Manifestation/ Resulting Deficit	Treatment
Constructional apraxia-graphic, 2-D or 3-D	Occipitoparietal lobe of either hemisphere	Inability to produce designs in 2 or 3 dimensions either on command or spontaneously; patient will be limited in his or her ability to perform purposeful tasks which require use of objects in environment	Transfer of training approach, i.e., practice copying or constructional tasks; sensory integrative (multisensory), i.e., provide additional proprioceptive and kinesthetic input by having patient draw in a clayboard[3]
Dressing apraxia	Occipital or parietal lobe (generally of nondominant hemisphere)	Inability to dress oneself due to disordered body scheme and/or spatial relations; deficit will be manifest by mistakes of orientation of putting clothes on, or neglect[12]	Functional approach with auditory, visual, and/or tactile cueing, and structured repetition; neurodevelopmental techniques (i.e., weight bearing, bilateral tasks, and so on) prior to dressing
Ideomotor apraxia	Parietal lobe of dominant hemisphere; supramarginal gyrus	Inability to imitate gestures or perform purposeful motor tasks while patient fully understands the idea behind the task; patient can carry out habitual tasks automatically	Place tasks on a subcortical level; identify which body parts are affected (i.e., unilateral limb, bilateral limb, total body, and/or buccofacial). Provide proprioceptive, kinesthetic, and tactile input before and during the required task
Ideational apraxia		Inability to perform purposeful motor tasks because the patient has lost the understanding of the concept/idea related to the task	Use visualization techniques; use functional approach

a separate entity from objects such as the T-shirt.

To summarize, no matter what type of apraxia is apparent, analyze underlying mechanisms and subskills of tasks in which deficits are demonstrated. Although there may be instances in which one particular approach is indicated, generally a combination of techniques and approaches is most effective. Examples of specific types of apraxia, underlying mechanisms, clinical manifestations, and sample treatment ideas are presented in Table 24–2.

VISUAL-PERCEPTUAL DEFICITS

Visual perceptual deficits can include body scheme disorders and/or disorders of higher-level visual discrimination or spatial relations skills. Any degree or combination of deficits can occur, and rarely are deficits seen in isolation. Body scheme deficits and visual discrimination deficits, their underlying mechanisms, clinical manifestations, and treatment suggestions are outlined in Tables 24–3 and 24–4, respectively.

Body Scheme Deficits

An intact body scheme serves as a postural model one has of body parts and their interrelationships. This model in turn serves to guide the individual in his or her external environmental interactions. An individual's body scheme is separate from body image. The body image is a mental representation of one's body that relates to feelings and ideas rather than a factual picture of the actual physical model. After sustaining a head injury a person's body scheme is almost always affected. Components that can be altered include somatognosia, unilateral neglect, finger agnosia, and impaired right-left discrimination.[9]

Generally, a combination of techniques from the neurodevelopmental, sensory integrative, functional, and transfer of training approaches is appropriate for body scheme deficits. A sensory integrative approach for somatognosia, for example, would utilize techniques such as having patients use their hand or a rough cloth to rub a specific body part while naming it. A transfer of training approach to this deficit would incorporate such techniques as quizzing the patient on

Table 24–3. BODY SCHEME DISORDERS

Deficit	Underlying Mechanism Lesion Site	Clinical Manifestation/ Resulting Deficit	Treatment
Somatognosia	Parietal lobe/dominant hemisphere	Lack of awareness of the body's structure and the relationship of body parts	Neurodevelopmental (i.e., bilateral tasks, handling techniques to educate patient to normal movement, sensory integrative, functional, transfer of training)
Right/left discrimination	Parietal lobe/either hemisphere	Inability to comprehend and use the concepts of right and left	Sensory integrative, transfer of training, functional
Finger agnosia	Parietal lobe/dominant hemisphere, angular gyrus	Hesitation or confusion in naming fingers on command or knowing which one was touched	Sensory integrative, transfer of training
Unilateral neglect	Inferior parietal lobe of right nondominant hemisphere	Inability to integrate perceptions from side of the body or environment	Transfer of training sensory integrative, neurodevelopmental, functional

Table 24–4. VISUAL DISCRIMINATION/SPATIAL RELATIONS DISORDERS

Deficit	Underlying Mechanism Lesion Site	Clinical Manifestation/ Resulting Deficit	Treatment
Form perception/ constancy	Parietal lobe/nondominant hemisphere	Inability to judge variations in form	Transfer of training, functional
Depth perception	Occiputal, occiputotemporal, occiputoparietal	Inability to judge depths and distances; may show up in areas such as navigating stairs and architectural barriers	Functional, transfer of training
Topographic orientation	Occiputoparietal lobe/nondominant hemisphere	Inability to understand and remember relationships between places causing difficulty finding his/her way in space	Functional, transfer of training
Figure-ground perception	Parietal lobe/nondominant hemisphere	Inability to distinguish foreground from background, may have difficulty finding one item from cluttered drawer or an item on a grocery shelf	Functional, transfer of training
Position in space	Parietal lobe/nondominant hemisphere	Inability to understand and deal with concepts related to spatial positioning of object, i.e., up/down, in front of/ behind	Functional, transfer of training
Spatial relations	Parietal lobe/nondominant hemisphere	Inability to perceive the position of two or more objects in relation to self and in relation to each other	Functional, transfer of training

body parts or putting together a body puzzle. Finally, if using a neurodevelopmental approach, the patient would be involved in bilateral activities, with weight bearing and handling techniques that facilitate normal movement. Any or all of these and numerous other techniques can be used effectively in treating any type of body scheme deficit.

Visual Discrimination and Spatial Relations

Once an individual has a consistent point of origin through an established body scheme, continued environmental exploration leads to the perception of areas such as objects and their relationships to the individual or to each other. The individual is able to judge distances, distinguish forms, and separate objects from a surrounding background. These and other skills fall under the general category of visual discrimination or spatial relations. Within this general category, specific skills that are most often altered after a head injury are form perception/constancy, depth perception, topographic orientation, figure-ground perception, position in space, and spatial relations. Table 24–4 outlines underlying mechanisms, clinical manifestations, and general treatment ideas. Specific treatment ideas pertaining to individual deficits are subsequently described.

FORM PERCEPTION/CONSTANCY

Treatment of impaired form perception usually falls under the auspices of a transfer of training or a functional approach. Tabletop activities can include matching similar parquetry forms, blocks, or graphic designs. Additionally, the therapist can type a row of random letters and have the patient search for and find one particular letter that has been typed numerous times.[9] Using a functional approach, the therapist can instruct the patient to sort clothes by category—i.e., shirt, pants, socks, and so on—and discuss the form perception cues or aspect used to complete the task.[13]

DEPTH PERCEPTION

The head injured patient should always be made aware of any depth perception deficits as a safety precaution against potentially hazardous situations (kitchen tasks, navigating stairs, and the like).

A combination of a transfer of training and functional approach can be used for decreased depth perception by having the patient practice depth or distance-related tasks within the functional realm. For example, the therapist can have patients practice slowly moving their foot up and down on a high step and then on a low step to feel the difference. The use of an obstacle course wherein patients must walk under and step over obstacles can also be very effective. Finally, the therapist should incorporate tactile cues as much as possible. For example, the therapist can have the patient reach and feel the depth, distance, and size of a wheelchair prior to a bed-to-wheelchair transfer.

TOPOGRAPHIC ORIENTATION

Topographic disorientation will likely show up in daily functional skills, rather than on standardized testing. Rarely, if ever, is this deficit seen in isolation but rather in conjunction with additional spatial relations and cognitive deficits.

Treatment for topographic disorientation falls under the realm of the functional and transfer of training approaches. Believing that improvement in one task will transfer to similar tasks, the therapist can practice with the patient getting from one treatment gym to another, or from the patient's room to the hospital cafeteria, and the like. The compensation or adaptation methods of the functional approach can also be used. To assist patients in compensating for their deficit, routine routes should be used repeti-

tively and learning should be done by rote memorization. Safety issues (i.e., not to drive, not to go out alone) should be emphasized. To adapt the patient's environment, markers, landmarks, and/or colored dots can be strategically placed. Eventually the cues can be lessened or removed altogether as the patient improves or has memorized the route.

FIGURE-GROUND PERCEPTION

An individual's center of attention at any given time creates a field of perception that is considered the "figure," or foreground. Stimuli not at the center of attention form a dimly perceived background.[14] This ability to separate out the necessary foreground of perception from extraneous background is often lost with the head injured patient. The head injured patient with a figure-ground deficit may have difficulty finding a hairbrush in a cluttered drawer or finding a particular item on a grocery store shelf.

Treatment for a figure-ground deficit can require a functional and/or a transfer of training approach. Transfer of training techniques can include "hidden objects" worksheets, or scattering objects or a deck of cards in front of the patient and having the patient point to or retrieve a certain item. As the patient improves, the complexity of the task is increased by increasing the background distractions.

The patient with a figure-ground deficit can be taught to functionally compensate for the problem. For example, the patient is made cognitively aware of the problem and how it interferes with functioning independently. He or she is then taught compensation strategies such as slowly and systematically examining small areas and not being impulsive. In the kitchen, for instance, the therapist can have the patient look and feel around the countertop to identify what items are there and where they are located.[9]

A functional adaptation approach can also be effective in treating a figure-ground deficit. Drawers can be organized, separating all items. Only a few items can be placed on the patient's nightstand. Meal trays can be arranged with only a few items presented at a time, with the patient eating in several courses as necessary.[9] Finally, items such as wheelchair brakes or hygiene items can be marked with red tape for ease in identification. The underlying concept for these and other techniques that fall into the category of a functional adaptation approach for a figure-ground deficit is to make the patient's environment simple and uncluttered.[15]

POSITION IN SPACE

Perception of position in space is the ability to interpret and act on concepts of spatial positioning of objects such as in-out, up-down, and front-back. The patient with a position-in-space deficit may not, for example, be able to locate his or her food tray if told it was on the table behind the desk, or would be unable to locate the dishwasher soap if told it was in the cabinet under the sink.

Assuming that improvement in one task will transfer to similar tasks, the therapist can have the patient with a position-in-space deficit practice a variety of tasks for which he or she has to discriminate different spatial orientations. Worksheets on which the patient must point out the figure or object that looks different (reversed) in a row of identical figures can also be useful. Alternatively, two 1-inch-cube blocks can be used in having the patient practice putting one on top of, behind, or in front of the other, in response to the therapist's request.[9]

SPATIAL RELATIONS

The patient with a spatial-relations deficit will have difficulty perceiving the position of two or more objects in relation to himself or herself as well as in relation to each other.[9] Developmentally, individuals must orient themselves in space before they can conquer an object-to-object orientation. This developmental concept can be incorporated into treatment when appropriate. An obstacle course or furniture maze can assist patients in orienting themselves to space. Concurrently or subsequently, object-to-object orientation tasks can be implemented. These tasks primarily would involve tabletop use of block designs, pegboard designs, connecting-dot worksheets, and/or puzzles. In these exercises, the patient copies patterns or designs done by the therapist. As the patient progresses, he or she may be asked to convert a two-dimensional paper design into a three-dimensional one using blocks, pegboard, and so forth.[16]

INTERRELATIONSHIPS AMONG VISION, PERCEPTION, AND COGNITION

Understanding the interrelationships among vision, perception, and cognition is mandatory to effective evaluation and treatment of specific deficit areas. At the most basic level, there exists a hierarchical relationship with vision (along with movement and sensation) as a basis for perception, which, in turn, is a foundation for higher level cognitive skills.

The human eye, through retinal cone cells, distinguishes different wavelengths and contrasts of light as well as differences in tone or texture. Impulses are encoded through skeletal, visceral, cortical, and subcortical processes by the functional visual components of fixation, tracking, focusing, and fusion.[17, 18] The end product of this encoding and subsequent integration is the brain's ability to understand what is seen according to size, shape, distance, and form. This understanding is perception.[8]

Vision, then, involves more than merely the activation of sensory receptors but rather is a complex process that leads to perceptual development. If a component of the visual processing system is impaired, an associated perceptual loss will likely occur.

At the base of perceptual development, through vision, movement, and our remaining senses, we develop a body scheme and a resultant stable space structure. It is important to note that accurate and precise control of extraocular muscles is essential to the development of this stable space structure. Subsequently, the individual can begin to discover and understand relationships and objects in the outside environment. We can begin to judge distances, identify spatial relationships, and/or separate a figure from the surrounding background. By perceiving object relationships in space, we can begin to identify similarities and differences between them. As our skill in this area increases, we are able to handle numerous elements within groups of objects. Knowledge of similarities and differences between objects leads to skills such as categorization and grouping of these objects. It is such categorization that leads to generalization and abstraction. In other words, basic perceptual skills provide the foundation for basic "conceptual" or cognitive skills.

Applying these and other theoretical concepts to practice will provide a rationale for evaluation and treatment of deficit areas. Without successful application of the concepts pertaining to interrelationships among vision, perception, and cognition, the effectiveness of treatment may be less than optimal. No deficit area can be treated without consideration of related areas.

Transfer of Training Approach

The transfer of training approach was a popular form of treatment 5 to 10 years ago and is still being used effectively today. The approach is based on the theory that repetitive practice of tabletop perceptual tasks will result in improvement that will transfer or carry over into similar perceptual tasks and ultimately generalize to daily function.[19] This approach has been used successfully in treating perceptual deficits in children.[14]

All visual-perceptual or perceptual-motor deficits can be treated with the transfer of training approach. For instance, patients with a body scheme deficit may be asked to name their own or others' body parts or to put together a body puzzle. Patients with a spatial relations deficit may be asked to perform paper and pencil tasks, or pegboard designs.[16]

The efficacy of the transfer of training approach remains controversial. Some clinicians believe the approach encourages splinter skills with no carry over into function. Taylor[13] conducted a 2-year study of left hemiplegics with three patient groups receiving treatment as follows: Group I— Sensory Integration, Group II—Transfer of Training, and Group III (Control Group)— Standard gross motor activities. Study results indicated no significant differences in outcome among the three groups. However, close examination of study methodology indicates treatment overlap between groups, therefore raising doubts as to the study's overall reliability.

Leonard Diller conducted a study on stroke patients examining the approach.[20] In his study, the experimental group received 10 one hour sessions in copying block designs, with a systematic, hierarchical cueing system. The control group, on the other hand, received the standard therapy treatment. The results of the study indicated sig-

nificant improvement on the performance of the experimental group in block designs as well as in five areas of occupational therapy (i.e., attitude/mood, consistency/attention, eye-hand coordination, degree of assistance for self-care, and additional special problems such as unilateral neglect).

The limited studies presented are insufficient evidence to strongly endorse a given approach. In addition, the studies described deal predominantly with stroke patients. Similar studies related to head injury patients are at present unavailable. A great deal of research is needed to scientifically support the use of the transfer of training approach with the head injury patient or, for that matter, the stroke patient.

Functional Approach

As with the transfer of training approach, the functional approach utilizes repetitive practice. The major difference in this approach is that the practice occurs on a functional level. For instance, a patient with a figure-ground deficit will practice retrieving items from a cluttered drawer or cabinet shelf. A patient with a body scheme deficit will practice daily dressing with cueing techniques, with environmental adaptations provided as needed. The functional approach is geared toward making the patient more independent, emphasizing treatment of the symptom rather than the cause of the problem.[9]

The functional approach uses two important concepts, those of compensation and of adaptation. The compensation method teaches the patient to be aware of a given problem and to work around it or compensate for it. For example, a patient with a visual field cut may be taught to compensate by more effective scanning or making sure items are placed within his or her field of vision.

Adaptation, which is often utilized in conjunction with compensation, creates changes or adaptations in the patient's environment to increase function.[9] Patients with a visual field loss or neglect, for instance, would use a red marker at the left side of a page to cue them to begin reading. A patient with acalculia could be taught to use a calculator.

Given recent pressures to decrease the length of hospital stays and measure functional outcomes, the functional approach continues to gain appeal with clinicians as the most practical treatment approach.

Neurodevelopmental Treatment

Through an infant's initial movements and kinesthetic awareness, perception is developed.[21] The infant moves from bilateral symmetrical movements to developing, as a child, an internal awareness of two sides of the body and their differences. As part of continued development and specifically through postural mechanisms, the child develops a sense of directionality. The ongoing orientation of the body to the external environment, provided by postural mechanisms, enables the child to project his or her internal laterality into external space.[9] A stable self- and body-image is developed, which in turn functions as a reliable, consistent point of origin for future sensations and perceptions.[21]

As just outlined, postural mechanisms play a crucial role in the development of a normal body scheme and subsequent perceptual skills. The individual who has sustained a head injury will have abnormal changes in postural mechanisms. Spasticity and other abnormal tone create an exaggerated static function rather than normal, dynamic postural control.[23] Additionally, visual, sensory and motor impairments cause patients to lose their sense of laterality as well as their sense of directionality.

Neurodevelopmental treatment (NDT) is a popular method of treatment used with the brain damaged adult to inhibit abnormal postural reflex mechanisms and facilitate normal movement. Tactile and kinesthetic stimulation through handling and movement is provided to encourage contact between the individual and the environment.[22] The ultimate goal of therapy is to teach the patient how to control his or her movements without the assistance of others.[22] A normal variety of postural sets are developed for smooth, easy, automatic movements. Once this is accomplished, the patient relearns his or her body scheme and develops a more normal body image. As previously described, the development of a normal body scheme in turn facilitates the redevelopment of higher-level visual perceptual or discrimination skills. Clinicians are discovering that NDT is not only an effective means of optimizing motor recovery, but one that will have an effect on perceptual-motor recovery as well. As just described, this effect lies mainly in the redevelopment of a normal body scheme, which in turn serves as a reliable, consistent point of origin for continued, future perceptual responses and development.[21]

Sensory Integration

Sensory integration therapy is a treatment approach traditionally used with learning disabled children. In recent years, however, there has been a great deal of interest and use of its theory and techniques with the brain damaged adult. Sensory integrative treatment is based on both neurophysiological and developmental principles and is defined as organization of sensation for use by the individual in interacting with his or her environment.[17] Sensory integration occurs at all levels of the central nervous system and converts our sensations into meaningful perceptions. Sensory integration occurs through an adaptive purposeful response as follows:[9]

> During sensory integrative therapy the therapist provides and controls sensory input, especially the input from the vestibular system, muscles, joints and skin. This controlled sensory stimulation is then followed by an adaptive response by the patient, which will integrate those sensations provided and controlled by the therapist.

The brain damaged adult has deficits at all levels of sensory integrative functioning. Table 24–5 summarizes sensory integrative functioning in normal subjects and in brain damaged adults.

Two additional theoretical constructs, related to the use of sensory integrative therapy with the brain damaged adult, are plasticity and the importance of environmental stimulation to normal development. Plasticity is related to the central nervous system's adaptive capacity, involving functional and structural changes when needed, to increase function.[23] Research has supported the concept that a child's normal development is tied into environmental interaction, which causes functional and structural brain

**Table 24–5. SUMMARY OF NORMAL SENSORY INTEGRATIVE
FUNCTION AND THAT OF THE HEAD INJURED PATIENT**

Normal	Brain Damaged
Sensory stimulation from the environment	Sensory stimulation from the environment
Normal sensory registration and processing	Abnormal sensory registration and processing due to impaired primary sensory systems (i.e., visual, auditory, tactile, olfactory, and gustatory)
Normal sensory integration and interpretation	Abnormal sensory integration and interpretation due to impaired primary sensory systems and impaired autonomic, proprioceptive, and vestibular systems
Appropriate functional adaptive response	Poor and inappropriate adaptive response due to impaired primary sensory systems, impaired autonomic, proprioceptive, and vestibular systems and disability-related mobility impairment

Adapted from Zoltan et al.,[9] with permission.

changes. These changes are possible because of the brain's adaptive or "plastic" capabilities. Although the concept of plasticity in children is almost universally accepted, its presence in adults is more controversial. Some professionals believe brain plasticity in adults is limited, whereas others believe there is sufficient potential for plasticity for therapeutic intervention. These professionals feel evidence of plasticity exists when observing that functional recovery does occur in brain damaged adults even when the lesion is massive and the patient is elderly.[24] If one believes that brain plasticity does exist in adults, then sensory integrative therapy is an appropriate treatment tool to be used with adults.

A second, related concept to brain plasticity is the use and importance of the environment. Environmental deprivation studies indicate severe loss of cognitive abilities as the result of deprivation.[25, 26] Although the head injured patient is not placed in a deprived environment, the patient's severe cognitive, sensory, mobility, and perceptual problems result in limited or no access to the environment. This limited access prevents the patient from receiving adequate tactile, proprioceptive, and kinesthetic stimulation. The therapist, therefore, provides an enriched environment through controlled sensory stimulation to facilitate the necessary environmental interaction.

Computer Use in Perceptual Retraining

The application of computer technology to health care has become popular in recent years. The use of computer treatment in direct patient care has come to the forefront, with its use ranging from prevocational applications and environmental control to visual, perceptual, and/or cognitive retraining.[27, 28] As with most new treatment modalities, there are mixed reviews of computer use in direct patient care. Smith[29] and Bracy[30] note that computers allow handicapped patients access to much more of the environment than was previously possible. Gianutsos[31] states that computer use in cognitive retraining increases the individual's flexibility and efficiency. In addition, computers provide immediate and consistent feedback, objectivity, convenient data storage, short presentation time, and standardized training.[32-34] Many clinicians advocate the importance of remembering that the computer is just a tool and not a replacement for human intervention or contact.[35, 36]

Several disadvantages of computer based treatment which have been identified include aggressive violent themes,[32] software limitations, computer anxiety, and the fact that the computer is probably unnecessary for basic perceptual and cognitive retraining.[33] Additionally, there are few published studies measuring the efficacy of computer retraining upon perceptual-motor, cognitive, or ADL tasks.[32]

Despite the described disadvantages and limited efficacy research, clinical experts indicate a strong potential for successful application. Successful application, however, depends on choosing software appropriately and remaining abreast of state-of-the-art software. For examples of videogames and computer programs that require visual, spatial, and perceptual-motor skills, refer to Table 24-6.

The following are two case studies that represent examples of how the theoretical information provided is applied to clinical practice.

Case 1. Michael is a 33-year-old male who sustained a gunshot wound to the right parietal lobe. He displays a moderate left hemiplegia, left homonymous hemianopsia, constructional apraxia for 3-D and graphic tasks, and requires moderate physical and minimal verbal assistance for dressing.

Problem No. 1: Constructional Apraxia
Treatment Approach: Transfer of training

Rationale: Research has indicated a strong correlation between performance on constructional tasks and activities of daily living.[2, 37, 38] It is believed, therefore, that improvement in constructional abilities through repetitive graded tabletop tasks will also result in an associated improvement in functional abilities.

Specific Techniques: Graded repetitive tabletop 3-D and graphic constructional tasks. Grade activities as needed depending on the patient's level of function.

1. 3-D: Block designs
   a. Begin with solid-color blocks creating designs requiring only two to four blocks.
   b. Demonstrate/build the design as the patient watches.
   c. Utilize "chaining" techniques, i.e., break the activity down into functional components. For example, in a four-block design, the therapist builds three blocks in the design and the patient places the remaining block. Next the therapist places two, the patient two, and so on.
   d. Build the design without the patient looking and have the patient replicate (use chaining technique as needed).
   e. Progress to more complex designs.
2. Graphic
   a. Begin with prewriting tasks and sim-

Table 24-6. EXAMPLES OF VIDEO AND COMPUTER SOFTWARE FOR PERCEPTUAL RETRAINING

Software	Company	Description
Video Olympics	Atari	Includes pong, soccer, hockey, foozpong, handball, and so on; players must intercept a moving light by manipulating paddles[35]
Target games (e.g., Space Invaders, Outlaw, Sky Diver)	Atari	Games involve coordination of visual and motor output involving the location and hitting a target[35]
Superman	Atari	Player searches out a missing villain; useful for visual scanning/search, and so on[35]
Squares	Tri Sensory Co.	Simple block design task to be used with moderate to severe dysfunction[9, 36]
Perception	Eduware	Set of advanced/difficult perceptual tasks with an important speed component[9, 36]
Ribbit	Picadilly Software, Inc.	Visual spatial game in which player avoids and seeks out objects that cross in front[9, 36]

ple designs; use clayboard tracing or the blackboard for added proprioceptive and kinesthetic input.

b. If using designs bear in mind that research with the head injured patient has indicated the following designs to be good discriminators of performance: circle, diamond, cube, house, and clock.[9]

c. As the patient progresses move to paper and pencil tasks without the additional proprioceptive and kinesthetic input. In addition move into more complex designs, dot-to-dot exercises, writing skills, and so forth.

Problem No. 2: Left Homonymous Hemianopsia

Treatment Approach: Functional and/ or transfer of training
Specific Techniques:

1. Depending on the long-term prognosis and goals, either of the following approaches could be used:

a. Adaptation: The environment would be adapted to the deficit—i.e., place items, talk to the patient, and the like, *within* the patient's field of vision

b. Compensation: Teach the patient how to compensate for the deficit—i.e., place items, talk to the patient, and the like, *outside* of the patient's visual field cut to force visual scanning

2. Repetitive tabletop activities. Activities used for the treatment of visual scanning have been found to be effective in teaching the patient to compensate for a visual field loss.

3. a. The patient may be asked to cross out target letters, numbers, and so on, using the following cues as needed:[39, 40]

Anchoring—cueing the patient as to where to begin the visual search with a colored marker or tape

Pacing—controlling the patient's speed of scanning, i.e., patient calls out or places a sticker under a number or letter as he sees it, thereby controlling the spacing and density of the visual stimuli (e.g., distance between stimuli, size, distracting elements)

b. Use the aforementioned techniques as needed with puzzles, mazes, and so on.

c. Lessen and remove these, or any additional, cueing techniques as the patient improves.

d. Progress to multicolor (e.g., Kohs, WAIS) designs and use the same progression as needed.

Case 2. Susan is a 16-year-old who sustained a severe closed head injury as the re-

sult of a motor vehicle accident. CT scan revealed brainstem and frontal-parietal lobe damage.

Perceptual problems include decreased visual scanning, ideomotor apraxia, impaired body scheme, decreased right/left discrimination, and inability to cross midline.

Sensory problems include decreased proprioception, decreased kinesthesia, and impaired tactile discrimination.

Motor deficits include poor sitting balance, decreased head control, and impaired equilibrium reactions.

Treatment Approach: Sensory integration

Rationale: Susan's medical history and clinical picture indicate diffuse brain stem or subcortical damage. If one analyzes her clinical deficits as a whole versus in isolation, the deficit areas are indicative of an underlying dysfunction of the somatosensory and vestibular systems. For example, at the most basic level of integration, vestibular and proprioceptive inputs give us control over eye movement.[17] At the next level of integration, the tactile, proprioceptive, and vestibular systems serve to develop a body scheme or percept which in turn leads to effective motor planning.[21]

Specific Techniques:

1. Controlled stimulation of the somatosensory (proprioceptive and kinesthetic systems) to improve body scheme and motor planning

2. Controlled stimulation of the vestibular system to improve vestibular ocular functioning, increase sitting balance and head control, and improve equilibrium reactions. Vestibular stimulation will also result in improved postural and bilateral integration, which will enhance the patient's ability to cross mid-line, her body scheme, and her overall motor planning abilities. Specific suggested vestibular based activities for this case would include inversion over a large therapy ball, use of tilt-table and large equilibrium board, and the like.

Note: For all vestibular stimulation activities watch for nausea, dizziness, change in skin tone. Monitor blood pressure and pulse before, immediately after and up to 24 hours as needed after any rotatory stimulation. Also monitor vital signs the first time the patient is inverted or placed on the tilt-table, and any other time during vestibular treatment as indicated.

SUMMARY

The preceding information provides a basis for understanding the visual, perceptual, and perceptual-motor deficits associated with head injury and related treatment approaches for those deficits. The head injury patient may suffer from visual impairments ranging from decreased visual attention or scanning and visual field cuts, to nystagmus, poor convergence, or double vision. Visual-perceptual deficits can include poor body scheme and/or disorders of higher-level visual discrimination skills. Related perceptual-motor deficits can include several types of apraxias ranging from dressing apraxia to constructional apraxia to ideomotor apraxia.

Vision, perception, and higher-level conceptual or cognitive skills are all interrelated; consequently deficit areas should be treated with this concept in mind. Treatment of visual, visual-perceptual, and perceptual-motor deficits can fall under the sensory integrative, neurodevelopmental, functional, and/or transfer of training approaches. The application of recent technologic advances and computer applications should also be considered as an adjunct therapeutic tool.

Effective therapy demands the appropriate application of relevant theory and practical techniques. Incorporating theoretical constructs into treatment is used in conjunction with the integration of the therapist's past clinical experience and observations. The difficulty arises in deciding which approach, or combination of approaches, will be effective for a given patient. Although there is no "cookbook" method for making these decisions, some guidelines can be used. Always employ relevant research literature and theory to back up decision making. Remain cognizant that the patient with a diffuse injury with brainstem damage will benefit most from a subcortical approach. Finally, no matter what approach is used, it should almost always be used in conjunction with a functional approach.

Although we have made advances in the remediation of visual-perceptual deficits, there is a strong need for continued research, particularly efficacy research. Research measuring specific outcomes of various therapeutic approaches and techniques is highly indicated. In addition, identification of factors that correlate with the ultimate functional outcome (such as when or how often the therapy is provided) would be helpful. Research studies devoted to these and other questions can only ultimately assist the clinician in clinical decision making and the refinement of evaluation and treatment procedures.

REFERENCES

1. Berrol, S et al: Head Injury Rehabilitation Project, Final Report. Santa Clara Valley Medical Center, San Jose, CA, November, 1982.
2. Baum, B and Hall, K: Relationship between constructional praxis and dressing in the head injured adult. Am J Occup Ther 35(7):438, 1981.
3. Sivak, M et al: Drawing and perceptual/cognitive skills: Behavioral consequences of brain damage. Arch Phys Med Rehabil 62:476, 1981.
4. Umphred, DA: Neurological Rehabilitation. CV Mosby, St Louis, MO, 1985.
5. Young, F: Early Experience and Visual Information Processing in Perceptual and Reading Disorders. National Academy of Sciences, Washington, DC, 1970.
6. Heilman, K and Velestrein, E: Frontal lobe neglect in man. Neurology 22:660, 1972.
7. Critchley, M: The Parietal Lobes. Edward Arnold Co, London, 1953.
8. Pigott, R and Brickett, F: Visual neglect. Am J Nurs 66:101, 1966.
9. Zoltan, B, Siev, E and Freishtat, B: Perceptual and Cognitive Dysfunction in the Adult Stroke Patient. Slack, Inc, Thorofare, NJ, 1986.
10. Solet, J: The Solet Test for Apraxia. Boston, 1975, Copyright by author.
11. Miller, N: Dyspraxia and its Management. Aspen Publications, Rockville, MD, 1986.
12. Archibald, YM and Wepman, JM: Language disturbance and non-verbal cognitive performance in eight patients following injury to the right hemisphere. Brain 91:117, 1968.
13. Taylor, MM: Controlled Evaluation of Percept-Concept-Motor Training Therapy After Stroke Resulting in Left Hemiplegia. Research Grant Rd, 2215-M, sponsored by Rehabilitation Institute, Detroit, September, 1969.
14. Frostig, M and Horne, D: Frostig Program for the Development of Visual Perception, rev ed. Follett Publishing, Chicago, 1973.
15. Burt, M: Perceptual deficits in hemiplegia. Am J Nurs 70:1026, 1970.
16. Adams, GF: Treatment of hemiplegia complicated by sensory defects. Physiotherapy 52:345, 1966.

17. Ayres, AJ: Sensory Integration and the Child. Los Angeles, Western Psychological Services, 1980.
18. Cohen, SA: A dynamic theory of vision. J Dev Read 6(1):15, 1962.
19. Cratty, BJ: Movement Behavior and Motor Learning, ed 2. Lea and Febiger, Philadelphia, 1967.
20. Diller, L: Studies in Cognition and Rehabilitation in Hemiplegia. Research Grant Rd, 2666-P, New York, Institute of Rehabilitation Medicine, July, 1971.
21. Kephart, N: Slow Learner in the Classroom. Charles E Merrill, Columbus, OH, 1960.
22. Bobath, B: Adult Hemiplegia, Evaluation and Treatment. William Hennemann Medical Books, London, 1978.
23. Restak, R: The Brain. Bantum Books, Toronto, 1984.
24. Layton, B: Perceptual noise and aging. Psychol Bull 82(6):875, 1975.
25. Sawtell, R and Martin, G: Perceptual problems of the hemiplegic patient. Lancet 1:193, 1967.
26. Soloman P et al: Sensory Deprivation. Cambridge, Harvard University Press, 1961.
27. Milner, D: Use of microcomputers in the treatment of patients with physical disabilities. Physical Disabilities Special Interest Section Newsletter 7(2):1, 1984.
28. Bair, J et al: Computer. Am Occup Ther Assoc Practice Division, 1383 Piccard Dr, Suite 300, Rockville, MD, 20850.
29. Smith, C: Computer update: Special Education TWA Ambassador, 86, June, 1984.
30. Bracy, O: Computer based cognitive rehabilitation. Cognitive Rehabilitation 1(1):7, 1983.
31. Gianutsos, R: What Is cognitive rehabilitation? J Rehabil July/Aug/Sept: 36, 1980.
32. Lynch, WJ: The use of electronic games in cognitive rehabilitation. In Trexler, LE (ed): Cognitive Rehabilitation—Conceptualization and Intervention. Plenum Press, New York, 1982.
33. Parente, R: Cognitive Rehabilitation and the use of Computers. Paper presented to Baltimore Adult Communications Disorders Interest Group, 1984.
34. Parente, R and Anderson, JD: Techniques for improving cognitive rehabilitation: Teaching organization and encoding skills. Cognitive Rehabilitation 4(1):20, 1983.
35. Lynch, WT: Video Games in the Remediation of Cognitive and Perceptual-Motor Disorders: Experience, Problems and Prospects. Presented at Symposium on Video Games and Human Development: A Research Agenda for the 80s, Harvard Graduate School of Education, May, 1983.
36. Wilson, PG: Software selection and use in language and cognitive retraining. Cognitive Rehabilitation 1(1):9, 1983.
37. Lorenze, EJ and Cancro, R: Dysfunction in visual perception with hemiplegia: Its relation to activities of daily living. Arch Phys Med 43:514, 1962.
38. Williams, N: Correlations between copying ability and dressing activities in hemiplegia. Am J Phys Med 46:1332, 1967.
39. Diller, L and Gordon, W: Interventions for cognitive deficits in brain injured adults. J Cons Clin Psychol 49(6):822, 1981.
40. Piasetsky, E, Ben-Yishay, Y and Weinberg, J: The systematic remediation of specific disorders: Selected application of methods derived in a clinical research setting. In Trexler, LE (ed): Cognitive Rehabilitation, Conceptualization, and Intervention. Plenum Press, New York, 1982.

Chapter 25

Reality Orientation Therapy

ROBIN McNENY, O.T.R.
JEAN DISE, M.S., O.T.R.

Upon awakening from a period of unconsciousness following head injury, most individuals are confused, disoriented, socially withdrawn, and unable to respond appropriately and effectively to their environment. Reality orientation therapy can help these head injured individuals begin to understand themselves and the environment. The best reality orientation programs are those with an interdisciplinary approach to frequent, nonthreatening reorientation offered continuously throughout the day. It is vital that identification of disoriented patients be made early and that a complete evaluation be done. As therapy is then begun, both environmental management and structured group sessions should be used to improve orientation.

Impaired memory further complicates the problem of disorientation by eliminating or diminishing a good compensatory strategy.[1] Disoriented patients with poor memory often repeatedly ask questions about meals, rest periods, and visiting hours. Reality orientation has been mentioned as a technique to aid in improving memory.[2] However, research has not established reality orientation as a modality for improving memory. Nevertheless, the opinion exists that reality orientation should be included in a program for head injured adults.

GOALS OF THE REALITY ORIENTATION PROGRAM

Disorientation is one of the most common neuropsychologic sequelae following head injury.[3] Disoriented patients lack knowledge of themselves, of time, and/or of their environment. Kreutzer and coworkers,[4] have divided the spheres of orientation as follows:

Personal Orientation: Basic knowledge of oneself, including facts regarding date of birth, age, name, and home

Temporal Orientation: Knowledge of the current day, date, month, and year, as well as knowledge of pertinent facts related to time of day

Environmental Orientation: Knowledge regarding the surrounding environment

Obviously, possessing information about who you are, where you are, and the passage of time is critically important to effective rehabilitation.

There are two primary goals in a reality orientation program. First, the team should help the patient develop oriented behavior. This includes an awareness of time, place, and person as well as appropriate interaction with the environment. Disoriented patients display a variety of maladaptive and inappropriate behaviors, including roaming into other patients' rooms, aggressiveness, poor personal hygiene, and uncooperativeness. Many of these behaviors stem from inadequate understanding of themselves and of the treatment environment.

Through reality orientation, disoriented patients begin to understand where they are and perhaps why they are in such an unfamiliar place. They begin to recognize the staff, other patients, and frequent visitors; often abusiveness toward others rapidly declines as they feel more secure in their new surroundings. In addition, the passage of time becomes increasingly meaningful to patients; therapy routines, regular meal-times, and scheduled rest periods will pro-vide patients with the structure needed to help them function more independently. Thus, more oriented behavior should result from an effective reorientation program.[5] Needless to say, the extent of recovery de-pends on the nature of injury and the level of recovery they have achieved.

The second goal should be to improve the individual's social awareness and social skills. Often, disoriented patients display bi-zarre and unacceptable behavior such as taking off their clothing in public places. So-cial isolation, such as hiding in the bath-room or sitting alone in a darkened room often occurs. When attempts are made to engage these patients in conversation, they may fail to verbalize, lack eye contact, or use profanity. As a result of their poor social skills, they suffer greater isolation as other patients, families, visitors, and often hospital personnel avoid them.

Through reality orientation, staff and fam-ily model and encourage appropriate social interaction. Preserving self-esteem is of the utmost importance during this process. Quizzing obviously confused patients is al-ways avoided. When patients respond or be-have inappropriately, they are offered the correct response without ridicule or re-proof. In this way, patients find the experi-ence of reorientation pleasant and reas-suring.

EVALUATION: AN OCCUPATIONAL BEHAVIOR APPROACH

Complete evaluation of the head injured patient involves more than assessment of the patient's awareness of the immediate envi-ronment, usually termed "person," "place," and "time." Frequently, various members of the rehabilitation team include this brief as-sessment in their initial contacts with the pa-tient. Because occupational therapists are concerned with a patient's ability to effec-tively interact with the environment, other information about the patient's premorbid lifestyle should also be obtained during the occupational therapy evaluation process (see Chapter 20).[6] This information can

guide the selection of modalities offered in a treatment plan and provides an appropriate base from which to begin the reorientation process.

Premorbid Information

Improvement of social awareness and skills is one of the goals of a reality orienta-tion program and the assessment process must reflect this goal. Many "social" skills can be considered universal; however, cul-tural and socioeconomic influences dictate what is "appropriate" behavior to each of us. A thorough understanding of a disori-ented patient's premorbid personal goals, skills, routines, habits, and role performance enables the therapist to structure the envi-ronment for optimal arousal and reinforce-ment of what is "appropriate."

There are a number of assessments avail-able to occupational therapists, which can be used to glean premorbid information about the patient. These include the *Occu-pational Therapy Functional Screening Tool,*[7] the *Occupational History,*[8] *Interest Checklist,*[9] and the *Role Checklist.*[10] Because the disoriented patient is an unreliable his-torian, families are usually contacted to ob-tain this information. Assessment of present functional status and the patient's immedi-ate environment is added to premorbid in-formation for an overall view of the patient's assets and limitations. The disoriented pa-tient experiences disruption in nearly all spheres of function. In the acute and early rehabilitation phases of recovery, the most immediate disruptions appear in the areas of personal care and daily living skills. For the disoriented patient, tasks such as feeding oneself or performing simple hygiene activi-ties (e.g., brushing teeth) are no longer au-tomatic, self-regulated, or time-appropriate unless structure is imposed. Other cognitive impairments such as inattention and mem-ory deficits further limit the patient's suc-cess experiences with basic self-care activi-ties. The reorientation process must include monitoring or periodic reevaluation of the amount of structure that must continue to be provided for the patient.

All head injured patients experience a major disruption of lifestyle, regardless of the age at which the trauma occurs. The ex-tent of long-term disruption to one's per-sonal goals, skills, routines, habits, and role performance is determined by the severity of the brain damage incurred. However, accurate assessment of the premorbid history is necessary in order to facilitate future progress in treatment. For the disoriented patient, accurate and complete assessment is dependent on input from reliable resources such as family and friends.

Present Orientation

Standardized tools such as the Galveston Orientation and Amnesia Test (GOAT)[11] are used to assess post-traumatic amnesia but may not be useful as an ongoing monitor of orientation. Corrigan and associates[5] suggested a standardized rating scale of observed behaviors as a method of assessing and monitoring orientation over time. This suggested method provides a weekly aggregate picture of performance in a reality orientation program. In addition, the system purports to represent the dynamic qualities of cognitive behaviors rather than reflecting performance of specific, nongeneralized behaviors and skills such as repetition of day, date, and place. Whatever instrument or method of orientation assessment is used as a data base, periodic re-evaluation of the patient's orientation status is necessary to monitor progress of the treatment program.

In sum, the reality orientation evaluation process must be comprehensive in order to plan a treatment program designed to reinforce oriented behavior and to reinforce social awareness and skills. Background or premorbid information is best obtained from reliable resources such as family and friends. A number of assessment tools that help provide this information are available to the occupational therapist. When patients are considered for inclusion in a group treatment program, rehabilitation team members must devise a mechanism for communicating baseline information and ongoing progress regarding the patient's orientation status.

THE TREATMENT PROGRAM: A TEAM APPROACH

Environmental Considerations

The head injured patient is typically first seen by the rehabilitation team at bedside. Depending on the level of recovery to date, the patient may or may not be responsive to others or to the environment. Nevertheless, it is to be expected that as arousal increases, the first interactions will be with someone nearby or something in the environment. For this reason, reality orientation must begin early and is best accomplished through the use of environmental management techniques.

It is difficult to alter the environment of an intensive care unit to control stimuli and clarify its meaning for the patient. However, once the patient is moved to the rehabilitation ward, efforts should begin to reorient the patient. Family members are recruited to assist staff. Measures taken to improve the environment need not be complicated or expensive.

Mobiles can be hung over the bed of a low-level patient. Decorated with pictures, the name of the hospital, the names and pictures of family, friends, and favorite activities, they are an excellent source of visual stimulation. Cards on the mobile should be changed at intervals.

Personal orientation boards with changeable strips of days, dates, months, and weather provide a resource for frequent re-orientation. In addition, patients can benefit from having their own calendar hung in the room each month. These reminders are best done in large print using eye-catching colors and designs. Marking off each day as it passes is beneficial.

Family members should be encouraged to bring in items familiar to the patient. It is advisable to avoid cluttering the room with too many items. Instead, families should rotate items brought from home. The following could be given as suggestions to the family interested in bringing in appropriate items:

Photographs: Included in this category should be preinjury photographs of the patient as well as those of family, friends, home, parties, pets, and special events. Photographs can either be mounted on poster board or be placed in album pages. To assist staff in using the pictures in therapy, the family should label each picture.

Favorite possessions: Wall posters, stuffed animals, clothing, quilts, pillows, and calendars help familiarize the patient with the environment and are useful in stimulating the patient's memory.

Radio and/or television: Radios can be

tuned to favorite stations and played for short periods. Because of the nature of most radio programming, the date, time, news updates, and weather are broadcast frequently and therefore enhance orientation. A tape player with several favorite tapes can be used at intervals for relaxation, and in therapy. For patients in a sensory stimulation program, tapes of family members talking, singing, or reading favorite poems or stories should be available. Some television can be permitted, particularly if the patient premorbidly enjoyed a few special programs. It is important, though, that there be periods when radio, television, and music are turned off to avoid both accommodation to the sound and overstimulation.

As patients become more mobile, they begin to explore the environment more and require supervision for safety, frequent orientation, and perhaps some environmental manipulation to foster independence and decrease confusion. Some techniques useful in modifying the environment for confused patients include labeling the doors to important places—i.e., the patient's room, the bathroom, therapy areas, and the dining room—painting colored lines along hallways to mark routes, placing hazardous items safely out of reach, and posting schedules and calendars in strategic places.

The daily routine of the disoriented patient should be well organized and as consistent as possible. Changes in the patient's day-to-day routine should be kept to a minimum. As the staff plans the schedule for the disoriented patient, consideration should be given to spacing therapy sessions, providing rest periods, and allowing time for toileting. Family input during this process is often helpful.

In addition to environmental manipulation, specific orientation aids can be used to supplement reorientation sessions. Of utmost importance is the placement of an individualized patient schedule in a spot where it is convenient for ready reference, such as on the armrest of the wheelchair, on the lapboard, or in a shirt pocket. Staff and family should use this schedule to orient the patient prior to each change in activity. Initially, the patient may require considerable assistance. However, as orientation improves, the patient should be encouraged to use greater initiative in following his or her schedule. Journals and notebooks can aid patients in improving their orientation.

While providing a record of activities and events, it can also be utilized to orient the patient. Whenever possible, patients should be responsible for recording daily events in their journal, seeking assistance only as needed. Teaching patients to keep the journal faithfully and to rely upon it as a resource can be helpful for those who have lingering memory deficits.

Throughout the reorientation process, the interactions among staff, family members, and patient are vital. All efforts must be placed on providing reorientation in a dignified and adult manner. Questions posed by the patient should be answered politely and directly. Conversations should be casual and calm. Appropriate behavior should be modeled for patients. Great care should be taken by staff and family to be empathetic, encouraging, and supportive; disoriented individuals often recognize that something is "wrong" with their "thinking" and may well resent others laughing at their errors. To maximize the benefit of environmental manipulation during orientation therapy, all staff should use a standard approach and provide consistent feedback to patients. For this reason, staff education is vitally important. All staff should provide repetition and consistency during encounters with the patient.

STRUCTURED GROUP SESSIONS

The second component of a reality orientation program is the structured reality orientation group. These sessions are held "classroom style" one to three times a day and are led by one or more professionals on the team. Typically, occupational therapy, nursing, and psychology are involved in these sessions.

Selection of Members

The selection of members for a reality orientation group should be done carefully. Use of the following guidelines might prove helpful:

1. Groups should number no more than five to six members to ensure good interaction and allow the leader to comfortably maintain control.

2. The attention span of members should be long enough to allow them to participate with a minimum of redirection from the leader. Generally, an attention span of five to seven minutes allows the patient to participate and minimizes the frequency of interruption of the group for redirection.

3. The behavior of members should be reasonably appropriate. Agitated and combative patients typically cannot benefit from group treatment and are disruptive during group sessions. However, mildly disinhibited patients should be included to provide them with opportunities for feedback regarding their verbal expansiveness or their rude interruptions. Patients who only occasionally become agitated may show improved behavior after inclusion in an orientation program. At times, the agitated patient is reacting to feelings of confusion and frustration.

4. The ability to speak articulately is not a criterion for inclusion in the group. Patients experiencing mild expression problems seem to benefit from the structured sessions and contact with other patients. However, there should be some indication that the patient will benefit from a passive role in the group. Severely language-impaired patients appear not to benefit from group treatment.

Frequency

The frequency with which group sessions are held should depend on the type of program offered, patient needs, and availability of staff to lead groups. Some programs offer group sessions in the mornings to give patients a good start in their day. Other programs have morning and evening classes. Evening sessions are helpful in providing a summary of and closure to the day. Holden and Woods[12] suggested having three groups divided according to their level of orientation, each meeting once daily.

Other Factors

As the planning for the reality orientation group proceeds, several other factors should be considered:

1. **Meeting Place:** A quiet place that will accommodate several wheelchairs should be chosen. The group should always meet in the same place if possible. The entire staff should understand the importance of minimizing distractions and interruptions during group sessions.

2. **Treatment Media:** The group will need a reality orientation board, which is the focal point of group sessions and should be displayed in a prominent place. In addition, the leader will need a variety of props for group sessions. Large colorful pictures are available commercially or can be secured from magazines. Sensory stimulation materials such as flavors, textures, and sounds should be obtained.

3. **Staff and Family Education:** All members of the treatment team, including families, should have some idea of what the reality orientation group involves. While only a few staff members actually lead the group sessions, the entire staff and family should support the group's efforts. Staff inservices on reality orientation as well as frequent updates on patient progress will aid staff as they provide individual orientation. Family education as to the purpose and format of the sessions should be provided by the group leaders through handouts or patient education classes and manuals.

Format

The actual group sessions should follow a consistent format from day-to-day. Such a format has been proposed by Barns and colleagues[13] and has been successfully adapted for use with the head injured population. When this format is used, orientation, promotion of self-esteem, and group interaction are encouraged.

Stage 1: The Climate of Acceptance. Introductions by the group leader of self and others present are done during the first few minutes of the session. New members are given special recognition; the leader or the patient, if able, shares information about the patient's family, work, home, and interests. When members are ready to "graduate" from the group or are leaving the group for other reasons, the opportunity is given for the remaining members to say "goodbye." Throughout these first few minutes, a warm, comfortable atmosphere is developed.

Stage 2: A Bridge to Reality. The focus of attention during this stage is the reality orientation board. To achieve the goal of re-orienting the group members to reality, the leader uses the board to stimulate a discussion among members of where they are, what day it is, what the weather is like, and what holiday is approaching. Members unable to spontaneously recall information are encouraged to read from the board. An atmosphere of testing should be avoided; incorrect responses made by patients should be met with a correct response given by the leader. Frequent repetition of orientation information should be made during this stage to aid memory-impaired patients.

Stage 3: Sharing the World We Live in. The next 10 to 15 minutes of the session should be spent discussing a topic or engaging in a task of interest to the members. The leader is typically responsible for planning this section, although higher-level patients can be assigned some of the preparation as "homework" (e.g., bringing a family photograph to the next group meeting). The topic may focus on basic concepts, holidays, weather, individuals in the group, the treatment setting, or current events. The possibilities for topics are limited only by the leader's imagination. Audiovisual aids are essential and may include pictures, objects, sensory items, nature items, or art materials. The leader facilitates attention through a discussion of the topic. All comments by all members regardless of their relevancy are recognized by the leader, and appropriate feedback is offered.

Stage 4: Climate of Appreciation. During the last 5 minutes, the leader summarizes the group meeting with a review of the reality orientation board. Reminders about the day's events are given. Comments by members are welcomed. Each patient's schedule for the day is reviewed. Members leave the group with a direction for the day ahead.

Throughout the group session, the leader is continually assessing the performance of each patient while facilitating attention and appropriate behavior and encouraging verbalization. Patients who are easily distracted benefit from being seated close to the leader; this allows the leader to gently and quietly redirect their attention. Patients lacking in social skills are given reminders when they behave inappropriately. Care

must be taken, however, that these reminders do not reinforce the undesired behavior by providing the patient with a "stage" and an "audience." Poor impulse control is best handled by calling on patients by name in turn and providing verbal or nonverbal cues to those who answer out of turn.

Occasionally the group may include patients who are nonverbal. Efforts should be made to include these patients in the discussions. While they may be less spontaneous, they may be able to answer direct questions with gestures or head nods. An effort should be made to awaken patients who fall asleep during orientation group; however, if they seem soundly asleep, it is usually best to allow them to doze and proceed with the group rather than risk further disruption of the session. The patients who indicate an intense desire to leave the session should be redirected by the leader and engaged in the task. However, if they continue to disrupt the group with their requests and efforts to leave, then they should be helped from the room as quickly and quietly as possible.

Documenting the performance and participation of group members is vital. It allows the leader to see if progress toward orientation is proceeding. In addition, the primary therapist is given feedback about the patient's performance. Daily documentation is ideal, although for large groups this may be an unwieldy task for a busy leader. Weekly summaries, therefore, may suffice.

Patients are ready for discharge from group sessions when they demonstrate consistent orientation to time, place, and person. This does not mean that the patients know every answer to every question but rather that they have a working concept of who they are, where they are, what time of year it is, and grossly what they are doing in therapy. The patients' orientation continues to be refined after they are discharged from the group.

The time required for patients to reach this point varies. For some patients, orientation is achieved in a matter of a few weeks. Other patients require months of group and individual therapy to reach a state of orientation. These patients naturally require patience, repetition, and consistency. We prefer that patients not be discontinued from orientation group sessions unless behavioral problems are limiting benefit for other patients. Those patients who remain disoriented despite months of participation in the orientation group continue to benefit from the routine beginning of their day and exposure to orienting information. Unless some other factor prohibits it, these individuals should continue attending the group until discharge from the facility. At that time, recommendations should be made to family or the staff at the new facility regarding management of the patient's orientation.

IMPLICATIONS FOR RESEARCH

There is a paucity of research regarding the effectiveness of reality orientation as a treatment modality. A number of factors limit "traditional" research methods with this modality. Ethical issues, such as deciding which patients will or will not be offered treatment, prohibit research efforts using control groups. Even with the best efforts to structure environments, there are a number of external factors present in a busy rehabilitation facility that may influence a patient's exposure to orientation information.

Nevertheless, investigative research could be attempted. For example, for patients participating in a reality orientation program data could be collected that compares demographic information with type of injury, number of treatment sessions, and rate of reorientation. Efforts to assess the effectiveness of a reorientation program with patients in various levels of function (e.g., Rancho levels[14]) could also be investigated. Increasing demands for professional accountability and the importance of measuring outcomes and treatment effectiveness for quality assurance necessitate the pursuit of research efforts for treatments used with the brain injured patient.

SUMMARY

Reality orientation therapy is provided in rehabilitation programs for head injured adults. The goal of treatment is to reacquaint disoriented patients with the environment, to maximize interaction with the environment, to reinforce oriented behavior, and to improve social awareness and social skills. The orientation evaluation process should include a comprehensive history of the patient's personal goals, habits, role responsibilities, and skills. In addition, assessment should include one's present state of awareness and orientation to the environment. With this broad data base, a treatment can be planned and provided that maximizes the patient's abilities to appropriately interact with persons and objects in the environment. Therapy is offered individually and in group programs. Group sessions provide a structured setting for repetition and consistent management of treatment modalities offered to the disoriented individual. Routine monitoring and documentation of performance is necessary for communication among rehabilitation team members regarding patient progress and program effectiveness.

Case 1. V.P. was a 29-year-old divorced mother of one, injured in a single-vehicle crash. V.P. entered the head injury unit still comatose and essentially unresponsive. Her environment was filled with familiar, orienting items including a calendar, pictures of her son, a radio, and posters.

Within 2 weeks, V.P. was responding to sensory stimulation consistently with eye opening, tracking, oral reflexes, and body posturing. Restlessness increased. At the same time, V.P. became more purposeful, pulling at restraints and pushing treatment items away.

Gradually, she began to verbalize, chiefly answering questions posed by staff. On formal evaluation of orientation, V.P. demonstrated impaired awareness of time, place, and person. She was also very impulsive in answers to questions and demonstrated poor problem-solving capabilities.

V.P. began orientation sessions. She talked out of turn, was restless, and had great difficulty maintaining attention. She initially responded poorly to cues to inhibit comments. Within 3 weeks, V.P. was able to attend a full orientation group session and sit quietly.

She was unable to follow a written schedule and could not locate therapy areas or her room. The treatment team and V.P.'s family worked together to provide V.P. with consistent cueing to check her schedule and look for signs to therapy rooms. Two weeks later, she was spontaneously consulting her watch, then her schedule throughout the day. She then was able to find most therapy areas independently. V.P. also demonstrated good orientation to time, place, and person and consequently was discharged from the orientation group. Reaching this point took approximately 3½ months.

Case 2. S.H. was a 20-year-old right-handed white male who, as a result of a motorcycle accident, had a skull fracture, resulting subdural hematoma, and contusion of the left temporal and parietal lobes. Following surgical removal of the clot, he remained comatose. Two months after admission, he regained consciousness and was transferred to the rehabilitation service for intensive physical, occupational, and speech therapies.

Premorbid History. S.H. was the third of four children. He had completed high school and taken a 2-month car maintenance course prior to the accident. His plans had been to consider college attendance, but he wanted to work for a couple of years first. His interests included swimming, boating, chess, guitar, and social events with his friends. His mother was active in the rehabilitation process. His father was less than supportive, and appeared to have difficulty accepting his son's limitations.

Level of Orientation. S.H. was disoriented as to time, place, and person. His impulsiveness and impaired memory and problem-solving abilities made him a safety risk. He lacked the ability to understand the expectations of the treatment team. He was unable to remember his past or to set goals for the future.

Treatment. S.H. was seen in daily orientation group sessions and was provided with items in his immediate environment to reinforce group efforts: calendar, clock, radio, and pictures of family and close friends. He was given a daily schedule of events, including all self-care tasks, meals, rest breaks, and therapies, and was directed to refer to the schedule and his personal watch throughout the day. After 2 weeks, he was requiring six reminders throughout the day to refer to his schedule. By four weeks, his knowledge of time, place, and person was accurate 90 percent of the time. Self-monitoring of his daily schedule had improved to needing, at most, two reminders each day.

REFERENCES

1. Moffat, N: Strategies of Memory Therapy. In Wilson, B and Moffat, N (eds): Clinical Management of Memory Problems. Aspen Publications, Rockville, MD, 1984.
2. Wilson, B and Moffat, N: Running a Memory Group. In Wilson, B and Moffat, N (eds): Clinical Management of Memory Problems. Aspen Publications, Rockville, MD, 1984.
3. Levin, H and Grossman, R: Behavioral sequelae of closed head injury. Arch Neurol 35:720, 1978.
4. Kreutzer, J et al: A Glossary of Cognitive Rehabilitation Terminology. Cognitive Rehabilitation, May–June, 1986.
5. Corrigan, J et al: Reality orientation for brain injured patients: Group treatment and monitoring of recovery. Arch Phys Med Rehabil 66:626, 1985.
6. Cerny, J and McNeny, R: Reality Orientation Therapy. In Rosenthal, M et al: (eds): Rehabilitation of the Head Injured Adult. FA Davis, Philadelphia, 1983.
7. Occupational Therapy Functional Screening Tool. Available from Occupational Therapy Services, Department of Rehabilitation Medicine, Clinical Center, Building 10, Rm 5D37, National Institutes of Health, Bethesda, MD 20205.
8. Harlan, B: Determining the Reliability of the Occupational Role History when used with Physically Disabled Persons. Unpublished Masters thesis. Richmond, Virginia Commonwealth University, 1983.
9. Neville, A and Kielhofner, G: Modified Interest Checklist. Unpublished workbook, National Institutes of Health, Washington, DC, 1983.
10. Oakley, F: The Model of Human Occupation in Psychiatry. Unpublished masters research project. Richmond, Virginia Commonwealth University, 1982.
11. Levin, HS, O'Donnell, VM and Grossman, RG: Galveston Orientation and Amnesia Test: Practical scale to assess cognition after head injury. Nerv Ment Dis 167:675, 1979.
12. Holden, UP and Woods, R: Reality Orientation: Psychological Approaches to the Confused Elderly. Churchill-Livingstone, London, 1982.
13. Barns, K, Sack, A and Shore, H: Guidelines to treatment approaches: Modalities and methods for use with the aged. Gerontologist Winter:513, 1973.
14. Hagen, C, Malkmus, D and Durham, P: Levels of Cognitive Functioning. In Rehabilitation of the Head Injured Adult: Comprehensive Physical Management. From Professional Staff Association of Rancho Los Amigos Hospital, Inc, Downey, CA, 1979.

Chapter 26

Treatment of Communication and Swallowing Disorders

BRENDA B. ADAMOVICH, Ph.D.

Various types of communication disturbances occur following traumatic head injury. Focal lesions may occur, resulting in language and speech disturbances similar to those that occur following cerebrovascular accidents (e.g., aphasia, apraxia, and dysarthria). Widespread, diffuse brain damage, which most often occurs following closed head injury, generally causes communication disorders as a result of impaired cognition, information processing, and attention. The ability to communicate or to exchange information between individuals requires attention, information processing, cognition, and language. Attentional deficits range from the ability to initiate attention to the ability to attend to the most salient features in a situation, or conversation. Necessary information processing skills range from the recognition of information to the use of internal or external feedback to generate responses most appropriate to a particular situation.

Cognitive skills include the ability to discriminate information such as that which pertains to a situation or conversation, the ability to meaningfully organize information presented or received from others, the ability to generate appropriate responses, and the ability to problem solve in logical steps. These processes directly affect communication. For example, a person will not be able to convey information or to comprehend it if he or she cannot remember the first part of a conversation by the time the conversation has been completed.

The section that follows describes methods of treating the various communication disturbances that result from closed head injury.

SPEECH

A variety of speech disturbances have been reported following closed head injury. Speech processes include articulation, phonation, resonation, vocalization, and fluency. Speech disturbances that reportedly occur following closed head injury include stuttering and cluttering behaviors;[1] echolalia and paralalia;[2] dysarthrias and apraxia;[3] and mutism.[4] Piller and Gordon[5] suggested that neuromotor disorders following closed head trauma are not different from those associated with brain damage from other causes. Furthermore, they observed that spastic states are usual, ataxia is common, and "Parkinson-like" states with various patterns of tremor and rigidity are all seen in closed head injured patients.

Disorders of speech volume, especially speaking too loudly, and abnormally rapid rates of speech often occur due to inadequate self-monitoring secondary to attentional deficits following closed head injury.

The dysarthrias are neurogenic motor speech impairments characterized by slow, weak, imprecise, and/or uncoordinated movements of the speech musculature. They represent a group of disorders caused by disturbed muscular control over the speech mechanism due to paralysis, weakness, abnormal tone, or incoordination of the muscles used in speech.[6] The dysarthrias may result in slow, restricted, weak, or uncoordinated muscle activity used in breathing for speech (respiration); producing sound in the larynx (phonation); selectively amplifying sound by changing the size, shape, and number of cavities through which it must pass (resonance); and varying intonation, stress, and rhythm during speech (prosody).[7] Paralysis of the lips, tongue, mandible, velum, laryngeal musculature, and/or respiratory system may occur. The localization of brain damage includes cortical and subcortical areas, the cerebellum, the brainstem, or the peripheral nervous system which includes the cranial and spinal nerves with their associated ganglia.[8] The specific dysarthrias that may result following closed head injury, according to the Mayo Clinic perceptual classification of dysarthrias,[9] include (1) flaccid dysarthria, characterized by breathy voice quality, hypernasality, and consonant imprecision secondary to a lower motor neuron lesion; (2) spastic dysarthria, exhibiting a strained-strangled-harsh voice quality, hypernasality, slow rate, and consonant imprecision secondary to an upper motor neuron lesion; (3) ataxic dysarthria, which features imprecise consonants, excess and equal stress, and irregular articulatory breakdown secondary to a cerebellar system lesion; and (4) mixed dysarthria (i.e., spastic and flaccid) characterized by imprecise consonants, hypernasality, harsh voice quality, slow rate, monopitch, short phrases, distorted vowels, low pitch, monoloudness, excess and equal stress, and prolonged intervals secondary to an upper and lower motor neuron lesion.

Apraxia refers to an articulatory deficit generally resulting from a unilateral left hemisphere lesion involving the third frontal convolution; however, cases of apraxia have been reported following more posterior, probably parietal, lesions.[7] Apraxia refers to difficulty programming the positioning of speech muscles and sequencing muscle movements to produce phonemes. There is no significant weakness, slowness, or incoordination of these muscles in reflective or automatic acts.[9]

The symptoms of apraxia are impaired volitional production of normal articulation and prosody that do not result from muscle weakness or slowness, nor from aphasia, confusion, general intellectual deficit, or hearing loss. Rather, these symptoms result from inhibition or impairment of central nervous system programming of skilled oral movements.[10] Examination of apraxia generally reveals intact vowel production and repetition of single phonemes. However, there is impaired repetition of combined monosyllables, multisyllabic words, words of increasing length, words with the same initial and final phoneme (e.g., coke and gag); with more errors on the initial phoneme than on the final phoneme and with repetition of sentences.[7]

Johns and Darley[11] listed the significant criteria for differentiating apraxia of speech from dysarthria. These include more substitution errors in apraxia compared with more consistency of error type in dysarthria; a greater effect of nonphonetic variables in apraxia compared with lesser effect on nonphonetic variables in dysarthria; more normal reasonable balance in dysarthria; typical absence of consistent dysphonia in apraxia compared with the frequent presence of consistent dysphonia in dysarthria; and cranial nerves nearly or wholly intact in apraxia compared with involvement of cranial nerves in dysarthria.

Assessment of dysarthria entails the evaluation of the extent of the disability including ratings of speech intelligibility, rate, and naturalness, as well as specific evaluations of respiration, phonation, resonation, articulation, and prosody. The purpose of the assessment is to identify the nature of the impairment and features that can be modified. Treatment focuses on the following areas: (1) prespeech, including the use of augmentative communication devices and increased physiologic support; (2) the establishment of respiratory support based on predetermined perceptual measures, subglottal air pressure, lung volume, and respiratory patterns; (3) velopharyngeal management utilizing behavioral and prosthetic (i.e., palatal lifts) treatment approaches according to assessments of hypernasality, nasal emission, articulatory patterns, aerodynamic measures, radiographic measures, and direct visualization; and (4) speaking rate, including rigid rate control, rhythmic cueing, phrase pacing, delayed auditory feedback, and computer approaches based on determination of optimum rate.[12]

Treatment for ideomotor apraxia generally emphasizes drills. Specific treatment techniques include imitation, phonetic derivation, phonetic placement, melodic intonation therapy, gesture, and augmentative communication devices.[7] Phonetic derivation refers to a method of deriving target sounds from intact nonspeech or speech gestures such as biting the lower lip and gently exhaling to produce an s.[13] Phonetic placement refers to the assumption of the correct position for producing a specific speech sound.

Augmentative Communication Devices

Nonvocal communication devices/prostheses for speech and language functions provide for an alternative, nonoral language communication mode. With early communication prostheses, disabled persons would point to letters, numbers, and words on language boards; however, restrictions in range of motion or degree of motor control limited the use of these boards. Today a number of mechanical and electronic communication devices are available. Initially these devices were automated language boards or motor-drive pointers attached to language boards that clients activated by switches that started or stopped the motor (Fig. 26–1). Newer devices significantly increase functioning and decrease usage restrictions.[14]

A general model for speech and language prostheses, as outlined by the Assistive De-

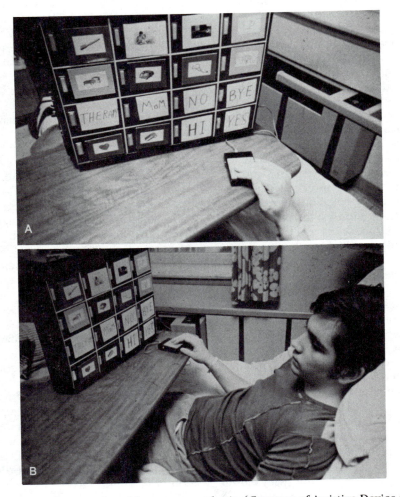

Figure 26–1. Model for speech and language prosthesis. (Courtesy of Assistive Device Center of California State University, Sacramento.)

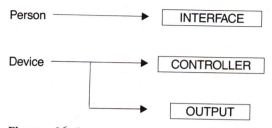

Figure 26–2. Communication board (motor-driven pointer activated by switch plate).

vice Center of California State University,[14] is presented in Figure 26–2. An individual interacts with the interface to make the device work. Interfaces include switches such as buttons or pedals activated by overt motor activity, the change of air flow caused by puffing or sipping air, or contractions of single muscles as measured by the myoelectric recorder. The controller connects the interface to an output device that generates communication. Output is the visual, auditory, or written message that both the receiver and the communicator can perceive such as a printed copy, alphanumeric display, or synthesized speech. Feedback is an important function of the output to allow the user to evaluate the message.[14]

Decisions regarding the type of device selected and the feasibility of device usage require a detailed evaluation of the patient's physical and cognitive limitations. Specific considerations include the assessment of attention, matching skills, memory, sequencing abilities, categorization abilities, vocabulary, grammar, semantics and pragmatics, or selection of usable items for each patient's communication system.

HEARING

A pure tone and audiometric hearing screening should be completed for all head injured persons. If the patient is difficult to test or if the screening reveals potential audiologic dysfunction, a referral should be made to an audiologist who is familiar with the behaviors that typically result from closed head injury. Complete audiometric testing may include auditory evoked potential measurements.

Particularly susceptible to injuries following basal skull fractures are the olfactory, oculomotor, and branches of the trigeminal, facial, and auditory nerves. Injury to the eighth cranial nerve can cause loss of hearing or dizziness immediately after injury. Other hearing disturbances can be caused by the rupture of the tympanic membrane (eardrum) or the presence of blood in the middle ear.

VISION

Much of the stimulus material utilized during therapy is presented visually. It is extremely important that visual acuity as well as visual processing be adequately assessed. Specific problems of head injured persons may be misdiagnosed if a patient lacks visual skills, including the ability to recognize and discriminate visual information (e.g., figure-ground information) and the ability to organize stimuli (e.g., part versus whole analysis). There are various visual diagnostic tests designed to evaluate visual skills, including the Weigl-Goldstein-Scheerer Color Form Sorting Test;[15] the Block Design, Object Assembly, and Picture Arrangement Subtest of the Wechsler Adult Intelligence Scale-Revised (WAIS-R);[16] the Developmental Test of Visual Perception;[17] the Southern California Figure-Ground Visual Perception Test;[18] and the Hooper Visual Organization Test.[19]

LANGUAGE

Many language deficits following closed head injury may actually be secondary to more generalized cognitive attentional and/or information-processing problems. For example, confabulation, tangential speech, and perseveration may actually be due to an attentional disturbance. Ordering errors may be due to organizational problems and word-finding problems, and comprehension deficits may actually be due to memory disturbances.

An aphasic disturbance is extremely difficult to assess when it coexists with cognitive and/or information-processing disturbances, as these disturbances may mask a language disturbance. On the other hand, what appears to be a language disturbance may also be due to a disruption in cognitive and/or information processing.

According to Luria,[20] the purpose of aphasia treatment is the deinhibition of temporarily depressed function, substitutions of the opposite hemisphere, and the radical reorganization of functional systems. General therapy considerations include the use of alerting statements to ensure that the patient is attending, lead-in informational statements that help patients focus their attention, and finally the use of rich, contextual, and life-like materials that help to maintain an individual's potential.[21] The selection of specific therapy tasks should be done after careful consideration of syntactic and semantic complexity. The more intact input modality (e.g., visual, auditory, gestural, and graphic) should be utilized first, and the rate of both the presentation and the response should be considered.[21]

There are four general categories of aphasia treatment: stimulation/facilitation approaches; behavior modification approaches; psycholinguistic approaches; and pragmatic approaches. Specific treatment programs in each of these categories are reviewed subsequently.

Stimulation/Facilitation Approaches

The stimulation approach generally uses intensive auditory stimulation, meaningful material, varied clinical material, repetitive sensory stimulation, requiring a response to each stimulus, eliciting rather than forcing responses, allowing incorrect or defective responses to go uncorrected, and searching for the most adequate stimulus. Schuell and coworkers[22] suggested that one language modality should be used to stimulate another in a program carefully graded for complexity, and treatment should begin where the patient starts to have difficulty.

The Porch Index of Communicative Ability (PICA) theory[23] regards aphasia as a cybernetic disturbance of information processing (e.g., tuning in, tuning out, dealing with noise build-up). PICA therapy includes work in several areas: verbal, auditory, reading, writing, object manipulation, visual matching, and copying. Each area is divided into more specific treatment areas.

The Clinician Controlled Auditory Stimulation for Aphasic Adults[24] provides 360 object pictures. Patients choose from two, four, or six pictures. Response decisions may involve a semantic, phonemic, or no relationship between words represented by the pictures. Other therapy progams designed for comprehension deficits include Language Rehabilitation: Auditory Comprehension[25] and the Graduated Language Training for Patients with Aphasia and Children with Language Deficiencies.[26]

Verbal production or self-cueing word retrieval strategies involve the use of an imposed delay, associations with the word to be retrieved, description of the item, phonologic associations, gesturing, and the use of written language.

Melodic Intonation Therapy (MIT)[27] is an approach in which functional language is taught in association with rhythm and melody in an attempt to utilize an intact right hemisphere. The program is taught in five steps. Patient requirements for participation in this program include good auditory comprehension, facility for self-correction, limited verbal output, good attention span, and emotional stability.[27]

The Voluntary Control of Involuntary Utterances (VCIU)[28] approach can be used with patients who have limited speech output with better comprehension. This program consists of the use of a written presentation of any real word the patient utters during an oral reading task. The patient completes a self-review of the words read correctly. The final stage is the production of words in confrontation or responsive-naming tasks.

Behavior Modification Approaches

B. F. Skinner, in his operant conditioning theory, suggested that desired behavior exists in the organism.[29] Such behavior can be manipulated to occur in response to a specific stimulus or reinforcer or both. The primary difficulty lies in the clinician's ability to select appropriate stimuli as well as reinforcers, which result in the attainment of the desired response. Behavior modification steps include analysis of undesirable behaviors, establishment of baselines, determination of the acceptable responses, identification of positive reinforcers, determination of scoring method, fading of reinforcers, use of time-out when necessary, and elimination of the reinforcement of undesirable behavior.[30-32]

Gestural Therapy

Gestural therapy includes the facilitation of natural gestures commonly used when communicating: head nods to signal yes and no, facial expressions suggesting disagreement, anger, agreement, surprise, and the like; pantomime; sign language; and the use of nonverbal symbols (such as holding an imaginary cup and raising that cup to the lips to signal a desire for a drink). It has been suggested that the central impairment of symbol function in aphasia extends to all symbol systems, including gesture.[33]

The Visual Communication Therapy (VCT) approach was developed by Gardner and colleagues[34] as a gestural treatment approach. This program requires the utilization of an index card system in which arbitrary symbols representing syntactic and lexical components are recorded. Slowly, aphasic patients learn to recognize these symbols and ultimately use them spontaneously.

Visual Action Therapy (VAT) is another gestural treatment approach designed by Helm-Estabrooks and associates[35] to develop limb and face gesturing. This therapy program uses eight objects consisting of both large and small drawings and action pictures. The program begins with training the ability to trace objects followed by the matching of large pictures of objects to the objects themselves, matching small pictures of objects, pantomime training, spontaneous production of the action of each object on request, and finally representational gestures.

Psycholinguistic Approaches

Psycholinguistic approaches incorporate generalizations about the decreased number, variety, and complexity of linguistic operation available to each patient both receptively and expressively.

Helm-Estabrooks developed the Helm Elicited Language Program for Syntax Stimulations (HELPSS),[36] which was designed to improve the use of syntactic forms of five sentence types: imperative intransitive; imperative transitive; WH interrogative (who, when, what, why, and where statements); declarative transitive; declarative intransitive; comparative; passive; yes/no question; direct and indirect object; embedded sentences; and future. The first level of this program requires a patient to report target sentences after delay. At the second level, patients complete stories with accompanying pictures.

Pragmatic Approaches

Pragmatic approaches require considerations of language and context as well as functional uses of language. The environmental language intervention program outlined by Lubinski[37] is based on the theory that communication effectiveness will increase with changed communicative settings and varied partners.

Brookshire[38] suggested the use of real-life situations in which aphasic subjects are to use knowledge of the world to decipher meanings of messages, if cognitive abilities are intact. Holland[39] indicated that exercises and drills can be constructed with semantic content and materials that the patient confronts in everyday experience. She suggested that if these considerations take place, therapy will be much more productive and beneficial.

Promoting Aphasics' Communicative Effectiveness (PACE), as developed by Davis and Wilcox,[40] utilizes more natural conversations with conveyance of ideas, not linguistic accuracy. In this program, the clinician and patient are equal senders and receivers of messages. Patients and clinicians take turns drawing from a stack of stimulus cards that lie face down on a table. Each takes turns acting as senders and receivers of information. The receiver must decipher the sender's message. As new information is exchanged, the modality (e.g., speech-writing, gesturing, drawing, or pointing to picture words) used by patients to convey information is of their own choice. The clinicians provide feedback regarding the patient's success in conveying a message.

ATTENTION

In order to communicate effectively, an individual must possess attentional skills that afford the ability to appropriately deal with information in the environment, in specific situations, and in conversations both as a speaker and as a listener. As information becomes more complex, greater attentional skills are necessary.

Treatment of attentional disturbances includes the following considerations:

1. Limiting aural and visual distractions or competing cues in the environment

2. Gradually adding distractions as attentional skills improve

3. Limiting and gradually increasing the length and intensity of work periods

4. Using techniques that focus attention such as addressing the patient by name before initiating a task, waiting for eye contact, touching the patient, or using phrases like "Are you ready?"

5. Using pertinent, meaningful stimuli, moving gradually from self-related, familiar items to external, less familiar items

6. Varying treatment concepts, rates, and sequences in an attempt to expand attentional skills (e.g., if a person is capable of attending for 5 minutes, change tasks at the end of each 5-minute period, and continue the treatment session for as many 5-minute periods as the patient is capable of tolerating). Varying the sequence of therapy activities and the therapy concepts themselves creates novel situations, which generally result in better attention to the situation.

The performance of high-level head injured persons deteriorates when distractions occur or when they are given too much information or stimulation, causing the individual to become overwhelmed and unable to effectively proceed. Tasks to test for difficulties in this area would be to observe the individual's performance while answering the telephone in the clinic, or while working at other jobs that require the completion of several tasks simultaneously such as those of receptionist or secretary.

INFORMATION PROCESSING

Information processing refers to the analysis and synthesis of information in sequential steps. Information processing theorists suggest that various stages of information processing are necessary for information to be learned or to become mean-

ingful. Several information processing theories exist. According to Parrill-Bernstein's information processing model of problem solving,[41] a stimulus is integrated with stored information based on past experiences and prior knowledge; a response is generated; the response is executed; and based on feedback, the response is revised accordingly. Atkinson and Shiffrin[42] hypothesized that information analysis is sequential rather than hierarchical, involving the moving of information from one memory store to another. Sensory information is registered or received. If further analyzed, the sensory information takes one meaning, primarily verbal, and progresses to the short-term store. To enter the long-term memory store, the information in the short-term memory store is further analyzed, organized, and rehearsed. Head injured patients may break down at any step in the information-processing continuum. Clinicians must determine where the breakdown occurs and begin to treat at this level. Better encoding can be facilitated by imposing delays before allowing patients to respond. This allows for the registering and analysis of sensory information. Visual and auditory rehearsal strategies facilitate comparison of stimuli to past events and better short-term storage. Cues to assist in the recognition and utilization of feedback are extremely important. Various stimulus factors that influence information processing include meaningfulness, verbal versus nonverbal, and mode of stimulus presentation (e.g., simultaneous versus sequential).

It is generally accepted that information is processed differently in the right hemisphere than in the left hemisphere of the brain such that the right hemisphere processes information in a more holistic, gestalt, or simultaneous fashion, whereas the left hemisphere is responsible for more analytical, linear, or sequential processing. Team members must be aware of the way each patient best processes information. For example, if teaching a transfer to a person who processes best from a right hemisphere perspective, the overall concept should be presented first (e.g., "We are now going to move from this chair to the bed") before all the individual steps are presented. On the other hand, if left hemisphere information processing is more intact, or preferred, each individual step might be given (e.g., "Lock your brake," "Stand up," "Turn around," "Sit down"), after which the overall purpose of the activity is emphasized. Treatment will be most successful in all areas if clinicians determine each patient's most effective method of information processing, and modify therapy tasks accordingly.

COGNITIVE-COMMUNICATIVE DISORDERS

General Treatment Considerations

AN INTERDISCIPLINARY TEAM APPROACH

A coordinated interdisciplinary treatment approach often works best when working on cognitive-communicative processes. Several disciplines might be working on sequencing skills: occupational therapy as it relates to the correct placement of a sling, physical therapy as it pertains to transferring from a wheelchair to a bed, and speech-language pathology with regard to the ordering of words to make sentences or thoughts to communicate. Any compensatory strategies used should be consistent among team members. Good communication and joint treatment sessions are often extremely helpful.

All individuals who come in contact with a head injured patient should be knowledgable of the patient's current cognitive level of functioning. This includes the professional as well as the support staff (e.g., housekeepers, dietary staff, and aides).

ESTABLISHING FUNCTIONAL GOALS

Clinicians working with head injured persons must be able to identify and develop treatment regimens for functional goals that focus on behaviors that would make a difference in the way each person functions in his home, community, or workplace.

The level of cognitive functioning must be communicated between disciplines and must continually be applied to functional activities. For example, if a person is capable of discriminating only two stimuli, a tray of six or seven items of food would create frustration and possibly agitation. A great deal more success would be experienced in this situation if only two items of food were presented at any one time during the task of eating.

This example would carry over to other functional activities such as washing. If a person was only capable of discriminating between two items, only two items such as the washcloth and the soap should be presented at one time, with the provision of additional items hinging on the removal of the same number of items from the patient's stimulus array. This task might be further complicated by the use of white soap, white washcloth, and white towels, a difficult discriminatory task. Items of different colors would be easier to discriminate.

The effect of sequencing on functional activities can be illustrated via the act of taking a shower which requires the sequencing of numerous steps. If a patient can sequence only three steps, he or she will be far more successful at completing the task if cues are provided after every three steps.

Patients tend to be more motivated to participate in the therapy program if they are working toward a goal that is meaningful to them. Both patients and families gain a better understanding of the significance of the cognitive deficits when the impact of the deficits are related to functional activities. It is hoped that this better understanding will lead to increased cooperation and motivation in treatment. Focusing on functional activities also helps clinicians separate the meaningless from the meaningful therapy goals, discarding those goals that do not make a difference in the way a person performs in activities of daily living.

GENERALIZATION

The primary purpose of therapy is to provide for the generalization of skills to functional settings. In addition to formalized or informal testing, all evaluations should include behavioral observations to determine functional consequences of cognitive deficits. This can occur on the unit, in the home (e.g., cooking, self-care, dressing), in the community (e.g., use of public transportation, shopping), and/or on the work site (e.g., appropriate behavior, task completion). Only after these observations and analyses of premorbid abilities and behavior patterns should therapeutic goal setting be completed. Problems with the generalization of learned clinical skills arise when head injured persons are treated in one setting and returned home to a different setting. Before discharge, assessment should occur in the patient's natural, ultimate environment and treatment should focus on the results of this assessment. Drabman and co-workers[43] reported that some individuals did not generalize cooking skills taught on a gas stove to an electric stove or cleaning and organizing skills from one room to another. Failure to generalize to novel settings has its origin, in part, in an incomplete behavior analysis of these novel settings. Treatment of problematic response in only one setting may lead to difficulties in other environments. It was suggested that the influence of training environments (e.g., setting, materials, and personnel) be considered. The setting may be *artificial,* such as the practice of money exchange with the therapist in the therapy room; *simulated,* such as the practice of money exchange in a role-playing group situation; or *natural,* as in the practice of money exchange at a department or grocery store. Stimulus material may be *simulated,* such as the use of a pretend stove during the teaching of cooking; *modified natural,* such as the use of a burner or clinic stove; or *natural,* such as practicing on the stove in the person's own home. These investigators suggested that techniques helpful for acquistion and transfer of stimulus control include (1) prompts such as verbal instruction, modeling, and physical guidance; and (2) response contingencies including time-out, response cost, and correction.

Specific Diagnostic/Treatment Considerations

A diagnostic/treatment hierarchy of cognitive-communicative processes as proposed by Adamovich and colleagues[44-46] is presented in Table 26-1. The hierarchy was designed in an attempt to establish an organized approach to the rehabilitation of attention, information processing, and cognition, progressing from easy to difficult levels of processing in a gradual, step-by-step fashion. However, a division between the levels is somewhat artificial in that the cli-

Table 26–1. HIERARCHY OF COGNITIVE-COMMUNICATIVE PROCESSES

Arousal/alerting
Perception/low-level selective attention
Discrimination
Organization
Recall
High-level thought processing
    Convergent thinking
    Deductive reasoning
    Inductive reasoning
    Divergent thinking
    Multiprocess reasoning

cian may be working on the most difficult tasks at one level and the easiest activities at the next level. Attention is the focus of early treatment; yet it is essential that the attentional skills continue to improve as the patient moves through the treatment continuum. Memory skills must also continually improve as more complex processing places a greater load on memory. Information processing considerations during all levels of treatment include the stimuli selected to accomplish each task; the mode of presentation of the stimuli (e.g., simultaneous versus sequential); the stimulus presentation rate, response time, and the use of feedback to modify responses.

The purpose of the hierarchy was to establish a diagnostic battery that is directly applicable to treatment. Clinicians would begin treatment at the level in the hierarchy where the patient began to have difficulty and would progress in a step-by-step fashion through the hierarchy of processes as listed in Table 26-1. Specific diagnostic tasks will be described that are recommended for each cognitive process. Clinicians should use therapeutic tasks that are similar but not identical to the diagnostic tasks to avoid contamination of retest performances due to practice effects. Examples of diagnostic and therapy tasks will be presented for each cognitive level. Additional therapy suggestions and materials appropriate at each cognitive level were described by Adamovich and associates[46] Normative, validity, and reliability data are currently under study regarding the test battery. The initial scoring system is under revision and therefore will not be addressed.

AROUSAL AND ALERTING

Patients at this cognitive level, if responding at all, respond reflexively. Factors to be considered are arousal, attentiveness, and vigilance. Arousal refers to a continuum extending from sleep to wakefulness. Attentiveness is the readiness of the organism to perceive incoming stimulation. Vigilance is the ability to maintain attentiveness.

Diagnostic tasks were designed to elicit startle, bite, and rooting reflexes. Treatment should include multi-modality stimulation (e.g., tactile, visual, gustatory, oral-verbal, auditory, and vestibular), to achieve reflexive responding that is gradually brought under voluntary control.

The initial goals should be the activation of any response to any stimulus. The frequency, type, and duration of the response should be gradually increased. One modality (e.g., auditory or visual) should be stimulated at a time. Each patient's tolerance level and ability to attend must be considered when a stimulation program is established. Programs begin with 5 minutes of stimulation each hour and are gradually extended as the patient is able to tolerate longer treatment periods. The short, frequent treatment sessions often pose scheduling difficulties for the treatment team. Quite often, patients at this level must be treated at bedside. Portable stimulation kits are convenient therapy tools. Small glass vials can be obtained from the hospital pharmacy to organize liquids of various smells and tastes. Items with various textures can be organized in another kit. Individuals often respond best to familiar items. Therefore, care should be taken to organize meaningful stimuli for each sensory modality.

Specific therapy activities include auditory stimulation and tracking tasks that progress from the use of gross, nonspeech sounds (bells, buzzers, musical instruments) to more finely discriminated speech sounds of familiar followed by unfamiliar voices; oral peripheral stimulation, including passive stretching and the use of facilitative exercises for increasing the range of the articulators (e.g., licking a lollipop or placing food at the corner of the mouth for tongue control or sipping liquid through a straw for lip control); verbal stimulation ranging from the production of gross, reflexive sounds to appropriate situation specific vocalizations; tactile stimulation using hot and cold temperatures and a variety of textures; visual stimulation using bright lights, colors, familiar pictures, and familiar objects; gustatory stimulation using foods that include bitter, sour, sweet, salty, and bland flavors; olfactory stimulation beginning with strong noxious smells (e.g., ammonia or sulphur) followed by strong pleasant smells (e.g., perfume, coffee) and finally external environmental smells; and vestibular stimulation using rocker boards, balancing balls, and other devices used to work on positioning and balance.

Treatment initially focuses on eliciting reflexive responses for hyporeflexive patients. Some patients do exhibit hyper-reflexive behaviors. Stimulation of these individuals, particularly with regard to strong, noxious olfactory stimuli, may trigger seizures. The presence of hyper-reflexive behaviors is quite obvious as patients exhibit extreme movement in response to slight stimulation. The focus of treatment with a hyper-reflexive individual is to lessen the amount and degree of responding. These individuals often require an environment that is as quiet and as uncluttered as possible. Visual and auditory distractions must be eliminated, or at least reduced, and gradually increased as the patient's tolerance allows. Potential distractors include anything in the patient's auditory and visual environment—pictures on the wall, flowers in the room, family members visiting, audible overhead pages, clocks ticking and so on.

PERCEPTION/LOW-LEVEL SELECTION ATTENTION

Diagnostic tasks include visual tracking of lights; auditory tracking of bells; recognition of gross sounds such as a horn presented randomly with other environmental sounds; shape recognition (e.g., line, circle, square); and recognition of words in paragraphs presented aurally with and without background noise.

Specific therapy activities include visual and auditory tasks such as

1. Tracking an auditory stimulus or scanning a visual stimulus such as a line
2. Perceiving and recognizing environmental sounds and words and pointing to corresponding pictures

3. Tracing or copying a figure followed by a word

4. Drawing within boundaries (e.g., drawing two parallel lines with a dotted line between them)

5. Bisecting lines by drawing a line through the mid-point of the horizontal lines (begin with one line per page and gradually add more lines)

6. Following simple commands (e.g., "open your eyes," "close your mouth")

7. Naming objects or familiar items beginning with meaningful stimuli such as pictures of a person's home, animals, family, friends, school, or neighborhood, as well as familiar sounds such as the person's dog barking, and voices of familiar people.

DISCRIMINATION

Diagnostic tasks include visual discriminations of geometric forms by color, shape, and size; auditory discrimination of words in word strings; discrimination of pictures of objects and sentences; and two-step discriminations (e.g., identification of numbers immediately followed by colors in word strings).

Treatment of discrimination should focus on gradually increasing the number and degree of similarity of stimuli. The clinician should present only two items to begin with, which differ only in one salient feature (color, shape, or size). The number of items is gradually increased. Next, three items are presented with two discriminating variables, such as color plus shape, and the number of items is gradually increased. This process is repeated—that is, increasing the number of discriminating variables, then increasing the number of stimuli. Treatment should begin with the discrimination of geometric forms because the number and type of discriminations are fairly obvious. Clinicians should then progress through the hierarchy of tasks as outlined in the previous paragraph.

ORGANIZATION

Organizational skills include categorization, closure, and sequencing. Categorization diagnostic subtests assess the ability to: (1) sort items into categories based on visual features (e.g., color, shape, and size), semantic relationships, and function; and (2) describe likenesses and differences of items that exhibit relationships ranging from concrete to abstract. Functional treatment activities should be used whenever possible (e.g., preparation of a grocery list in which the foods are categorized according to food type or location in the grocery store). Initially, clinicians must supply the framework for categorization such as providing a list which is already divided into categories. Eventually the patient should be required to supply the framework necessary to categorize information.

Closure diagnostic subtests require the completion of incomplete visual formation (e.g., h__t) and aural information (e.g., sounds are presented one at a time, and the patient must mentally combine the sounds to form a word). Additional nonlinguistic closure treatment tasks include the use of geometric forms with sections missing or pictures with parts or objects missing. Visual linguistic closure tasks include letters with portions missing, words with letters missing, and sentences with words missing.

Sequencing diagnostic subtests evaluate the ability to temporally or spatially order information. Nonlinguistic tasks include the sequencing of colors from light to dark. Linguistic tasks include the sequencing of letters, words, and sentences. Functional diagnostic tasks assess the ability to sequence the steps of activities of daily living such as washing, eating, and shopping. Additional sequencing treatment tasks include nonlinguistic tasks requiring the patient to sequence objects from small to large. Linguistic sequencing tasks include (1) connecting dots in a numerical or alphabetical order; (2) reordering strings of numbers, letters, days of the week, and months of the year; (3) visually or auditorially sequencing letters, words, and sentences; (4) sequencing the steps of activities of daily living; and (5) following and giving written directions.

MEMORY

Memory disturbances occur due to ineffective encoding, inadequate storage, retrieval difficulties, or lack of strategies to deal with interferences.

Diagnostic tasks measure immediate recall, delayed recall, recall with interference, cued recall, free recall/word fluency, recall of directions given aurally, and recall of information in paragraphs presented aurally and visually.

Memory treatment should focus on the

provision of compensatory strategies to cope with lasting memory difficulties. Specific internal retrieval strategies consist of the following: verbal description; visual imagery; chunking activities in which information is visually or aurally organized into segments that coincide with the patient's memory span; categorization or appropriate grouping of information to be recalled; rehearsal in which information to be recalled is drilled or practiced; use of associations based on semantic relationships (e.g., cane-crutches and day-night), acoustic relationships (dew-shoe), or visual relationships (desk-dresser); temporal or spatial ordering in which events in episodic and semantic memory are recalled by remembering certain landmark events associated with the event to be recalled or those that occurred at a similar point in time; primacy and recency benefits; and the PQRST approach (i.e., *p*review, *q*uestion, *r*ead, *s*tate, and *t*est). Mnemonic devices consist of specific memory tricks used to increase associative learning through paired association. During encoding, new words or bits of information are chained or paired to a pre-established set of key words and phrases or a familiar sequence of known locations. This can be referred to as a peg system in which new items are pegged to existing items; for example, rhyming peg (one = bun); phonetic peg (two = n because *n* has two down strokes); or loci peg (items are linked to familiar locations). The substitute word system is based on linking a visual image with a word (e.g., to remember the name Cameron, visualize a camera on his balding head [outstanding facial feature]). The link system links lists of items together in a funny way to facilitate retrieval (e.g., to remember bologna and milk, picture a cow eating bologna as the farmer milks it).

Generally, closed head injured persons must learn to rely on external memory aids to assist memory including calendars, appointment books, notepads, daily logs or diaries, memo books, lists, structure/routines, alarms to remind them to refer to their appointment book, tape recorders that deliver sequences of instructions to be followed, and microcomputers such as the Sharp Memo Writer E 6200 or the Toshiba Memo Note II. Other computers may be costly and difficult to program. Harris and Morris[47] suggested that memory cues should be given close to the time of the required action, should be active rather than passive (e.g., an alarm versus a book reminder), and should be specific to each situation. Glisky and Schacter[48] suggested that memory remediation could be divided into three main categories: (1) practice and exercise drills; (2) strategy learning; (3) and external aids. These investigators suggested that external aids were the most beneficial with the head injured population including (1) storage devices (diaries, notebooks, lists, calendars, and computers); (2) cueing devices (alarms, watches, and bell timers); and (3) structuring the environment to decrease the memory load (e.g., labeled cupboards and drawers).

Early on, visual charts showing progress toward therapy goals are helpful (Fig. 26–3). Each functional task (e.g., showering) can be divided into a series of steps necessary to accomplish that task. The progress chart provides two important reminders for patients with memory deficits: (1) that the activities they are asked to complete in daily therapy sessions are important to achieve successes on a functional task, and (2) that progress toward the functional goal is occurring. The visual chart also serves as a reminder of what is happening in therapy when the patient is asked to convey this to a family member.

REASONING/PROBLEM SOLVING

Head injured persons tend to experience problem-solving difficulties primarily due to a narrow perspective, concrete and incomplete analyses of the problems, an impulsive approach that does not allow them to think through the problem, a lack of an organized approach to the problem, and a tendency not to recognize when additional information is needed. Types of reasoning/problem solving include convergent thinking, deductive reasoning, inductive reasoning, divergent thinking, and multipurpose reasoning.

CONVERGENT THINKING

Convergent thinking refers to the recognition and analysis of relevant information to identify the central theme or main point. Diagnostic tasks include the identification of central themes and missing facts in paragraphs and stories.

Additional convergent thinking treatment

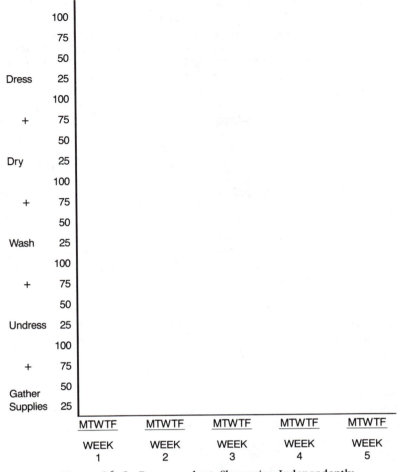

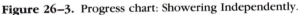

Figure 26–3. Progress chart: Showering Independently.

tasks could entail the identification of a common theme in a group of objects (e.g., shoes and bread—both have heels); the identification of one word that could be combined with four other words to form another set of words (e.g., saddle, stroke, track, and show could all be combined with the word side to form sidesaddle, sidestroke, and so forth); and the identification of relevant information in visually or auditorially presented sentences, paragraphs, and conversations with respect to who did what, when, and where.

DEDUCTIVE REASONING

Deductive reasoning refers to problem solving in a step-by-step fashion such that individuals must utilize or eliminate various clues sequentially. Diagnostic tasks include

the selection of a correct item from a list of items by elimination according to clues regarding function; the selection of matching items such as individuals and their vehicles through the elimination of other items according to cues or descriptions which qualify the items (e.g., Donna must haul large containers in her line of work).

Additional deductive reasoning therapy tasks may include forward or backward chaining in which the patient is to deal with the relevant information and devise solutions in a progressive (forward) or regressive (backward) step-by-step process until the final solution is reached; the identification of missing premises, in which two facts are necessary to reach a conclusion (e.g., given "All children must go to school and Bob and Jane are children," the patient is to deduce the Bob and Jane must go to school); and the analysis of sentences and paragraphs to determine punctuation, spelling, and other grammatical errors.

INDUCTIVE REASONING

Inductive reasoning refers to the formulation of solutions based on details that lead to, but do not necessarily support, a standard conclusion. Diagnostic tasks include the identification of antonyms and analogies.

Additional inductive reasoning therapy tasks may include the formulation of synonyms; the recognition of cause-and-effect relationships in which either the cause or the effect of a situation is presented; and open-ended problem solving such as story-completion tasks.

DIVERGENT THINKING

Divergent thinking refers to the generation of unique abstract concepts or hypotheses that deviate from standard concepts or ideas. Diagnostic tasks include the recognition and interpretation of homographs, idioms, absurdities, and proverbs.

Other divergent thinking therapy tasks include: multifunction stimuli (simile and metaphor formulation and interpretation) requiring the analysis of a figure of speech in which one object or event is described in terms usually denoting another object or event (e.g., "The ship plowed the sea"); responding to "realism" questions (e.g., "Is a bigger tree also an older tree?" or "If you didn't have that name, would you still be the same person?"); and the interpretation of poetry, fables, puns, jokes, and riddles, which require the patient to consider abstract relations, double meanings, paradoxes, and nonstandard meanings.

MULTIPROCESS REASONING

Multiprocess reasoning requires the use of two or more reasoning processes. Diagnostic tasks include the evaluation of task specific insight, and the recognition of whether or not sufficient information is available to solve a problem.

Other multiprocess reasoning therapy tasks include the mediation of an argument requiring analysis and synthesis of information. Two points of view in a specific argument should be presented. Using deductive reasoning, the premise or assumptions of each person must be considered in order to arrive at a solution. Once this is accomplished, the solution must be tested by analyzing the truth of the premises. Finally, using complementary reasoning, a compromise must be negotiated based on the premises that are accepted and agreed to by both parties.

Generally, the steps of problem solving include problem analysis, the formulation of a strategy and alternatives based on past experience or previous knowledge, selection of a solution that is generalized and executed, and finally, solution evaluation. When designing therapy tasks, clinicians must define a skill, analyze all segments or properties of the skill, develop a hierarchy of steps to accomplish the skill, plan techniques to achieve each step with consideration of the patient's style of learning, train the patient to a criterion as established for each segment in the hierarchy until the goal for the target ability is reached, and finally, evaluate the program continually and revise it when indicated. Clinicians should begin with nonlinguistic stimuli that can be controlled for physical features such as color, shape, and size. Complexity of these tasks should be gradually increased by increasing the number of stimuli, the number of different dimensions of the stimuli (e.g., color plus shape), and the rate and duration of stimuli presentation. Next, linguistic stimuli should be introduced, and the clinician should present a similar task complexity hierarchy. Ben-Yishay advises clinicians working on problem solving to teach the patient to ask the right questions, break the task down into meaningful units, and establish a system of gradual cueing (see Chapter 27).

Use of Computers

Computers can be helpful in the treatment of attention, concentration/persistence, visual localization, visual scanning, visual tracking, reaction time, memory, hand-eye coordinatioin, and specific cognitive tasks including perception, discrimination, and language.[49–51] Specific benefits of computers include the following:

1. A single stimulus can be presented in a highly controlled manner.

2. The patient is required to compete only with himself or herself, providing for a sense of control over therapy and progress which leads to increased motivation and feelings of self-worth.

3. Accurate, objective, and immediate feedback is received.

4. Patients often enjoy using computers.

According to Wilson and Moffat,[52] clinicians should consider the following when selecting computer programs:

1. Consistent, controlled levels of difficulty within a task
2. Lesson- or file-generating capability
3. Concise, easy-to-follow instructions
4. Consistent response format
5. Accurate, age-appropriate content
6. Degree of supervision required
7. Friendly, unambiguous, and informative feedback
8. Control of variables or parameters (i.e., length of time the stimulus is displayed, length of response-delay time, task speed, number of trials per set, level of difficulty, type of prompts, size of stimuli, timing, and type of reinforcements)
9. Method of keeping and reporting data

All computer training should be selected and monitored by professional clinicians as part of a comprehensive treatment program for each patient. Computers should never be used as a substitute for the clinician. Since aides are often used to work with patients during computer treatments, clinicians should also know how to appropriately utilize aides. Cognitive remediation cannot occur using only a computer and an aide. Computers, like workbooks, are merely tools. All computer treatments designed to assist in the overall cognitive rehabilitation program should be under the direction and supervision of professional rehabilitation specialists. Third party payors have and will continue to look for cost-effective ways to provide treatment. It would be extremely unfortunate if third party payors would cover the cost of cognitive rehabilitation only if it were done by an aide with a computer.

Group Therapy

Group treatment creates a communicative environment that is more natural than the individual therapy setting. Group therapy provides individuals with opportunities to (1) increase social interaction and self-monitoring skills, (2) increase self-esteem and self-motivation, (3) increase the ability to develop short- and long-term meaningful goals, (4) share feelings and needs, and (5) provide and receive peer review of behaviors.

Specific group therapy goals include interpersonal interaction in which speakers and listeners are both evaluated; pragmatic skills (e.g., situational appropriate behavior, eye contact, turn-taking); social skills; empathic abilities; personal and social adjustment; and life skills (e.g., shopping, utilizing public transportation, emergency skills). Community outings are particularly helpful to test skills in real-life settings.

SWALLOWING DISTURBANCES/DYSPHAGIA

Description

Swallowing disturbances which occur following closed head trauma are generally secondary to brainstem or anterior cortical lesions. Resulting behavioral effects include (1) a delay in the triggering of a swallowing reflex and (2) a malfunction of the cricopharyngeal muscle at the junction of the pharynx and the esophagus. If the cricopharyngeal function shows no improvement over a 3-month post-trauma period, a cricopharyngeal myotomy may be indicated. Other swallowing difficulties may be due to the paralysis of one or more structures in the vocal tract including the tongue, pharynx or larynx.[53]

Winstein[53] conducted a retrospective review of 201 charts of patients admitted to the rehabilitation program at the Adult Head Trauma Service at Rancho Los Amigos Hospital. Of the patients studied, 54 patients or 27 percent evidenced swallowing problems or neurogenic dysphagia. Of this group, 44 patients or 82 percent were nonoral feeders who were fed via nasogastric tube (39 patients) or gastrostomy tube (5 patients). The nonoral feeders were more cognitively impaired than were the oral feeders; this tended to be the major interfering factor. Half of the nonoral feeders had a good reflexive swallow and the majority had a good voluntary cough with a hypoactive gag reflex.

According to Logemann[54] the stages of swallowing include (1) the preparatory stage, in which food is masticated and manipulated by the lips, teeth, mandible, tongue, cheek musculature, hard palate, and soft palate; (2) the oral or voluntary stage, when the tongue propels food posteriorly to trigger a swallowing reflex; (3) the pharyngeal stage, when the reflex carries the bolus through the pharynx; and (4) the esophageal stage, when esophageal peristalsis carries the bolus through the cervical and thoracic esophagus to the stomach.

Swallowing disorders may be diagnosed through radiographic studies and clinical observation. One radiographic procedure used is cinefluoroscopy, in which a fluoroscopic image is recorded on movie film to allow for the examination of swallowing and of swallowing structures in slow motion and frame by frame. Video fluoroscopy, known as the modified barium swallow (or cookie swallow), is a newer development in which a video taperecorder is attached to fluoroscopic equipment. Compared with cinefluoroscopy, this procedure allows for greater flexibility in swallow analysis, less exposure to radiation, and simultaneous voice recording. The primary purpose of these procedures is to determine the aspiration of food into the lungs, as well as the cause of aspiration (e.g., decreased tongue function, decreased swallowing reflex, impaired laryngeal closure, and/or cricopharyngeal hypertonicity). Materials used during the test include liquid barium, barium paste, and a cookie coated with barium paste.[54]

A behavioral evaluation of swallowing should include the assessment of normal reflexes (gag and cough), abnormal reflexes (e.g., bite, rooting, suck-swallow); head control; jaw control; tongue control; sensation of tongue, palate, face, and lips to touch and temperature; taste evaluations (bitter, sour, sweet, and salty in all four quadrants of the tongue); pulmonary function to determine whether the patient can tolerate any amount of aspiration; and actual swallowing of various appropriate food consistencies (solids, semisolids, soft foods, and liquids). Special notes during swallowing evaluation should be made as to the pocketing of food inside the mouth, drooling, choking, and denture fit. As a result of the evaluation, safety issues must be addressed immediately regarding the patient's ability to handle hot liquids and various food types without choking. Other recommendations should include the food consistency tolerated such as solids (e.g., crackers, meat), applesauce and puréed foods, soft foods (e.g., jello, pudding), and hot and cold liquids. The best posture for swallowing should also be assessed. Usually, foods are most successfully managed while a patient is sitting up at 90 degrees with the head slightly forward. The best position of the food in the mouth should be recommended. Generally, placing the food on the more intact side results in the best swallow.

Treatment

The purpose of swallowing therapy is to (1) eliminate the need for nonoral feeding (such as by nasogastric [NG] tube, pharyngostomy, esophagostomy, gastrostomy, or jejunostomy) for those who are unable to take food by mouth or (2) to improve the oral swallowing of a variety of food consistencies.[54] Dysphagia treatment is particularly important to avoid aspiration, which may lead to aspiration pneumonia.

Dysphagia may be treated directly or indirectly. Direct treatment involves the introduction of food into the mouth with the reinforcement of appropriate swallowing behaviors. The general sequence of oral feeding begins with soft foods followed by semisolids, solids, and finally liquids.

Indirect treatment includes (1) oral-motor exercises for the lips, tongue, cheek musculature, soft palate, and laryngeal musculature; (2) stimulation of the swallowing reflex via thermal stimulation of the anterior faucial arch or laryngeal elevation; and (3) exercises to increase abduction of the true vocal folds to prevent aspiration including pushing and pulling exercises. Head injured persons may have difficulty with swallowing therapy due to an inability to follow directions, an inability to remember the directions, difficulty concentrating during treatment, and/or a lack of motivation.

Swallowing disorders are probably best treated by a team of professionals. Generally, the speech-language pathologist or occupational therapist, or both, assume primary responsibility for the swallowing evaluation and treatment. The nurse is particularly important to help identify patients with swallowing disorders, to notify the patient's physician of the swallowing difficulties, to ensure that the recommended procedures and precautions are adhered to during feeding when other team members are not present, and to suction patients as necessary during feeding. The respiratory therapist should assume responsibility for evaluating the respiratory status of the patient and should participate on the dysphagia team in the treatment of patients with respiratory complications which may require tracheostomy tubes either permanently or temporarily. Since physical therapists often treat patients with pulmonary problems, they may also be members of the treatment team. The dietician should assist in the establishment of an appropriate dietary plan and documentation of the ongoing nutritional status of each patient.

Patients with persistent neurogenic dysphagia often improve more quickly after gastrostomy and removal of the NG tube. Possible reasons for this include alleviation of the irritation caused by the NG tube, allowance of normal pharyngeal closure not permitted with the tube in place and resolution of pharyngeal dysesthesia caused by accommodation of the tube. Accommodation of the NG tube was supported by Winstein's[53] incongruent findings that the majority of nonoral feeders who were NG tubefed had a hypoactive gag but demonstrated good cough.

CONCLUSION

In this chapter, the nature of communication and swallowing disorders that may oc-cur secondary to closed head trauma were reviewed and specific treatment methods were suggested. Processes critical to effective communication are speech, hearing, vision, language, attention, information processing, and cognition. Attempts were made to demonstrate the intrinsic relationships among attention, information processing, cognition, and language. General treatment considerations encompass goal-setting appropriate to a variety of treatment programs and patient situations; the importance of an interdisciplinary treatment team; the need to establish functional, meaningful treatment goals; and the importance of working toward the generalization of treatment strategies to each patient's home and community. Discussion of specific treatment activities included commentary regarding the use of computers during cognitive-communicative rehabilitation as well as augmentative communication devices and group therapy.

Although research investigating problems resulting from closed head injury and corresponding treatment approaches has increased recently, much more information is still needed. Due to the variety of neurologic lesions that tend to produce idiosyncratic problems following closed head injury, single-subject research designs may prove to be of particular value when evaluating the effects of specific treatment protocols. All clinicians must accept the responsibility of scientifically evaluating the effectiveness of their treatment as an obligation to patients, families, and the parties responsible for paying for services provided.

REFERENCES

1. Helm, NA, Butler, RB and Benson, DF: Acquired stuttering. Neurology 27:349, 1977.
2. Levin, HS: Aphasia in closed head injury. In Sarno, MT (ed): Acquired Aphasia. Academic Press, New York, 1981.
3. Beukelman, DR: Management of Dysarthric Speakers. Presentation at the American Speech-Language-Hearing Annual Convention, Detroit, 1986.
4. Von Cramon, D: Traumatic mutism and the subsequent reorganization of speech functions. Neuropsychologia (19)6:801, 1981.
5. Diller, L and Gordon, W: Interventions for cognitive deficits in brain injured adults. J Consult Clin Psychol 49(6):822, 1981.
6. Rosenbek, JC and LaPointe, LL: The dysarthrias: description, diagnosis and treatment. In Johns, DF (ed): Clinical Management of Neurogenic Communicative Disorders. Little, Brown, Boston, 1978, p 251.
7. Wertz, RT: Neuropathologies of speech and language: an introduction to patient management. In Johns, DF (ed): Clinical Management of Neurogenic Communicative Disorders. Little, Brown, Boston, 1978, p 1.
8. LaPointe, LL and Johns, DF: Some phonemic characteristics in apraxia of speech. J Commun Dis 8:259, 1975.
9. Darley, FL, Aronson, AE and Brown, JR: Motor Speech Disorders. Philadelphia, WB Saunders, 1975, p 193.

10. Rosenbeck, JC and Wertz, RT: Treatment of apraxia of speech in adults. In Wertz, RT and Collins, MJ (eds): Proceedings of the Conference: Clinical Aphasiology, 1972. Veterans Administration Hospital, Madison, WI, 1976.

11. Johns, DR and Darley, FL: Phoenemic variability in apraxia of speech. J Speech Hear Res 13:556, 1970.

12. Yorkston, K and Beukelman, D: Ataxic dysarthria: Treatment sequences based on intelligibility and prosodic considerations. J Speech Hear Dis 46:398, 1981.

13. Rosenbek, JC: Treating apraxia of speech. In Johns, DF (ed): Clinical Management of Neurogenic Communicative Disorders. Little, Brown, Boston, 1978, p 191.

14. Coleman, CL, Cook, AM and Meyers, LS: Assessing non-oral clients for assistive communication devices. J Speech Hear Dis 45:515, 1980.

15. Weigl, E, Goldstein, K and Scheerer, M: Color Form Sorting Test. Psychological Corp, New York, 1945.

16. Wechsler, D: Wechsler Adult Intelligence Scale. Psychological Corp, New York, 1981.

17. Frostig, M: Developmental Test of Visual Perception. Follett, Chicago, 1963.

18. Ayers, AJ: The Southern California Figure-Ground Visual Perception Test. Western Psychological Services, Los Angeles, 1966.

19. Hooper, R: Patterns of Acute Head Injury. Williams & Wilkins, Baltimore, 1969.

20. Luria, AR: Higher Cortical Functions in Man. Basic Books, New York, 1966.

21. Darley, FL: Aphasia. WB Saunders, Philadelphia, 1982.

22. Schuell, HM: Differential Diagnosis of Aphasia with the Minnesota Test, ed 2, rev by Sefer, JW. University of Minnesota Press, Minneapolis, 1973.

23. Porch, BE: Porch Index of Communicative Ability. Vol II: Administration, Scoring, and Interpretation, rev ed. Consulting Psychologists Press, Palo Alto, CA, 1971.

24. Marshall, RC: The Clinician Controlled Auditory Stimulation of Aphasic Adults. CC Publications, Tigard, OR, 1978.

25. Martinoff, JT, Martinoff, R and Stokke, V: Language Rehabilitation: Auditory Comprehension. CC Publications, Tigard, OR, 1980.

26. Keith, RL: Graduated Language Training for Patients with Aphasia and Children with Language Deficiencies. College-Hill Press, Houston, 1980.

27. Sparks, R, Helm NA and Albert, ML: Aphasia rehabilitation resulting from melodic intonation therapy. Cortex 10:303, 1974.

28. Helm, NA and Barresi, B: Voluntary control of involuntary utterances: A treatment approach for severe aphasia. In Brookshire, RH (ed): Clinical Aphasiology Conference Proceedings. BRK, Minneapolis, 1980.

29. Skinner, BF: The Behavior of Organisms: An Experimental Analysis. Prentice Hall, Englewood Cliffs, NJ, 1938.

30. Holland, A: Case studies in aphasia rehabilitation. J Speech Hear Dis 37:3, 1972.

31. Brookshire, RH: Speech pathology and the experimental analysis of behavior. J Speech Hear Dis 32:215, 1967.

33. Duffy, RJ, Duffy, JR and Pearson, KL: Pantomimic recognition in aphasics. J Speech Hear Res 18:115, 1975.

34. Gardner, H et al: Visual communication in aphasia. Neuropsychologia 14:275, 1976.

35. Helm-Estabrooks, N, Fitzpatrick, PM and Barresi, B: Response of an agrammatic patient to a syntax stimulation program for aphasia. J Speech Hear Dis 46:422, 1981.

36. Helm-Estabrooks, N: Helm Elicited Language Program for Syntax Stimulation. Pro-Ed, Austin, TX, 1981.

37. Lubinski, R: Environmental language intervention. In Chapey, R (ed): Language Intervention Strategies in Adult Aphasia. Williams & Wilkins, Baltimore, 1981.

38. Brookshire, RH: Auditory comprehension and aphasia. In Johns, DF (ed): Clinical Management of Neurogenic Communicative Disorders. Little, Brown, Boston, 1978.

39. Holland, AL: Functional communication in the treatment of aphasia. In Bradford, LJ (ed): Communicative Disorders: An Audio Journal for Continuing Education. Grune & Stratton, New York, 1978.

40. Davis, GA and Wilcox, MJ: Incorporating parameters of natural conversation in aphasia treatment. In Chapey, R (ed): Language Intervention Strategies in Adult Aphasia. Williams & Wilkins, Baltimore, 1981.

41. Parrill-Bernstein, M: Problem Solving and Learning Disabilities: An Information Processing Approach. Grune & Stratton, New York, 1981.

42. Atkinson, RC and Shiffrin, RM: Human memory: A proposed system and its control processes. In Spence, KN and Spence, JN (eds): The Psychology of Learning and Motivation: Advances in Research and Theory. Vol 2. Academic Press, New York, 1968.

43. Drabman, RS, Hammer, D and Rosenbaum, MS: Assessing generalization in behavior modification with children. The generalization map. Behav Assess 1:203, 1979.

44. Adamovich, BB and Henderson, JA: An Investigation of the Cognitive Changes of Head Trauma Patients Following a Treatment Period. Paper presented at American Speech-Language-Hearing Association Convention, Toronto, 1982.

45. Adamovich, BB and Henderson, JA: Cognitive Deficits Post Traumatic Head Injury: Diagnostic and Treatment Implications. Paper presented at ASHA Annual Convention, Cincinnati, November, 1983.

46. Adamovich, BB, Henderson, JA and Auerbach, S: Cognitive Rehabilitation of Closed Head Injured Patients. College-Hill Publications, San Diego, 1985.

47. Harris, JE and Morris, PE (eds): Everyday Memory, Actions, and Absent-Mindedness. Academic Press, New York, 1984.

48. Glisky, EL and Schacter, DL: Remediation of organic memory disorders: current status and future prospects. J Head Trauma Rehabil 1:3, 1986.

49. Bracy, O et al: Cognitive retraining through computers, fact or fad? Cognitive Rehabilitation 2, 1985.

50. Skilbeck, C: Computer assistance in the management of memory and cognitive impairment. In Wilson, BA and Moffat, N (eds): Clinical Management of Memory Problems. Aspen Systems Corp, Rockville, MD, 1984.

51. Adamovich, BB: Entry and Discharge Criteria: How

Do We Know When We're Coming or Going. Invited participation at the Third Annual Southwest Head Injury Symposium: "Bridging the Gaps in the Head Injury Care System," sponsored by the Center for Rehabilitation Medicine, Northridge Hospital Medical Center, Northridge, CA, Jan 31, Feb 1–3, 1985.

52. Wilson, BA and Moffat, N: Rehabilitation of memory for everyday life. In Harris, J and Morris, P (eds): Everyday Memory: Actions and Absentmindedness. Academic Press, London, 1984.

53. Winstein, CJ: Neurogenic dysphagia, frequency, progression, and outcome in adults following head injury. Phys Ther (63)12:1992, 1983.

54. Logemann, JA: Evaluation and Treatment of Swallowing Disorders. College-Hill Press, San Diego, 1983.

Chapter 27

Cognitive Remediation

YEHUDA BEN-YISHAY, Ph.D.
GEORGE P. PRIGATANO, Ph.D.

Since the publication of Ben-Yishay's and Diller's chapters in the first edition of this volume on cognitive deficits and remediation,[1,2] there have been some new and significant additions to the literature on the subject.[3-10] Therefore, rather than merely restating the ideas that have been presented in those chapters, though we feel that in the main they are still valid, our aim is to examine the concept of cognitive remediation in the light of the newer insights gained from the more recent publications.

Our understanding of cognitive remediation can best be explained by examining (1) some of the implications of the coming together of rehabilitation and neuropsychology; (2) the role of cognitive remediation in the wider context of the interventions taking place in the rehabilitation process; and (3) the reasons why, in the case of most typical individuals with a closed head injury, the neuropsychological rehabilitation endeavor must follow a holistic, or multifaceted, approach in order to attain optimal functional outcomes.

THE COMING TOGETHER OF REHABILITATION AND NEUROPSYCHOLOGY

Traditionally, the fields of rehabilitation and neuropsychology were two separate disciplines. In recent years a gradual coming together of the two disciplines has been taking place, especially in the care of persons who suffer closed head trauma. The relationship between the two disciplines has

not been an easy one, however. As Diller has recently shown,[7] the existing gaps between rehabilitation and traditional neuropsychology are the result of considerable conceptual, methodological, and clinical differences; and more work must be done before the two disciplines can be integrated. In the present context, we wish to restate the most salient arguments only, from Diller's insights.[7]

First, the primary focus of traditional clinical neuropsychology has been on diagnostic issues—namely, the attempt to sort patients into pathological entities and identify underlying cognitive impairments. Thus, the language of neuropsychology is the language of generic cognitive deficits which are identified by responses to standardized tests. Neuropsychology as a discipline has conceptual and empirical ties to the neurosciences and its main body of knowledge is derived from the laboratory.

Second, the primary concern of rehabilitation is the management of disabilities, which are limitations in the functional abilities of the head injured individual, as they unfold in the course of daily living. For example, a successful real estate agent following a head injury retained the "gift of gab" and remained capable of communicating in a friendly, enthusiastic, and "persuasive" style. However, he was unable to continue in his job because he neglected (a) to properly examine and evaluate which zoning laws or city ordinances applied in the case of certain properties and (b) to inform prospective clients, due to memory deficits and impairment in analytic-synthetic reasoning.

On the strength of his reputation in the community and his excellent "salesman's techniques," he had managed to consummate attractive deals, only to be sued later for misleading his customers or misrepresenting the facts. Issues of management are too complex to be addressed by the mere identification of the underlying cognitive pathology of an individual. Rehabilitation as a discipline has, therefore, been traditionally strongly allied with the social sciences.

Third, there is as yet an insufficient body of empirical data to make possible the identification, much less the accurate prediction, of when and to what extent a diagnosed cognitive deficit (i.e., a statistically significant decrement from the normatively expected test score) will translate into a clinically significant functional disability (see also Prigatano and colleagues[11]). Hence, to move the newly emerging field of neuropsychological rehabilitation forward it is necessary to develop the conceptual and methodological tools to bridge the existing gaps between rehabilitation and neuropsychology.

Fourth, the challenge, accordingly, for neuropsychological rehabilitation is (1) to demonstrate that neuropsychological assessment techniques can predict clinical outcomes of rehabilitation interventions; (2) to demonstrate that such measurement techniques can be expanded so as to suggest specific remedial treatments; (3) to link these neuropsychological assessment methods with systematic remedial training techniques; and thereby (4) to establish continuity among the diagnosis, rehabilitation, and postrehabilitation, clinical adjustment phases.

THE ROLE OF REMEDIAL INTERVENTIONS IN NEUROPSYCHOLOGICAL REHABILITATION

Since the cognitive remedial activities are part of the wider context of the total rehabilitation process, it is necessary to consider some of the distinguishing characteristics of rehabilitation interventions and the more narrowly focused cognitive remedial interventions.

The head injury rehabilitation process is complex and multifaceted and is usually a more prolonged affair than is the case in most other types of disability. With the head injured patient, the development of a systematic (as opposed to a "seat of the pants") approach to rehabilitation interventions depends on integrating the following: (1) considering the inherent potentials, as well as limitations, of the spontaneous processes of recovery of functions; (2) possibly optimizing the recovery process—within the boundaries of the person's zone of potential for recovery—by means of active, remedial training techniques; and (3) doing so in a timely, suitable, and efficacious manner. As Grimm and Bleiberg[6] and Diller[7] have recently pointed out, a closer integration of these three dimensions is necessary in order to advance the field of head trauma rehabilitation. Hence, those interventions which are usually referred to as "cognitive remediation" must be properly aligned with the other two dimensions—natural recovery and clinical management.

Considering the state of the art of cognitive remediation in neuropsychological rehabilitation, we are faced with four basic issues or concerns:

1. Lack of an universally accepted operational definition of the objectives of cognitive remediation, including the absence of a clear delineation of the scope of activities falling into this remedial category

2. Lack of sufficient empirical support that various teaching or remedial training exercises (suggested for the amelioration of different "generic" cognitive deficits) improve functional readaptation in patients with head trauma

3. Lack of sufficient data base (although one is growing) that cognitive remediation combined with different forms of psychotherapeutic intervention can substantially, cost-effectively, and sustainedly raise the level of psychosocial adjustment of traumatically head injured individuals[4, 5]

4. Lack of a theoretical model to guide clinical practice and systematic applied research in this area. Models are also needed to specify which patients have a reasonable chance of benefiting from different types of remedial intervention programs[12]

These questions are important and have been addressed in a number of recent papers. It is not our intention to pursue them in detail. However, we will briefly address each of these questions as they relate to the points made in the present and previous chapters.

Defining Cognitive Remediation

The term *cognitive remediation* "does not refer to a standard set of therapeutic activities prescribed to someone with a particular generic deficit."[6] Although many rehabilitation programs for the traumatically head injured routinely advertise that "cognitive remediation" is an integral component of their treatment "package," it has been difficult to establish exactly what is meant by the term. In most instances there is a lack of explicit mention of what techniques to employ, with what rationale and expected outcomes.

The various definitions that have been suggested share—at least implicitly—some common elements, but differ from one another in other respects. Thus, for example, Gianutsos and Gianutsos[13] define cognitive rehabilitation as "a service designed to remediate disorders of perception, memory and language." This is a much narrower definition than the ones suggested by Ben-Yishay[14] and by Prigatano and associates,[5] who define the aim of cognitive rehabilitation following a traumatic head injury as being the amelioration of deficits in problem-solving abilities in order to improve functional competence in everyday life situations. Ben-Yishay's[14] and Prigatano's[5] definition of problem solving is consistent with Luria's[15] conception of the logical reasoning (problem-solving) cycle, which extends equally to both verbal and nonverbal domains. (For a further discussion of this, see Grimm and Bleiberg[6] and Goldstein and Levin.[9])

Granted that the purpose of cognitive remediation is the amelioration of deficits in problem-solving ability, where does one begin? How does one choose which specific aspects of the deficient problem-solving skills to target for remedial intervention? And finally, according to what guidelines does one construct appropriate remedial techniques?

A Rehabilitation-Relevant Model for Cognitive Remediation

A rehabilitation-relevant model was proposed by the New York University group.[16, 17] According to this model, the targets of cognitive remedial intervention should be those areas of functioning that have been found to predict best postrehabilitation outcomes in (1) self-care and daily life functional competence, (2) vocational attainment, and (3) interpersonal skills and social adjustment. It is in keeping with this model that various cognitive remedial techniques were proposed during the past decade by the NYU group. These techniques were published in a monograph series edited by Ben-Yishay.[18]

As previously mentioned, Luria's[15, 19] formulations provide the most articulate (neuropsychological) conceptual basis for a model of cognitive remediation, or retraining, after brain injury. His ideas are particularly well suited as a conceptual basis for a rehabilitation system, since Luria was interested in the notion of facilitating restoration of function via teaching methods. (Luria's ideas were heavily influenced by Hughlings Jackson. For a further discussion of Jackson's contributions to the rehabilitation of higher cerebral functions; see Prigatano.[20])

In the following sections Luria's main ideas, as they pertain to rehabilitation, are briefly summarized and discussed. Luria and coworkers[19] state:

> There is a reason to suppose that the degree of replaceability of the damaged area of the cerebral cortex by neighboring areas may vary. If the lesion is in a highly differentiated zone (motor, sensory, speech, etc.), the possibility of such transfer of disturbed function to neighboring areas is minimal. If the lesion is in a newer or less differentiated area, the possibility may be maximal.

Luria's theory is essentially the theory of restoration of higher cerebral brain functions by reorganization of functional (biopsychological) systems.[19] Four principles guided his clinical work. The first is the principle of differential restoration of functional systems. Luria argues that a detailed neuropsychological examination is needed to delineate which aspects of the higher cerebral processes have been impaired and which remain intact. While most clinicians would agree that this should be accomplished, in clinical practice it may be very difficult to achieve via our present neuropsychological assessment methods. Often we define areas as being grossly intact versus grossly impaired. For example, one frequently sees in neuropsychological reports that verbal short-term memory is intact, as opposed to an impairment of nonverbal, visuospatial short-term memory. The specific underlying cognitive deficit(s) responsible for this type of statement is (are) often not easily determined. Certainly Luria's[7] and Christensen's[21] diagnostic work have contributed significantly in this regard. But, as Prigatano and associates[5] have pointed out, more is required for the purposes of developing a rational system of remedial interventions.

The second principle that Luria[19] espouses is taking advantage of the intact cognitive processes; namely, that one should teach through systems of information processing that have not been affected. (This kind of substitution or compensation training idea was also suggested by Zangwill.[22])

The third principle is complete, extended programming of the restorative activity. By this, Luria means that the training task should be broken down into a series of highly articulated routines and subroutines capable of making the underlying mental processes of the problem-solving task fully explicit (hence, comprehensible) to the patient.[19] This is necessary since, due to the brain injury, these patients cannot, on their own, perceive the subtle gradations and transitions in the chain of reasoning that are implicit in the usually more condensed ways in which most nonimpaired individuals solve problems. The "short cuts" (or mental algorithms) we normally develop over the years condense what were once complex action or thought sequences. The extended programming principle, at its core, is the idea that the retraining should follow the logical course of the origins of the reasoning chain, before it became condensed, thus aiding the patient's present disturbed function.

The fourth principle is that of constant signalization of the defect and the effect of the actions. This simply emphasizes the importance of providing explicit cueing and feedback to guide the behavior of the brain injured patients who often lack the adequate ability to monitor and evaluate the correctness of their actions.

These four principles are often embodied in many forms of cognitive retraining. Unfortunately, however, the treatment teams fail to adequately extend and program the remedial activities and do not coordinate and systematize their remedial inputs to meet the requirements of efficacious retraining as suggested by Luria.[19]

Even more important is that many cognitive remediation therapists do not fully appreciate how personality and especially motivational factors influence the rehabilitative process. The patients' reactions to cognitive and motor deficits and how this dimension interacts with higher cerebral deficits to produce the ultimate level of psychosocial adjustment is often neither adequately understood nor adequately assessed. Furthermore, as a number of investigators have pointed out,[3, 5, 11] the importance of personality and motivational variables in the cognitive remedial and rehabilitation process of the traumatically head injured patient is paramount and may not be ignored. Thus, a holistic approach to the neuropsychological rehabilitation of brain injured patients is frequently necessary.

Self-Awareness in Cognitive Remediation

Luria's[19] four principles of re-education or restoration of higher cerebral functioning after brain injury seem necessary but insufficient conditions to achieve maximum rehabilitation gains.

There is no doubt that a thorough neuropsychological assessment of the patient's weaknesses and strengths is vital, but the clarification of the specific importance of these in the patient's functional life requires additional situational evaluation, not just the administration of neuropsychological tests.

We have already alluded to the importance of clarifying the nature of the patient's personality difficulties, as they interact with the cognitive sequelae of the head injury. This, too, can be reasonably understood only by working with a patient in many different settings: for example, in one-to-one interpersonal situations; under conditions of formal testing and/or problem solving; in unstructured social situations.*

The need for extended programming and for signalization (i.e., systematic cueing and feedback) in our view, cannot be done only in a one-to-one individual therapy session. The patient must be worked within a variety of settings, including both individual and group activities in order for extended programming to have a chance to take place. Moreover, these should also be extended, in close coordination with the remedial rehabilitation program interventions, to the patient's home and work environments.

Finally, a point that Luria did not emphasize in the context of discussing remedial retraining is the problem of self-awareness after brain injury. (Yet in the clinical examination of the patient, Luria was one of the first to emphasize the importance of asking patients about their own insights into their neuropsychological limitations; see Christensen.[21]) The problem of self-awareness, despite its importance, has been poorly researched and even less assessed in clinical practice. Present neuropsychological test measurements do not even include an assessment of this function.

Stuss and Benson,[24] in their recent summary of the literature on the frontal lobes, emphasize the importance of self-consciousness (or self-awareness) for guiding behavior. They state:

> A strong argument can be made for self-consciousness as a function of the prefrontal area of the human brain. One striking finding in some (but not all) frontally damaged patients is an apparent decrease in normal self-awareness. Variously described as shallowness of interest, loss of self-concern, impairment of self-monitoring, and so on, this alteration suggests prefrontal dysfunction to the experienced clinician. A fair amount of evidence links self-awareness to the executive control functions just described. Self-awareness is necessary for controlling, via a feedback loop, the perceived discrepancy between a present state and a mental comparison . . . without this ability, there would be decreased self-regu-

lation, a frequently observed phenomenon after frontal lobe damage (p. 247) (Fig. 27–1)

The importance of dealing with problems in self-awareness in the neuropsychological rehabilitation of head injured individuals has been recognized by those who adopt a holistic approach to remedial intervention.[4, 5, 11] It is recognized that a lack of sufficient self-awareness (and understanding) of one's deficits, as well as residual abilities, is a significant factor in the lack of sufficient motivation to engage in remedial activities and to the lack of realistic assessment of one's future prospects. Often this accounts for a patient's insistence on pursuing impossible rehabilitation goals. Hence, the best model for achieving meaningful results after cognitive remediation is the holistic (or social milieu) model, which, as will be further discussed, has inherent methods of fostering self-awareness.

Evidence Concerning the Efficacy of Cognitive Remediation

Several recent review articles on this subject[3, 6, 25, 26] have examined the findings to date on the efficacy of cognitive rehabilitation. The conclusions from these reviews of the literature can be summarized as follows:

1. There is a lack of empirical evidence to support the notion that cognitive remedial interventions can result in the restoration of damaged generic, cognitive functions to their preinjury states.

2. There is a lack of empirical evidence that various forms of "direct" cognitive retraining (e.g., to remediate "generic" memory functions) can restore impaired higher cerebral functions in the brain injured patient past certain timeframes.

3. There is, however, cautious optimism regarding the ability to improve, via systematic remedial interventions, patients' attentional and problem-solving abilities.

4. In certain instances, cognitive remedial interventions can and do lead to the attainment of different degrees of compensations for what essentially remain permanent generic impairments of brain functioning. The compensation comes about as a result of the amelioration of the effects of the generic

---

*In his early writings Luria actually recognized the importance of motivation and personality factors in the rehabilitation process.[23] This, however, was not emphasized in subsequent publications by him or his colleagues.

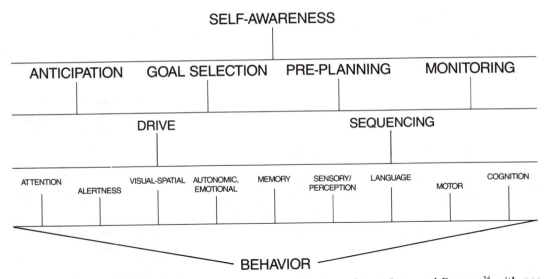

Figure 27–1. Hypothesized hierarchy of frontal lobe functions. (From Stuss and Benson,[24] with permission.)

deficits, to the point where the person's functional adjustment in daily life and/or learning situations improves.

5. Most of the highly specialized and so-called purely "cognitive" remedial techniques (e.g., techniques for eliminating hemivisuospatial inattention) may be useful in those brain injured individuals who exhibit isolated and highly circumscribed deficits. Yet even here it is necessary to exercise caution as Prigatano and coworkers[5] and Gazzaniga[27] have pointed out.

The cognitive interpersonal, and vocational outcomes of holistic neuropsychological remedial programs are summarized and discussed further on in this chapter.

Typical Problems Encountered in Persons With Traumatic Brain Injury

Many long-term cognitive, emotional, and motivational sequelae of traumatic brain injuries have been described in the literature. In the present context, therefore, we merely wish to summarize some of the more salient "generic" deficits, as they manifest themselves in clinical rehabilitation settings. Table 27–1 summarizes the most frequently encountered sequelae.

Several points must be emphasized in connection with the list of problems outlined in Table 27–1:

1. Despite individual differences, in terms of both prevalence and extent of involvement, various combinations of these problems do exist in patients with closed head injuries who are referred for rehabilitation.

2. A specific neurobehavioral manifestation is often the result of interactions among several generic deficits. Thus, for example, an observed deficiency in memory functioning is often the result of the interactions between attention and concentration deficits, coupled with adynamic or impulse control problems, with memory deficits; all of these in turn can be further exacerbated by the patient's coexisting thought or personality disorders. Thus, an observed or test-determined failure to perform competently in persons with diffuse brain injuries is often a multidetermined event.

3. In a rehabilitation context, it is important to estimate (a) which of the patient's generic deficits is most likely to produce a particular behavioral or test-determined inadequacy; (b) which of these are of primary or secondary importance; (c) under what environmental circumstances is the patient likely to experience a similar failure; and conversely, (d) under what circumstances is the patient likely to succeed, despite the existence of these "generic" deficits, due to

**Table 27–1. SOME OF THE COMMON SEQUELAE OF
MODERATE AND SEVERE TRAUMATIC BRAIN DAMAGE**

Assumed Generic Deficits	Clinical Variants
Disturbances in the balance between excitatory and inhibitory processes	a. Adynamic or impulse control problems b. Reduced stamina and/or energy levels c. Organically based tendencies to "flood" emotionally, even when engaged in emotionally "neutral" (i.e., cognitive or problem-solving) tasks d. Lowered tolerance for frustration and/or "irritability"
Disturbances in basic attentional functions	a. Suboptimal alertness and/or arousal b. Inadequate focusing of attention and/or c. Inadequate concentration (i.e., ability to sustain train of thought) d. Psychomotor impersistence
Impaired memory functions	a. Problems in registering and coding, hence, in the acquisition and retention of new verbal or nonverbal information b. Problems in the retrieval (free recall; cued or context-bound recall; in recall by recognition of newly acquired or old verbal or non-verbal information)
Impaired "integrative" functions	Problems in the adequate or time efficient execution of various perceptual-motor-spatial-sequential tasks
Impaired speed of information processing	Impaired or slowed down sensory-motor-skills; i.e., disrupted "kinetic melodies" and/or habituated functional "algorithms"
Impaired language and communications skills	a. Problems in comprehension of word meaning or "labeling," i.e., word finding, in oral communications b. Impaired academic skills (reading, spelling, writing, arithmetic) c. Impaired ability to "stick" to the topic and tendency to become fragmented in free speech
Thinking disorders	a. Problems in convergent reasoning; e.g., abstracting the core or main idea b. Problems in divergent reasoning; e.g., ability to flexibly shift one's perspective and consider alternatives c. Problems in the area of "executive functions," e.g., ability to plan, prioritize, formulate "action plans" implement, self-monitor and self-correct actions, and evaluate results
Inadequate awareness	a. Problems related to unrealistic expectations* concerning the recovery of functions and the possibility and/or prospects of resuming one's preinjury lifestyle b. Problems in assessing severity of one's deficits, i.e., understanding their implications c. Problems related to poor compliance in treatments and/or resistance to inputs/guidance by rehabilitation professionals
Reactive affective responses	a. Agitation and/or depression in response to perceived "losses" b. Poor morale and/or sense of "hopelessness" regarding the future
Damaged self-esteem and "ego-identity"	Low self-esteem and impaired sense of "self"; i.e., viewing oneself as "diminished" or "devalued" by the injury; inability to deal with/accept the situation with a measure of "calm resignation"; inability to find any solace in present life

*Naturally, unrealistic expectations or resistance to undergo rehabilitation can be caused by purely psychologic factors (e.g., "denial") as well. But in the traumatically head injured person, the underlying causes are very frequently the result of interactions between organic and psychogenic factors.

the attenuating influences of the environment or compensatory factors.

Such questions are at the root of any serious differential diagnostic and remedial endeavor. Perhaps Kurt Goldstein[28] has addressed these issues most articulately. While he emphasized that in the brain injured person "changes in consciousness come with changes in mood and emotional attitude,"

Goldstein also pointed out that the "individual life history and the emotional constitution are of equal importance." The importance of premorbid personality factors in the rehabilitation of brain injured persons has been recently shown by Prigatano and others.[5, 11]

THE NEED FOR A HOLISTIC APPROACH

In the sections that follow, we will attempt to illustrate why a holistic approach is frequently the most suitable one for the neuropsychological rehabilitation of persons with traumatic closed head injuries, and to explicate the role of cognitive remediation within the framework of a holistic approach.

Considering the array of problems with which most persons with traumatic brain injuries present in rehabilitation settings and that such an array of problems demands virtually simultaneous and multifaceted remedial solutions, we are led to the following conclusions:

1. Rehabilitation programs for traumatically head injured individuals must consist of well-integrated interventions that exceed in scope, as well as in kind, those highly specific and circumscribed interventions which are usually subsumed under the term "cognitive remediation."

2. An adequate, effective program of neuropsychological rehabilitation must, of necessity, be organized and operated along holistic lines.

3. Efforts at cognitive remediation must be completely embedded in the totality of the rehabilitation endeavor, wherein its expected outcomes, the specific techniques it employs, and the process of their application must be subservient to the wider goals of the rehabilitation endeavor.

4. Cognitive rehabilitation programs in which the "treatment" is *primarily* focused on computer-assisted cognitive retraining are unlikely to achieve successful treatment outcomes. This may be a consequence of the lack of generalization of treatment effects, narrowness of the "computer" approach, and failure to consider the context in which cognitive and interpersonal deficits occur.

An Operational Definition of the Holistic Context

One way to define the overall objective of the holistic neuropsychological rehabilitation endeavor is to define, operationally, the clinical challenges that must be met by any neuropsychological rehabilitation program for the traumatically head injured individual. Such a definition was recently advanced by Ben-Yishay and coworkers.[4] Figure 27–2 presents this definition.

Reduced to essentials, our postulate is that patients must advance through a hierarchy of six distinct stages in the remedial process. The first, *the engagement*, refers to those remedial interventions which are designed to optimize alertness, basic attention, and concentration. The second, *awareness*, refers to those therapeutic interventions whose principal focus is to make the patient

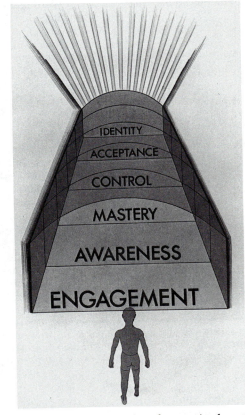

Figure 27–2. A hierarchy of stages in the rehabilitation of the head injured adult. (From Ben-Yishay, et al,[4] with permission.)

sufficiently aware and capable of understanding the consequences of the brain injury, and to be willing to undergo intensive rehabilitation while at the same time helping the patient retain the will to go on striving to overcome handicaps. The third and fourth, respectively, *mastery and control,* refer to two corollary stages in the rehabilitation process during which the focus of interventions is on the amelioration of those cognitive and personality deficits that lend themselves to remediation. This also refers to the stage in which patients attempt to use compensatory techniques for daily problem solving. The fifth, *acceptance,* is arrived at when the preceding challenges have been successfully met. The patient then attains a sense of realization that the limits of compensation, via remedial retraining, have been reached and that the "better part of valor" is to accept the results as the best possible outcome under the circumstances. The acceptance of this fact is an indication that the patient has reoriented his or her thinking about the future; that the patient is prepared to undertake, to pursue as practical goals, those functional outcomes within his or her grasp rather than continue, unrealistically, to hold onto preinjury career and life goals. Finally, the sixth, *identity,* refers to the culmination of the successful resolution of all the preceding stages; when the patient becomes reintegrated in the community and practices the level of productivity permitted by his or her residual limitations with a renewed sense of "ego-identity."

From Concepts to Practice

The original pilot program of holistic neuropsychological rehabilitation for outpatient head injured war veterans was established by Ben-Yishay and associates[29] in Israel in 1974. This was followed in 1977 by the NYU Head Trauma Program.[4, 18] Then Prigatano's[5] and Scherzer's[30] programs were established in 1980 and 1983, respectively. The following discussion focuses on the NYU program because (1) it has been in existence for the longest period; (2) it has been operating, since its inception, according to a precise protocol that has remained virtually unchanged; and (3) it has served as a model for the development of other programs. (For a discussion of a variant of this program, see Prigatano and others.[5])

THE NYU HEAD TRAUMA PROGRAM:
A BRIEF OVERVIEW

The NYU Head Trauma Program was designed to serve, by virtue of its structure, methods, and procedures, as a vehicle for holistic neuropsychological rehabilitation of out-patient traumatically head injured young adults who have reached a neurological plateau. These patients had not been able to return to work after conventional rehabilitation intervention.

The program delivers its rehabilitation interventions in two phases. The first phase is devoted to assessment and intensive remedial treatments. These take place in the setting of a "therapeutic community." The therapeutic community consists of 10 patients plus their families and close friends, and the treatment team (consisting of five to six psychologists and two vocational counselors, a ratio of less than two patients to one staff member). Treatments are administered in 20-week cycles. Occasionally, there is a need in some individual cases to repeat a second cycle of phase one before advancing the patient to phase two of the program.

Phase two of the program is the individualized "tailored-designed" phase of the treatments. During phase two, each patient receives some further individualized extensions of the treatments. They are specifically geared to prepare the patient for productive work, commensurate with the patient's current abilities. Patients are then placed at actual work sites, where they undergo in vivo guided occupational trials. At the successful conclusion of the occupational trials, the actual employment and the postdischarge follow-up stages ensue.

Each 20-week cycle consists of (1) the initial evaluation, (2) the remedial treatments, and (3) the postremedial evaluation of the outcomes.

The Initial Evaluation Period. The initial evaluation process was especially designed to (1) obtain a comprehensive picture of which areas of cognition have remained intact and which have become impaired; (2) obtain, via special remedial probes, reliable diagnostic/prognostic information concerning the patient's readiness for and potential to benefit from systematic cognitive remedial interventions; (3) assess the patient's current interpersonal skills/repertoires; (4) assess the extent of the patient's awareness of the consequences of the injury, and the extent of the patient's "malleability" (i.e., ability to respond to various therapeutic interventions and to modify one's maladaptive behaviors); and (5) assess the patient's social network.

The evaluation takes place over a period of 1 to 2 weeks, totaling 20 to 35 hours. Typically, a patient in evaluation undergoes the tests, the various clinical observations, plus the special remedial probes, in proximity to and/or direct contact with a group of patients whose treatments are unfolding at the same time. This affords the staff opportunities for assessing the new candidate's remedial rehabilitation potential in vivo in the setting of an ongoing mini–"therapeutic community" program. Furthermore, it allows the patient and family members to experience, first hand, what it would entail to participate in a day program such as this. Hence, the assessment provides many indices of intactness and deficiencies in capacities in various domains of functional life, and it provides directly observed/measured prognostic indices of the ability to cooperate in and benefit from a holistic program of rehabilitation.

Intensive Remedial Period. The intensive remedial treatments are given over a period of 18 consecutive weeks, during which a carefully coordinated package of "individual" (1:1 patient-to-staff ratio), "individualized" (2:1 ratio), and "small-group" (3:1 ratio) cognitive and/or interpersonal remedial treatments are delivered to the 10 patients who start and end the treatments together. Of the 20-week cycle, 1 week is devoted to the baseline and 1 week to the postremedial assessments.

During the intensive remedial phase, the treatments are delivered routinely 4 days a week, 5 hours a day (including peer lunch), according to a set schedule and following a preplanned curriculum. In addition to the daily routines, patients and/or their family members also receive a variety of additional cognitive or therapeutic interventions which are scheduled at weekly or longer intervals over the 20-week cycle.

The combined total number of hours of treatment received during one cycle is 400 hours. Broken down into three categories of treatment, each patient thus receives: 46 hours of individual, 167 hours of individualized, and 187 hours of small-group remedial treatments.

To concretize matters, Figure 27–3 presents the program "clock" as it unfolds over a 20-week cycle of treatments. The following is a brief description of the content of each component:

The Team. Members of the team (whose number, including the predoctoral and postdoctoral fellows, usually exceeds the 2:1 patients-to-staff ratio) operate as a "therapeutic cooperative." This means that (1) the entire team is responsible to formulate jointly the treatment plans; (2) all members of the team perform all tasks, i.e., their roles are interchangeable; and (3) each member of the team comes in daily contact with all of the patients in the group. Within this highly coordinated system, one third of a staff member's time is devoted to preparations, conferences, and deliberations with the rest of the team.

Daily Orientation. Consisting of one-half hour each day, at the beginning of treatments, this is a small-group procedure, designed to foster the individual patient's (1) orientation to the objectives and procedures of the program and the motivation to apply self; (2) awareness and acceptance of

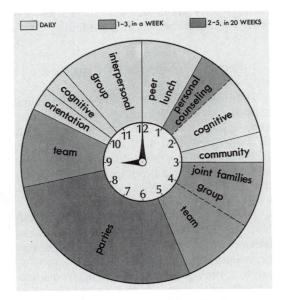

Figure 27–3. Activity schedule of holistic neuropsychologic rehabilitation program.

deficiencies; (3) habitual use of necessary compensatory mnemonic aids; and (4) capacity to objectively assess daily progress and set concrete goals in the presence of peers and staff.

Daily Cognitive Remedial Training. For 2 hours each day, individual or individualized (systematic) remedial training exercises are carried out, in accordance with a set curriculum and using five training modules. Training is provided in the areas of (1) attention, concentration, and psychomotor speed of response; (2) eye-hand coordination and fine-motor dexterity; (3) visuoconstructional abilities; (4) visual information processing (perceptual analysis, spatial organization plus visual problem solving); and (5) logical reasoning. These remedial modules and the rationale for their administration have been described in detail elsewhere.[18]

Daily Interpersonal Communications Skills. This is primarily an individualized cognitive-interpersonal exercise. The training, carried out for 1 hour daily with each individual patient in the presence of peers and staff, has been designed to improve interpersonal communications skills and emphatic ability. Each patient, in turn, is coached and receives organized feedback, from peers and staff alike, on how to determine relevant content, organize facts for presentation, monitor adherence to a planned presentation format, employ appropriate affective tone and body posture in communicating, and receive and synthesize verbal feedback. While acting as observer/listener, the patient is coached on how to define appropriate parameters for critique, critically analyze a presentation, and communicate constructive criticism in an interpersonally appropriate manner.

Daily Community Meeting. This daily small-group procedure lasting one-half hour ends each day. It was designed to (1) foster a sense of "belonging," (2) improve appropriateness of social behavior, (3) foster sociability, (4) enhance ability and willingness to comply with social rules of conduct, and (5) increase self-esteem and realistic acceptance of the patient's own situation. Community sessions are attended by the entire patient group, significant others, staff, and visitors (i.e., visiting professionals and/or family members of prospective candidates for treatment).

Weekly, Multiple Family Group. This weekly 2-hour group session is attended by all the significant others and the staff. It is designed to provide (1) guidelines for managing the patient at home; (2) in-depth understanding of the purpose, techniques, and results of the program; and (3) mutual support among families.

Conjoint Patient-Family Counseling. The number of hours spent in conjoint patient-family counseling over the 18-week treatment period varies from patient to patient, according to need. At the minimum, each family is seen for four to five consecutive conjoint and counseling sessions, with or without the patient present.

Special Presentations. Twice during a cycle of treatments (e.g., the 9th and 19th weeks) patients and staff prepare a special "party" for the significant others. Each patient prepares, with assistance from the staff, a personal statement to be presented along with his or her peers in front of the entire therapeutic community. These presentations serve an important therapeutic purpose in that they constitute vehicles for demonstrating and consolidating social competence and poise in interpersonal communications and the area of applied cognition. These special presentations also serve as a means for demonstrating openness, a willingness to "come to grips" with one's situation in the presence of one's community. The presentations are videotaped and are used clinically during individual counseling to further enhance each patient's self-esteem and reinforce the commitment to adopting a realistic attitude about the rehabilitation process.

The Re-evaluation Period. The last week of each cycle is devoted to (1) reassessment of the patient, (2) presentation of treatment results to the patient and the family, (3) recommendations for the next phase, and (4) preparation of the patient prior to discharge from the highly structured and psychologically supportive program to a less structured environment (e.g., the guided occupational trials).

PHASE TWO: THE GUIDED OCCUPATIONAL TRIALS

The guided occupational trials phase lasts typically from 3 to 6 months and is designed according to each individual's special abilities and needs. It involves (1) intensive, individual prevocational remedial explorations and training; followed by (2) in vivo guided work trials (usually within the setting of the medical center); in conjunction with (3) personal and/or small group counseling, for the duration of the trials.

Although individual patients differ in the extent of their need for (and the frequency of) personal supervision/training during this phase of the treatment, virtually all receive a minimum of 2 hours a week of personal counseling, 1 hour of small-group counseling, plus the equivalent of three or more small-group sessions in the form of "on the job" inspections. These treatments are provided by the program's vocational counselors, often in conjunction with other team members.

The Nature of Cognitive Remedial Interventions in a Holistic Setting

As mentioned earlier the overall aim of cognitive remediation is to improve problem solving ability, consistent with Luria's[19] conception of the problem-solving cycle. In the work by Ben-Yishay and Diller[2] the underlying logical of derivation of specific cognitive remedial modules was spelled out in detail. Briefly restated, it is this:

Step 1: Establishing the predictive power of test procedures. In determining which neuropsychological test procedures are particularly relevant for rehabilitation considerations, the first step is to establish empirically, by correlational studies, their power to predict important aspects of the patients' recovery process in the neurological, behavioral, cognitive, and interpersonal spheres. It should also predict important outcomes of rehabilitation: degree of self-sufficiency attained in living conditions, personal adjustment, and vocational adjustment following systematic rehabilitation interventions.

Step 2: Establishing reliability of testing procedures. Having established that certain standardized or specially designed tests are rehabilitation relevant—that they predict important aspects of patients' functioning—the next step is to ascertain which of these tests are best suited to reliably sample patients' competence, or the lack of it, in the given domains of functioning.

Step 3: Analyzing the stimulus and performance properties of tests. The third step is to analyze the stimulus and the performance properties of these tests and establish the hierarchy of complexity of the various component functions, from the least to the most complex, cognitively demanding component.

Step 4: Converting the hierarchies of component functions into training modules. The conversion of a scaled hierarchy of task components into a cognitive remedial module is finalized by methodically incorporating into the task hierarchy: (1) a step-wise cueing methodology, to make possible its use as a good teaching device; (2) special provisions (e.g., modes of displaying, rates of presenting, and ways of "modeling" the task) aimed at accommodating typical head injured individuals' problems in the area of information processing; and (3) suitable clinical management techniques to effectively neutralize the ever-present interferences with the learning process of attentional disturbances and "catastrophic" reactions: various manifestations of anxiety caused by the perception of the inability to adequately cope/perform.

Thus, in keeping with these guidelines, five cognitive remedial modules were developed by the NYU Head Trauma Program.[18]

Underlying the modular approach to cognitive remediation were three corollary assumptions: (1) that systematic training on a module would result in the amelioration of the generic cognitive deficit which this module was designed to tap and address remedially; (2) that the improvement in functioning following the remedial training would generalize to other tasks which share in common with the module the same underlying ability/skill structure; and (3) that if the right number and "mix" of remedial modules is effectively employed within the program, this would inevitably result in the material enhancement of the patient's problem-solving skills, hence his or her ultimate rehabilitation.

It is not in the scope of this chapter to outline in detail the many clinical-didactic issues involved in the actual administration of cognitive remedial training in a holistic rehabilitation setting. We will, therefore, confine ourselves to briefly identifying some of the more salient features of the cognitive remedial endeavor.

Figure 27–4 presents schematically the six principal aspects of performance of the remedial tasks that are systematically emphasized by the staff:

1. *Order of cognitive functions singled out for remedial training.* At the NYU Medical Center Head Trauma Program, the order of remedial training is basic attention, followed by eye-hand coordination with finger dexterity, followed by constructional praxis, visual information processing, and (verbal) logical reasoning, respectively. (See Ben-Yishay and Diller[2] for a more detailed discussion of the rationale.)

2. *Strategy.* The heart of any remedial instruction, irrespective of which module is employed, is to show the patient, explicitly and using concrete details, the most efficacious strategy he or she ought to pursue in order to arrive at the correct solution.

3. *Process.* Facilitating the process of the problem-solving task is another central feature of an optimal cognitive remedial training exercise. This refers to the manner in which the cueing methodology is applied. In the case of brain injured individuals, "saturation cueing," or the gradual fading of cues, from the most to the least explicit is the most effective procedure. In addition to the timing and the manner in which the cueing methodology is applied, the problem-solving process is facilitated by the judicious application of clinical management techniques to maintain attention at optimum levels and to prevent catastrophic reactions. Thus, process facilitation renders the problem-solving task as free as possible of interruptions that are deleterious to optimal learning and, worse yet, of aborted and/or stymied efforts at accomplishing tasks. The latter are the inevitable results of negative emotional responses such as anxiety and frustration in the face of an experienced failure to cope.

4. *Efficiency.* For best effect, the remedial exercise must be carried out by the patient not only correctly but also efficiently. This requires that special attention be paid, during the training, to ensuring that (1) the patient exercises good "housekeeping" procedures: effectively organizes the materials and the work space; (2) the various components of the task sequence are properly planned and prioritized; and (3) the entire problem-solving task sequence is executed in a "smooth" and time-efficient manner. This is achieved by repeating remedial tasks that have already been mastered by the patient but this time with an emphasis on "doing it faster and faster."

5. *Closure.* In addition to teaching a patient how to solve problems correctly and efficiently, a further sought-after byproduct of the cognitive remedial training endeavor is to impart to the patient a sense of closure, or the feeling that he or she can once again successfully begin and end problem-solving tasks. This is necessary if one wishes to undo the damage that was caused to the patient's self-confidence and self-esteem by the many experiences of failure to cope (due to aborted or deflected problem-solving efforts) since the injury.

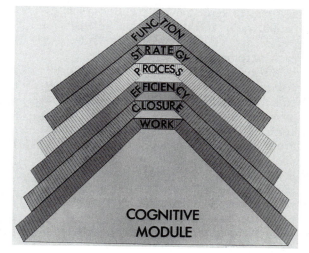

Figure 27–4. Expected benefits of the modular approach to cognitive remedial training.

6. *The cognitive training experience as a "work" sample.* Within the context of holistic neuropsychological rehabilitation, the cognitive remedial training experience is also referred to by the staff as a "work" experience (preparatory to the actual work experiences to follow during the second stage of the program). In that context, the patient is constantly exhorted to view the remedial training materials as "tools" and to view the various procedures designed to ensure good housekeeping and efficient execution of the tasks as samples of good "workmanship"; to view his or her interactions with the other patients and the staff as opportunities to practice "good work relations"; and, finally, to gauge his or her behaviors in this area in order to obtain practical indices of progress toward work readiness.

Outcomes of Cognitive Remediation in Holistic Settings

To date, three programs, organized and operated along nearly identical holistic lines, have published group data on various aspects of cognitive remedial training.[5, 30–36] In these programs, cognitive remedial training was embedded in and systematically coordinated with other types of rehabilitation interventions such as personal counseling functions; small-group therapeutic interventions specially modified for head injured individuals; and various types of social, "community," activities.

Owing to the great similarity of the three programs in terms of patient selection, types and mix of remedial interventions, staff-to-patient ratio, and duration and intensity of treatments, we may consider the findings of each as roughly comparable.

Three specific questions concerning outcomes are relevant in this context: (1) How effective did the cognitive retraining efforts prove to be? (2) What were the relative contributions of the cognitive retraining and the modified small-group therapeutic interventions to patients' ultimate vocational adjustment? (3) Given an equal chance to compete in a multivariate study designed to retrospectively predict the level of employment that was attained by patients at the end of their programs of rehabilitation, which of the following categories of predictor variables accounted for greater amounts of the total variance: (a) clinical demographic variables, (b) cognitive measures, at the end of the remedial interventions, or (c) "process" variables (i.e., indices of compliance, cooperation, and awareness and acceptance of one's existential situation, in the course of the remedial-rehabilitation program)?

Effectiveness of Cognitive Retraining. All three studies[5, 30–36] reported statistically significant improvements in the patients' performance scores on a number of the tests comprising the respective criterion batteries of cognitive measures. However, the cognitive improvements were uniformly modest, rarely amounting to dramatic, clinically meaningful changes in the patients' overall capacity levels, in the given domains of functioning sampled. Furthermore, the improvements in performance scores were relatively circumscribed; that is, the degree of generalizability of the training effects remained relatively limited.

Relative Contribution of Cognitive Remedial Training and Small-Group Therapy. Results of one of the series of studies (n = 20) by Ben-Yishay and coworkers[32] are particularly relevant here. First they examined the question of the relationships between patients' initial (baseline) competence (measured by an extensive battery of neuropsychological tests plus measures of competency in daily life functions), and their ability to benefit from cognitive training compared with the ability to benefit from a modified small-group therapeutic procedure (designed to improve interpersonal communication skills, self-awareness, and acceptance of one's disability).

It was found that (a) both the cognitive learning and the small-group assimilation indexes could be predicted from some of the same or different baseline test performances; (b) the ability to benefit from cognitive training and the ability to assimilate small-group therapy "messages" correlated highly with one another (n = 20; r_s = 77). Hence, the results have shown that one may predict rehabilitation "process" variables (learning in cognitive training and improved self-awareness and acceptance of one's existential predicament in a small-group/special therapeutic procedure) from baseline competence measures.

The analysis was then extended further to test whether an outcome variable — postrehabilitation employment level — could be predicted from the cognitive learning and the group assimilation indexes, and if so, which of the two indexes contributed the most to that prediction. It was found that the ultimate employment level could be predicted very well from both (vocational outcome from learning index; $r_s = 75$; vocational outcome from group assimilation index; $r_s = 0.91$).

However, since the cognitive learning index and the group assimilation index correlated with one another as well ($r_s = 0.77$) partial correlations were performed. Following the partial correlations it was found that when the mediating effects of small-group assimilation were removed from the correlation between cognitive learning and vocational outcome, there was a significant drop in the magnitude of the correlation (i.e., from the previous $r_s = 0.77$ to an $r_s = 0.35$, which was significant at p 0.05 level only). On the other hand, when the mediating effects of cognitive learning were removed from the correlation between vocational outcome and the group assimilation index, the resulting correlation coefficient remained, still, very high (from the previous $r_s = 0.91$ there was a slight reduction only to $r_s = 0.74$).

It was concluded, therefore, that of the two process variables — learning index on cognitive training tasks and group assimilation index — the ability to benefit from small-group interventions (i.e., improved self-awareness and acceptance) is the most potent predictor of postrehabilitation vocational attainments.

Results of Retrospective Prediction Studies. At the end of a 5-year study on holistic neuropsychological rehabilitation involving 70 chronic traumatically head injured young adults,[34, 35] several retrospective prediction analyses were undertaken. The question under scrutiny was what best predicts vocational outcome following intensive rehabilitation. Results of two of these retrospective prediction analyses are particularly relevant here.

In the first study an attempt was made to predict the ultimate employment level attained from certain demographic indices (e.g., age at injury, years of schooling), injury related indices (e.g., duration of coma,

time since injury), and a wide spectrum of pretreatment assessment indices. The indices included 67 test scores assessing neuropsychologic integrity, lower and higher level cognitive functions, academic skills, a wide range of functional daily life competencies, and a number of interpersonal skills which were statistically collapsed into 20 factor scores, or "marker" predictor variables.

It was found that by using the aforementioned set of predictor variables, vocational outcome could be predicted but only with relatively low accuracy (multiple R = 0.56; the total amount of variance accounted for being 31 percent only). The four predictor variables that contributed to this prediction were duration of coma, the verbal memory factor (the "marker" of all verbal memory test scores), the regulation of affect factor (the "marker" of several measures of the ability to control and modulate affective responses in daily life situations), and the visual information processing factor (the "marker" of tests assessing aspects of visual information processing ability).

In the second retrospective prediction study, prediction of ultimate vocational rehabilitation was attempted by using the same demographic and injury related variables as in the first study. But, this time, instead of the pretreatment assessment variables the "markers" for the cognitive and the interpersonal post-treatment test scores (which were similarly factored) were introduced into the equation. An "acceptance" index was also added to the equation. This consisted of a cumulative weighted scale score assigned by the staff for patients' compliance/cooperation, self-awareness, and self-acceptance during the remedial interventions phase.

Thus, in the second prediction study, the demographic and injury related indexes were allowed to compete with indexes of post-treatment gains in the various cognitive and interpersonal domains sampled by the original assessment battery, plus with a number of "process" variables: measures of the degree of patients' success, as judged by the staff, in assimilating the remedial interventions.

Results of the second retrospective prediction analysis have shown that by using the latter set of predictor variables it was possible to predict ultimate vocational adjustment with a relatively high degree of accuracy (multiple R = 0.81, amount of variance accounted for totaling 65 percent, correct classification of the subjects being 75 percent). The number of variables that contributed to this prediction were: (1) duration of coma; (2) the involvement with others factor: a "marker" of several measures assessing the patients' ability to relate to and empathize with others in daily life and family situations; (3) the regulation of affect factor: a "marker" of the patients' ability to regulate and modulate the expression of emotions in daily life situations; (4) the verbal categoric reasoning factor: a "marker" of all tests of abstract and inferential reasoning; (5) the visual information processing factor: a "marker" of all test scores assessing different aspects of visual information processing ability; and (6) the acceptance factor: the "marker" for the process measures. When each of these six predictor variables was looked at in terms of how much each contributed to the total amount of variance that was accounted for in this prediction equation, it was found that duration of coma accounted for only 7 percent of the total amount of variance, whereas categorical reasoning and visual information processing combined (the two predictor variables which in effect measured post-treatment gains in the cognitive sphere) accounted for an additional 12 percent of the total variance. On the other hand, involvement with others, regulation of affect, and acceptance accounted for 46 percent of the total amount of variance. These three predictor variables reflected the patients' ability to relate to others, to effectively regulate the expression of their emotions in everyday functional life situations, and to assimilate various remedial therapeutic interventions designed to improve self-awareness and self-acceptance.

CONCLUSIONS

Based on our review of the current state of the art of cognitive remediation and results of empirical studies on the application of cognitive remedial techniques for rehabilitation purposes, several conclusions appear to be obvious:

1. Cognitive remediation, as a concept as well as a set of remedial techniques, is meaningful only if (a) it is embedded in and systematically coordinated with other neuropsychological rehabilitation interventions, and if (b) the administration of cognitive remedial exercises is done in a manner designed to improve problem-solving abilities in traumatically head injured persons.

2. Even when applied under optimal conditions, such as in the setting of holistic day programs (wherein the patients are exposed, simultaneously with the cognitive retraining exercises, to a host of other rehabilitation interventions and to intensive motivating and supportive experiences), cognitive remedial training has resulted in only very modest improvements in the generic cognitive functions which were the targets of the remedial training, plus the degree of generalization of the effects of the remedial remained circumscribed. Furthermore, when the power of cognitive remedial training effects to predict an important functional rehabilitation outcome, such as vocational rehabilitation, was compared with the predictive powers of intrapersonal and interpersonal skills and the effects of small-group therapeutic interventions designed to foster self-awareness and -acceptance, the predictive power of cognitive remediation was found to be significant but negligible.

3. Finally, despite the promising beginnings in the direction of basing the cognitive remedial endeavor in neuropsychological rehabilitation on sound conceptual foundations and the evidence from empirical studies that supports the suggested processes of generating specific remedial modules, cognitive remedial training remains an evolving hypothesis.[5, 37] Much more remains to be done to elucidate both its fiducial limits, as well as to develop and validate its remedial methodologies.

REFERENCES

1. Ben-Yishay, Y and Diller, L: Cognitive deficits. In Rosenthal, M et al (eds): Rehabilitation of the Head Injured Adult. FA Davis, Philadelphia, 1983.

2. Ben-Yishay, Y and Diller, L: Cognitive remediation. In Rosenthal, M et al (eds): Rehabilitation of the Head Injured Adult. FA Davis, Philadelphia, 1983.

3. Miller, E: Recovery and management of neuropsychological impairments. John Wiley & Sons, New York, 1984.

4. Ben-Yishay, Y et al: Neuropsychologic rehabilitation: Quest for a holistic approach. Semin Neurol 5(3):252, 1985.

5. Prigatano, GP et al: Neuropsychological Rehabilitation After Brain Injury. Johns Hopkins University Press, Baltimore, 1986.

6. Grimm, BH and Bleiberg, J: Psychological rehabilitation in traumatic brain injury. In Filskov, SB and Boll, TJ (eds): Handbook of Clinical Neuropsychology, Vol 2. John Wiley & Sons, New York, 1986, p 495.

7. Diller, L: Neuropsychological rehabilitation. In Meier, MJ, Benton, AL and Diller, L (eds): Neuropsychological rehabilitation. Churchill Livingstone, New York, 1987, p 3.

8. Diller, L and Ben-Yishay, Y: Outcomes and evidence in neuropsychological rehabilitation in closed head injury. In Levin, HS, Graffman, J and Eisenberg, HM (eds): Neurobehavioral recovery from head injury. Oxford University Press, 1987, p 146.

9. Goldstein, FC and Levin, HS: Disorders of reasoning and problem solving. In Meier, MJ, Benton, AL and Diller, L (eds): Neuropsychological Rehabilitation. Churchill Livingstone, New York, 1987, p 327.

10. Diller, L and Ben-Yishay, Y: Analyzing rehabilitation outcomes of persons with head injury. In Fuhrer, MJ (ed): Rehabilitation Outcomes: Analysis and Measurement. Paul H. Brookes, Baltimore, 1987, p 209.

11. Prigatano, GP et al: Cognitive, personality and psychosocial factors in the neuropsychological assessment of brain injured patients. In Uzell, B and Gross, Y (eds): Clinical Neuropsychology of Intervention. Martinus Nijhoff, Boston, 1986, p 135.

12. Prigatano, GP et al: Psychosocial adjustment associated with traumatic brain injury: Statistics. BNI Quarterly, 1987, pp 3, 10.

13. Gianutsos, R and Gianutsos, J: Rehabilitating the verbal recall of brain injured patients by mnemonic training: An experimental demonstration using single case methodology. J Clin Neuropsychol 1:117, 1979.

14. Ben-Yishay, Y: Cognitive remediation after TBD: Toward a definition of its objectives, tasks and conditions. In Ben-Yishay, Y (ed:) NYU, Rehabilitation Monograph No. 62. 1981, p 14.

15. Luria, AR: The Working Brain. Basic Books, New York, 1973, p 323.

16. Diller, L: A model for cognitive retraining in rehabilitation. Clin Psychol 29(2):13, 1976.

17. Ben-Yishay, Y: Rehabilitating the severely head injured individual: Plain answers to complicated questions. In Ben-Yishay, Y (ed): NYU Rehabilitation Monograph No. 61. 1980, p 1.

18. Ben-Yishay, Y (ed): Working Approaches to Remediation of Cognitive Deficits in Brain Damages. NYU Rehabilitation Monographs: No. 59 (1978); No. 60 (1979), No. 61 (1980), No. 62 (1981), No. 64 (1982), No. 66 (1983).

19. Luria, AR et al: Restoration of higher critical function following local brain damage. In Vinken, RJ and Bruyn, GW (eds): Handbook of Clinical Neurology, Vol 3. Elsevier–North Holland, Amsterdam, 1969.

20. Prigatano, GP: Higher cerebral deficits: The history of methods of assessment and approaches to rehabilitation. Part II, BNI Quarterly, Vol 2, 1986, p 9.

21. Christensen, AL: Luria's Neuropsychological Investigation Text. Munksgaard, Copenhagen, 1974.

22. Zangwill, OL: Psychological aspects of rehabilitation in cases of brain injury. Br J Psychol 37:60, 1947.

23. Luria, AR: Restoration of Function After Brain Injury. Macmillan, New York, 1963.

24. Stuss, DT and Benson, DF: The Frontal Lobes. Raven Press, New York, 1986.

25. Schachter, DL and Glisky, EL: Memory remediation: Restoration, alleviation and acquisition of domain specific knowledge. In Uzzell, BP and Gross, Y (eds): Clinical Neuropsychology of Intervention. Martinus Nijhoff, Boston, 1986, p 257.

26. Newcombe, F. Rehabilitation in clinical neurology: Neuropsychological aspects. In Vinken, P, Bruyn, GW and Klawans, HH (eds): Handbook of Clinical Neurology. Elsevier Science Publishers, Amsterdam, 1985, p 609.

27. Gazzaniga, MS: Is seeing believing: Notes on clinical recovery. In Finger, S (ed): Recovery From Brain Damage. Plenum Press, New York, 1978, p 409.

28. Goldstein, K: The effects of brain damage on the personality. Psychiatry 15:245, 1952.

29. Ben-Yishay, Y et al: Digest of a two year comprehensive clinical rehabilitation research program for out-patient head injured Israeli veterans. In NYU Rehabilitation Monograph, No. 59, 1978, p 1.

30. Scherzer, BP: Rehabilitation following severe head trauma: Results of a three year program. Arch Phys Med Rehabil 67:366, 1986.

31. Ben-Yishay, Y et al: Relationships between aspects of anterograde amnesia and vocational aptitude in traumatically brain damaged patients: Preliminary findings. In Ben-Yishay, Y (ed): NYU Rehabilitation Monograph, No. 61. 1980, p 55.

32. Ben-Yishay, Y et al: Rehabilitation of cognitive and perceptual defects in people with traumatic brain damage: A five year clinical research study. In Ben-Yishay, Y (ed): NYU Rehabilitation Monograph, No. 64. 1982, p 127.

33. Ezrachi, O et al: Rehabilitation of cognitive and perceptual defects in people with traumatic brain damage: A five year clinical research study: Results of the second phase. In Ben-Yishay, Y (ed): NYU Rehabilitation Monograph, No. 66. 1983, p 53.

34. Ben-Yishay, Y and Piasetsky, E: Rehabilitation of cognitive and perceptual deficits in persons with chronic brain damage—A comparative study. In Diller, L et al (eds): Annual Progress Report. RT Center, NIHR Grant No. G008300039, 1985, p 4.

35. Ben-Yishay, Y and Piasetsky, E: Rehabilitation of cognitive and perceptual deficits in persons with chronic brain damage—A comparative study. In Diller, L et al (eds): Annual Progress Report. RT Center, NIHR Grant No. G008300039, 1986, p 4.

36. Prigatano, GP et al: Neuropsychological rehabilitation after closed head injury in young adults. J Neurol Neurosurg Psychiatry 47:505, 1984.

37. Prigatano, GP: Recovery and cognitive retraining after craniocerebral trauma. J Learn Disabil 20(10):603, 1987.

Chapter 28

Treatment of Behavioral Disorders

PETER EAMES, M.D.
WILLIAM J. HAFFEY, Ph.D.
D. NATHAN COPE, M.D.

Although many behaviors may be disordered following head injury (e.g., walking, dressing, remembering information, communicating with others), socially unacceptable or socially deviant actions present very serious management problems for carers and treatment personnel. Such actions may be so severe as to preclude the individual from rehabilitation. Moreover, if these conduct disorders persist, they are formidable barriers to acceptance in the community, which is the ultimate aim of rehabilitation.

This chapter is designed to provide a practical set of guidelines for dealing with behavioral disorders in brain injured patients. Since the aims of management and the issues involved in achieving those aims vary throughout the course of recovery, we shall define and consider four somewhat arbitrary periods in the recovery process: (1) the period of medical instability and post-traumatic confusion, (2) the period of formal rehabilitation, (3) the period of community resettlement, and (4) the extended care period. We conclude by presenting five clinical vignettes which illustrate the points made in the chapter.

TREATMENT OPTIONS

A comprehensive approach to the management and treatment of behavioral disorders involves the coordinated use of the following:

1. Normalization and manipulation of the physical environment

2. Physical management techniques
3. Medical treatments, especially pharmacological
4. Systematic application of behavior management principles and techniques
5. Strategies designed to remedy individual cognitive deficits
6. Educational and supportive counseling

The selection of specific methods is dictated by the nature and source of the behavioral disorder, management goals, and the potential benefits and disadvantages (both short- and long-term) of the method. This selection process is guided by the results of the detailed assessments made by the rehabilitation team.

CONTEXTUAL ASSESSMENT

As with any aspect of medical or rehabilitation treatment, assessment involves observing the disordered behavior, considering all potential sources of the problem, and pinpointing the actual sources in each individual case. To do this accurately, the total context in which the disordered behaviors are occurring must be examined. In brain injured patients, this context includes the brain, the body, the person, and the environment.

The Brain

Behavior is often conceived of as resulting from the interaction between the organism and the environment. With this patient population, it is essential to remember that the organism is brain injured such that specific neuropathological abnormalities may be the main source of the observed behavioral disorder.

Examples include epilepsy,[1, 2] temporo-limbic syndromes,[3] hypothalamic, hormonal, or metabolic disturbances,[4] hydrocephalus, and intracranial bleeding.[5] Disordered behavior associated with post-traumatic psychosis may result from temporal lobe impairments. Global confusion or specific cognitive deficits, resulting from the brain injury itself or from secondary complications (including drug intoxications), can provoke such disorders of behavior as agitation, aggression, or other dangerous activity.

Disorders may also result primarily from the brain's inability to direct or control behavioral output. For example, impaired inhibitory mechanisms can lead to quite excessive and socially maladaptive behaviors.

Conversely, a major barrier to adaptive behavior can be a lack of responsiveness. When the brainstem reticular activating systems are impaired, underarousal reduces all forms of behavior. Similarly, impaired limbic function can result in disruptions in the motivational mechanisms. Both processes may prevent the person from expending the effort needed for adaptive behavior.

Therefore, the first step in contextual assessment is a careful analysis of the state of the brain itself, the organ of behavioral control that is now damaged. In most cases, treatments designed to overcome the constraints imposed by brain disorders (e.g., correction of seizure disorders, hydrocephalus, underarousal) must have first priority in planning overall management strategy.

The Body

Restlessness, agitation, screaming, or other forms of disordered behavior may be the patient's means of communicating physical discomfort from a full bladder, constipation, or other physical sources. This is particularly a danger in patients with severe communication disorders or confusion. A patient with heterotopic bone formation may almost reflexly strike out at the therapist or nurse who is exercising a painful joint. More attentive medical and nursing

care may be the prime need in such situations, rather than behavioral or pharmacological treatment.

The Person

It is essential to know enough about the individual whose behavior is disturbed to ensure that he or she is seen in true perspective. Investigation of preinjury behavior patterns is often extremely helpful for understanding current behavior. Of particular relevance is discovering how the person previously reacted to frustrating and stressful situations. Identification of "red flags" which previously provoked excessive or socially inappropriate behavior is often valuable in structuring interactions with the person. For example, knowledge of the person's attitudes and actions when dealing with authority figures (e.g., parents, teachers, supervisors) is sometimes useful in predicting what might be expected under current conditions. A psychological profile of the person's assets and liabilities should be obtained to help interpret current behavior and plan management.

The Environment

The brain injured patient's behavior is greatly influenced by the external environment. This has two main elements — other persons and the physical surroundings. When analyzing specific instances of disordered behavior, it is essential to investigate those actions of other persons which preceded the patient's behavior, to try to discover what they may have done to elicit the disordered response. Examination of the circumstances which preceded the disordered behavior (antecedents) may reveal a variety of patterns. For example, incidents of aggression may prove to be associated primarily with specific tasks or individuals. This is a qualitatively different situation from one in which the patient behaves aggressively whenever any demand is made. Absence of traceable antecedents, especially to episodic explosive behavior, increases the likelihood of neuropsychiatric sources (e.g., command hallucinations, episodic dyscontrol[3]) as the cause.

Even more important to contextual assessment and treatment planning is an examination of what others did (or did not do) immediately after the disordered behavior. Behavior is largely determined by its consequences. If the actions (or lack of action) of those in the environment reinforce the patient who is behaving maladaptively, the probability of the disordered behavior recurring is increased. Alternatively, if those in the environment withhold or withdraw reinforcement following a disordered behavior, the eventual outcome will usually be a reduction in the frequency of that behavior. If they present an unpleasant consequence, the likelihood is increased that the patient will refrain from acting in that manner under similar conditions in the future. This interaction between those in the environment and the person who has acted in a maladaptive manner is central to designing appropriate behavioral management.

The physical setting is a part of the environment that is too often overlooked. Unfamiliar environments stimulate a range of negative emotions. In some cases, the physical environment enhances confusion in the acutely brain injured patient. In other cases, the alien nature of the environment can provoke escape-related aggression. (This will be elaborated on later in the chapter.) Clearly it is important to examine whether aspects of the physical environment are contributing to the patient's disordered behavior.

Sampling Period

When a patient is exhibiting a range of excessive or potentially dangerous behaviors, *it is essential, before embarking on a course of treatment, to collect sufficient samples of the behaviors to allow identification of the probable causes.* For some types of disordered behavior, a brief sampling period (24 hours) may provide sufficient data to arrive at a contextual diagnosis and a management plan. In other cases, a longer sampling period may be required. Without an adequate understanding of the sources of the observed behaviors, it is impossible to construct a coherent, coordinated plan. By examining the frequency, intensity, and duration of the full range of disordered behaviors, and the circum-

stances associated with their occurrence, the treatment team can select those that need to be dealt with first. This selection is based on the impacts of the behaviors (on the patient and on others) and also on the probabilities of successfully effecting changes through interventions specifically aimed at the identified sources.

There are pressures that militate against such an approach. Baseline recording is often inaccurately perceived by clinicians, administrators, family members, and reimbursement agents (e.g., insurance companies) as "doing nothing." Thus, the belief is that treatment is not occurring, which raises questions about the appropriateness of placing a patient in such a program. Instead of explaining how essential such observation is to rehabilitation and how such baseline measurement is typically longer than the observations conducted in curative medicine settings the temptation is to begin a course of intervention. In this way, it is obvious to all that treatment is occurring. Documentation of observed behaviors is often perceived as superfluous activity, especially by clinicians who are already feeling overwhelmed by documentation requirements and who believe that the nature of the problem is obvious. Moreover, clinicians whose prime focus is physical rehabilitation and functional skill training can view such activity as the responsibility of the "behavior therapists" or "psychologists." Another pressure is the desire to quickly alleviate the behavioral disorders, usually through drug intervention, so as to permit the rest of the team to get on with the business of rehabilitation. Finally, there is a belief that progress is evident when it occurs, and thus the systematic collection of baseline data that serves as the benchmark against which the effectiveness of interventions can be measured is seen as unnecessary.

We would argue that the disadvantages of inadequate baseline measurement are twofold. First, there is the risk that treatment is misdirected. This results in ineffective and inefficient allocation of resources and can often lead clinicians to assume that the problem is intractable. Second, the data necessary to investigate the merits of treatment methods and thus to discriminate effective and efficient treatments from incidental ones are never properly collected. This hampers the improvement of rehabilitative technology and interferes with developing ways of improving program accountability.

MANAGEMENT OF DANGEROUS BEHAVIOR DURING ASSESSMENT

Dangerous behavior occurring during the assessment period must be controlled. The methods used to protect everyone's safety and welfare should, as far as possible, have three aims. The principal aim is to prevent harm to everyone involved. Additional aims should be the avoidance of methods which interfere with the assessment process, or which may prove counterproductive in the long run. Physical or chemical restraint may be necessary in emergencies. However, to discontinue the assessment and continue to use drugs as the primary treatment after the emergency has been handled effectively is ill-advised. This usually happens when other treatment options are not explored, simply *because* the drug intervention has decreased the dangerous behavior. What is usually overlooked is that it has also decreased most adaptive behavior. Thus, the full range of options (including drugs) must be explored if the long-term welfare of the patient is to be served.

SUMMARY

Contextual assessment should result in a comprehensive picture of the origins, natures, and impacts of the patient's behavioral disorders. It should include a clear idea of the relative importance of each type of behavior as a barrier to achieving the desired medical and rehabilitative goals. The management plan should evolve from the results of the assessment, and the probabilities of effecting positive changes in each disorder. Typically, brain-based constraints such as epilepsy, temporolimbic syndromes, hypothalamic disorders, intracranial hematoma, and toxic or metabolic disturbances should be dealt with primarily. Once these types of constraints have been treated as extensively as possible, other treatment options must be planned through a coordinated, interdisciplinary team approach.

PRACTICAL MANAGEMENT IN DIFFERENT PHASES OF RECOVERY

Period of Medical Instability and Post-traumatic Confusion

TYPES OF BEHAVIORAL DISORDERS

The principal behavioral disorders in the initial recovery phase are:

1. Apparently non–goal-directed body movements, and agitation (e.g., thrashing limbs, rocking)
2. Inappropriate goal-directed behaviors such as attempting to remove own or other patients' life-sustaining tubes or other apparatus, trying to get out of bed to care for personal hygiene needs when circumstances make it clearly inappropriate, wandering, and so on
3. Screaming, moaning, or incoherent, disorganized, or bizarre verbalizations
4. Disinhibited behavior such as uncontrolled laughter unrelated to environmental stimuli, or inappropriate sexual behavior
5. Accusations of neglect or abuse by staff

SOURCES OF BEHAVIORAL DISORDERS

The principal source of these disorders is post-traumatic confusion resulting from inability to process information accurately. Specific symptoms such as blindness (cortical, peripheral, or from severe periorbital swelling), aphasia, or deafness can contribute to some of these behavioral disturbances, even in those who are not globally confused.

Rarely, behavioral disorders in the early recovery phase may be related to post-traumatic psychosis (delirium). Levin and colleagues[6] review this topic, and describe a subsample of 10 patients, in a sample of 800 neurosurgical admissions, who showed agitated or disinhibited behavioral disturbances associated with acute psychotic manifestations. The median interval from onset to examination was 19 days. Only one of these patients had a preinjury psychiatric disorder or evidence of drug abuse. Symptoms included confabulation, delusions, paranoid ideation, hallucinations, agitation, aggressiveness, reduplicative paramnesia (a belief that they were in a place other than the neurosurgery unit), and sexually explicit behavior. These symptoms were transient, and none of the patients was considered psychotic at follow-up at a median interval of 206 days.

The role of preinjury psychological factors in determining early post-traumatic psychosis is not entirely clear. Levin and colleagues,[6] citing an earlier study by two of the authors,[7] noted that head injury patients showing agitated and disinhibited behavior in the acute confusional state were "heterogeneous with respect to pre-injury personality and demographic characteristics." Similar discrepancies exist in relation to later developing psychotic states. Hillbom[8] concluded that only a very small number of patients showing post-traumatic schizophrenic-like symptoms had a pre-existing schizoid personality disorder. He attributed the symptoms to temporal lobe neurological impairments. In contrast, Lishman[9] found that preinjury constitutional predisposition was a major factor in the development of major psychosis post-traumatically. It would appear that examination of the preinjury psychiatric and psychological history is likely to be important in selecting treatment, since neurologicalally and psychiatrically determined disorders are likely to have different prognoses and to respond to different sorts of treatment.

ASSOCIATED DANGERS

The main danger associated with behavioral disorders in the early recovery phase is the threat to the physical welfare or, indeed, survival of the patient. The safety and well-being of other patients and of staff may also be at some risk.

AIMS OF MANAGEMENT

The management objectives are to ensure the continuation of necessary medical treatments and to protect everyone's safety. These should be accomplished in ways that do as little as possible to impede the natural processes of recovery.

MANAGEMENT

Normalization and Manipulation of the Environment. Acute hospital wards are alien environments to most lay persons. The experience of alienation is undoubtedly more intense for a patient who emerges from coma with only a fragmentary awareness of what has happened and is happening. Such a patient usually has no recollection of the circumstances that have lead to the present moment. Thus, finding oneself connected to various machines, with tubes attached to various parts of one's body, and unable to sit up because of physical restraints, can evoke a range of negative emotions that may provoke behavioral disturbances.

Normalization and manipulation of the physical environment may be very helpful in decreasing these disturbances. Acknowledging that hospital rules and procedures may place limitations on environmental changes, we believe that conscious attention to such factors can contribute greatly to decreasing the alien character of the patient's surroundings. For example, putting by the bedside items obtained from family which may help reorientate the patient to a more understandable reality is a relatively simple adjustment to the physical environment. Pictures of relatives and friends (especially ones that include the patient), and personal possessions (e.g., a favorite toy, a cap or shirt from a sports team the patient supported, a fishing or hunting license) are simple examples.

Staffing patterns rarely permit hospital personnel to spend long periods of time at the bedside. Nevertheless, whenever staff members are caring for the patient, conscious attention to normalizing the interaction (even with apparently comatose patients) can be valuable. For example, taking a few moments to introduce yourself, telling patients where they are and what you are going to do, and extending the same courtesies you would ordinarily give to patients without brain impairments, are all ways of helping to orient the patient to the current situation.

Adjusting one's interaction with the patient to reduce the possibility of adverse reactions is another frequently overlooked environmental manipulation. For example, for a patient with unilateral spatial neglect or sensory-perceptual deficits, staff can make a deliberate effort to approach from the part of the environment most accurately perceived by the patient. To help staff who interact only occasionally with the patient (e.g., laboratory technicians), a sign can be placed in a prominent place saying, for example: "(Patient's name) may be startled if you approach from (his/her) left side. Please approach from the right, introduce yourself, and say what you intend to do."

In attempts to normalize the social environment, the most underemployed resource is the family. Relatives often keep vigil at the patient's bedside. There appears to be a growing sensitivity to the family's needs, and many medical centers now employ nurses or social workers to attend specifically to these needs. Relatives often undertake their own methods of eliciting responses from their loved ones. Allowing them as much access to the bedside as possible, and educating them in ways to help reduce the patient's confusion is potentially valuable for both the patient and the family. The patient's surroundings become more normal (i.e., the family unit). Relatives know the patient and his or her ways, and are often more sensitive to subtle but important indications of progress or regression. Confused agitated patients often respond better to reassurances and corrections from a relative than from a staff member. In such circumstances, the family members are performing a useful role, and this is often of great psychologic benefit to them also. Feelings of helplessness are lessened when the relatives feel that they are vital members of the treatment team. Educating the family and promoting their participation in this way is a primary means of decreasing conflicts which may arise between them and the staff, particularly over questions of interpretation of the patient's behavior.

Appropriate Physical Management Methods. In the early phase of recovery, a primary management objective is protection of the agitated, confused patient from physical harm. This may result from falling out of bed or from attempts to disconnect equipment, remove infusions, and so on. Typically, mechanical restraints are used to prevent such occurrences; however, these may increase confusion, agitation, and resistiveness.

A useful alternative to arm and wrist restraints to prevent resistance to nursing care is to place the patient's hands in large mittens, secured like boxing gloves, and preferably without a separate thumb section. For extremely agitated patients, a much better

alternative to mechanical restraints is to place the patient at floor level in an enclosed protected environment. A mattress surrounded by portable walls lined with therapy mat equipment permits greater freedom of movement. Although such a restraint enclosure may seem unusual, once staff and families see the benefits to the patient and once the equipment becomes routine, it will generally be acceptable.

For patients in the acute confusional period who are ambulatory or wheelchair-mobile, wandering is a major safety risk. There is even greater risk for those who attempt to run away. Such patients often dissipate pent-up energy in this way. Restricting them increases the probability of agitated or aggressive behavior, both because of the restriction itself and because of the closing off of an avenue for release of energy. A novel solution is to adapt a wheelchair with long extension bars that prevent movement through doorways and anti-tip bars that reduce the chance of overturning the wheelchair. The patient can be secured with a belt and can then be allowed access to an area that permits maximal movement while preventing unauthorized exit and risks to safety. Of course, this option cannot be used with patients who need to be connected to monitors or some other devices, but for other confused patients it allows release of energy without compromising safety or requiring constant one-to-one supervision.

Use of Drugs. Given the range of life-threatening factors that initially require intensive monitoring and medical care, it is not surprising that relatively minor physical problems may receive less attention. The development of behavioral disturbances may begin at this early stage as a response to pain or physical discomfort from minor ailments. This is more likely when the patient's ability to communicate with staff is reduced. Vigilant nursing care can identify such problems and eliminate potential sources of the behavioral disorder. In this way, more intrusive procedures, such as physical or chemical restraint, may be avoided.

Many medical and nursing staff consider pharmacologic interventions to be the most effective means of managing behavioral disorders in this early phase. As a basic rule, however, we advise use of drug treatments only after all other available approaches have been properly considered as alternatives. In many acutely brain injured patients, agitation is transient. Because most drugs typically used to treat behavior disorders have significant unwanted effects ("side effects") (Table 28–1), unless a true behavioral emergency exists all methods of normalizing and manipulating the environment should be thoroughly explored before embarking on a trial of drug treatment. Compromising natural recovery processes to manage transient disturbances is difficult to justify.

The first step in considering drug treatment for disordered behavior, as indeed with any treatment, is to exclude treatable underlying pathologic conditions that may be the cause of the behavior. Examples are hydrocephalus, intracranial hemorrhage, and meningitis. In some such cases, neurosurgical, rather than pharmacologic, intervention may be indicated. The behavioral

disturbance may be related to epilepsy, which can be managed with a drug with fewer adverse effects on recovery (e.g., carbamazepine).

It is generally not appreciated how frequently behavior disorders are due to the misuse of drugs in the clinical setting. In other words, drugs currently being administered may be the inadvertent cause or contributor to the disorder. Trying an alternative drug with fewer unwanted effects, or eliminating drugs altogether for a trial period, surprisingly often leads to improvement. Other sorts of management (e.g., a catheter, or passive stretching procedures) that may be provoking aggressive responses might be discontinued temporarily to assess whether the withdrawal is followed by a decrease in the frequency or intensity of the behavioral disturbance.

Evaluation of possible psychiatric causes of the behavioral disturbance may reveal the

Table 28–1. ADVERSE EFFECTS OF SOME COMMONLY USED DRUGS

Name	Trade Name	Impaired Arousal	Impaired Movement	Epilepsy	Impaired Cognition
Major Tranquilizers					
Chlorpromazine	Thorazine	+	+	+	+
Thioridazine	Mellaril	+	(+)	+	+
Trifluoperazine	Stelazine	−	+	+	+
Haloperidol	Haldol/Serenace	+	+	(+)	+
Fluphenazine	Modecate	(+)	+	+	+
Minor Tranquilizers					
Diazepam	Valium	+	−	(+)	+
Lorazepam	Ativan	+	−	(+)	+
Chlordiazepoxide	Librium	(+)	−	−	+
Antihistamines					
Chlorpheniramine	Piriton	+	−	+	+
Diphenhydramine	Benadryl	+	−	+	+
Prochlorperazine	Compazine/Stemetil	+	+	+	+
Antidepressants					
Amitriptyline	Elavil/Tryptizol	+	+	+	+
Imipramine	Tofranil	(+)	(+)	+	+
Phenelzine	Nardil	−	(+)	+	+
Anticonvulsants					
Carbamazepine	Tegretol	−	−	−	−
Phenobarbitone	Luminal	+	+	−	+
Phenytoin	Dilantin/Epanutin	+	+	−	+
Sodium valproate	Depacote/Epilin	−	−	−	+
Primidone	Mysoline	+	−	−	+

+ = occurs
(+) = occurs rarely
− = does not occur

presence of a psychotic or manic disorder. Specific pharmacologic treatment can then be directed at the underlying disorder, rather than drugs being used as a nonspecific chemical restraint.

When symptomatic drug treatment of a behavioral disorder is indicated, it is important first to consider the pharmacology of the drug and its potential interactions with other drugs currently being used. An exhaustive discussion of the pharmacologic management of brain injured patients is beyond the scope of this chapter but is available elsewhere.[10, 11] It is important to remember that no drug acts in precisely the same fashion in all cases and that the same neuroactive drug may have different effects in different patients, according to the nature and distribution of the damage to the brain. Indeed, there appear to be some positive indications of drug use that are quite atypical in brain injured patients. Each drug trial should be thought of as an experiment in which the specific effects and associated unwanted effects must be continuously monitored and possible long-term consequences considered. With this caveat, we list target

problems and some appropriate drugs with minimal adverse effects in Table 28–2. Nevertheless, we recognize that in individual cases circumstances may dictate the use of drugs with known adverse effects. Decisions of this sort must be made only after careful risk-benefit analysis. The unwanted effects of greatest concern in brain injured patients are sedation, interference with cognitive processes, interference with the speed and control of motor functions, the production of movement disorders, and above all, the precipitation of epilepsy.

Evaluating the efficacy of a drug treatment requires careful observation and documentation of the patient's behavior. This is equally true for behavioral treatments. Data on the frequency, intensity, and duration of behavioral disturbances following intervention must be compared with data collected before the initiation of the treatment (i.e., baseline data). Even if the intended effect of decrease in the behavior occurs, it is still necessary to determine whether the treatment was responsible. We recommend the use of single-case methods in the evaluation of a trial of treatment, whether pharmaco-

Table 28–2. USEFUL DRUGS WITH MINIMAL ADVERSE EFFECTS

Problem	Drug	Trade Name
Epilepsy	Carbamazepine	Tegretol
	Acetazolamide	Diamox
	Clobazam*	Frisium
Aggression/Agitation	Carbamazepine	Tegretol
	Propranolol	Inderal
	Lithium	Priadel/Camcolit
(low dose)	Meprobromate	Miltown/Equanil
(low dose — and caution)	Amitriptyline	Elavil/Tryptizol
(caution — addictive)	Chlormethiazole*	Heminevrin
Night Sedation	L-Tryptophan	Optimax/Pacitron
	(Give anticonvulsant at night)	
Depression	L-Tryptophan	Optimax/Pacitron
	Viloxazine*	Vivalan
Psychosis/Paranoid State	Sulpiride*	Dolmatil
	Pimozide	Orap
Hypomania	Carbamazepine	Tegretol
	Lithium	Priadel/Camcolit
	Pimozide	Orap
(if absolutely necessary)	Haloperidol	Haldol/Serenace
Drivelessness/Slowness	Bromocriptine	Parlodel
	L-Dopa	Sinemet
	Pemoline	Cylert/Ronyl
	Amphetamines	
	Methylphenidate	Ritalin

*Not available in United States.

logic or behavioral. (See Barlow and Hersen[12] for discussion of the various single-case designs that can be used.)

Single-case designs help to overcome common flaws in clinical practice. One such flaw is to continue with a treatment without a trial withdrawal. Another is to continue with one particular treatment without considering the possibility that another could be equally effective while having some other advantage over the first (e.g., potency, pharmacokinetics, route of administration, fewer interactions with other needed drugs, fewer unwanted effects). When comparing the effects of different drugs, it is important to ensure that the period of return to baseline ("washout") is sufficiently long to allow the first drug to be completely eliminated before a second is tried and assessed. A third common flaw is the continuation of a drug beyond the point when it is required.

When the patient's behavior is so dangerous that other management methods are insufficient, chemical restraint may be the only alternative. If the patient is still in the intensive care unit, and especially if intracranial pressure monitoring is available, then the safest procedure is to return the individual to a state of controlled coma. This requires very careful and skilled observation, of course, since the drug effects may obscure the development of an intracerebral complication.

In less medically controlled environments, the most often-neglected rule is to give a sufficient dose to secure proper sedation. If oral administration is feasible, our experience indicates that meprobamate or chlormethiazole, or possibly lorazepam, should be used. If a parenterally administered drug is required, current standard recommendations are for the use of high-potency neuroleptics such as haloperidol. An alternative is a parenteral benzodiazepine such as lorazepam. Such treatment must, however, be considered very short-term chemical restraint. If frequent repetition seems to be needed, serious consideration should be given to referral to a specialist unit for behaviorally disturbed brain injured patients.

Application of Behavior Management Principles and Techniques. Behavior management approaches often cannot be used in the presence of medical instability and severe post-traumatic confusion, but as the patient comes to interact more with the environment, even though a degree of confusion may still be present, simple conditioning trials can be instituted. Although these will have little effect on controlling the observed behavioral disturbances, their purpose is to lay the foundation for later therapeutic interventions.

Learning is central to rehabilitation. Early efforts, even in the intensive care unit, designed to evoke consistent responses by the patient to environmental stimuli have the potential in theory to establish associations that could facilitate later learning. A simple conditioning paradigm can be attempted. An example would be presenting a confused patient with a small portion of food, which is then given as soon as there is an appropriate expression of a desire to eat it. For a less confused patient, providing a small amount of food at predetermined intervals which have passed without any sign of agitation may help to establish a learning model that can be employed more completely at later stages. The main purpose is to lay the foundation for subsequent contingency management. However, such procedures are also useful in training the patient to focus attention, and so prepare the way for later cognitive treatments.

Educational and Supportive Counseling. We have already mentioned the importance of encouraging staff and family to examine the ways they interact with the confused patient, in order to make the incoming signals from the environment more readily interpretable. This requires continuous staff training and family education. Training the family to understand that disordered and occasionally bizarre behaviors are a natural feature of recovery can often allay their fears and reduce well-intentioned but misdirected responses on their part. Advising them on how best to help the patient in this early stage is equally important. In the period of medical instability, a nurse or social worker whose role is to provide education and emotional support to the family members can be invaluable in helping them through the emotional peaks and troughs that characterize this phase.

Period of Formal Rehabilitation

Formal rehabilitation typically begins with the resolution of post-traumatic confusion and extends until regular progress toward achievable goals is no longer apparent. In brain injury rehabilitation, this period may last several years.

TYPES OF BEHAVIORAL DISORDERS

As confusion resolves, so too do some behavioral disorders. Disorders that persist, however, acquire more distinct and identifiable forms. Initially, the main problem is their impact on rehabilitation efforts. There are two classes of such behaviors: positive behavioral disorders, which actively affect others, and negative disorders, which involve a lack of behavior. The main behaviors in these classes are shown in Table 28–3. Behaviors associated with psychiatric syndromes can also impede rehabilitative efforts.

Positive disorders tend to interfere with active therapies, and present a substantial management challenge to staff. Negative disorders lead to reduced behavioral output, and impede the acquisition of adaptive responses. Unless both types of disorder are managed effectively, rehabilitation goals cannot be fully achieved (see Wood and Eames[13] for further discussion).

Some behavioral disorders may make life exceedingly difficult for staff and other patients without necessarily interfering with treatment. Examples are crude, obscene, or sexually aggressive gestures or speech, verbal abusiveness, restlessness and irritability, emotional lability, outbursts of anger, odd or peculiar mannerisms, excessive demands for attention, hypomania, and suicidal gestures or talk. However, if they persist, these disorders can effectively block the primary goal of rehabilitation—namely, reintegration in the community. This reintegration may also be prevented by inadequate levels of prosocial behavior, even if positive disorders are absent.

SOURCES OF BEHAVIORAL DISORDERS

As in the period of medical instability, a number of factors may be primarily responsible for disorders of behavior. Some may be directly associated with or are late complications of the brain injury itself. Examples are neurologic conditions such as late-developing epilepsy, intracranial bleeding, or hydrocephalus; neuropsychiatric disorders such as temporolimbic syndromes; and cognitive impairments, especially those that reduce the individual's ability to understand the requirements of normal situations, to predict the likely consequences of an action, or to inhibit impulses.

There are also secondary psychological factors associated with the individual's experience of being injured. Frustration or reactive depression are potent causes of aggression. Incompetence in ordinary tasks, like basic toileting, dressing, eating, or walking can be very distressing and frustrating. Hostility, anger, and aggression are common responses to this awareness of incompetence. Alternatively, the person who seeks to avoid situations that highlight incompetence may have learned that therapists, caretakers, and relatives withdraw their demands for performance in the face of that person's angry responses. Such maladaptive learning can become an ever-increasing source of continued behavioral disorder.

Exacerbation of pre-existing personality weaknesses or the emergence of previously latent psychopathic tendencies may occur either as a direct consequence of the brain injury or as a secondary response to perceived or actual incompetence.

ASSOCIATED DANGERS

The risk to personal health at this stage is mainly related to poor judgment. A typical

Table 28–3. CLASSES OF BEHAVIOR DISORDERS

Class	Description
Positive	Aggressive
	Impulsive
	Disinhibited
	Childish
	Antisocial
	Manipulative
	Perseverative
Negative	Insightless
	Driveless
	Amotivational
	Slow
Syndromal	Depressive
	Paranoid
	Obsessive-compulsive
	Cyclothymic
	Labile
	Hysterical

example is refusal to take medications deemed necessary for health (e.g., drug treatments for hypertension, diabetes, or epilepsy). In later stages of rehabilitation, when the person may be in a residential community re-entry (resettlement) program, this risk to personal safety increases because of the reduction in external controls on the person's behavior. Drug abuse (especially by those who are also taking prescribed drugs), engaging in sexual encounters with multiple partners without regard to health risks, and self-imposed secret restriction of food or liquid intake are further examples of risks to personal safety.

A secondary source of harm to brain injured patients arises when their disordered behavior results in their exclusion from rehabilitation settings. Because of the scarcity of brain injury rehabilitation units that specialize in the management of severe behavioral disorders, such patients may be placed in psychiatric, geriatric, or mental handicap settings, which usually lack adequate rehabilitation services and are almost always socially inappropriate for the brain injured person. Moreover, they typically manage the disordered behavior with only physical and pharmacological restraints, which may compromise the recovery process.

In the rehabilitation phase there may also be a danger to other patients, staff, and relatives of being injured by the aggressive individual.

AIMS OF MANAGEMENT

As in the earlier stage of recovery, everyone's safety must be ensured. Management must be directed also at reducing the barriers to rehabilitation. Since the primary aim of rehabilitation is a return to the community, simple containment or toleration of disordered behavior within the rehabilitation setting is inadequate because the community at large will not adopt a lenient attitude toward such behavior. The aim of treatment must therefore be twofold: the elimination of socially unacceptable behavior and the promotion of prosocial, adaptive behavior.

MANAGEMENT

Normalization and Manipulation of the Environment. A principal goal in the

rehabilitation of the brain injured person whose disordered behavior is a fundamental barrier to return to the community is the restoration of self-regulated, socially acceptable responses to environmental demands.

Proponents of the independent living movement[14] have pointed to the dangers inherent in a medical model in which the patient receives services that are selected and directed by persons other than the patient. A major problem with this model is that the patient is assumed to be incapable and is often excused from personal responsibility for his or her actions. Patients learn that the expectation upon them is compliance with demands established by others, and that their future well-being is directly associated with dependence on others. Everything in the caretaker-patient relationship, including physical aspects of the environment (e.g., uniforms and patients' hospital clothing), reinforces the dependency.

An alternative model is to acknowledge injured patients' limitations, but to assume nevertheless that with sufficient structure and guidance they can gain control over their behavior. The interaction between injured persons and caretakers should be guided by the premise that these persons are responsible for their own actions.

In this sense the less the physical environment looks like a hospital, the better. This is because in our culture the "sick role" and the associated reduced culpability for one's actions are reinforced by being in a hospital. Rehabilitation settings should look more like normal environments where the person is expected to behave in accordance with accepted norms. An environment in which staff and patients wear "civilian" rather than "hospital" clothes is a more normal one, and it subtly communicates the fact that the same standards of social behavior will apply to all.

The social environment is central to the reinforcing of self-directed, responsible behavior. Patients are continually exposed to the staff's interpersonal interactions, whether with the patients, the family, fellow staff members, or clinical or administrative supervisors. The nature of these interactions can model and reinforce self-directed, responsible behavior and so provide powerful opportunities for appropriate learning. By contrast, patients are likely to learn ineffective, passive-aggressive, or other maladaptive ways of responding to stressful or frustrating situations if the staff behave in such ways themselves.

Appropriate Physical Management Methods. Psychiatric nurses have been dealing with physically dangerous patients for generations. Physical management techniques used in psychiatric settings are relevant for rehabilitation staff, who are typically undertrained in this important aspect of management. Books and training guides about physical intervention are potentially useful.[15–18] However, the range of techniques cannot be effectively learned solely from a manual or video cassette, because the most important part of the process is the development of confidence through experience. An appropriate way of introducing these skills into a rehabilitation setting is to employ or hire a small number of skilled psychiatric nurses or technicians. In this way, learning is practical, continuous, specific to the setting, and immediately visible.

Physical management techniques are designed to contain dangerous behavior. It is important that they be employed only when necessary, and that careful safeguards be practiced to ensure that they are not abused by staff. It is also very important not to reinforce the behaviorally disturbed patient through the social attention that can be provided inadvertently during a physical intervention. This point will be elaborated in the section on behavioral techniques (also see Haffey and Scibak[19]).

Use of Drugs. As noted earlier, the development of behavioral disorders may be due to late-developing medical conditions. It is unwise to assume that a person who has been medically stable and who begins to manifest disordered behavior, is doing so for psychological reasons. A thorough medical reassessment should be conducted, regardless of the length of time from injury (see Case 1 at the end of this chapter). It should include consideration of the possible contributions of current drug or other medical treatments.

The pharmacological management of post-traumatic epilepsy (either prophylactic or of actual seizures) is a common but complex medical management problem, and cannot be dealt with here. Trimble,[20] Eames,[2] and Cope[10, 11] have recently addressed this topic.

Two particular points covered by these authors deserve mention. First, there is increasing evidence that the commonly prescribed anticonvulsants phenobarbital (phenobarbitone), phenytoin (Dilantin), and clonazepam (Clonopin, Rivotril) have significant ill effects on speed and control of motor functions, cognition, and affective functions compared with carbamazepine (Tegretol) and valproic acid derivatives (Depakote, Epilim). Second, many psychoactive drugs (e.g., neuroleptics and antidepressants) often used to treat behavioral and affective disorders after brain injury, in addition to adversely affecting cognition and motor control, can precipitate epilepsy. Thus, whenever possible, nonpharmacological methods of management are preferable. When drug treatment is considered, the selection of agents least likely to provoke seizures or interfere with motor, cognitive, or affective functions is recommended (see Table 28–2).

Immediate or exclusive reliance on drug treatments for behavioral disorders is an unacceptable substitute for a well-trained rehabilitation team skilled in physical and behavioral management techniques. However, to avoid drug treatments simply because of philosophical or clinical bias is equally inappropriate. The sensible solution is the essential one of incorporating physicians skilled in pharmacology into a comprehensive team approach to rehabilitation. Published applications of successful pharmacological treatments of behavioral disorders in head injured patients include the works of Sheard and colleagues,[21–23] Monroe,[24] Tunks and Dermer,[25] Rao, Jellinek, and Woolston,[26] and Jackson, Corrigan, and Arnett.[27] Cope's review[10] is particularly valuable.

Efforts aimed at eliminating maladaptive behaviors must be complemented by others designed to promote and stabilize prosocial adaptive behaviors. Attentional and memory deficits can be a major barrier to eliciting and training such behaviors. Cope[10, 28] noted that evidence derived from other populations indicates that neuropharmacological remediation of information processing deficits associated with arousal, attention, and memory disturbances may be possible with cholinergic drugs, and that psychostimulants like amphetamine and methylphenidate may be helpful in decreasing aggression and overcoming attentional deficits, minor motor abnormalities, and overactivity in those with attention deficit disorder (ADD). Lipper and Tuchman[29] reported control of post-traumatic agitation with amphetamine.

The use of pharmacological treatments to enhance information-processing capacity is an underdeveloped aspect of medical management in this field. Drug studies using rigorous single case designs should be conducted. The findings could lead to better integration of the pharmacological, behavioral, and cognitive rehabilitation of those with head injury.

Application of Behavior Management Principles and Techniques. There is a large body of literature demonstrating the effectiveness of applying social learning principles and techniques for the reduction of maladaptive behaviors and the promotion and stabilization of prosocial adaptive behaviors. Social learning theorists maintain that behavior is largely determined by its consequences. According to Thorndike's law of effect, a behavior that is immediately followed by a rewarding consequence is likely to be repeated. On the other hand, a behavior that is followed by a consequence that the recipient finds undesirable is likely to be suppressed. Behavior is maintained by rewards. If a reward is no longer forthcoming, the likelihood is that the behavior will gradually be eliminated.

When the goal of treatment is to reduce or eliminate a behavior, the following hierarchical steps should be followed:

1. Reward all instances of adaptive behavior (positive reinforcement of a competing behavior).

2. Withhold rewards that are currently maintaining the maladaptive behavior (extinction).

3. Withhold all sources of positive reinforcement for a brief period after each instance of the maladaptive behavior (time-out from positive reinforcement).

4. Apply a predeclared penalty following the maladaptive behavior (response-cost, positive restitution, and overcorrection procedures).

5. Apply an aversive consequence following extremely severe or resistant maladaptive behavior (aversive conditioning).

Detailed descriptions and explanations of the specific techniques designed to implement this social learning approach are available in standard texts.[30-32] Haffey and Scibak[19] and Wood[33] discuss the implementation of these procedures in brain injury rehabilitation. Here we will simply highlight some observations made in the course of our clinical experience.

The most important observation is that the positive reinforcement of adaptive behaviors tends to happen too infrequently and is rarely incorporated into the routine conduct of rehabilitation practice. Because study of human behavior and learning is rarely extensively included in their training programs, nurses and other health professionals are usually unaware of the potential value of social learning principles and techniques. The systematic application of these techniques requires a considerable degree of operational and administrative organization. Even when staff are committed to this approach, continuing to provide adequate positive reinforcement is difficult. More often than not, the behavior that needs to be reinforced is, in real-life terms, quite ordinary. Staff may find it difficult to produce effusive social reinforcement for such ordinary behavior. Moreover, it is difficult to sustain when the patient is at other times abusive or aggressive toward the person who is supposed to provide the positive reinforcement. Finally, such an approach is often counterintuitive: a "natural" response is to reprimand a person who is behaving inappropriately, rather than to give a reward for merely refraining from such behavior. Nonetheless, when applied with skill, this simple approach is often a very powerful means of changing behavior.

The second observation is that withholding positive reinforcement will be effective only if the learning environment is generally reinforcing. "Time-out" is an abbreviation of "Time-out from positive reinforcement." If the usual experience is not one of reinforcement, there is nothing to withhold. Removing a person from an unrewarding environment will do nothing to reduce the frequency of a maladaptive behavior. Indeed, removal may inadvertently reinforce such behavior if the person thereby achieves a desired state (e.g., reduction of demands to perform) or is moved to an environment in which reinforcement is available (e.g., a room with a television or radio).

At times, the achievement of time-out requires that the person be removed physically to an environment that contains no source of reinforcement. To be effective, staff must be trained in physical management techniques and in methods of instant, nonverbal communication. To be effective, interventions must be made promptly, by an adequate number of staff, yet smoothly, and without apparent hustle and bustle. The removal is achieved by beginning a calm but firm movement of staff at some distance, which simply carries the patient along with it. Since attention can be reinforcing in itself, the move must be made mechanically and without social contact. One behavioral unit has coined the term "PUNT," an ingenious acronym for "*Physical Unemotionally Navigated Time-out.*"

The application of predetermined penalties implies that rewards are being earned that can be cashed in for desired material goods, activities, privileges, and so on. Without such a conscious structuring of the rehabilitation unit as a social learning environment (or token economy), the application of these procedures is unsystematic, arbitrary, and potentially open to abuse by staff. There must be clear specification of the behaviors that merit a particular penalty, the nature of the penalty, and the methods of applying it, if effective learning is to occur in a manner that ensures that the patient's legal, civil, and human rights are respected. With the possible exception of extreme self-destructive behavior, use of aversive penalties is unwarranted.

Learning control over maladaptive behavior is only one step in the process of achieving acceptance in the community. Learning stable prosocial behaviors is also essential. Social learning principles and techniques have proved successful in achieving this end with very severely disturbed and cognitively impaired groups.[34–36] The techniques can also be a potent addition to the rehabilitation of the brain injured individual.

We do not mean to imply that the social learning approach can simply be grafted on to existing rehabilitation units with a minimum of effort. On the contrary, considerable time, effort, and training are required to establish the appropriate environment. However, this is not to say that units that deal with a reasonable number of head injury patients cannot achieve such an environment.

There is a need for units that specialize in the treatment of patients with very severe behavioral disorders. The organization and methods of one such unit are described by Eames and Wood.[37] Their outcomes suggest that such units play an important part in the continuum of brain injury rehabilitation services.[38]

The social learning approach may not be universally applicable. There is a group of brain injured individuals who appear to be unable to learn through conditioning.[13, 33, 38] This inability may be because of preinjury personality factors (psychopathic or hysterical) or damage to brain structures involved in conditioning or reinforcement (typically from the very diffuse brain insults of anoxia or hypoglycemia) (see Case 5 at the end of the chapter). These individuals are likely to show progressive worsening of both skills and behavior if treated in very structured behavior modification settings, especially if the structure is explicit.

Strategies Designed to Remedy Individual Cognitive Deficits. As the posttraumatic confusional state resolves, the constellation of the individual's cognitive deficits becomes apparent. These deficits often interfere with the performance of a range of tasks and activities. This incompetence in everyday living activities that were performed almost automatically before the injury often gives rise to feelings of frustration, anger, and poor self-esteem. At the same time, the individual's tolerance of frustration and ability to use cognitive defense mechanisms are impaired. Thus, the potential for these feelings to provoke socially unacceptable behaviors is high. Specific cognitive deficits can also lead to misinterpretation of environmental events. The patient who misinterprets another's actions may strike out in self-defense against what is perceived as a threat. Malec[39] has demonstrated how high-level cognitive deficits can result in maladaptive behavior.

Rehabilitation efforts that increase the individual's cognitive competence can thus play a crucial part in improving behavioral competence. Wood[40] showed that patients were more attentive in skills training sessions with physical, occupational, and speech therapists following systematic attention training. Improvements in the individual's performance deficits can potentially reduce the incidence of maladaptive behavior by eliminating a source of frustration, anger, or poor self-esteem.

Malec[39] argued that social behavioral competence could be enhanced through specific training. This includes teaching the person to examine in advance the social appropriateness and likely consequences of an intended action. Social skills training that incorporates strategies designed to compensate for cognitive deficits seems intuitively sound. Ben-Yishay and associates,[41, 42] Prigatano and his colleagues,[43] and Scherzer[44] have published results of outpatient day rehabilitation programs that focus on cognitive and personality disturbances. Prigatano concluded that "... substantial improvement in interpersonal skills and reduction of emotional distress is possible.... These improvements appear to be related to reducing cognitive confusion and teaching patients to compensate for neuropsychological impairments."

Cognitive impairments that preclude a person's return to preinjury roles and responsibilities are also potent precursors of maladaptive behavior. If one's cognitive deficits exclude one from meaningful activities (e.g., work, school, or performing family, household, or financial duties), then the potential for self-destructive or socially maladaptive behavior is increased. This is particularly a problem with the young, who are more prone to drug or alcohol abuse, indiscriminate sexual behavior, or antisocial acts. The rehabilitation team that successfully designs cognitive prostheses (e.g., diaries, alarms, communication aids) that allow the patient to engage in rewarding activities despite the cognitive deficits is contributing significantly to the reduction in emotional distress and its results. Fryer and Haffey[45] reported the positive effects of two different models of cognitive rehabilitation on community reintegration.

Educational and Supportive Counseling. The psychological challenges faced by brain injured individuals and their personal social networks (families and significant others) are very great. Muir and Haffey[46] described features that seem to be specific to traumatic brain injury, as compared with other catastrophic injuries.

Educational interventions should focus on helping patients and the members of their personal relationship system to understand the effects of the brain injury. This can reduce the distress and confusion which naturally result from experiencing something as complex and frightening as traumatic brain injury. It is equally important to provide

suggestions about what each individual can do to contribute to the recovery process.

Psychological distress is particularly severe when the family sees their loved one acting in bizarre or socially aberrant ways. Explanation of the reasons for such behaviors is an important prerequisite for an understanding of the management methods used by the rehabilitation team. This understanding also helps the family to grasp the reasons for the team's requests that they respond in particular ways, and avoid responding in other ways, to maladaptive behaviors. Explaining social learning principles and techniques in a way that helps the family to become an effective agent for change is one of the most beneficial contributions the team can make to the patient and the family. This is not easy, because, among other things, it often requires the family to act in ways that do not come naturally to them, and that may mean radical changes in their preinjury patterns of interaction with each other.

This process must be an integral part of the rehabilitation services. If family members are actually incorporated into the rehabilitation team, they are likely to feel more confident that their loved one is receiving the best possible treatment. This often helps to reduce their own distress, and also better prepares them for the time when they will be the main caretakers. In most cases, waiting until a few weeks before discharge is too late.

Counseling may also help the patient develop better coping strategies. Disordered behavior may come from psychological reaction to the stresses of injury. As with the family, supportive counseling that provides an opportunity to express one's distress to an empathetic person is very important. In a psychologicalally supportive climate, the counselor can communicate to the patient the undesirable consequences of continuing to behave in disordered ways and can provide specific guidelines and training in how to deal with distress in more productive ways.

Period of Community Resettlement

TYPES OF BEHAVIORAL DISORDERS

The period of community resettlement begins in the treatment center as the main focus becomes preparation for return to the community. The primary problem at this stage is the potential recurrence of those maladaptive behaviors that were brought under control during treatment. The second phase of community resettlement begins when the individual actually returns to the community and attempts to meet the demands of everyday life. The pressures associated with community resettlement can lead to a recurrence of maladaptive behaviors. In other instances, maladaptive behaviors not previously observed may become evident.

SOURCES OF BEHAVIORAL DISORDERS

In the preparation phase, two main sources are of concern. The first is reduction in external controls (e.g., environmental, pharmacological, and behavioral); the second is anxiety associated with the return to the community. When individuals actually return to everyday living in the community, they typically face increased performance demands, which often require the expenditure of significant amounts of energy and effort to succeed. Unless these persons feel a reasonable degree of satisfaction with daily life, there is an increasing likelihood of maladaptive behavior associated with depression or other forms of psychological distress.

DANGERS OF BEHAVIORAL DISORDERS

One principal risk is that the achievements of active rehabilitation may break down under the stresses of an unstructured, relatively less supportive, and definitely less externally controlled way of life. Another risk is that the person may despair of ever achieving a meaningful existence. This may initially be manifested by involvement in nonproductive and potentially harmful behaviors such as drug and alcohol abuse or indiscriminant sexual activity. The person simply may stop exerting the effort necessary to succeed. In the extreme, the person may engage in more potent self-destructive activity including attempting suicide.

AIMS OF MANAGEMENT

While the person is still in the treatment program, management strategies are mainly designed to ensure the transfer of skills (behavioral control and prosocial behaviors) from the treatment to the discharge setting. An additional aim is to prevent or reduce the negative consequences of the patient's or the family's anxiety about resettlement.

Discharge planning should also focus on establishing support networks for both the patient and family which should include mechanisms to respond to crises that may periodically arise.

MANAGEMENT

Once desired levels of performance have become stable in the treatment setting, the external controls and supports that have helped to achieve and maintain them can be gradually withdrawn. If maladaptive behaviors re-emerge, or if the frequency of prosocial behaviors decreases, then the likelihood of satisfactory performance in the discharge environment is low. In this event, the rehabilitation team must reintroduce some external controls, choosing procedures that can most easily be continued by those in the discharge environment. Once the necessary levels of performance have been reestablished and sustained, the team must focus its efforts on setting up the transfer of these procedures to the discharge caretakers.

This will usually include training them in how to use the behavioral techiques that seem likely to be needed and is often best accomplished through a series of therapeutic home leaves. During the leaves, the caretakers and the patient test out their skills, and after each visit, a detailed debriefing allows the identification of continuing training needs. This usually involves very careful probing of day-to-day events during the visit to identify specific problem situations and the behaviors in which the patient and caretakers are engaged during these situations. This process facilitates the learning of person- and setting-specific response patterns that will increase the probability of a successful discharge.

Another important aspect of such training is assisting caretakers in recognizing early warning signs of problems that, if not addressed, can develop into serious crises. Alerting the caretakers to be vigilant for even subtle alterations in the head injured patient's behavior is central to prevention.

These observations are particularly important in situations in which the person experiences frustration in attempts at establishing meaningful activities and relationships. Review of early indications of depression or of involvement in self-defeating activities arising from dissatisfaction with life is one of the best means of preventing potentially harmful occurrences. All too often, the burden of providing meaningful activity and emotional support falls heavily upon the caretakers.[47–49] Alerting them to such dangers and helping them identify community resources to respond to psychological crises is a valuable source that the treatment team can provide.

Though often difficult to initiate, frank discussion of the possible risk of suicide is, we believe, a primary means of prevention. Little systematic study of the incidence of suicide attempts and actual suicides in head injured persons has been conducted. Brooks[50] noted that of 42 severely injured patients at 1-year follow-up, 10 percent had talked about suicide and 2 percent had attempted suicide. At 5-year follow-up, these percentages had increased (17 percent had talked about suicide and 15 percent had attempted it). There were no actual suicides over 5 years for this group. Shneidman and his associates[51] concluded that suicide is an act designed to stop an "intolerable" existence as contrasted with an intent to die. Since social isolation is a serious problem for many head injured persons who return to community living,[47, 52] it is possible to discuss suicide potential in the context of continued disconnection from the types of meaningful activities (work, school, friendships, intimate relationships, leisure, and so on) which make life worth living. The point is to alert caretakers to possible signs of psychological distress and to advise them about ways to respond to such distress, including initiating a psychiatric consultation.

Helping caretakers find ways to communicate with their injured loved ones about their feelings is very important, for Shneidman's data indicate that the decision to attempt suicide is typically given long consideration. Unfortunately, in our own experience with head injured persons who committed suicide, in all but one of nine cases, there was little evidence of warning signs (prodromal clues), which Shneidman indicates precede suicide, even in patients who

were receiving psychiatric or psychological support. Nonetheless, caretakers who are on the watch for behavioral changes and other indications of depression or psychological distress may be better equipped than professionals who have limited opportunity to observe the person and whose primary source of information is the patient's self-report. Finally, emphasizing the importance of trying to keep the head injured person engaged in meaningful activity, even when enduring impairments and disabilities preclude involvement in preferred activities, is another means by which treatment personnel can help reduce the chances of existential despair.

In those situations when such a systematic transition from the treatment center to the community is not possible, an alternative approach is to provide written guidelines in the form of a discharge notebook for use by both the patient and the caretakers, and to make an explicit offer to provide advice at anytime, for example, by telephone. A home visit by a member of the rehabilitation team to review the use of the procedures can be valuable in ensuring their proper application. Prearranged regular telephone contacts can be especially valuable, since they increase the likelihood that the caretakers will actually seek help whenever they perceive the need. Just knowing that this is available can be very reassuring, even if continuing care is provided by other community-based agencies. Finally, establishing the availability of short-term readmission to the unit, either for respite or for a "refresher course," can prevent the need for long-term institutional care.

The rehabilitation team must also help to establish connections with a local support network. On a professional level, this may include making sure that the person's primary or family physician is fully informed of the details of ongoing treatment and of the need for pharmacological review. It also includes close liaison with employers, schools, and so on, according to the discharge circumstances. These contacts should be used to help those in the community to understand how best to structure the environment to ensure the greatest likelihood of success as well as to how to respond in problem situations before they develop into full-blown crises. A useful strategy is to establish a relationship between the employer or teacher and a particular member of the team. This can be the key to sustaining the patient's place in the community, which might otherwise be endangered by a breakdown of adequate performance.

The rehabilitation team should also provide the patient and the family with information about meetings of head injury support groups such as the state chapters of the National Head Injury Foundation in the United States, or Headway groups in the United Kingdom. These groups provide a wealth of information and emotional support which is especially important for carers, as Kozloff's findings indicate.[47]

Period of Extended Care

There are some patients whose behavior does not achieve the level of control necessary for acceptance in the community. There are also persons with enduring severe physical or cognitive impairments for whom there are no community living options. Both of these will need long-term care settings.

TYPES AND SOURCES OF BEHAVIORAL DISORDERS

The behavioral disorders that typically preclude return to the community include

1. Behaviors that appear dangerous (to self or others)
2. Behaviors associated with intractable psychosis
3. Behaviors related to extreme dissociative disorders
4. Severe social disinhibition, especially of sexual behavior
5. Other intractable antisocial behaviors

For those with enduring physical and cognitive deficits, early problems usually concern their safety. However, in the longer term they may develop a range of disorders of behavior in response to the lack of meaning and purposeful activities in their daily lives.

ASSOCIATED DANGERS

The dangers of the most extreme of these behavioral disorders are to society at large, as well as to the individual, unless the pa-

tient is appropriately accommodated and contained. In less extreme cases, in the absence of an appropriate placement, the dangers include risks to personal safety and welfare; institutionalization in inappropriate settings or even imprisonment; social rejection and isolation; and atrophy of regained physical, practical, cognitive, and social skills. Moreover, a frequent fate is that the person's behavioral disorders are managed with large doses of drugs, which remove them even further from contact with a meaningful existence, and may also have long-term ill effects on their health.

AIMS OF MANAGEMENT

The aim must be to find or establish settings that provide security, supervision, and structure, in an atmosphere that is conducive to the best possible quality of life and that safeguards the individual's dignity.

MANAGEMENT

Psychiatric facilities providing secure custodial care remain at present the only option for the most seriously disturbed and dangerous. However, the majority of head injured persons who require extended care placement need an alternative to convalescent or nursing homes, which can manage them only through excessive reliance on psychoactive drugs and physical restraint. There is a need to develop long-term care settings in which the untrained staff receive training in physical and behavioral management techniques. Design of the physical plant and use of electronic monitoring devices can enhance security without uneconomically high staffing ratios. The development of a range of choices of meaningful and rewarding activities tailored to the individual's capacity will decrease the incidence of behavioral disorders whose principal source is boredom or psychological distress of an existential kind. Moreover, participation in such activities may promote positive feelings of self-esteem, and so contribute directly to improvements in the quality of life.

Case 1. The Importance of Identifying and Treating Late-Developing Neuropathologic Conditions. A boy of 18 suffered severe head injury in a motorcycle accident. He was in a coma for 3 weeks, and subsequently had PTA of 30 weeks. For 10 months after emergence from the coma, he was almost continuously sedated with phenothiazines: each time sedation was reduced, he became too agitated and aggressive to be managed in the accident ward. He was then admitted to a behavior modification unit. Sedation was discontinued, and phenytoin replaced with carbamazepine. He made steady improvement.

Four months later, progress became punctuated by episodes of irritability and confusion lasting for several hours at a time. After a while, it was noticed that clear fluid flowed from his nose whenever he leant over the billiards table. Investigation revealed multiple dural tears. The neurosurgeon did not believe this could be connected to his behavior, but repaired the leaks to avoid meningitis. The episodes of confusion and irritability ceased, and the patient continued his general progress.

This case highlights the need for periodic evaluation of the underlying sources of behavioral disturbances, especially in situations in which there is an alteration in the nature or frequency of existent behavioral disorders. In particular, it emphasizes the need for assessing possible neuropathological sources.

Case 2. The Importance of Pharmacological Management of Temporolimbic Syndromes.
A man of 22 suffered a severe diffuse injury in a car accident. He was in a coma 8 days, and had PTA of 6 weeks. He had no neurological abnormality, though CT scan showed right frontoparietal contusion, and neuropsychological assessment disclosed some performance and memory deficits. A few months after injury he showed evidence of persistent quasidelusional self-identification with a rock star of his teen years. Nine months after injury he was described as intermittently withdrawn, confused, aggressive, and uncooperative.

Two years after injury, the patient was admitted to a behavioral modification program. He made steady progress in skills and behavior but continued to have episodes of confused and aggressive behavior. After 3 years, these episodes became longer and more frequent, and during them he showed clear evidence of full paranoid delusions and formal thought disorder; nevertheless, between epidoses he continued to progress in personal, social, and occupational skills. Although carbamazepine had been recommended from shortly after admission, it was

not prescribed until a year later. Because of his psychotic state, it took 3 months to persuade him to try the drug. Within 3 weeks his aggressive behavior ceased, and there were no further episodes of psychosis; he was fully insightful about his previous delusions. Moreover, it became apparent that his underlying progress had indeed been excellent: within 2 months he was working in the community and soon afterward obtained independent lodgings. A year and a half later, he had changed jobs three times but was still working. Because of an auto accident while drunk, he had lost his driver's license and was walking 2 miles each way to work. He had continued with carbamazepine, regularly obtaining prescriptions from a local physician.

This case demonstrates that diagnosis and appropriate drug management of temporolimbic syndromes can decrease episodic, explosive behavior and psychotic states that otherwise would have negated the learning of functional skills which occurred during rehabilitation in a behavior modification program.

Case 3. The Importance of Systematic, Highly Structured Behavioral Programming.
An 18-year-old girl suffered severe brainstem damage complicated by hydrocephalus and ventriculitis, in a car accident. She was in a coma for 24 weeks. She was very dysarthric, spoke in an almost autistic, telegrammatic, and ritualistic way, and had a marked left hemiparesis. She behaved in very ritualistic, obsessive-compulsive ways, and persistently hit out, threw objects around, and banged any available surfaces with her hand or fist. These behaviors seriously impeded attempts at rehabilitation.

For the first year and a half after emergence from coma, the patient was treated in a number of head injury rehabilitation programs, several of which claimed to use "behavior modification techniques," but without any change in her behaviors or accessibility to therapies. She was then admitted to a fully structured behavioral unit with token economy, where aberrant behaviors were dealt with in a systematic and consistent way, and cooperation with therapists was constantly reinforced. Interfering behaviors gradually reduced—at first only within the unit, but later generalizing to other settings. After 15 months, she spent a holiday in her home area; she was seen by several professionals previously involved in attempts at her rehabilitation, who were agreeably surprised at her control and cooperativeness, and also at her gains in speech and language and in the quality of her mobility and dexterity. Nine months later, she was discharged home. Behavioral control remained appropriate except in a day center, where her skills at petty theft proved a problem. A year later, there had been some recurrence of the behavioral disorders, though her personal care skills had been maintained. During a further 1 month stay in the unit she rapidly regained the lost ground, which she fully maintained 2 years later.

This case illustrates the need for specialized brain injury rehabilitation units employing intensive, highly structured behavioral management methods to treat severe maladaptive behaviors which otherwise prove an insurmountable barrier to rehabilitation efforts. It also points out the difference between a behavior management program and a treatment facility that simply attempts to employ selective behavior modification techniques in problem cases.

Case 4. The Importance of a Trial of Systematic Behavioral Programming Even With Frontal Lobe Syndrome.
A garage owner aged 33 suffered very severe diffuse brain injury in a car accident. He was in a coma for 2 weeks, had PTA of 20 weeks, but was neurologically normal at 24 weeks. Four years later, his IQ matched preinjury estimates, and MQ matched IQ, but he had shown gradually increasing frontal lobe behavioral disorder, with functional memory problems, gross deficits of planning and judgment, marked social disinhibition, and increasingly bizarre insightless behavior. For example, he pretended to run his "office" from a local cafe; he opened three bank accounts in different variations of his name; he fraudulently obtained three driving licenses in false names; he spent several days and nights in the pouring rain in a cul-de-sac "doing a motor vehicle census"; when visited at home by two physicians for medicolegal examinations, he hid under the bedclothes throughout their stay.

He was admitted (4½ years after injury) to a behavior modification unit, where socially inappropriate behaviors were systematically ignored and prosocial performances positively reinforced. He made a gradual transition to hostel accommodation. After 1 year of treatment, he had selected, negotiated, and furnished an appropriate house for himself, and having surrendered his false driving licenses, had submitted to a driving assessment and successfully passed the test for a new license. He was then discharged, and at 1-year follow-up he was working as a part-time garage attendant. He kept his house in good condition (he left his "daily help" almost nothing to do except the ironing), and prepared at least seven sensible meals a week at home. Five years later, he sent an appropriate postcard from Monte Carlo, where he had driven to see the Rally.

This case emphasizes the efficacy of a systematic behavioral approach even when severe psychiatric disorders related to organic brain damage would lead most treatment personnel and reimbursement agents to doubt the merits of embarking on such a course of treatment due to their estimation of the low probability of success. It is also noteworthy that these results were accomplished with a person 4½ years after injury who was becoming more dysfunctional as time progressed.

Case 5. The Importance of Recognizing the Limits of Behavioral Programming.
A woman of 34 suffered a subarachnoid hemorrhage, with a partial destructive lesion of the left hemisphere, a mild degree of secondary brainstem compression, and more severe, very diffuse, ischemic anoxia, in the last month of her first pregnancy. She was in a coma for 6 weeks. She had a background of good higher educational achievement despite moderate developmental learning disabilities, strong personality traits of "independent-mindedness bordering on obstinacy," and a family history of poor interpersonal relationships, and of histrionic traits.

Two years after her brain injury, on admission from a nursing home to a behavior modification program, she was conscious, and dependent for almost all personal care activities; she had been persistently uncooperative with attempts at active rehabilitation. She had moderate left brachial monoplegia and what was described as "marked bilateral lower limb spasticity" but was in fact classic hysterical contracture. She appeared to have no retrograde memories for some 10 years and to be persistently and totally disoriented. Nevertheless, analysis of her behavior revealed the skillful use of recently acquired information in manipulative ploys. Interview under amylobarbitone and methedrine revealed full orientation in time and place, accurate knowledge about her husband and son (including his birth date and age), and the capability of normal movement except for a mild spastic paresis and dyspraxia of the left arm. Within 4 hours she reverted to her usual state, and further attempts with the technique produced increasingly brief responses which disappeared after the third occasion.

During 3 months of structured behavior modification it was apparent that the tighter the system was, the more aberrant and manipulative her behavior became. Discharge arrangements took 3 months more to complete, and during this time, despite the use of minimal system pressures, her behavior remained extremely aberrant and manipulative, including successfully hidden avoidance of anticonvulsant medication, and the self-infliction of a third degree burn to her foot, achieved by actively wedging it underneath a radiator. On return to the original nursing home, she suffered what appeared to be almost intractable status epilepticus for a week; however, EEG and other evidence showed this to be a "pseudo-seizure" disorder. She remained stably dependent for the next 6 months, but then started refusing to eat and inducing vomiting, and was diagnosed as suffering from anorexia nervosa. Within 3 months she starved herself to death.

This tragic story is an extreme example of the dissociative disorder that may follow very diffuse brain injury and demonstrates the inappropriateness of a behavioral approach in such circumstances. It is also a salutary reminder that even modest success cannot always be achieved despite the most careful attention to the principles discussed in this chapter.

CONCLUSION

This chapter has focused on practical issues related to the assessment and treatment of behavior disorders following head injury. We have emphasized the importance of conducting a systematic assessment of the multiple possible origins of the observed maladaptive behaviors so that treatments selected have the greatest probability of accomplishing medical and rehabilitative goals.

Since the origins of behavioral disorders and the aims of management vary throughout the course of recovery, we have examined issues most germane to the period of medical instability and post-traumatic confusion, the period of formal rehabilitation, the period of community resettlement, and the extended care period.

We have emphasized the need for an integrated approach in which the interdisciplinary rehabilitation team systematically employs a range of options including normalization of the physical environment, use of appropriate physical management strategies, medical management techniques including pharmacological interventions, behavior management principles and techniques, cognitive remediation strategies, and educative and supportive counseling interventions to achieve therapeutic goals. We have argued that professionals skilled in pharmacology and behavior management are indispensible members of such an interdisciplinary team. We have also discussed the value of integrating the family into the rehabilitative team.

We have attempted to integrate practical suggestions that have emerged in the course of our clinical experience with information from the clinical research literature while providing references for readers interested in exploring any particular point in greater depth than could be covered in this brief chapter.

REFERENCES

1. Willmore, LJ: Mechanisms and management of posttraumatic epilepsy. In Miner, M and Wagner, K (eds): Neurotrauma: Treatment, Rehabilitation and Related Issues. Butterworths, Boston, 1986, p 99.
2. Eames, P: Risk benefit considerations in drug treatment. In Wood, R, and Eames, P (eds): Models of Brain Injury Rehabilitation. Chapman & Hall, London, 1989, p 164.
3. Maletsky, BM: The episodic dyscontrol syndrome. Dis Nerv Sys 34:178, 1973.
4. Horn, L and Garland, D: Medical and orthopedic problems. In Rosenthal, M, et al (eds): Rehabilitation of the Adult and Child with Traumatic Brain Injury. FA Davis, Philadelphia, 1989.
5. Cope, DN, Date, E and Mar, E: Serial computerized tomographic evaluations in traumatic head injury. Arch Phys Med Rehabil 69:483, 1988.
6. Levin, HS, Benton, AL and Grossman, RG: Neurobehavioral Consequences of Closed Head Injury. Oxford University Press, Oxford, 1982.

7. Levin, HS and Grossman, RG: Behavioral sequelae of closed head injury: A quantitative study. Arch Neurol 35:720, 1978.

8. Hillbom, E: Schizophrenia-like psychoses after brain trauma. Acta Psychiatr Scand 60:36, 1951.

9. Lishman, WA: The psychiatric sequelae of head injury: A review. Psychol Med 3:304, 1973.

10. Cope, DN: Neuropharmacology and brain damage. In Christensen, AL and Uzzell, BP (eds): Neuropsychological Rehabilitation. Kluwers Academic Publishers, Boston, 1987, p 19.

11. Cope, DN (ed): Neuropharmacology. J Head Trauma Rehabil 2(4), 1987.

12. Barlow, DH and Hersen, M: Single Case Experimental Designs: Strategies for Studying Behavior Change, ed 2. Pergamon Press, New York, 1984.

13. Wood, RL and Eames, P: Application of behaviour modification in the treatment of traumatically brain-injured adults. In Davey, G (ed): Applications of Conditioning Theory. Methuen, London, 1981, p 81.

14. Condeluci, A and Gretz-Lasky, S: Social role valorization: A model for community re-entry. J Head Trauma Rehabil 2(1):49, 1987.

15. Thackrey, M: Therapeutics for Aggression: Psychological/Physical Crisis Intervention. Human Sciences Press, New York, 1986.

16. New York State Office of Mental Retardation and Developmental Disabilities: Physical Intervention Techniques. Bureau of Staff Development and Training, New York State Office of Mental Retardation and Developmental Disabilities, Albany, NY, 1980.

17. Florida Department of Health and Rehabilitative Services: Aggression Control Techniques: Instructor's Guide. State of Florida, Department of Health and Rehabilitative Services, Tallahassee, FL, 1983.

18. Belanger, N and Mullen, JK: Safe Physical Management. Safe Physical Management Associates, New Bloomfield, PA, 1984.

19. Haffey, WJ and Scibak, JW: Management of aggressive behavior following traumatic brain injury. In Ellis, DW and Christensen, AL (eds): Neuropsychologicalal Treatment of Head Injury. Martinus Nijhoff, The Hague, 1989, p 317.

20. Trimble, MR: Psychopharmacology of Epilepsy. John Wiley & Sons, New York, 1985.

21. Sheard, MH: Lithium in the treatment of aggression. J Nerv Ment Dis 160:108, 1975.

22. Sheard, MH and Marini, JL: Treatment of human aggressive behavior: 4 case studies of the effect of lithium. Comprehensive Psychiatry 19:37, 1978.

23. Sheard, MH et al: The effect of lithium on impulsive aggressive behavior in man. Am J Psychiatry 133:1409, 1976.

24. Monroe, RR: Anticonvulsants in the treatment of aggression. J Nerv Ment Dis 160:119, 1975.

25. Tunks, ER and Dermer, SW; Carbamazepine in the dyscontrol syndrome associated with limbic system dysfunction. J Nerv Ment Dis 164:56, 1977.

26. Rao, N, Jellinek, HM and Woolston, DC: Agitation in closed head injury: Haloperidol effects on rehabilitation outcome. Arch Phys Med Rehabil 66:30, 1985.

27. Jackson, RD, Corrigan, JD and Arnett, JA: Amitriptyline for agitation in head injury. Arch Phys Med Rehabil 66:180, 1985.

28. Cope, DN: The Pharmacology of Attention and Memory. J Head Trauma Rehabil 1(3):34, 1986.

29. Lipper, S and Tuchman, M: Treatment of chronic post-traumatic organic brain syndrome with dextroamphetamine: First reported case. J Nerv Ment Dis 162:366, 1976.

30. Bandura, A: Principles of Behavior Modification. Holt, Rinehart and Winston, New York, 1969.

31. Kazdin, AE: Behavior Modification in Applied Settings. Dorsey, Homewood, IL, 1980.

32. Sulzer-Azaroff, B and Mayer, GR: Applying Behavior-Analysis Procedures with Children and Youth. Holt, Rinehart and Winston, New York, 1977.

33. Wood, RL: Behaviour disorders following severe brain injury: Their presentation and psychological management. In Brooks, N (ed): Closed Head Injury: Psychological, Social and Family Consequences. Oxford University Press, Oxford, 1984, p 195.

34. Whitman, TL, Scibak, JW and Reid, DH: Behavior Modification with the Severely and Profoundly Retarded. Academic Press, New York, 1983.

35. Bernstein, GS et al: Behavioral Habilitation Through Proactive Programming. Brookes, Baltimore, 1981.

36. Foxx, RM: Increasing Behavior of Severely Retarded and Autistic Persons. Research Press, Champaign, IL, 1984.

37. Eames, P and Wood, RL: Rehabilitation after severe brain injury: A special unit approach to behaviour disorders. Int Rehabil Med 7:130, 1985.

38. Eames, P and Wood, RL: Rehabilitation after severe brain injury: A follow-up study of a behaviour modification approach. J Neurol Neurosurg Psychiatry 48:613, 1985.

39. Malec, J: Training the brain-injured client in behavioral self-management skills. In Edelstein, B and Couture, G (eds): Behavioral Assessment and Rehabilitation of the Traumatically Brain-Damaged. Plenum Press, New York, 1984, p 121.

40. Wood, RL: Management of attention disorders following brain injury. In Wilson, BA and Moffat, N (eds): Clinical Management of Memory Problems. Croom Helm, London, 1984, p 148.

41. Ben-Yishay, Y et al: Neuropsychologic rehabilitation: Quest for a holistic approach. Semin Neurol 5:252, 1985.

42. Ben-Yishay, Y et al: Relationship between employability and vocational outcome after intensive holistic cognitive rehabilitation. J Head Trauma Rehabil 2(1):35, 1987.

43. Prigatano, GP et al: Neuropsychological rehabilitation after closed head injury in young adults. J Neurol Neurosurg Psychiatry 47:505, 1984.

44. Scherzer, BP: Rehabilitation following severe head trauma: Results of a three-year program. Arch Phys Med Rehabil 67:366, 1986.

45. Fryer, LJ and Haffey, W: Cognitive rehabilitation and community readaptation: Outcomes from two program models. J Head Trauma Rehabil 2(3):51, 1987.

46. Muir, CA and Haffey, WJ: Psychological and neuropsychological interventions in the mobile mourning process. In Edelstein, B and Couture, G (eds): Behavioral Assessment and Rehabilitation of the Traumatically Brain-Damaged. Plenum Press, New York, 1984, p 247.

47. Kozloff, R: Networks of social support and the outcome from severe head injury. J Head Trauma Rehabil 2(3):14, 1987.

48. Brooks, N et al: The five year outcome of severe

blunt head injury: A relative's view. J Neurol Neurosurg Psychiatry 49:764, 1986.

49. Brooks, N et al: The effects of severe head injury on patient and relative within seven years of injury. J Head Trauma Rehabil 2(3):1, 1987.

50. Brooks, N: Personal Communication, May 7, 1987.

51. Shneidman, E, Farberow, N and Litman, R: The Psychology of Suicide. Jason Aronson, New York, 1976.

52. Lezak, M: Relationships between personality disorders, social disturbances, and physical disability following traumatic brain injury. J Head Trauma Rehabil 2(1):57, 1987.

Chapter 29

Methods of Family Intervention

CRAIG A. MUIR, Ph.D.
MITCHELL ROSENTHAL, Ph.D.
LINDA N. DIEHL, R.N., M.S.

The true impact of a traumatic head injury is a collison between the head injury and all the survivor's loved ones. A primary focus of rehabilitation must be to limit the number of victims and the amount of victimization that stems from each head injury. The family members and other loved ones of the traumatic head injury survivor are crucial partners in the comprehensive rehabilitation of the head injured adult.

It has been well documented that families experience extensive behavioral and psychologic burden as a result of traumatic head injuries.[1] Furthermore, it is becoming clear that for many survivors the family will often be the final or at least long-term home for many survivors. Because the physical, cognitive, and behavioral sequelae of head injury are so numerous and diverse, the rehabilitation effort cannot be considered satisfactory if it is confined to the survivor alone. The treatment program must include the home environment and the community to which the survivor usually returns.

This chapter briefly reviews the effects of traumatic head injury on families. The review is followed by a conceptualization of the family as a system and a description of the head injury as an event in the family life cycle. Types of interventions with families and family members are described and research methods surveyed.

EFFECTS ON THE FAMILY

The facts that traumatic head injury is burdensome to many families and that the burden persists have become increasingly clear. As early as 1972, Panting and Merry[2] found that 60 percent of the relatives of head injured survivors needed some stress-related medication, which they had not needed previously, as a direct result of emotional burdens placed on them by the head injury sequelae. Bond[3] and Brooks and McKinlay[4] found that family stress was more related to patients' mental disabilities than to physical disabilities.

The stresses attendant upon traumatic brain injury apparently do not decrease over time like the stresses related to other taumatic injuries. Rosenbaum and Najenson[5] found that wives of spinal cord injured men experienced significantly less depression and emotional strain by the end of 1 year than they had at 6 months postinjury, but there was no similar decrease in emotional stress for the wives of traumatic brain injury survivors. Brooks and colleagues in Glasgow[6-8] reported on types and levels of burden experienced by the relatives of 55 patients at 3, 6, and 12 months postinjury. Their findings supported the notion that the degree and intensity of burden does not significantly decrease over the first year. More recently, Brooks and associates[9] surveyed families up to 7 years after head injury and did not find a significant reduction of reported family burden.

Data also strongly suggest that survivors of severe head injury will frequently become more dependent on their families for finances and services. Families must often assume the major responsibility for the survivors' long-term care.[10]

433

It may be concluded that the head injury traumatizes the entire family, not just the identified patient. The families of traumatic head injury survivors must therefore be considered integral to the rehabilitation process. The following is a model for understanding families' responses to head injury and some of the methods of including them in rehabilitation.

THEORETICAL FRAMEWORK FOR FAMILY INTERVENTIONS

Our theoretical model is based on conceptualizing each person's family as a personal system which experiences traumatic head injury to one of its members as a partial death and reacts with a complex mourning process.[11-13]

Personal System

The family may be conceptualized as a "system" in many ways:[14, 15]

1. All of the individuals are psychologically and behaviorally connected to each other.

2. These connections develop over the life cycle of the family and can be clearly described.

3. A significant change in the behavior of any member produces changes for all the members of the system.

4. Most events result in changes of individual parameters in continuous manner ("first-order" changes), but other events alter the way the entire system functions ("second-order" changes).

5. Family systems may be grouped along various dimensions, but each is in some ways unique.

We have chosen to call the family system of a head injury survivor a "personal system" to emphasize the inclusion of friends and other important nonrelatives. Relationships with nonrelatives help to define each family. Close friendships, for example, are an important but often neglected part of family systems interventions.[16] Interactions with friends often change significantly after a severe head injury; the immediate family frequently becomes the primary resource for the head injured person.[10, 17]

Important elements of personal systems are (1) the developmental life cycle, (2) roles, and (3) changes.

Each personal system is composed of individuals who interact with each other in characteristic ways. These interaction patterns have evolved over the entire developmental life cycle.[18-20] The patterns are affected by natural changes that occur along the family's life cycle such as having children and being promoted at work. In Western cultures a major culmination occurs when the children become individuated enough to separate from the original family unit. Traditionally, they develop a subsystem and carry on the cycle.

The uniqueness of each person and the uniqueness of the relationships that develop guarantee that each personal system is somewhat different from any other, as well as being somewhat the same. It is this unique set of people and their long-developed, characteristic ways of interacting, that comprise the personal system.

Roles and role changes are common topics in the head injury literature and in clinical experience.[17, 21] "Roles refer to the entirety of the expectations and norms that a group (for example, a family) has in regard to an individual's position and behavior within the group. A role is thus equivalent to the behavioral expectations that are directed toward an individual within a given situation or social context"[22] (p. 301). Two established roles in a nuclear family system are those of husband and wife. However, the expectations for the persons in those roles will vary somewhat from family to family. For example, in some families the husband is expected to be the primary generator of income for necessities. If the wife works outside the home she is expected only to earn "extra" money for things the family could not ordinarily afford. In other families, both spouses are expected to be full-time wage earners.

Another very important area of role definition is between parents and children. Generational roles and the boundaries between them are crucial for the development of children's individual personalities so that they may separate from their parents.[23]

The magnitude of a change in a personal system may be measured in many ways.

These include the effects on individuals and effects on the personal system itself. Most system parameters are flexible enough to accommodate ordinary events in the family life cycle. These "first-order" changes can be managed by the personal system as it is. Adaptation to first-order changes do not compromise the structure of the personal system itself. "Second-order" changes are those that interact with general family system rules, or with rules of a specific family, in ways that do require alteration of the structure or internal order of the personal system.[24, 25]

An example of first-order change is when a wife who has only been expected to earn money for "extras" has to work briefly outside the home to supplement income, or to become the sole wage earner, because the husband is temporarily unemployed. Although the situation may be stressful for individuals, no changes in the ways the husband and wife relate are required, and the children maintain their roles as well. When the husband is employed again the other family members go back to their customary behaviors.

The necessity for the wife to have a permanent job outside the home, however, would represent a major shift in role expectations within this family. This "second-order" change will usually produce other alterations in the family system, such as the wife feeling guilty about not spending enough time with the children and the husband feeling that he has permanently lost an important part of his role as provider. If the role shift is of greater magnitude relative to the particular family system, the subsequent impact on the system will also be greater. The most common example after severe head injury is that the husband is "reduced" to earning only "extra" money, while the wife must earn the necessities. The systemic changes are even more drastic if the husband cannot maintain "gainful" employment at all. Words like "reduced" and "gainful" reflect role expectations in the broader culture; inability to fulfill those expectations causes a significant loss of value for the individual.

A change of even greater relative magnitude occurs if the husband not only loses his income-generating capacity but also changes behavioral repertoires so completely that generational boundaries are blurred or permanently altered. The person who previously held a spouse/parent role is then reduced to a child role within the marriage, and may even reverse roles with the children in the family. Blurring or reversing of generational roles is considered to be evidence of a pathologic family system and may be most often found in families with severely disturbed offspring.[26] This degree of damage to the family system is not uncommon after a severe head injury.[27, 28] These second-order changes can be catastrophic. The entire family system may destabilize and break down, requiring extensive restructuring of roles before even a semblance of equilibrium is reached. A more common result is permanent emotional deprivation for all members of the family system.

The majority of traumatic head injuries are neurologically subtle, and therefore are labeled "mild" or "minor." The neurobehavioral sequelae may be so mild that they are not perceived by casual friends. Close friends and family members are more likely to be aware of differences in the person's abilities and behaviors but not of the underlying causes or of their ramifications for patient and family. Recognizing that neurologically minor head injuries can have major consequences, Boll and Kay[29] suggested that the best indicator of the "severity" of a head injury may be the severity of the resulting dysfunction. In a family systems formulation, the "severity" of the dysfunction is defined by preinjury role expectations. The following case is an example of a "minor" injury with severe family system consequences.

Case 1. A 29-year-old woman had a motor vehicle accident, after which she suffered about 1 hour of coma and several days of post-traumatic amnesia. She recovered so well that she could return to her job at a bank, but it became clear over the next 6 months that she could not handle the same level of complex tasks as before the injury. She returned for outpatient cognitive rehabilitation and counseling, then went on to a local college and eventually earned a business degree. With help from her supervisor and many others she was finally able to do the same job that she had been doing before her injury. Her family and friends were very pleased, and her supervisor felt justly satisfied. The patient became profoundly depressed and began to drink heavily. After a crisis she entered psychotherapy. She had secretly held onto the hope that she would once again be competitive at a very high level, just as she had as a child in a family system which placed great value on intellectual achievement. Before the accident she had been a rising star in her profession, with superior performance ratings and offers from the corporation of advanced schooling. Afterward she was faced with the final verdict that she was as high in the company as she would ever go. This required second-order changes in the way she valued people (including herself) and in her relationships with her family, which had shifted its achievement hopes to her younger brother and treated her with the solicitude reserved for the ill.

Partial Death

The losses suffered by a head injured survivor can be conceptualized as a "partial death."[30, 31] Partial deaths can consist of those first-order changes everyone experiences as they move from what they once were to what they are becoming. Change in itself produces loss, regardless of the positive or negative nature of the change.[32] Major losses are partial deaths of a more serious nature; they may produce extreme stress on the members of the personal system and require second-order role restructuring.

The partial deaths that result from head injury vary from "minor" residual symptoms to virtually complete characterologic change in the survivor and subsequent major changes in what is expected of the other family members. In some cases, the survivor's family members report that fundamental aspects of the survivor's personality have changed, that the person they could depend on to fulfill their expectations and needs no longer exists. In other words, that the person they knew and loved is "dead." Since the recovery process is an uncertain one, filled with many reasons for hope and despair, feelings about the changes may continue to be in turmoil for months and years. This uncertainty and the concomitant disorganization of the grieving process have led to the coining of the term "mobile mourning."

Mobile Mourning

Complete death is comparatively frequent and straightforward. Ritualized means of coping with it have been developed in the culture and in the family life cycle. Unlike the finality that accompanies an actual death, partial death leaves the members of the personal system in a state of extended turmoil. In effect, they are uncertain what losses to mourn because it is not clear which losses in physical and mental function are permanent and which are transient. In contrast to the classic formulations of the mourning process—that is, a progression through stages of denial, euphoric hope, despair, and resignation[33, 34]—the uncertainties about the nature of the losses from head injury produce long-term disorganization of the mourning process.[35–38] Fluctuations along continua from euphoria to despair and from mild resentment to rage may go on indefinitely because the patient continues to change from time to time. Although the terminology used to describe this process varies,[28] three things seem clear: (1) family reactions are highly stressful because of the nature of "recovery" from head injury; (2) family system responses are more variable than they would be after complete deaths; (3) families do not necessarily progress through stages or emotional reactions in an invariant sequence.

Initial refusal to acknowledge severe loss is an adaptive mechanism that prevents complete disruption of the family system.[39] However, if denial persists as the primary response there is greater likelihood that a pathologic condition will be created—that is, one in which longstanding role expectations are tenaciously maintained about a person who can no longer fulfill them. A salient problem with traumatic head injury survival is that often there are enough indications of improvement over several years to allow denial or "unrealistic" expectations to persist unchecked for months—or even years—after the injury.

The mourning process after head injury is intense and disorganized. Professional intervention is often required to facilitate grieving and bring some degree of equilibrium back to the personal system. Since head injury rehabilitation requires an interdisciplinary effort over a prolonged period of time, most members of the rehabilitation team at any given stage of the process are likely to have frequent contact with the survivor and his or her personal system. Consequently, there is a need for all of the members of the treatment team to be aware of the complexities of the issues involved and to be prepared to participate in what will hopefully be a process of adaptation.

ASSESSING THE NEED FOR INTERVENTION

Mental health interventions were initially developed for people who were voluntarily coming to a professional for help and had a fairly high level of sophistication. More recently a multiplicity of therapeutic modalities have been developed. Research and polemics have focused on finding out which interventions work best with different patient groups, including those who come for help involuntarily. Types of interventions are typically compared as to their effectiveness with groups of patients who have the same diagnosis or type of diagnosis. For example, drug therapy using high doses of phenothiazines has been compared to psychotherapy, with schizophrenic patients. But these data would not be considered applicable to patients with a diagnosis of anxiety neurosis or of manic-depressive disorder. There are now many techniques to deal with a wide variety of diagnostic groups.

Family members of head trauma survivors do not necessarily fit any of these patient groups, however. More precisely, some of the members may fit into standard diagnostic categories, while others do not. As we have seen, traumatic brain injury can produce upsetting reactions in family members who were more or less well adjusted before the injury. Many of their problems are due to the profound effects of a traumatic event rather than longstanding difficulties in their everyday lives. Furthermore, family members generally come to rehabilitation programs expecting help for their injured relative, not for themselves. If invited to see a mental health professional, many family members will resist because they do not view themselves as the identified patient or in need of counseling. These differences between traditional psychotherapy patients and the members of a head injured family system must be kept in mind even when a family member presents a traditional symptom picture. For example, sending a family member to a traditional mental health clinic may be ineffective.

There is an assumption that certain attributes of family systems cause (or at least contribute to) certain types of psychological problems. While there may be data to support this concept in traditional mental health research, that is not the case with traumatic head injury. Rather, the grouping is simply based on the existence of a common trauma. There are a few studies that indicate that head injury is more common in some family contexts than in others—for example, in familial alcoholism.[40] However, these interesting beginnings are not yet helpful in identifying traits of head injury family systems. When data suggest that "families of the head injured" behave in particular ways, care must be taken not to make implicit or unwarranted assumptions about homogeneity or causality.

Grouping head injury families together for treatment and research is helpful to the extent that there are some needs or responses which are common enough to form the basis of therapeutic approaches. However, we must expect large amounts of unexplained variance in theoretical formulations and research that categorize families only according to the head injury variable. For example, Lezak[28] makes it clear that families will vary widely in their passage through response stages, and that some families will not go through some of the stages at all.

The *meaning* of a head injury is defined by each personal system. The interventions for each family must also fit each personal system. Some needs are exhibited or expressed by a large percentage of families, while other needs may exist in a small percentage. Considerable variation among families, and among members of a given family, in the use and valuing of intervention modalities is to be expected and is not necessarily a negative outcome. Rather, the rehabilitation team should decide what to offer families based on explicit criteria and then derive outcome goals from those criteria.

A team may decide to offer families what most of them seem to want and need, or to provide treatment for those who are most distressed. If a family intervention is provided in the belief that the majority of families want and need it, then outcome criteria should include attendance by a majority of families and the meeting of their explicit needs. If, on the other hand, a treatment is designed to assist those families that are most disturbed by the head injury, then the percentage of families attending is less important than that the program meets the needs of that identified group of families.

Intervention strategies have been developed with a wide variety of criteria. Examples of these groupings are families who expressed severe systemic problems 1 to 7 years postinjury and who volunteered for a 20-week family training project;[41] families of head injured persons who came to a clinic several months or years after injury;[2, 9] and families who agreed to be interviewed or otherwise studied because the survivor was having ongoing problems several months after a "minor" head injury.[42] These groupings have usually been based on extensive clinical experience and research, and should not be lightly discarded. Rather, the needs of the families that attend each type of intervention must be assessed explicitly, and evaluation criteria must be based on those assessments.

Examples of needs that are very frequently expressed by families after traumatic head injury are information about head injury and better communication with the rehabilitation program. All but one of the 16 families who volunteered for a 16- to 20-week training program also wanted more education about brain injury despite having experienced formal rehabilitation programs.[43] Other research also indicates that roughly half of responding family members are dissatisfied with the communication between themselves and clinicians caring for the survivor. Thomsen[44] found that of 40 relatives interviewed, 22 were favorably disposed but 18 were dissatisfied with the information they had received. Oddy and colleagues[45] found that 40 percent of the relatives in their study were somewhat critical of services received, and the most common criticism involved communication between themselves and medical staff. Panting and Merry[2] also indicated that about 50 percent of the relatives were dissatisfied with services or with "communication."

Rehabilitation is the interaction of two highly developed systems: the personal system of the patient and the human system of the rehabilitation team. Each system has defined roles and expectations for its members, but also has expectations about the members of the other system. When these intersystem expectations differ or for other reasons are not met, confusing conflicts often result which will impede therapy unless they are untangled.

Life within a rehabilitation team would be less complicated if "psychological" and "family" issues were always readily identifiable as such and could then be passed on to the person in the system whose role is to treat these sorts of problems. Family system issues frequently do not present in such a clear-cut manner. Furthermore, family members may identify a non–mental health team member with a more obviously helpful role (for example, nurse, physical therapist) to trust with their concerns. Rehabilitation team members are rarely asked "simple" questions.

Case 2. A nurse in a rehabilitation program was asked by a patient's brother if people should generally maintain positive attitudes around the patients. The nurse replied affirmatively and the brother soon left. Two hours later the nurse found herself being berated by the patient's wife for taking sides with the patient's family against her. The situation that underlay this bewildering encounter was that the parents and siblings of the patient were responding to his injury as they would have to a child who has been hurt and needs to be protected; the wife was responding to the drastic change in her role from primary child-raiser to primary income-producer and family financial manager. The patient's brother saw the wife talking earnestly to the patient, who was crying; that was when he talked to the nurse. He then proceeded to call his mother and father and tell them that the wife was making the patient cry by upsetting him about financial matters and, further, that a staff member had agreed that the wife should not do such a thing. The mother proceeded to call the wife and there was an angry exchange. Actually, it turned out that the patient had been sitting in his wheelchair on the patio and had tried to move himself more into the sunshine but ended up tipping himself into the bushes instead. Someone had just rescued him and he was still crying when his wife came out and sat down next to him.

In this incident a patient's personal system is in a state of disarray. The various members chose reasonable explanations of observed behavior in their attempts to move toward greater comfort, or equilibrium. They then tried to gather evidence to bolster their positions. Every rehabilitation team member thus becomes part of the personal system processes whether intending to or not, merely by interacting with the patient.

Since every team member is potentially involved with the family system, the issue is not who should be involved but rather how the various team members can optimize family adjustment. It is not feasible for all rehabilitation professionals to be equally trained in family interventions, or to take large amounts of time to deal with families. The issue, then, is which members of the team are comfortable and competent to perform various types of family interventions. The four-level PLISSIT model, originally developed by Annon for sexual counseling,[46] may provide a helpful framework.

In the PLISSIT model, the four increasingly intensive interventions are termed *Permission, Limited Information, Specific Suggestions,* and *Intensive Therapy*. To apply this model to family interventions with brain injury, one might say that all staff should be trained to give "permission" for family members to vent their concerns about their loved one and to handle these emotional events supportively. "Limited information" may be conceptualized as a continuum. On one end of the continuum are the specific details of the patient's daily behaviors such as schedule, compliance with therapies, bowel and bladder program, and food intake. At the other end of the information spectrum are educational materials and programs which encompass more general or more difficult questions about the nature of brain injury and the patient's progress and prognosis. All team members should be able to provide the more specific details about a given patient or be able to locate the information fairly quickly for a family member. Educational interventions such as those described below might be the appropriate vehicles for more complex information. The third level, "specific suggestions," would best be handled by each patient's core team members who could provide some focused information about the patient's prognosis, transfer techniques, and so forth. Finally, the fourth level, "intensive therapy," would be provided by team members trained to engage in family counseling or family therapy.

TYPES OF FAMILY INTERVENTIONS

Family intervention techniques may be discussed in two broad categories: those in which the lead is taken by rehabilitation professionals and those conducted by non-professionals (i.e., by peers/family members). Given the striking growth of family-initiated support groups, there may soon be a third category of interventions in which some portions of the intervention are provided by trained family members and other portions by professionals. For example, the technical details of neurobehavioral sequelae may best be provided by professionals, while mutual support and confrontation may best be provided by other family members.

Six categories of interventions will be considered below: (1) patient-family education, (2) family counseling, (3) family therapy, (4) behavioral family training, (5) respite care, and (6) family support groups.

Patient-Family Education

Data that large numbers of survivors' family members want information about head injury have been responded to with enthusiasm. Patient-family education has become an established technique for improving communication and giving information in head injury rehabilitation programs throughout the United States. It is currently the most prevalent format for family intervention.

FAMILY CONFERENCES

Family conferences may be interdisciplinary meetings that include virtually all of the team members or are limited to selected professionals. The purposes of these conferences are to share information among survivor, family, and rehabilitation staff and to provide a valuable forum for jointly defining and modifying goals. The conference is also a forum in which the members of the rehabilitation system interact directly with the members of the personal system. Priorities and expectations of each system are displayed and may be discussed openly. As an ongoing part of the rehabilitation program these sessions may also provide the opportunity for enhanced goal and role negotiation between the two systems. For example, a family system that takes a passive role vis-à-vis medical professionals may be encouraged to be more assertive; conversely, family members who expect all their questions to be answered may be helped to become students of head injury rehabilitation.

EDUCATIONAL GROUP APPROACHES

Group learning activities can be used to provide specific information, promote socialization, and reinforce what family members are learning in the various therapeutic programs. Adults have traditionally been exposed to educational activities in the group setting. This structure may be used to strengthen family members' active participation in the rehabilitation program as a learning activity rather than taking on more passive roles as recipients of a treatment activity.[47-50]

A prototype for educating patients and families about head injury was developed by Diehl and colleagues[51] at the Medical College of Virginia. In this program, head injured individuals and their families attended a series of 10 to 12 sessions. Content of the sessions typically included some or all of the following topics:

1. The nature of traumatic brain injury
2. The rehabilitation process
3. Coping with change
4. The role of siblings in rehabilitation
5. Self-care
6. Use of community resources
7. Safety and risk factors
8. Use of leisure time
9. Vocational rehabilitation
10. Sexuality

The groups generally consisted of six to eight survivors and their families, and were held once or twice weekly for up to 10 weeks. Active participation, role negotiation, and mutual goal-setting were major objectives for the groups, in addition to passing on information. Patients and family members became more involved in the rehabilitation process and increased their knowledge of head injury, its implications, and its management. Benefits for the rehabilitation program included increased awareness of patient and family needs, more standardized descriptions of health care procedures, and increased sensitivity to family systems' expectations.

Family Counseling

The purpose of supportive family counseling is to help a family deal with feelings of loss and helplessness. It may also help family members understand and resign themselves to the disability and its potential consequences. If the counseling is conducted with one family at a time (as opposed to multiple-family group counseling), there is ample opportunity for assessment of the family system and subsequent tailoring of treatment to meet specific system needs. Family members are given the opportunity to express their feelings of guilt, anguish, anger, sadness, and loss. As discharge from a rehabilitation program approaches, many families express apprehension because they have been given an implicit message that a plateau has been reached. During the transition from hospital or rehabilitation program to community, the family counselor can play a key role in helping the family anticipate future problems and be more psychologically and physically prepared to assume the burden of care. This is particularly true if the counselor has identified the areas of most probable stress for the particular family. If, for example, a particular family system rejects expressions of disability or of potential family burden because of a commitment to "positive thinking," the counselor can know that and be available after discharge to help the family deal with realities that are not amenable to positive thinking.

Brief counseling may also be appropriate for groups that are smaller than the entire family but involve more than one person. The most typical family subgroup in head injury rehabilitation involves the parents or spouse of the survivor, though at other times the siblings may want to come in as a small group without parental oversight, or the blood relatives may want to talk without the presence of in-laws.

It should be emphasized that this level of counseling is primarily for the purpose of improving day-to-day functioning rather than for delving into long-term or severe conflicts. For example, communications may be clarified, differing interpretations of specialists' statements may be resolved, or first-order role changes may be agreed upon. It is not a setting in which the participants may be given permission—explicitly or implicitly—to express whatever pent-up feelings they have been suppressing. The participants usually have to get along together after the sessions, so it is important that a mild, supportive atmosphere be established by the therapist. It is not unusual for family members to take counseling sessions as an opportunity to say things that are destructive of family relationships, feeling that this is a forum where "anything goes" as long as it is honest. Firm control of the group process is sometimes necessary to prevent harm from being done.

Individual family members often express, or otherwise demonstrate, the need for individual counseling sessions. This may occur for a variety of reasons, such as greater acceptance of professional counseling help by one individual than by the rest of the family members, the need to express feelings that would be too uncomfortable in the presence of other family members, or simply greater comfort with individual counseling than with group process. The following is a case example of brief, supportive intervention.

Case 3. The family member was a 26-year-old woman who was obviously distraught during family conference and requested individual counseling. She expressed intense internal, family, and community pressures to maintain her severely head injured husband in their home. They had three small children; the patient needed complete physical care and was aggressive with the wife and children. Three successive rehabilitation programs had been unable to help him and had recommended placement in a skilled nursing facility. The wife's resources were exhausted, emotionally and physically, by the task of caring for her husband and children. She was acutely aware of the effects of this situation on the children. But her community church had held prayer meetings and charity events to fund additional rehabilitation and to request divine intervention on the patient's behalf. Being a deeply religious person, she could not reconcile herself to placing her husband outside the family home lest "Our Lord Jesus comes to heal him and he's not there." After several sessions, she was asked why, if Jesus could find the family home, He could not locate the patient in a nursing home. She responded that "No one ever put it that way before," and proceeded rapidly to the decision that she had not been "trusting in the Lord enough. I just have to leave it in His hands and take care of our children." She was able to use the funds that had been donated for her husband to provide some rehabilitation within the nursing home.

This family member's willingness to make such a dramatic decision was due primarily to her being in crisis; that is, the situation had stressed her to the point that she was ready to make second-order changes in her role expectations. Assessment of the structure and internal rules of this particular family system was necessary to identify the primary needs and conflicts. For example, the reactions of her church, community, and the rest of the patient's family had to be considered carefully, particularly because nursing home placement is a very controversial topic in head injury rehabilitation.

Family Therapy

Family therapy may be defined as "a professionally organized attempt to produce behavioral change in a disturbed marital or family unit by essentially interactive, nonphysical methods."[52] In the case of traumatic brain injury, family therapy can be useful for families with a premorbid history of dysfunction or those in which the presence of a head injured relative has created catastrophic reactions, maladaptive communication, and dysfunction interaction patterns within the family system.

The goals of family therapy are to (1) assess the family system in depth and tailor intervention methods accordingly; (2) provide supportive environments in which family members can freely verbalize feelings about the trauma and its effects upon them; (3) educate the family about the nature of their communication or interaction problems and develop methods for resolving conflicts within the relationship patterns of the family system; and (4) examine, clarify, and try to restructure roles and responsibilities.

There are many ways of classifying family therapy approaches.[53, 54] Examples of approaches frequently used in head injury rehabilitation include (1) emphasizing the mutuality of responsibility for the family problems and shifting the burden of causality from the identified patient to the dysfunctional areas of the family system; (2) focusing on, and strengthening, the positive aspects of the family system; (3) exploring dysfunctional interaction patterns by reenacting family conflicts and assisting family members to substitute conflict-resolution strategies which are acceptable within their system; and (4) prescribing "homework assignments" for the family to practice outside the sessions to foster generalization of behavior change.[55, 56]

Psychotherapy for individual family members is used for roughly the same reasons as individual counseling sessions. The major difference is that it is best reserved for those individuals whose conflicts are not amenable to the briefer techniques or for those who are willing and able to explore their responses in greater depth.

> **Case 4.** The father of a 36-year-old woman suffered a head injury which severely limited his ability to experience or express any feelings beyond his own immediate, concrete needs. His speech was also compromised by dysarthria and extreme tangentiality. The woman had participated in family and individual counseling sessions during his in-patient rehabilitation program; she provided much of the transportation and home-therapy for him during out-patient treatment. The day he was discharged from out-patient treatment she became very distraught and ended up screaming at his speech therapist that her father couldn't even say "three little words."
>
> During psychotherapy sessions she was able to identify and eventually resolve long-standing conflicts centering on emotional deprivation and the need to do so much for her father that he would finally say "I love you" to her.

It is not uncommon for the spouse or partner of the brain injured survivor to experience great distress and have concerns about their marital relationship. The roles of relative equality may change dramatically to care-receiver and caregiver, and generational role expectations may result in the survivor being seen more as a child than as a peer. The spouse may then be unable to perceive the survivor as an appropriate person with whom to share intimacy and sexual relations. A spouse of a brain injured survivor may feel that "I am now living with a stranger."

Similarly, the head injured survivor may experience distress and discomfort in relating to the able-bodied spouse. Low self-esteem, impaired body image, and feelings of loss may permeate their existence and greatly limit their capacity to adopt anything besides an egocentric perspective. In addition, cognitive-communicative and be-

havioral impairments may further alter the way spouses relate to each other. The process of coping with the reality of neurological and psychological residuals, and determining future directions for the relationship may be aided by professional marital therapy.

Behavioral Family Training

Behavioral family training may be defined as the establishment of specific, operationalized goals and techniques for teaching family members or family systems to more effectively manage the problems presented by traumatic head injury. Work with families of other long-term disability groups has indicated the value of this approach in such difficult and diverse areas as training communication and problem-solving skills to the families of relapsing schizophrenics[57] and teaching behavior management skills to families of acting-out children.[58] The primary difference between family training and family counseling or therapy is that family training focuses on more behavioral methods of problem solving with specific, pretraining objectives.[59–61]

Family training in the field of head injury may take many forms. A multiple-family group model was adopted in a recent study.[62] An initial group of nine families was taken through a clearly defined training program consisting of 18 weeks of didactic presentations, homework, supportive and confrontive discussions, data gathering, and behavioral management interventions. The overall result was the creation of a problem-solving–oriented family support group. Behavioral changes of major or minor importance were observed in a majority of families and in the survivors.

Respite Care

Respite from caretaking activities has come to have a life of its own: many day treatment, day care, residential, and nursing home programs provide formal or de facto respite care. Respite care is increasingly an option for families and their settlements with insurance companies for the lifelong care of the survivor. Respite care can be an extremely valuable mode of family intervention, enabling families to continue their caretaking of the survivors in a somewhat less stressful fashion, and at times alleviating the need to place the survivor in a full-time residential or extended nursing home facility.

DAY TREATMENT PROGRAMS

Day treatment or day hospital programs aim to provide a therapeutic environment during daytime hours, following which the survivors return to their homes or other residential quarters. It is generally the purpose of these programs to provide active, therapeutic programming that results in documented progress in attaining daily living and vocational skills on the part of the survivor, as well as actively involving family members in the therapeutic program. The National Directory of Head Injury Rehabilitation Services[63] listed approximately 170 such programs in the United States, and new programs are developed on a frequent basis. Day treatment programs provide a therapeutic environment for the survivors at much lower cost than hospital or residential programs and allow family members time to continue with their own lives. In addition, many of these programs offer family education, counseling, and therapy.

Many families choose to use day care or residential programs periodically to meet the need for family rest or a family vacation from caretaking responsibilities. Other families and survivors choose to be involved with day care programs for 3 to 5 days per week on an extended basis. Many day programs provide a daily activity program for survivors whose progress toward therapeutic goals is inadequate to meet the requirements of various funding agencies. These day care or maintenance programs can provide a very positive environment for the survivors outside of the family home, and also provide respite and resources for the family members.

Family Support Groups

Some families who have experienced the trauma of head injury may be able to provide emotional support and information to each other that cannot be provided by rehabilitation professionals. The family-to-family support can be seen occurring informally in any trauma center or intensive care unit waiting room and particularly in rehabilitation settings. Many professionals in the field view this family-to-family support as a crucial element in helping families to work through the mourning process. More importantly, many family members themselves have found this type of mutual support and information exchange to be extremely valuable.[64]

This has led to the development of national organizations that are led and run by members of families who have been stricken by a traumatic head injury. The National Head Injury Foundation in the United States and Headway in Great Britain have become very extensive organizations that provide national, state, and local organization; information on programs for the head injured and for families; a network of family support groups led by family members and professionals; and a national directory of head injury rehabilitation programs.[65] Advocacy for more treatment programs, more funding to support research and program efforts, legislation to acknowledge the existence of traumatic head injury as a separate medical syndrome, and legislation to support prevention measures are also major interests of these family-oriented organizations.

EVALUATING FAMILY INTERVENTIONS

There are many dimensions along which interventions with families can be measured.[66] The primary question to be asked is whether the intervention accomplished what it was designed to accomplish. The second group of questions center around comparative analyses. For example, various interventions, aimed at accomplishing the same ends, may be compared with each other on a variety of measures such as success rates and costs. Another direction of comparison may be loosely labeled "cost-benefit" analysis: the monetary and other "costs" of interventions may be compared with the benefits derived from them. Implicit in this perspective are the issues of comparing different treatment models, or of comparing the "costs" of an intervention with the "costs" of not intervening. Validity and reliability of measurement techniques in this field are also of increasing importance.

A simple but powerful example of some cost-comparison issues is the increasingly common weighing of the dollar costs of an intervention against the dollar costs of leaving the family as it is. For instance, a health and accident insurance company that is responsible for a maximum number of dollars for the survivor's medical care may not be interested in paying for services to the family unless those services reduce the company's financial exposure for the patient. Likewise, workers' compensation carriers or vocational counselors may reasonably inquire how an intervention for which they are asked to pay is likely to improve the survivor's likelihood of returning to work or to otherwise reduce their virtual lifelong exposure for the patient. Nor is it unreasonable for a company to enter into a settlement with the patient and family that is less expensive than the proposed intervention plus postdischarge financial burden, even if rehabilitation professionals feel that the settlement creates nonmonetary "costs."

Evaluation of family education programs is still largely anecdotal and unsystematic. Rehabilitation professionals are used to focusing on the issues or problems that they see as most important, such as family adjustment, rather than on simpler issues. This is a natural consequence of the mission and resources of most rehabilitation systems. The result, however, is that there are very few data on such simple matters as whether family members learned concrete information that was presented to them. There is some evidence now that many family members have learned fairly complex information about head injury several years after the end of formal rehabilitation. However, the amount of knowledge possessed by these family members was fairly low despite the fact that most had participated in educational programs during the inpatient rehabilitation phase.[67] These findings are preliminary and incomplete; they are not reported to suggest that educational programs are ineffective but rather to point up the need for evaluation research in even this comparatively simple area.

Research on the effectiveness of family counseling and therapy in the field of traumatic head injury is beset by the same kinds of problems that are endemic to these interventions with other populations. Among the most troublesome issues are the difficulty in specifying and quantifying goals, the necessary tailoring of interventions to meet particular needs, and the difficulty in comparing the effectiveness of different techniques. The use of single-case and quasi-experimental research designs appears to be the most likely direction for this research. Suffice it to say that family therapists must work actively in the research arena to forestall the use of oversimplified, criterion-oriented methods.

There are few data yet available on the effectiveness of family support groups. Many family support groups do not have carefully developed goals and objectives which would lend themselves easily to research efforts. The overall goals are to provide emotional support and information to families in need of help. The remarkable growth of these support groups, and anecdotal reports, support the notion that these groups are fulfilling a vital role for large numbers of families. Some families do not find the groups helpful, but there is little systematic data regarding relevant family variables or outcomes.

One variable which appears to be of particular relevance is the severity of the head injury itself. Family support groups have tended to focus on severely injured survivors and their families. Since one of the major values of peer support is the sharing of common experiences, this focus has tended to leave out the families of survivors of "mild" or "moderate" head trauma. Their day-to-day experiences appear to be significantly different from those of families of a loved one with a severe head trauma.

Respite care is not usually directed at changes in a family system. However, within the context of first-order changes, it would be valuable to know if respite care decreases subjective burdens for the family. This would be an especially valuable direction for research if it included objective indicators of family distress such as use of stress-related medications, incidence of stress-related medical problems, and other monetary costs to the family and to society.

One of the potential advantages of behavioral family training is the applicability of quantitative research methods to this essentially clinical process. Ideally,

Clinical observations, whether systematic or serendipitous, prompt theoretical refinements and additional empirical study. Through continued empirical investigation, clinical procedures undergo considerable change over time. A self-corrective process thus ensues from this constant interplay between clinical and research endeavors.[68]

Preliminary results of one behavioral family training project suggest that behavioral change in the family member participants and their survivors is possible.[69] More research on this technique is needed, including the identification of necessary training components and relevant family system variables.

Evaluation Measures in Family Interventions

Methods of assessing family systems, and of evaluating the effects of family interventions, include informal observational techniques,[70, 71] formal observational techniques,[72–75] self-report measures,[76, 77] and behavioral response products.[78] (Reviews of the research literature in this area may be found in references 79 and 80.)

Formal observational methods have been used extensively in many areas of family systems research, but have just begun to be used in the area of traumatic head injury. Kozloff[81] and Lezak[82] used combinations of systematic observations and self-reports to investigate post-trauma patient and family functioning. Particular attention was paid to social and behavioral functioning.

Most assessments of head injured family systems have been by self-report. The techniques range from the identification of level of subjective burden on a seven-point Likert scale[83] to multipage questionnaires and established instruments such as the Family Assessment Device[84] and the Katz Adjustment Scale.[85] Many researchers have supplemented self-report questionnaires with direct interviews.

The findings of family assessment research with these various methods have been used briefly in this chapter and reviewed throughout this volume. Research has employed these measurement techniques and instruments to evaluate hypotheses and theories founded on clinical observations, and has thus begun to establish a viable body of knowledge about the effects of traumatic head injury on family systems.

Evaluating the effects of interventions with families appears to be more difficult. The traumatic head injury itself seems to be such a major event that its effects show up on most general assessment measures with most families. The effects of family interventions, however, frequently do not appear on general adjustment scales such as the Katz, or even on subjective evaluations of family burden. Preliminary studies suggest that even when intervention results in increased knowledge, better family interaction patterns, and observable behavioral changes, these beneficial effects do not appear on psychometric scales.[67] It would appear that adequately sensitive family inventories have not yet been constructed, or that they have not yet been applied to family intervention research in the field of head injury.

CONCLUSION

Traumatic head injury is an assault not just on the person who directly suffers the injury, but also on the entire personal system. The meaning of the injury is defined by the personal system. Changes required of family systems range from comparatively mild, first-order alterations to severe blows that compromise systemic functioning and result in significant, second-order changes in the way the systems themselves function. Individual roles and generational expectations may be blurred, altered, or even reversed.

Rehabilitation of the head injured adult involves all the members of the rehabilitation system and the entire personal system of each survivor. Intersystem conflicts, if not dealt with effectively, may subvert even the physical rehabilitation of the patient. Many types of interventions are in use with families, including family education, counseling, therapy, behavioral training, and respite care. Although research methodology continues to demonstrate the effects of the head injury on the long-term health of the family, measures of change are frequently not sensitive enough to establish the utility of family systems interventions. Research in this area should concentrate on the development of assessment measures which are thorough enough to reveal a broader spectrum of family systems issues throughout the family life cycle and sensitive enough to evaluate system change due to family interventions. Given the very large numbers of traumatized families and the long periods of mourning they undergo, it is essential that we identify the most effective and cost-beneficial intervention methods.

REFERENCES

1. Brooks, DN (ed): Closed Head Injury: Psychological, Social and Family Consequences. Oxford University Press, Oxford, 1984.
2. Panting, A and Merry, P: The long-term rehabilitation of severe head injuries with particular reference to the need for social and medical support for the patient's family. Rehabilitation 38:33, 1972.
3. Bond, MR: Assessment of the psychosocial outcome after severe head injury. In CIBA Foundation Symposium Number 34: Outcome of Severe Damage to the Central Nervous System. Elsevier Excerpta Medica, Amsterdam, 1975, p 141.
4. Brooks, DN and McKinlay, W: Personality and behavioral change after severe blunt head injury—a relative's view. J Neurol Neurosurg Psychiatry 46:336, 1983.
5. Rosenbaum, M and Najenson, T: Changes in life patterns and symptoms of low mood as reported by wives of severely brain injured soldiers. J Consult Clin Psychol 44(6):881, 1976.
6. Brooks, DN: Psychological deficits after severe blunt head injury: Their significance and rehabilitation. In Osborne, DJ, Greeneberg, MM and Eiser, JR (eds): Research in Psychology and Medicine. Academic Press, London, 1979, p 469.
7. Brooks, DN and Aughton, ME, Psychological consequences of severe blunt head injury. Int Rehabil Med 1:160, 1979.
8. McKinlay, WW et al: The short-term outcome of severe blunt head injury as reported by the relatives of the injured person. J Neurol Neurosurg Psychiatry 44:527, 1981.
9. Brooks, DN, et al: The effect of severe head injury on patient and relative within seven years of injury. J Head Trauma Rehabil 2(3):1, 1987.
10. Jacobs, HE: The Los Angeles head injury survey: Project rationale and design implications. J Head Trauma Rehabil 2(3):37, 1987.
11. Muir, CA: Mobile Mourning: Response of the personal system to partial death due to brain injury. Presented at the 2nd Annual Conference on the Rehabilitation of the Traumatic Brain Injured Adult, Medical College of Virginia, Richmond, VA, June, 1978.
12. Rosenthal, M and Muir, CA: Methods of family intervention. In Rosenthal, M et al (eds): Rehabilitation of the Head Injured Adult. FA Davis, Philadelphia, 1983, p 407.
13. Muir, CA and Haffey, WJ: Psychological and neuropsychological interventions in the mobile mourning process. In Edelstein, BA and Couture, ET (eds): Behavioral Assessment and Rehabilitation of the Traumatically Brain-Damaged. Plenum Press, New York, 1984, p 247.
14. Buckley, W (ed): Modern Systems Research for the Behavioral Scientist, A Sourcebook. Aldine, Chicago, 1968.
15. Hill, R: Modern systems theory and the family: A confrontation. Soc Sci Info 10:7, 1971.
16. Haber, R: Friends in family therapy: Use of a neglected resource. Fam Process 26(2):269, 1987.
17. Kozloff, R: Networks of social support and the outcome from severe head injury. J Head Trauma Rehabil 2(3):14, 1987.
18. Duvall, ER: Family Development. JB Lippincott, Philadelphia, 1967.
19. Hill, R: Family Development in Three Generations. Schenkman, Cambridge, 1970.
20. Wynne, LC: The epigenesis of relational systems: A model for understanding family development. Fam Process 23:97, 1984.
21. Condeluci, A and Gretz-Lasky, S: Social role valorization: A model for community reentry. J Head Trauma Rehabil 2(1):49, 1987.
22. Simon, F, Stierlin, H and Wynne, L: The Language of Family Therapy: A Systematic Vocabulary and Sourcebook. Family Process Press, New York, 1985.
23. Haley, J: Toward a theory of pathological systems. In Zuk, GH and Boszormenyi-Nagy, I (eds): Family therapy and disturbed families. Science and Behavioral Books, Palo Alto, CA, 1967, p 11.
24. Ashby, WR: Design for a Brain. Chapman & Hall, London, 1952.
25. Watzlawich, P, Weakland, JH and Fisch, R: Change: Principles of Problem Formation and Problem Resolution. W. W. Norton, New York, 1974.
26. Minuchin, S, Rosman, BL and Baker, L: Psychosomatic Families: Anorexia Nervosa in Context. Harvard University Press, Cambridge, 1978.
27. Lezak, MD: Living with the characterologically altered brain-injured patient. J Clin Psychiatry 39:592, 1978.
28. Lezak, MD: Psychological implications of traumatic brain damage for the patient's family. Rehabil Psychol 31(4):241, 1986.
29. Boll, TJ and Kay, TE: More complex and hardly mild: A new look at mild head injury. Presented at the Fifth Annual National Head Injury Symposium of the National Head Injury Foundation, Chicago, November, 1986.
30. Schneidman, ES: Deaths of Man. Penguin Books, Baltimore, 1974.
31. Schneidman, ES: Voices of Death. Harper & Row, New York, 1980.
32. Rochlin, G: Griefs and Discontents, the Forces of Change. Little, Brown, Boston, 1965.
33. Bowlby, J: Attachment theory, separation anxiety and mourning. In Arieti, S (ed): American Handbook of Psychiatry, Vol 6. Basic Books, New York, 1975.
34. Szalita, AB: Grief and bereavement. In Arieti, S (ed): American Handbook of Psychiatry, Vol 3. Basic Books, New York, 1975.
35. Romano, MD: Family response to traumatic head injury. Scand J Rehabil Med 6:1, 1974.
36. Krueger, DW: Emotional rehabilitation: An overview. In Krueger, DW (ed): Emotional Rehabilita-

tion of Physical Trauma and Disability. Spectrum Publications, New York, 1984.

37. Lezak, M et al: Relationship between personality disorders, social disturbances and physical disability following traumatic brain injury. Presented at the Eighth Annual Meeting of the International Neuropsychology Society, San Francisco, February, 1980.

38. Thomsen, IV: Late outcome of very severe blunt head trauma: A ten–fifteen year second follow-up. J Neurol Neurosurg Psychiatry 46:260, 1981.

39. Moos, RH: Coping with Physical Illness. Plenum Press, New York, 1977.

40. Alterman, AI and Tarter, RE: Relationship between familial alcoholism and head injury. J Stud Alcohol 46(3):236, 1985.

41. Muir, CA, Jacobs, HE and Martel, M: Family Training and Outcome. Presented at the Sixth Annual National Symposium of the National Head Injury Foundation, San Diego, CA, December, 1987.

42. Gronwall, D: Rehabilitation programs for patients with mild head injury: Components, problems, and evaluation. J Head Trauma Rehabil 1(1):1, 1986.

43. Muir, CA: Family needs and interventions. Workshop for Southern California Head Injury Foundation, February, 1987.

44. Thomsen, IV: The patient with severe head injury and his family. Scand J Rehabil Med 6:180, 1974.

45. Oddy, M, Humphrey, M and Uttley, D: Stresses upon the relatives of head-injured patients. Br J Psychiatry 133:507, 1978.

46. Annon, JS: The Behavioral Treatment of Sexual Problems, Vol 1. Enabling Systems, Inc, Honolulu, 1969.

47. Diehl, LN: Patient-family education. In Rosenthal, M et al (eds): Rehabilitation of the Head Injured Adult. FA Davis, Philadelphia, 1983, p 395.

48. Elliot, J and Smith, RD: Meeting family needs following severe head injury: A multidisciplinary approach. J Neurosurg Nurs 17(2):111, 1985.

49. Rogers, PM and Kreutzer, JS: Family crises following head injury: A network intervention strategy. J Neurosurg Nurs 16(6):343, 1984.

50. Mathis, M: Personal needs of family members of critically ill patients with and without acute brain injury. J Neurosurg Nurs 16(1):36, 1984.

51. Diehl, LN: Patient-family education. Presented at the Second Annual Conference on the Rehabilitation of the Traumatic Brain Injured Adult, Richmond, VA, June, 1978.

52. Glick, ID, and Kessler, DR: Marital and family therapy. Grune & Stratton, New York, 1974, p 1.

53. Mandanes, C and Haley, J: Dimensions of family therapy. J Nerv Ment Dis 165:88, 1977.

54. Gurman, AS and Kniskern, DP (eds): Handbook of Family Therapy. Brunner/Mazel, New York, 1981.

55. Rosenthal, M: Understanding and optimizing family adaptation to traumatic brain injury. In Bach-y-Rita, P (ed): Traumatic Brain Injury. Demos, New York (in press).

56. Rosenthal, M, and Greckler, C: Family therapy issues in neuropsychology. In Wedding, D, Horton, AM and Webster, J (eds): The Neuropsychology Handbook. Springer, New York, 1986.

57. Falloon, IRH et al: Family therapy with relapsing schizophrenics and their families: A pilot study. Fam Process 15:94, 1981.

58. Falloon, IRH and Liberman, R: Behavior therapy for families with child management problems. In Fal-

loon, IRH et al (eds): Families with Child Management Problems. Plenum Press, New York, 1976, p 121.

59. Barton, C and Alexander, JF: Functional family therapy. In Gurman, AS and Kniskern, DP (eds): Handbook of Family Therapy. Brunner/Mazel, New York, 1981.

60. Lieberman, RP et al: Handbook of Marital Therapy: A Positive Approach to Helping Troubled Relationships. Plenum Press, New York, 1980.

61. Stuart, RB: Helping Couples Change: A Social Learning Approach to Marital Therapy. Guilford Press, New York, 1980.

62. Jacobs, HE, Muir, CA and Wixom, C: Assessment and intervention in family training. Presented at Fifth Annual National Symposium of the National Head Injury Foundation, Chicago, IL, 1986.

63. National Directory of Head Injury Rehabilitation Services. National Head Injury Foundation, Framingham, MA, 1988.

64. Spivak, MP: Advocacy and legislative action for head-injured children and their families. J Head Trauma Rehabil 1:41, 1986.

65. Spivak, MP et al: The shake, rattle and role of the NHIF in influencing public policy. Presented at the Sixth Annual National Symposium of the National Head Injury Foundation, San Diego, December, 1987.

66. Grotevent, HD and Carlson, CI: Family interaction coding systems: A descriptive review. Fam Process 26:49, 1987.

67. Muir, C, Jacobs, H and Martel, M: Family training and outcome. Presented at National Head Injury Foundation, 6th Annual National Symposium, December, 1987.

68. Margolin, G: Behavioral marital therapy. In Wolman, BB and Stricker, G (eds): Handbook of Marital and Family Therapy, 1983, p 247.

69. Jacobs, H and Muir, C: Family training—an important solution. Presented at Sixth Annual Southwest Head Injury Symposium, Lake Tahoe, CA, January, 1988.

70. Baldwin, AL, Baldwin, CP and Cole, RE: Family free-play interaction: Setting and methods. In Parental pathology, family interaction, and the competence of the child in school. Monogr Soc Res Child Dev 47:36, 1982.

71. Watzlawick, PA: Structured family interview. Fam Process 5:256, 1966.

72. Bales, RF: Interaction Process Analysis: A Method for the Study of Small Groups. Addison-Wesley Press, Cambridge, MA, 1950.

73. Beavers, WR: Hierarchical issues in a systems approach to illness and health. Fam Syst Med 1:47, 1983.

74. Hahlweg, K et al: The Munich marital therapy study. In Hahlweg, K and Jacobson, NS (eds): Marital Interaction: Analysis and Modification. Guilford Press, New York, 1984, p 3.

75. Gurman, AS and Kniskern, DP (eds): Handbook of Family Therapy. Brunner/Mazel, New York, 1981.

76. Livingston, MG, Brooks, DN and Bond, M: Patient outcome in the year following severe head injury and relatives' psychiatric and social functioning. J Neurol Neurosurg Psychiatry 48:876, 1985.

77. Olson, DH et al: Family Inventories: Inventories Used in a National Survey of Families Across the Family Life Cycle. Family Social Science, 290 McNeal, University of Minnesota, St Paul, MN, 1985.

78. Haynes, SN: Behavioral assessment of adults. Handbook of Psychological Assessment. Behavioral Science Press, New York, 1985.

79. Moos, RH and Moos, BS: Manual for the Family Environment Scale. Consulting Psychologist Press, Palo Alto, CA, 1981.

80. Riskin, J and Faunce, EE: An evaluative review of family interaction research. Fam Process 11:365, 1972.

81. Kozloff, R: Networks of social support and the outcome from severe head injury. J Head Trauma Rehabil 2(3):14, 1987.

82. Lezak, MD: Relationships between personality disorders, social disturbances, and physical disability following traumatic brain injury. J Head Trauma Rehabil 2(1):57, 1987.

83. Bond, M: The psychiatry of closed head injury. In Brooks, DN (ed): Closed Head Injury: Psychological, Social and Family Consequences. Oxford University Press, Oxford, 1984, p 148.

84. Epstein, NB, Baldwin, LM and Bishop, DS: The McMaster Family Assessment Device. J Marital Fam Ther 9:171, 1983.

85. Katz, MM and Lyerly, SB: Methods for measuring adjustment and social behavior in the community. I. Rationale, description, discriminative validity and scale development. Psychol Rep 13:503, 1963.

Chapter 30

Therapeutic Recreation

JAMES P. BERGER, M.A., C.T.R.S.
ANNE E. REGALSKI, C.T.R.S.

In a study conducted by Oddy and co-workers, it was noted that "... work, leisure activities and contact with friends were the areas of life most affected after a severe head injury."[1] They reported in another study that the closed head injured engaged in fewer leisure activities two years post injury compared to pretrauma activity levels.[2] Similarly, Pollack and colleagues have illustrated cases of head injured who had poor re-establishment of peer relationships and lacked initiative to use leisure time effectively.[3] They concluded that a cognitive rehabilitation program cannot be truly effective unless it successfully assists its clients to re-establish a satisfactory lifestyle. Rehabilitation for the head injured patient should focus on improving all aspects of life—not only physical and cognitive skills, but also daily living skills including leisure, recreation, community re-entry, and social skills.

This chapter defines therapeutic recreation, its purpose, the scope of its services, and its potential outcomes, as applied to the head injured. The clinical application of therapeutic recreation intervention in the inpatient setting and its place in outpatient community-based treatment programs will also be addressed. Community-based treatment programs include transitional living, cognitive retraining, and day treatment programs.

THERAPEUTIC RECREATION

Therapeutic recreation can be described as "a process which utilizes recreational ser-vices for the purposive intervention in some physical, emotional, and/or social behavior to bring about a desired change in that behavior and to promote the growth and development of the individual."[4] There seems to exist a relationship between this definition of therapeutic recreation and the objective of rehabilitation as developed by Kottke, who states "the major objective of rehabilitation is the opportunity for each client to re-enter the community at an optimal level of functioning; to receive enough satisfaction and success within that environment; to desire to maintain physical/psychological health and thus reduce changes of regression and re-admission."[5]

The therapeutic recreation specialist working with the severely head injured individual must recognize the physical, cognitive, and behavioral changes that accompany the injury and the changes that occur within the family system to accomplish the above intent. Many head injured find aspects of "normal" life restricted not only physically but also socially and cognitively. To assist the therapeutic recreation specialist in addressing and prioritizing these aspects a model developed by Gunn and Peterson may be utilized.[6] The model, known as the therapeutic recreation services model, is based on a continuum of three phases through which each individual may pass.

The phases of this model are:

1. **Rehabilitation/Treatment:** Treatment to improve the patient's overall functional ability which is directed by a certified therapeutic recreation specialist

2. **Education:** Leisure education to assist the patient with the acquisition of leisure skills and attitudes through instruction and counseling, which is directed by a certified therapeutic recreation specialist

3. **Recreation Participation:** A patient's voluntary participation in organized leisure and recreational activities, which are made available and supervised by a certified therapeutic recreation specialist

Therapeutic recreation includes treatment, education, elements of counseling, family services, and referrals to community agencies. In many situations, the primary emphasis of therapeutic recreation is not on providing activities, but on developing a social climate or a living situation in which the head injured patient can function with satisfaction and increasing social capabilities.

LEVELS OF COGNITIVE FUNCTIONING

The "levels of cognitive functioning" rating scale, developed by Rancho Los Amigos Hospital in California, is often used and accepted as a guide for rehabilitation treatment of the head injured patient (scale is detailed in Table 20–1). The levels referred to throughout the remainder of this chapter are based on this scale.

HEAD INJURY TREATMENT TEAM

Therapeutic recreation is an integral part of the rehabilitation program. The therapeutic recreation specialist evaluates head injured patients and develops a treatment program to address their leisure needs and abilities. Consistency and repetition are key elements to effective rehabilitation of the head injured. Treatment team meetings are used to share information on the patient's functioning status and treatment approaches. The therapeutic recreation specialist notes the treatment focus of other disciplines (i.e., speech therapy's memory compensatory techniques, occupational therapy's emphasis on bilateral upper extremity activities, and physical therapy's

proper body positioning) and the therapeutic recreation specialist reinforces them in his or her treatment sessions (i.e., encouraging the patient to use memory compensatory techniques during community trip planning, and reminding the patient to use both upper extremities and proper body positioning in leisure activities). The therapeutic recreation specialist's report of the patient's social, leisure, and community functioning provides the treatment team with a reality mirror of the patient's everyday life experiences. It illustrates how the patient is carrying over skills developed in the structured clinical setting to practical activities of recreation, and community reintegration outings, which are less structured environments. This feedback assists the treatment team in evaluating the patient's total care program; if problem areas are identified, revisions can be made.

FAMILY INVOLVEMENT

The family is also a vital part of the therapeutic recreation process. In instructional sessions, the need to identify and modify the family's leisure interests and activities to include the patient is addressed and ideas are shared. Therapeutic recreation services further involve the family by including them in evening group recreation participation activities and community reintegration outings; the therapeutic recreation specialist functions as a role model in these situations. Active family involvement can be instrumental in facilitating a patient's progress and more importantly in assisting with the carryover skills acquired in therapeutic recreation services treatment to the home and community. Often, at discharge time, the head injured patient is still dependent upon the family to initiate, structure, and assist (verbally or physically or both) in leisure and recreation activity involvement. The family may also be needed to provide transportation and supervision for community involvement. This dependency necessitates the need for education and instruction in these areas.

The next section specifically identifies the therapeutic recreation intervention process that is used to guide the head injured toward optimal independence and a full leisure lifestyle.

TREATMENT INTERVENTION

Therapeutic recreation services often are not initiated until the head injured patient reaches cognitive level V. The two main reasons for this late introduction of services are (1) the low-level head injured patient's limited ability to tolerate a full rehabilitation program, and (2) the limited staffing in many rehabilitation settings of therapeutic recreation specialists. Criteria for rehabilitation admission usually allow for the admission of head injured patients at cognitive levels III and IV who present with minimal responses, limited tolerance, and agitation. These patients are not usually ready for an extensive treatment program; however, therapeutic recreation treatment may be indicated in some cases. If a therapeutic recreation specialist is available and given a cognitive level III patient with adequate tolerance and appropriate response to treatment, activities may be provided that focus on stimulation (i.e., tactile, auditory, olfactory, and visual) in addition to simple motor commands and orientation/attention activities. The head injured patient at level IV would be involved in similar activities, but a higher degree of structure would be utilized to minimize agitation. Those patients at cognitive level V and higher appear to be ready for an intense rehabilitation program including therapeutic recreation services to facilitate progress, thus allowing for a more dynamic therapeutic recreation approach.

ASSESSMENT OF THE HEAD INJURED PATIENT

As noted earlier, the patient should be functioning at a minimum of cognitive level III on the Rancho Los Amigos scale and possess sufficient physical tolerance for increased activity. The therapeutic recreation specialist begins the assessment by gathering background information through various techniques, including

1. Personal interview with the patient and family
2. Medical record review, which includes social history, medical status, and treatment team documentation such as neuropsychological test results and functional skills assessments

3. Clinical observation of functional performance in leisure and recreational activities
4. Informal observations of the patient in social situations with family, peers, and staff
5. Practical assessment of behavioral responses in relation to specific tasks presented by the therapist, which assists in determining social, cognitive, perceptual, and sensory motor skills
6. Leisure interest and lifestyle test batteries (Table 30–1)

The initial assessment conducted by the therapeutic recreation specialist includes the following information:

1. Identification of pretrauma lifestyle: the areas defined include work, school, family, and socioeconomic considerations
2. Identification of leisure, social, community, and daily living habits: the patient's activities, interests, and needs, and the identification of the patient's general understanding of each of the aforementioned areas
3. Identification of the patient's abilities and limitations in the areas of physical, cognitive, and social functioning
4. Identification of specific goals with measurable objectives and a defined treatment program based on all of the above information and the leisure ability continuum

Upon completion of the initial assessment, the specialist determines which phase or phases of the leisure ability continuum (see page 000) are the most important and appropriate to address. The therapist then identifies short- and long-range goals based on this information and patient needs. If services are provided to the head injured patients at levels III and IV, the emphasis of the treatment program is in the areas of physical and cognitive skill development. The head injured patient at level V would continue in these areas along with social skill development but with more structure and an increased level of difficulty. The level VI patient continues physical, cognitive, and social skill development at higher skill levels and may also be involved in community reintegration and education emphasizing leisure awareness and leisure identification activities. Head injured patients at levels VII and VIII would be involved in all three phases of the continuum as determined

Table 30–1. ASSESSMENT INSTRUMENTS

Miranda Leisure Interest Finder (Miranda, 1975)
Leisure Counseling
Milwaukee Public Schools
Director of Municipal Recreation and Adult Education
P.O. Drawer 10-K
Milwaukee, Wisconsin 53201

Leisure Activity Blank (McKechnie, 1975)
Consulting Psychologists Press
577 College Avenue
Palo Alto, California 94306

Leisure Attitude Scale; LAS (Crandall and Slivken, 1978, 1980)
Crandall, R and Slivken, K: Leisure attitudes and their measurement. In Iso-Ahola, S (ed): Social Psychological Perspectives on Leisure and Recreation. Springfield, IL, Charles C Thomas, 1980, p 261.

Ragheb, MG and Beard, JG: Measuring leisure attitudes. J Leisure Res 14(2):155, 1982.

Leisure Well-Being Inventory (McDowell, 1979)
C. F. McDowell
Leisure Lifestyle Consultants
P.O. Box 1516
Eugene, Oregon 97405

Leisure Diagnostic Battery (Ellis, Witt, 1984)
Ellis, GD and Witt, PA: The leisure diagnostic batteries: past, present and future. Therapeutic Recreation Journal 4:31, 1986.

Avocational Activities Interest Index (D'Agostini, 1972)
N. D'Agostini
Sutter Memorial Hospital
Sacramento, California 95819

Avocational Activities Inventory (Overs, Taylor, and Adkins, 1977)
Leisure Counseling
Milwaukee Public Schools
Director of Municipal Recreation and Adult Education
P.O. Drawer 10-K
Milwaukee, Wisconsin 53201

and prioritized by the therapist, team, and patient.

When developing a specific treatment program, the therapeutic recreation specialist must consider the skills that leisure and recreation activities demand. All activities have social, emotional, physical, cognitive, and/or creative components. The specialist must use a process called *activity analysis*. Each activity is broken down into its most basic components to identify their appropriateness and therapeutic value for the patient at his or her current level of functioning. Leisure and recreation activities that require skill development or enhancement in social, emotional, physical, cognitive, and creative skills are clearly therapeutic. Modification and adaptation of the activity or equipment

used may be helpful in selecting activities that meet the established goals of the program. Examples of adapted activities can be found in Table 30–2. Also, activities that stimulate interest and provide success opportunities should be selected.

THERAPEUTIC RECREATION TREATMENT PROGRAM

The therapist will develop a specific treatment program based on the head injured patient's current level of functioning, leisure interests, needs, and abilities. The program will include various forms of activity involvement including individual treatment, small- and large-group activities, and com-

**Table 30–2. EXAMPLES OF ADAPTED
RECREATION ACTIVITIES**

☐ Wheelchair bowling with armrest removed for individuals with adequate strength and range of motion, or wheelchair bowling with a metal ramp that individuals with limited strength and range of motion can position and roll the ball off

☐ Cards with a card holder (wooden block with rows of slits) for individuals with limited use and control of one or both upper extremities

☐ Cooking activities with (a) a rocker knife; (b) a grater with suction cups to stabilize it; (c) a cutting board with aluminum nails to secure food for peeling and cutting; and (d) a Dycem pad to stabilize bowls for individuals with limited use of one or both upper extremities and/or ataxia

☐ Ball activities with Nerf ball products for individuals with limited strength and/or coordination

☐ Billiards using a pool stick with two rollers at the end with which the individual pushes the ball, for individuals with limited use and control of one or both upper extremities

☐ Games with simplified rules for individuals with limited cognitive abilities

☐ Computer activities using a joy-stick and touch pads for individuals with limited use and control of one or both upper extremities

munity reintegration trips. Community reintegration is recommended when the following criteria are attained:

1. Cognitive level VI (exceptions are occasionally made for the cognitive level V patient for the purpose of increasing motivation—however, only if the patient does not have a behavior problem)
2. Therapeutic recreation specialist and treatment team recommendations for community activities
3. Adequate tolerance level
4. Appropriate cooperation and treatment program compliance

Through practical application of leisure activities and community reintegration participation, the specialist reinforces (1) appropriate leisure lifestyle management; (2) psychosocial adjustment issues dealt with by social work and psychology; (3) coordination, as well as motor and functional skills developed in physical and occupational therapies; (4) communication skills practiced in speech and language; and (5) cognitive skills addressed in psychology and speech and language therapies.

Prevocational skill development may be addressed in conjunction with the patient's leisure goals if the patient expresses a concern and interest at the time of the initial assessment and if the treatment team so recommends. Some of the prevocational activities the therapist may offer include computer training, typing, filing, categoriz-

ing, photocopying, photography, and woodworking.

Therapeutic recreation services are further described through the use of modules shown in Table 30–3. The modules are delineated into treatment areas of social skills, therapeutic games and leisure skills, leisure education, and community reintegration. Each module describes sample activities, treatment goals, and treatment objectives, and notes the appropriate cognitive levels at which to utilize the treatment activities.

TREATMENT ACTIVITY GUIDELINES

As previously noted, the Rancho Los Amigos Levels of Cognitive Functioning can serve as a guide for the treatment of the head injured. The eight stages describe the head injured's general behavior, abilities, and limitations at each level. Using these levels as a reference, the following special considerations can be helpful in the effective treatment and management of the head injured patient.

Cognitive Level III: Localized Response

1. Structure the environment. It should be quiet and distraction free to avoid overloading the patient.

Table 30–3. THERAPEUTIC RECREATION SERVICES TREATMENT MODULES FOR THE HEAD INJURED

Activity Examples	Cognitive Level*	Treatment Goal	Treatment Objectives
		Module 1: Social Skills	
Group Activities Wheel of Fortune Theme parties Current events Password Family Feud	*V–VIII* V Limited involvement for observation/stimulation or with 1:1 supervision for socialization on an automatic level VI Involvement with structure and verbal guidance for attention and direction VII Involvement with structure with increased emphasis on independence (verbal guidance as needed for judgment, for example) VIII Independent involvement with a leadership role for skill refinement	To provide activities that emphasize social skills redevelopment and that offer structure on an individual and group basis	**Group Focus** 1. To improve functional speech and communication skills in group leisure activities 2. To facilitate appropriate socialization and cooperation in a group setting **Group and Individual Focus** 3. To increase attention and memory skills 4. To increase initiation and assertion skills 5. To increase self-esteem through success opportunities
Individual Activities Speak 'n' Spell Memory—Names and faces Environmental awareness Various leisure and recreational activities	*V–VIII* V Involvement for reorientation and skill development with structure and verbal guidance VI Involvement for reorientation and skill development with increased complexity of the task, structure, and verbal guidance required VII Involvement for skill development with minimal structure and verbal guidance VIII Independent involvement for skill refinement		

454

Module 2: Therapeutic Games/Leisure Skills

Activities	Involvement	Goal	Objectives
Educational Flash cards Identification games Matching games Puzzles Computer Games Simon	**V–VI** V Involvement for reorientation and cognitive retraining, structure, and verbal guidance required VI Involvement for reorientation and cognitive retraining with increased complexity of task; structure and verbal guidance required	To provide activities that facilitate leisure skill development, cognitive remediation, and physical recovery	1. To develop leisure skills and adaptive leisure skills 2. To increase attention skills 3. To improve identification and recognition skills of color, numbers, objects, and shapes 4. To improve matching skills 5. To improve visual spatial relation skills 6. To improve strength and coordination 7. To increase initiation and assertive skills 8. To increase memory skills 9. To improve reading and direction following skills 10. To increase motivation
Computer games Sports Swimming Billiards Basketball Video arcade games Crafts Table games Cooking	**VII–VIII** VII Involvement for skill development with minimal structure and verbal guidance, for example, for attention to detail VIII Independent involvement for skill refinement		

Module 3: Leisure Education and Counseling

Activities	Involvement	Goal	Objectives
Leisure definition and identification Leisure awareness discussion Leisure value identification Leisure interest survey Leisure resource identification Leisure activity selection Leisure planning and lifestyle management	**VII–VIII** VII Involvement for skill development VIII Involvement for skill refinement and exploration	To provide the opportunity for the development of a personal knowledge and understanding of leisure, its potential utilization, and its benefits	1. To define leisure and recreation 2. To promote awareness of self, attitudes, values, and feelings related to leisure 3. To promote the development of decision-making and problem-solving skills related to leisure participation with self, others, and the environment 4. To identify curent leisure interests, needs, resources, and activities

Table 30–3. (Continued)

Activity Examples	Cognitive Level*	Treatment Goal	Treatment Objectives
		Module 3: Leisure Education and Counseling	
			5. To improve communication and socialization skills 6. To develop leisure planning and lifestyle management skills
		Module 4: Community Reintegration	
Restaurants Shopping malls Theaters Sporting events Parks and amusement centers Special community activity events Community recreation programs Support group meetings	**VI–VIII** VI Involvement for re-orientation to community with close supervision, structure, and verbal guidance VII Involvement with minimal structure and verbal guidance VIII Independent involvement for skill refinement	To provide organized community trips that offer opportunities to develop community participation skills and use rehabilitation re-education skills.	1. To practice and improve functional skills developed during all therapies in a non-structured community setting 2. To improve leisure planning skills 3. To improve psychosocial adjustment to the disability in the community 4. To practice and improve communication and assertion skills with the public 5. To improve safety and accessibility awareness skills 6. To introduce the concept of handicapped advocacy

*See pages 00, 00, 00, and 00, for information on therapeutic recreation services treatment intervention at cognitive levels III and IV.

2. Use a calm approach.

3. Orient the patient to self, therapist, and task.

4. Allow time for delayed responses.

5. See the patient often for short periods of time and provide familiar stimuli.

6. Use simple one-step commands (e.g., close your eyes, grasp this object).

Cognitive Level IV: Confused, Agitated

Continue 1 through 5 of cognitive level III treatment guidelines with increased emphasis on orientation and structure.

1. To increase activity tolerance and cooperation, set a criterion for a minimum of tasks to be completed by using a simple contingency (e.g., put these four puzzle pieces in their places and you will be done for today).

2. Use simple tasks in which the patient can succeed, and always praise task completion.

3. Do not point out mistakes; keep the activity positive, repeat directions, and demonstrate if necessary.

4. Repeating basic orientation and attention activities from treatment session to session will be necessary to improve these skills.

5. Use multiple short-term activities with frequent breaks. If the patient becomes agitated, give him or her a break and change activities. If the patient appears to be overloaded, give the patient a break or calmly end the treatment session.

Cognitive Level V: Confused, Inappropriate, Nonagitated

Continue 1 through 4 of cognitive level III and 1 through 5 of cognitive level IV treatment guidelines with increased complexity of tasks.

1. If the patient becomes distracted, redirect him or her to task.

2. Involve patient in reviewing orientation information (i.e., ask who, what, where, and when questions).

3. Provide maximum structure to aid initiation and completion of task (i.e., gestures and/or step-by-step verbal directions).

4. Ignore confabulation.

5. Use simple, brief, concrete directions and gestures as needed.

6. Provide close supervision, as patient may wander or get lost.

Cognitive Level VI: Confused-Appropriate

Continue 1 through 4 of cognitive level III, 1 through 4 of cognitive level IV and 1 through 6 of cognitive level V treatment guidelines.

1. Give the patient choices of activities to allow him or her some control over the environment.

2. Allow the patient time to process information and respond.

3. Emphasize activities to improve memory. Review treatment activities at end of sessions, and previous day's activities and community reintegration trips.

4. Make patient aware of impulsivity by gently noting how working fast affected his or her activity performance—remind patient to slow down.

5. Explain to the patient how it is beneficial to participate in therapeutic activities. Goal setting may be helpful.

Cognitive Level VII: Automatic-Appropriate

Continue 1 through 2 of cognitive level V and 1 through 5 of cognitive level IV treatment guidelines.

1. Increase sophistication of activity, as patient may not see relevance of simple activities.

2. Encourage independence and independent activity involvement with peers.

3. Emphasize safety precautions, as judgment is still impaired.

4. Challenge the patient, appeal to his or her competitive sense to increase motivation.

5. Give the patient a leadership role such as teaching therapist an activity, assisting a peer, or assisting with activity setup and cleanup.

6. Give the patient increased responsibility in activity initiation, selection, and planning.

7. Encourage independent problem solving.

8. Role-model appropriate social skills.

9. Give patient cues to focus his or her attention on details.

10. As deficits are demonstrated in the patient's activity performance, gently note to the patient how his or her deficits affect his or her activity performance, and offer suggestions to improve them.

Cognitive Level VIII: Purposeful and Appropriate

Continue cognitive level VII treatment guidelines with increased emphasis on independence.

1. Increase sophistication of activity, as patient may not see relevance of simple activities.

2. Encourage independence and independent activity involvement with peers.

3. Challenge the patient, appeal to his or her competitive sense to increase motivation.

4. Give the patient a leadership role such as teaching therapist an activity, assisting a peer, or assisting with activity setup and cleanup.

5. Give the patient increased responsibility in activity initiation, selection, and planning.

6. As deficits are demonstrated in the patient's activity performance, gently note to the patient how his or her deficits affect activity performance, and offer suggestions to improve them.

Many head injury rehabilitation treatment teams use basic behavior modification techniques for the management of patients who demonstrate behavior problems. The therapeutic recreation specialist, of course, is consistent with the team and uses these same techniques. If a specific behavior problem (i.e., taking objects, "skipping" therapy, or touching others inappropriately) occurs and persists during therapeutic recreation, the therapeutic recreation specialist would report it to the team. The team would then consult with the psychologist to develop a specific behavior modification program to address the problem. All team members would be instructed on the program for consistent administration. The program may focus on shaping a positive behavior by using reinforcement for each demonstration of the desired behavior. Examples of behavior modification programs include token economy programs and privilege earning programs which allow for the acquisition of extra telephone time, cigarettes, and even weekend home passes.

DISCHARGE PLANNING

Another aspect of therapeutic recreation services treatment that occurs near to the time of discharge is the provision of a home program and referrals to community and leisure resource agencies. This part of the program assists the patient in continuing their pursuit of an active, fulfilling leisure lifestyle post discharge.

The home program consists of home and community activity ideas and guidelines for use postdischarge. The home program indicates which activities will require some form of supervision or direction for the head injured due to safety concerns and functional abilities. It is also used to illustrate to head injured patients and their families how to structure activities to make them positive therapeutic experiences. Other guidelines in addition to those identified earlier include the following suggestions:

1. Schedule and structure each day's activities to include meals, self-care, leisure, recreation, and so forth.

2. Encourage the initiation of activities; offer choices if necessary.

3. Incorporate treatment recommendations such as encouraging scanning when a visual neglect is present or using impaired extremities as much as possible.

4. Use compensatory techniques such as visual imagery, appointment calendars, and daily records to aid recall.

Referrals to community agencies that provide leisure and recreation participation opportunities are also made prior to discharge. The referrals consist of the names of programs, agencies, and/or support groups, as well as their phone numbers, contact person, and a brief description of the program and/or services being recommended. Examples of referral sources include head injury support groups such as state branches and local chapters of the National Head Injury Foundation (NHIF), local parks and recreation departments, local schools and adult education programs, commercial recreation agencies located in the head injured individual's geographic area, transportation agencies, and various other resources related to the head injured individual's specific areas of interest. The therapeutic recreation specialist sometimes arranges for the head injured individual to directly contact the referral source or arranges for the placement of the head injured individual on the agency's mailing list. Participation in recommended community programs prior to discharge from the rehabilitation center is encouraged whenever possible.

COMMUNITY REHABILITATION PROGRAMS

Head injured individuals usually require continued multidisciplinary rehabilitation treatment after discharge from their initial inpatient rehabilitation hospitalization. In the past 3 years, there has been a surge of growth in community-based rehabilitation programs for the head injured. Some of the programs have been identified as cognitive retraining services, day treatment services, day care services, residential care services, and transitional living services. In general, the existing community programs, each are unique, all share some common characteristics. They provide opportunities for general physical fitness activities, interpersonal and social contact, continued development of daily living skills, and continued success. These programs use the medical-restorative model and the educational-action-training model; that is, the restoration of physical function and health and the maintenance/adaptation of social and living skill competencies.

Therapeutic recreation specialists in community treatment/residential programs perform many of the same functions and services that were described for clinical inpatient treatment. Greater emphasis is placed on community reintegration and independence, leisure education, leisure lifestyle management, and daily living activities.

The specialist establishes a treatment program based on information and input from the family, the head injured individual, the team members, and the insurance providers. Specific assessment areas are as follows.

Home Environment Assessments

☐ Family's current daily routine
☐ Head injured individual's daily routine
☐ Identification of significant blocks of structured time
☐ Identification of significant blocks of idle time
☐ Identification of available resources such as family, friends, financial, and transportation
☐ Home accessibility

Patient Assessment

☐ Identification of current functioning levels
☐ Identification of leisure and recreational interests
☐ Identification of past leisure interests, lifestyle, and functioning levels
☐ Identification of strengths and limitations

Community Environment Assessment

☐ Identification of potential leisure resource agencies
☐ Identification of services and programs offered at each agency
☐ Identification of accessibility of each agency .

Once the therapist has all this information, a comprehensive, goal-directed treatment program would be established and assimilated into the total treatment program.

When a head injured individual enters the community, attention can no longer be focused only on improvement of function but also on finding the head injured a satisfactory place in society. The client must take responsibility for interaction with the nondisabled community, and problem-solving toward achievement of personal goals. Execution of these tasks requires experience, practice, and confidence.[7] As head injured individuals become aware through community involvement that they are contributing to their own growth, they develop a sense of confidence in their ability to succeed in community tasks and living.

CASE STUDIES

The following case studies are presented as examples of therapeutic recreation intervention with head injured individuals and their behavioral responses to it.

Case 1. A 19-year-old male head injured patient, 2 months postinjury was at cognitive level VII. Prior to his injury, the patient was attending college, was working part-time, and was active in fitness-type sports. The therapeutic recreation specialist found him to be oriented, interactive, motivated, and progressing in his functional skills, including ambulation. His deficits included concreteness, decreased activity speed and problem-solving skills, social inappropriateness, and a lack of awareness of his deficits.

His therapeutic recreation treatment program included activities such as high-level board games, personal computer activities, group games, leisure education, and community reintegration trips for cognitive remediation and the redevelopment of social, leisure, and community lifestyle management skills. During therapeutic recreation treatment, he required reminders to slow down, attend to details, and consider alternative solutions. Competition with self, therapist, and peers seemed to motivate him. His deficits became apparent to him through his activity performance and feedback from the therapist. This insight seemed to further motivate him and he began to use his free time to improve his skills through frequent leisure involvement. The therapeutic recreation specialist gave him leadership roles which he responded to positively. The team worked together to monitor his socialization skills, and consistently gave feedback to discourage his inappropriateness.

As the patient's recreational therapy progressed, he met and exceeded all of the treatment goals, which included (1) to learn two new leisure skills with independent skill, including problem solving; (2) to participate on one community trip with independent skills in the areas of appropriate socialization, money management, and topographic orientation; and (3) to identify two leisure activities and two leisure resources for postdischarge involvement and use.

At discharge, he had progressed to cognitive level VIII and was independent in ambulation, leisure, and community skills. Overall, he seemed to have made a positive adjustment to his situation with improved self-esteem. He had made realistic plans to resume normal social, and leisure activities. Further plans included returning to school in a limited capacity with a lighter class load and the exploration of part-time employment opportunities.

Case 2. A 16-year-old female head injured patient, 3 months postinjury, was functioning at a cognitive level V. Prior to her injury, the patient was living with her parents and two siblings. She attended high school and worked part-time. Her leisure pursuits involved a small select group of friends and sport activities.

Upon initial assessment, she appeared anxious and scared. She talked with decreased voice volume and preferred to use gestures. She lacked affect and initiation, and was distractable and impulsive. Other deficits included decreased function in the right upper extremity, visual problems, and wheelchair dependency due to decreased coordination and strength. Ataxia of all extremities was also noted.

Her treatment program included therapeutic games, leisure skill development, and group activities for the purpose of increasing social activity involvement, cognitive remediation, and community reintegration trips for increasing physical, social, leisure, and community skills.

During treatment time, the patient was cooperative but required reminders to slow down, scan, and use her right upper extremity. She required encouragement for group activity involvement but with the continued support of her family and peers, she slowly became more comfortable with others while also making improvements in her deficit areas. Near discharge, she still required some encouragement to attend group programs, but she was initiating a few, select activities.

The patient's therapeutic recreation treatment goals were (1) to increase her activity involvement by attending three evening activities per week for at least 30 minutes in duration for a period of 2 consecutive weeks; (2) to initiate a conversation with at least one peer during the evening programs a total of six times over a 2-week period; (3) to spontaneously scan and use her right upper extremity in four consecutive treatment sessions; (4) to redevelop skills in one pretrauma leisure interest including independent initiation, setup, and physical ability. The patient met or partially met all of the therapeutic recreation treatment goals.

At discharge, she had reached cognitive level VII with a noted improvement in affect and all other deficit areas. Problems still existed in all areas but to smaller degrees. She required structure and physical assistance in most activities. Even though her ataxia continued to be a problem, she redeveloped independent skill in some activities such as rug-hooking, a preinjury leisure interest. Her plans at discharge included involvement in outdoor summer activities and returning to school in the fall.

CONCLUSION

The philosophy of leisure ability emphasized by therapeutic recreation provides a foundation from which treatment-oriented services can derive a logical and appropriate purpose. Simply stated, if independent leisure functioning is the overall purpose of therapeutic recreation services, then the treatment component can and should address functional behavioral areas that are prerequisite to, or a necessary part of, leisure involvement and lifestyle. Behavioral areas can be identified by using the commonly acknowledged domains of physical, mental, emotional, and social functioning. Each of these areas has obvious significance for leisure involvement. In most cases, therapeutic recreation is treating not the pathology itself, but the functional deficiency or limitation imposed by the pathology. The selection of the four areas of physical, mental, emotional, and social functioning enables an understanding of the actual results of an illness or disability and how these limitations may affect the living situation of the patient. The therapeutic recreation specialist is particularly concerned with how these limitations relate to and influence leisure functioning.[6]

All individuals have needs to be creative, productive, social, and physical, and to use cognitive functions. For head injured patients who may not be able to return to work, leisure and recreation involvement is especially important as it may be the only opportunity for these people to meet these needs.

While the physical sequelae of head injury tend to decrease over time, psychoso-

cial problems—including leisure-related issues and limitations—tend to become more prominent. Therapeutic recreation can play a major role in addressing many of these psychosocial limitations through the provision of relevant and appropriate services. Therapeutic recreation services should focus on

1. Planning services on an individual basis considering patient characteristics and needs
2. Emphasizing services in leisure education with the emphasis on social and leisure skill development
3. Programming for the complete patient unit which includes education and involvement of family and friends
4. Providing follow-up outpatient and/or community referral services focused on transition of needs which maximize adjustment and independence[8]

Mayberry notes that an important value of therapeutic recreation is that it increases a patient's self-confidence, with a positive carryover to other rehabilitation tasks.[9] For example, if a patient achieves success in a therapeutic recreation activity such as a chess match, then his or her mood, self-reliance, and drive will most likely be increased and have a positive effect on performance in other areas of therapy.

Social adjustment to a newly acquired disability and community reintegration are very difficult for the head injured. The development and maintenance of social contacts occur through many activities and aspects of life. It seems difficult to separate social development and leisure development at times. "Opportunities for social contact through leisure involvement should be emphasized both within and outside of the rehabilitation setting with the focus on eliminating or compensating for limitations. ..."[10] Weddell and associates indicated limitations in both areas of involvement for severe head injured individuals and that both areas should be addressed in the therapeutic recreation program.[11] Therapeutic recreation assists with these difficult areas by involving patients in social and community situations; these activities give head injured persons the opportunity to prepare for their return to home and community living. One of the important functions the therapeutic recreation specialist is responsible for is leisure discharge planning, which helps prepare the patient for continued therapeutic recreation involvement after discharge.

All disabled individuals, including the head injured, are entitled to a meaningful existence, which includes the pursuit of satisfying leisure and recreational experiences. The purpose and role of therapeutic recreation services is to provide for and facilitate the development and expression of an appropriate leisure lifestyle.

REFERENCES

1. Oddy M, Humphrey, M and Uttley, D: Subjective impairment and social recovery after closed head injury. J Neurol Neurosurg Psychiatry 41:611, 1978.
2. Oddy, M and Humphrey, M: Social recovery during the year following severe head injury. J Neurol Neurosurg Psychiatry 43:798, 1978.
3. Pollack, I, Kohn, H and Miller, M: Rehabilitation of cognitive function in brain-damaged persons. J Med Soc NJ 4:311, 1984.
4. Frye, V and Peters, M: Therapeutic Recreation: Its theory, philosophy and practice. Stackpole, Pennsylvania, 1972, p 41.
5. Kottke, FS: Future focus of rehabilitation medicine. Arch Phys Med Rehabil 6:1, 1980.
6. Gunn, S and Peterson, C: Therapeutic Recreation Program Design: Principles and Procedures. Prentice Hall, Englewood Cliffs, NJ, 1978, p 11.
7. Safilios-Rothschild, C: The Sociology and Social Psychology of Disability and Rehabilitation. Random House, New York, 1970.
8. Connolly, P: The importance of leisure and social skill development for individuals with severe head injury. Research into Action 4:33, 1984.
9. Mayberry, RP: The mystique of the horse in strong medicine. Riding as therapeutic recreation. Rehabil Lit 39:6, 192, 1978.
10. Rehab Brief: Bringing research into effective focus. 5(5):1, 1982.
11. Weddell, R, Oddy, M and Jenkins, D: Social adjustment after rehabilitation: A two year follow-up of patients with severe head injury. Psychol Med 10:257, 1980.

Chapter 31

Re-entry into the Community and Systems of Posthospital Care

LARRY CERVELLI, B.S., O.T.R.

Rehabilitation planning for people with brain injury now includes consideration of the potential for long-term recovery of functional capability and the need for a broad array of postacute services to support this recovery.[1–5]

Past research has identified the significant long-term deficits and disabilities resulting from traumatic brain injury.[6, 7] The inadequacy of traditional hospital settings for long-term management and remediation of cognitive and behavioral dysfunction is also clear. Acute service settings are generally not equipped to provide an adequate array of postacute services. Funding sources also appreciate the need for a broader spectrum of treatment and training settings and are supporting its development.[8, 9]

Families of brain injured individuals have participated in the creation of a national organization (National Head Injury Foundation) with state-level affiliates to exert the political influence necessary to foster development of a system of care that minimizes the gaps into which their loved ones can fall.[8]

In this chapter the problems resulting from a nonsystematic approach to longitudinal brain injury care are described. In addition, a methodology to approach the gaps in service delivery is addressed.

There are few tangible rewards for community service agencies to band together, share power and expertise, and share credit or blame for patient and family outcomes from the *entire* care system. Existing rewards or punishments are usually through political influence and budgetary allotment. Since a system of care, by definition, will cut across single agencies (hospital, college) or their larger systems (health, education) there are many *disincentives* to a systems approach. Cost containment, professional reputation, and community political pressure seem to be major driving forces for development of a systems approach.

An alternative to a "community" systems approach may be the vertical integration strategy in service development by the for-profit sector of rehabilitation and acute medical care. Offering a total care system within one "company"—thus decreasing the family's or insurer's need to shop for care in many places—is becoming a major theme in rehabilitation marketing.

NATURE OF THE PROBLEM

The high incidence, and male youth predominance, of brain injury in the United States have been cited elsewhere in this volume (see Chapter 2). Two startling additional findings further identify brain injury as a major national health problem. First, 93 percent of all people with brain injury admitted to hospitals alive were discharged alive.[10] Most people therefore *survive* their

463

brain injury if they get to an acute hospital. Second, the prevalence rate—those people actively being treated for the sequelae of the brain injury—was 437:100,000.[10] It is difficult to ascertain what percentage of brain injury survivors need comprehensive or extensive postacute rehabilitative services. Therefore, it is necessary to have available knowledgeable, trained service providers who are organized into effective networks that facilitate appropriate service provision in a timely and cost-effective fashion.

LIMITATIONS OF ACUTE HOSPITAL SETTINGS

The extended recovery from severe brain injury does not fit the traditional model of acute hospital care. With an average 7-day length of stay for many acute medical problems, the service design is for diagnosis; a "quick fix," rapid discharge; and perhaps follow-up care (from home) into an outpatient clinic. Medical stability and the ability to ambulate are frequently the discharge criteria.

Brain injury, by its very nature, does not fit this mold. Acute medical problems, including those associated with the original onset, may be resolved in the ICU and at the earliest stages of rehabilitation.[11] Chronic and late developing medical problems—heterotopic ossification, epilepsy, hydrocephalus, spasticity—may not require inpatient management except for surgical intervention, but do require considerable expertise for effective treatment.

Physical management is frequently complicated by problems, including stressful behavior disorders, that are beyond the capacity of hospital personnel.[6, 12] Aggressiveness, apathy, impulsive wandering from the facility, and generally disinhibited behavior can result in reliance on restraints, medication, and personal supervision that drains personnel resources, drives costs up, and can result in less than optimal patient outcomes.

Cognitive limitations (e.g., disorientation, poor memory, language dysfunction) result in time demands on personnel to repeatedly explain simple care procedures, reorient the patient to immediate events, and allay anxiety in a frightened, agitated patient. Delayed recovery of basic cognitive functioning distresses and frustrates staff members untrained in the nature of recovery from traumatic brain injury.

Finally, the physically capable but behaviorally and/or cognitively deficient patient presents physical security risks for the hospital. Disorientation, fear, lack of insight or appreciation of deficits, and the desire to "go home" results in elopement events that negatively influence discharge planning and timing. A secure environment is needed yet not readily available without extraordinary physical building modifications and special staffing for personal supervision. Civil rights laws and regulations make admitting the patient into locked psychiatric units increasingly more difficult and inappropriate. Brain injury recovery complicates the routine hospitalization process by having multiple deficits and disabilities occurring simultaneously and therefore requiring a large, professionally competent treatment staff that works harmoniously in an interdisciplinary fashion to achieve goals.[2] Unfortunately, the recovery process does not proceed at a uniformly rapid rate,[7] so that discharge and follow-up care is a complicated process of determining safety, physical, and personal care needs, identifying available community- or hospital-based outpatient treatment resources, and securing transportation to support a continuing program. In spite of these needs, the health care environment has been one of forced shorter length of stay, or limiting, by contract, the total amount of funding for hospitalization and care.

Diagnostically related groups (DRG's) are based upon a number of similar diagnostic categories, and the allowable length of stay (LOS) is an average of the number of hospital days necessary to provide acute care. Catastrophically disabled people will usually fall outside the average, thus making these patients unattractive for hospitals to care for. Although rehabilitation hospitals and acute hospital-distinct rehabilitation units are presently DRG-exempt, there is a real possibility that exemption will end in the future. This would make the brain injured a very risky group to care for since extra costs (e.g., costs for an attendant) and longer than average LOS costs are borne by the provider.

Finally, the care of the brain injured individual, although requiring active involvement of a physician skilled in rehabilitation, greatly relies on allied health professionals to address specific areas of patient deficit and disability. Rather than being the primary source of care, the rehabilitation physician becomes an integrated team member who facilitates care provision through team leadership, ordering treatment and providing cotreatment (e.g., behavioral management plus medication). This is substantially different from traditional medical care models.

In summary, care of the brain injured individual stresses traditional hospital and other inpatient-based care models. Deficits and disabilities are multiple and concurrent; require an extraordinary number of different specialists, and result in behavioral and cognitive as well as physical and medical problems. Rate of improvement is often unpredictable. The need for discharge prior to full recovery of potential function demands systematic and coordinated patient participation in many care programs.

PROBLEMS ADDRESSED OVER TIME

Studies done in California[13] and other areas[5, 12, 14, 15] have identified the long-term nature of deficits and disability following mild, moderate, and severe brain injury. They may be grouped into five patient performance areas: health, physical function, cognitive function, behavior, and role resumption. Examples of each are as follows:

Health: Deviation from ideal body weight, epilepsy, hydrocephalus, central nervous system instability

Physical Function: Vision, hearing, sensation, static positions, locomotor skills, ambulation, hand function, physical capacity

Cognitive Function: Concentration, memory, complex ideational skills, cognitive perceptual-motor skills, verbal and written expression, conceptual organization, reception, self-regulatory skills

Behavior: Emotional instability, low frustration tolerance, disinhibition, anxiety states

Role Resumption: Community, household, self-care, prevocational, and academic skills

According to Mackworth and coworkers,[7] the extrapolated improvement curves of these deficits and disabilities fall within timeframes of 6 months to 5 years. Clinical experience has also borne out that cognitive

and behavioral skills take far longer than physical skills to achieve an optimal level.

HOSPITAL DISCHARGE PROCESS AND PROBLEMS IMPEDING COMMUNITY RE-ENTRY

Acute medical hospitals and rehabilitation unit settings are highly structured to allow a few people to care for many. Since many facilities bill on a fee-for-service basis, there is an incentive for patients to have dense daily treatment schedules. Regimentation allows feeding, AM and PM care, bowel and bladder training programs, and room cleaning all to be done in a coordinated and staff-efficient fashion.

These pressures make it difficult to assess what *minimal* structure is actually necessary for patient safety and comfort following discharge. Someone is always vigilant regarding patient behavior on the ward. What amount of assistance and supervision is critically necessary in the home setting, and the exact times that they should be available, is frequently unknown.

Trained rehabilitation staff members have an experience and skill-based frame of reference and know how to interpret the seriousness of patient behaviors. Yet they frequently underestimate how a behavior (e.g., verbosity) might negatively affect the patient in a less structured environment such as a community college (class disruption, teacher exasperation). Sophistication and experience often results in therapists "automatically" structuring the environment and the patient behaviors (e.g., verbal cueing for word-finding problems; standing on the side of preserved vision) so that deficits and disabilities are frequently not expressed problems. These deficits frequently become factors in unsuccessful and costly community placement.

Rehabilitation programs need specific program components to allow patients the *structured* opportunity to perform in unforgiving, real-life environments. Brain injured people without physical deficits may provide no visual cues of disability for the public, frequently causing confused social interaction. Without a community skills assessment component, the discharge planning process is based upon clinical *estimation* of patient performance in less structured environments. Only the most sophisticated care provider feels at ease with this approach.

Lezak[15] and others have addressed the adjustment process that families experience following brain injury. The family plays a key role in facilitating and supporting the community re-entry process. "Technical support" such as making therapy appointments, following up on legal matters, handling monetary issues, providing transportation, and advocating for service provision are survival issues.

To move a brain injured person into community-based programming usually means identification of more than one care provider to address physical, cognitive, behavioral, vocational, and educational needs. In the past 8 years, post-acute transitional facilities have been developed to address many of these needs. Apart from these special centers, however, the training resources needed in most communities include (1) special education to facilitate further academic achievement; (2) vocational counseling, evaluation, and re-training; (3) resocialization programming to develop and maintain the establishment of social interactive skills; (4) recreation and leisure skills development; (5) cognitive skill development; and (6) independent living skills development.

Most community-based care providers— school teachers, mental health counselors, vocational rehabilitation counselors, therapists, and sheltered workshop employees— do not feel prepared or comfortable in providing services to the severely brain injured. This is frequently due to (1) inadequate basic educational preparation, (2) sparse coherent literature to guide their treatment approach, (3) inadequacy of their assessment tools to identify patient problems/needs, (4) lack of experience to guide their interpretation of patient behavior and responsiveness to care provided, and (5) lack of role models upon which to pattern their behavior.

COMMUNITY RE-ENTRY AND SYSTEMATIC CARE

Community re-entry is commonly spoken of in terms of living or getting treatment or training in a "community setting" other than a hospital or rehabilitation center. My view is that community re-entry really means that the service recipient receives different kinds of care from different providers, and therefore has to participate in more normalized daily living experiences to get those needed services. The disabled individual needs to somehow keep appointments, handle money, use transportation, and deal with unforgiving, impartial citizens who neither excuse nor compensate for poor memory or concrete thinking. Rather than rely on a protective, structured environment the patient faces hundreds of trivial and major challenges each day. Daily survival of these community challenges *is* the personal empowerment that results from possessing functional skills and a risk-taking attitude. Accomplishment, self-awareness, and adjustment to capability/disability should follow.

Defining a system of health care for the brain injured individual is not a simple task. Some factors making it particularly difficult are as follows:

1. Brain injury impacts all areas of human performance.
2. Brain injury impacts each person differently due to the nature of onset, specific types of neurologic injury, premorbid health, and premorbid functional and social status.
3. Brain injury sequelae change over a long timeframe in ways and degrees not yet clearly measured nor understood.
4. The technology and value structure for providing care to this population are relatively new in the past two decades; resources are just now being applied in significant amounts.
5. The social environment has undergone substantial values clarification and changes in the past 25 years, so receptiveness to the disabled population, including the brain injured, is still changing.[16, 17]
6. Health care providers, especially rehabilitationists, have only recently begun trying to define the components of a long term care system.[2] The development of posthospital components of care have been given an organized political boost in just the last several years.[8]
7. A consumer/care provider organization, the NHIF, has been organized for only 8 years to provide effective lobbying for political recognition of this population. Its state chapters have lobbied care providers

of all types for service development and expansion.

In spite of the recency of specific attention to the problems and needs of the brain injured population, general systems literature may help us understand what a system's characteristics are and identify why there currently is no organized system of care for brain injured adults.

"The most striking feature of the human service field is its non-systems character: lack of coordination of various service elements."[18] Systems for intervention and rehabilitation ideally have five primary characteristics:

1. Are immediately available, accessible, and affordable
2. Are flexible enough to meet special needs of the individual while still dealing with broad problem areas
3. Take place within the person's own social milieu where there is a firm link to family and friends
4. Are aimed at reducing risk of institutionalization and disenfranchisement from the community
5. Should be coordinated so that delivery systems make most effective and efficient use of existing and emerging community resources

With long recovery/improvement times expected in many performance areas, the issues of accessible and affordable services are substantial. To meet demands for service, most agencies have matriculation rate expectations. Funding usually flows to patients who have clear potential for benefiting relatively quickly from restorative versus "maintenance" services (e.g., behavioral control dysfunction makes educational agencies reluctant to provide educational service). Highly specialized techniques used by specially trained (and expensive) staff members make it difficult to provide specialized care in every neighborhood. Since few agencies are yet funded or staffed to coordinate services to the brain injured adult, there is only informal coordination occurring at the community level. The Massachusetts Statewide Head Injury Project (SHIP) is an exception, as is the California Family Survival Project. Both are relatively new agencies.

Community-oriented systems[18] should be guided by five principles:

1. Normalization
2. Most appropriate alternative
3. Developmental model
4. Equal human and legal rights as non-handicapped citizens
5. Mainstreaming

Certainly a system for brain injured people should and could adhere to these principles. Whether a developmental model—one that attempts to rehabilitate by developing progressively more simple to complex skills (cognition and behavioral control)—will be determined effective for this population remains to be seen. Training to specific tasks in specific environments versus relying on skill generalization is an area of dispute in brain injury rehabilitation. It can be said, however, that the entire rehabilitation process should attempt to developmentally empower and maximize self-direction in each patient.

Given these characteristics and principles, what are the system properties that govern its behavior? Ackoff[19] states that a system is two or more elements of any kind and that each has three properties:

1. Each element has an effect on all others as a whole system.
2. Each is affected by at least one other; none has an independent effect on the whole system.
3. Every possible subgroup has the first two properties and therefore the system cannot be further subdivided into independent subsystems.

In terms of an array of care for the brain injured adult, this would mean that acute physical rehabilitation care delivered to a patient in a medical rehabilitation program would be negatively affected if the mental health care delivered was inadequate. Conversely, poor physical rehabilitation care would negatively influence successful mental health services. "A system then, viewed structurally, is a divisible whole, but viewed functionally it is indivisible in the sense that some of its essential properties are lost taking it apart."[19] The essential "product" that is lost when the entire continuum of necessary care elements is lacking, inaccessible, or poorly coordinated is optimal empowerment and self-direction for each uniquely disabled and improving head injured person.

"System performance depends critically on how the parts fit and work together, not merely how well each performs independently; it depends on *interaction* rather than *actions*. Furthermore, a system's performance depends on how it relates to the environment—the larger system of which it is a part—and to other systems in that environment."[19] An example is how the rehabilitation system moves a patient from an acute medical rehabilitation program to a vocational training program, and how the funding of the entire human service system affects this movement.

The whole system has characteristics that subelements do not and loses some of them when disassembled. While a medical rehabilitation facility can offer a variety of physical, cognitive, behavioral, and role resumption therapeutic services, it cannot provide many hours of daily life experience in the community. Maximum patient empowerment will come from other system elements providing these community living opportunities.

System maintenance issues, such as management, problem solving, and planning cannot be addressed here. However, dealing with problems as a system, by all its elements, is an essential property of planning. An example might be the realization that the physically violent brain injured are unmanagable in *any* treatment setting in a regionally organized care system. Planning may yield the strategy of developing a new treatment facility or program that interfaces with existing treatment facilities.

In summary, the creation of a true system of care of the brain injured adult demands that each treatment element (medical, physical, cognitive, behavioral, vocational, educational, and so on) be coordinated so that each element is directly affected by what happens to the others. Additionally, there should be mechanisms for managing the entire system's effectiveness by guiding system-wide planning and problem-solving processes.

Given these requirements, it is clear that no "system" at present exists for caring for brain injured adults. Autonomous elements (e.g., medical rehabilitation facilities, educational institutions) identify patient needs and address them primarily within their own facility or sphere of influence. It is my view that the lack of an existing external or internal *demand* for *system* effectiveness (maximum patient empowerment and functional independence) makes this inefficient organizational behavior possible. Several new factors may, however, force change upon this behavior.

First, the political power of families and providers has dramatically increased in the last ten years. Creation of the National Institute of Handicapped Research (now National Institute of Disability and Rehabilitation Research) focused new rehabilitation research for the catastrophically disabled, including the brain injured. Modest initial funding for brain injury research has been expanded, and an increasing number of critical issues in head injury patient care are being clarified. Concurrently, the NHIF has organized chapters and affiliates in more than 35 states. It has provided families and friends of brain injured adults with advocacy education and a framework for political advocacy at the state and national levels. The signing in May 1985 of an Interagency Agreement[8] that linked the NHIF, Office of Special Education and Rehabilitation Services, United States Department of Education and Rehabilitation Services Administration, Office of Special Education Programs, National Institute of Disability and Rehabilitation Research, Council of State Administrators and Vocational Rehabilitation, and National Association of State Directors of Special Education was a major success in political activity. Furthermore, the possibility exists that *funding sources* and *consumers* of patient care services may gather enough information from their own data collection methods to focus their dissatisfaction on inefficient and ultimately less effective care processes and outcomes. Political/economic/consumer forces may drive local political groups and community service agencies to further organize their activities.[20]

Another new and powerful force in the brain injury rehabilitation and brain injury patient care environment is the entry of many new for-profit corporations.[21–23] They are horizontally and vertically integrating care services as a way of maximizing economic benefit; moreover, they are responding to dissatisfaction with existing service fragmentation and incompleteness by funding sources, case managers, and families. The dramatically heightened competitiveness in the health care market generally, and rehabilitation and long-term care specifically, has spawned the explosive expansion of comprehensive, inpatient acute treatment programs: transitional, residential, nonmedical, independent living training; coma management; and long-term custodial living programs. (The NHIF service directory has expanded from 150 to more than 500 brain injury program listings in less than 6 years.) The establishment of a variety of treatment services in many different settings frequently tied together with in-house case management services, all under the same corporate roof, is forcing independent single-care providers to re-examine their service array and ability to compete with these more diverse care provision systems. Whether data-driven analysis of patient outcomes and cost benefits actually shows better performance remains to be seen. From a marketing standpoint, these single corporate systems do appear to effectively address the demands of sophisticated service purchasers and individual families.

A system of care should ideally offer the entire range of needed services for all of its clients. It should move service recipients through efficiently (maximum result for least cost), and toward expected outcomes (maximum empowerment and functional independence). To accomplish this, the system should have components that are integrated via entry/exit criteria and provide a method for moving patients among elements effectively (case management).

Failure to meet these criteria results in the following common scenarios:

1. Lack of sufficient components

    a. A physically recovered adult with poor memory and attentional skills sits at home and watches television all day.

    b. An individual with adequate self-care and cognitive skills remains living with parents because no wheelchair accessible housing is available.

    c. An individual with a college degree but poor social skills cannot land his or her first competitive job.

    d. An individual with adequate physical and social skills gets cognitive rehabilitation on an outpatient basis at a hospital because the community college has no guided re-entry program.

2. Lack of matched entry/exit criteria

    a. The hospital-based rehabilitation center refers an individual who can work very well in structured 1:1 environments to the community vocational evaluation center. The vocational center does all evaluation and training in groups of ten students, and so the patient fails.

    b. The rehabilitation center refers a very depressed dysphasic patient to the local mental health center for supportive counseling. The mental health center counselor refuses to provide care, citing patient reluctance to verbalize feelings. The family refuses to attend counseling sessions because the counselor lacks credibility.

    c. The neurologic intensive care unit refers for rehabilitation care an acute comatose patient who is neurologically improving. The rehabilitation service refuses the transfer, citing no rehabilitation potential, and transfers the patient to a nursing facility for custodial care.

3. Lack of guided movement between components

    a. An individual is discharged from an acute care medical rehabilitation facility. Follow-up re-evaluation is scheduled but the patient fails to appear—the patient has forgotten the appointment and the family, exhausted from 90 days of continual patient supervision, has also neglected the appointment.

    b. A day care program develops an intense day program for an individual with brain injury. Both parents work nights and neglect to transport the patient to the program. Repeated telephone attempts to contact them fail and the individualized program dissolves.

    c. A patient is admitted to a locked psychiatric unit because of an explosive, destructive rage episode. Psychotropic medication calms the patient but the rehabilitation staff does not hear about this episode. A diagnosis of temporal lobe epilepsy is made three months later at a routine team re-evaluation.

Clearly, the ability of a single community-based agency to meet the many complex and diverse needs of the brain injured patient is limited. Many communities have a variety of services for the physically disabled but none specifically designed for brain injured individuals. To adequately meet all of the needs addressed earlier, a "system" is needed. That system generates the interactive processes between the elements of care. These interactive processes can be, in order of complexity and intensity,[24] (1) networking, (2) coordination, (3) cooperation, and (4) collaboration.

Each of these techniques potentially expands the service capability of each service provider by accessing the knowledge and experience of the others, and potentially improves system outcomes through more complete and efficient service delivery.

Networking can be conceptualized as interpersonal communication between *individuals*. It requires little or no agency commitment and is generally not noticed by the community at large. An advisory council is an example of this technique. Technical sharing between like-service providers (OT, psychologist) is another example of networking.

Interagency coordination strives to avoid service duplication while providing essential services. Members operate autonomously, but participate in additional joint activities. The cooperative nature is not highly visible to the community. The *entire coordinating agency* is represented but not necessarily involved. An efficient referral procedure between a medical rehabilitation facility and the local office of the department of vocational rehabilitation may be a coordinated activity. Another example of such activity would be the development of a local or state resource directory.

Interagency cooperation aims at integration among participating agencies rather than just parallel operation. Some autonomy is relinquished to obtain necessary benefits. A joint in-service training program, shared fund-raising, and publicity programs are examples of this technique. Community visibility is greater than in previously described techniques. The *entire agency* is represented.

Finally, collaboration is the most intense and complex technique. Agency personnel join together to accomplish a single goal, and relinquish agency autonomy to do so. There is intense structured personal interaction. The general community is very much aware of the activity and its participants. An example might be the establishment of a day care center for brain injured adults. Agencies may contribute space, staff, and program development expertise, and pro-

vide direct or consultative services.[3] Entire agencies are represented, but small groups or individuals are the ones who implement the plan.

The latter three linkage options have varied requirements of management leadership structures and styles. "The key skill is to be able to identify the best type of interaction for any particular purpose or project and then to be able to use the skills appropriate for that specific purpose."[24]

The common pitfalls of creating interagency linkages are[25]

1. Focusing prematurely on the program or the intended outcome, thereby channeling energy into developing structures or implementation procedures for the partnership before the participants have fully understood and committed themselves to the relationship

2. Not identifying and resolving power relationships (the result is conflicts over sources of influence and decision making among participating organizations)

3. Ignoring ideologic differences among partners coming from different "domains"—education, health, mental health, and businesses each have their own values and belief systems; identifying, understanding, and resolving differences among these values and beliefs is critically important; polarization and disintegration can easily result.

METHODS OF TREATMENT

Processes

Long-term systematic care of the brain injured individual includes evaluation, re-evaluation, treatment, and managed movement among different care settings. In brain injury rehabilitation, evaluation and re-evaluation are necessary in a variety of domains. A behavioral assessment, neuropsychologic evaluation, medical examination, and language assessment yield a comprehensive view of the needs of an individual at a given point in time. Performed serially, at least annually, such assessments define longer-term recovery trends so that planning and implementing changes in vocational, educational, and independent living arrangements can be determined from a comprehensive data base. Further, annual contact with a knowledgeable rehabilitation team can identify emerging problems and can prevent crises from occurring. For example, it is easier to make changes in living arrangements *before* families dissolve in conflict and physical violence than after a major incident of explosive or disinhibited behavior occurs.

An important element in the provision of high-quality, long-term care is the availability of well-trained, experienced staff members. To develop and maintain expertise, a given facility must treat a sufficient volume of brain injured patients to see *trends* in subgroupings of brain injured persons. The complexity of concurrent deficits and disabilities, number of complex treatment goals, and variety of different agencies providing simultaneous care can be a difficult challenge for all treatment staff.

Providing for efficient and effective patient movement among the various treatment settings and specialists is one of the most difficult aspects of long-term care. Third-party payors often complain about the financial resources wasted by placement of a client in a facility that cannot effectively manage a particular problem (e.g., behavior problem, surgical problem) or the need to hold a client in a facility longer than necessary due to the unavailability or inaccessibility (financial, geographic, or otherwise) of the next service program required in the continuum of care.

Case Management

More commonly, the problem of moving the disabled person from one care setting to another is hampered by the lack of a specific nonfacility individual who is responsible and accountable for the process of interaction between care system elements. The response to this deficit has been the rise to prominence, particularly for private sector patients, of the case manager. While not uniformly defined, the case management function has been described as "ensuring that individual members of a target population receive the service they need to function adequately in the least restrictive setting possible."[26] The case manager may fulfill this objective by identifying client needs, planning for meeting those needs, and linking

various service providers with each other to ensure coordinated and timely service.

Above all, case management is a strategy for guidance of the dynamic interactive elements of a care system. To be successful in this role the case manager must have authority to drive the system. This may come from administrative policies and agreements between service agencies, legal and legislative mandates, fiscal control and responsibility, and clinical expertise. Clearly the insurance industry uses its fiscal authority to drive the care system, whereas patient guardians and public sector agencies may use their legal authority. Many head injury care providers are now installing in-house case management systems in response to demand for a single contact person, readily available to external case managers, who can synthesize and coordinate the work and reporting of the many professional team members addressing the patient's myriad deficits and disabilities.

Care Settings

The notion of community re-entry and of a long-term care system mandated a variety of care agencies that dynamically interact through specific design. Figure 31–1 is a graphic display of residential services.

Though these options are generally self-explanatory, a brief discussion of our experience serving the head injured in a few specific community agencies may be helpful.

Community College. In Santa Clara County, California, community colleges were able to actively serve 5 to 25 severely disabled head injured students through several different strategies. All provided special van transportation services, specially trained guidance counselors, adaptive communication devices, educational aids, learning laboratories with student tutors, and specific educational/socialization goal-driven semester-long education plans. Architectural barriers for mobility impaired students were essentially absent.

These college programs liberally mixed resocialization activities (e.g., "rap" groups, clubs), preacademic tutoring (reading comprehension and recall drills), and basic academic classes. The designing and blending of these programs for individual students was done by guidance counselors who were

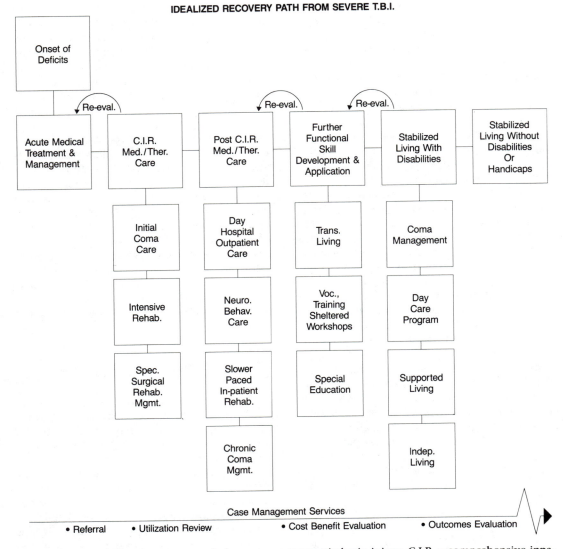

Figure 31–1. Idealized recovery path from severe traumatic brain injury. C.I.R. = comprehensive inpatient rehabilitation.

interested in serving disabled students generally, and head injured students specifically. They were trained in head injury issues by peers in the local medical rehabilitation hospital and State Department of Rehabilitation vocational counselors who had extensive experience in head injury rehabilitation. Ongoing peer support and joint service development and coordination was done through a Disabled Students Program Professional Advisory Board that routinely met.

Special problems that occurred frequently are listed in the table on page 473 with some responses that proved useful.

The success of head injured students, of course, varies due to their deficits and disabilities. It has been demonstrated that this agency, given creative and knowledgeable staff, can provide an effective service to some head injured people. Networking and coordination with other rehabilitation facilities and agencies makes this most effective.

Community Mental Health Centers. Serving head injured families has been difficult for many community mental health centers. A survey of mental health providers in Santa Cara County[27] revealed that most professional staff felt uneducated about head injury and uncertain or discouraged about

Problem	Response
Difficulty choosing classes	Counselor gets medical rehabilitation team patient evaluations and recommendations
Getting lost between classes	Route maps Between-class student guides Classes chosen for location
Conflct with teachers	Teachers hand picked by counselor for temperament and tolerance
Sensory overload in classes	Classes chosen by counselor for size and composition
Unresolved anger and upset from forgotten daily events	2× daily "rap group" to ventilate anger and re-establish calm approach to remainder of the day
Very slow new learning; learning disability	Tutoring by work-study students; special tutoring equipment
Poor self-esteem	Enrollment in physical exercise and conditioning classes that result in better grades and positive socialization

how their assessment and treatment techniques affected these patients, and stated they had seen very few head injured patients or their families. A concurrent survey of disabled people and their families, including head injured people, revealed that they were reluctant to seek service from mental health centers because they lacked confidence in the professional staff. They felt that the staff lacked knowledge about head injury and did not feel they could benefit from services offered. Families and patients continued to seek long-term mental health counseling from the medical or other rehabilitation agency at which they had been treated. Provider fears revolved around being influenced by long-term service demands.

The response to this survey resulted in an inter-agency collaborative effort to increase and improve mental health service to head injured people. Rehabilitation staff from the medical center provided extensive head injury education to a special multidisciplinary mental health team. The special team provided on-site direct and consultative services to a wide variety of community educational, vocational, and day care agencies. Services were substantially improved and interagency referrals increased.

Day Care Program. The gap between change-oriented, funded rehabilitation training programs and self-directed functionally independent living is a chasm into which many severely head injured adults fall. Too impaired to participate in community college, sheltered vocational evaluation and training, or other routine daily activity,

many people sit home or drift around the community in unstructured "play." Family frustration and anger is extreme when members are trapped into providing constant daily supervision.

Santa Clara County developed the Adult Development Center, a low-cost day care program housed in a local church and staffed by employees of the county adult education program and volunteers. The interagency collaboration that developed this resource is described in a publication.[3] Designed to provide cognitive, educational, and resocialization opportunities, the program had an important side effect of relieving family of constant supervision responsibilities, which improved the quality of life of all concerned. Strong interagency networking and collaboration with the State Department of Rehabilitation, community colleges, vocational training agencies, the community mental health center, a church, and the medical rehabilitation facility resulted in a low-cost resource that allowed long-term structured day activity. Individualized goals and long-term (typically more than 1 year) engagement facilitated slow-paced change to occur. Many students graduated to higher-level programs at other agencies.

A similar program has been designed through western Massachusetts interagency collaboration and involves a chronic care hospital, a medical rehabilitation skilled nursing facility specializing in care of the head injured, the Massachusetts Statewide Head Injury Program (SHIP), the Massachusetts Rehabilitation Commission, and the University of Massachusetts. The intent of the program is identical to that of the Adult Developmental Center. A major difference is that SHIP is funding patient attendance, and providing referral screening, patient intake, and follow-along case management services. Funding primarily is by a contract between SHIP and the chronic care hospital. It is anticipated that adequate initial funding and strong in-house case management should result in more efficient movement of clients in and out of the agency.

Day Treatment Centers.   When health and personal care needs do not require institutional placement, a day treatment center may provide one or several therapeutic services. Services are goal specific and improvement oriented. They are delivered under medical supervision. The head injured individual frequently has difficulty with effective use of public transportation, and missed appointments reduce treatment effectiveness. Unstructured time between appointments can magnify behavioral problems. These centers frequently make changes to accommodate these problems by increasing supervision and decreasing gaps in treatment schedules.

Transitional Living Centers.   There is a wide gap between learning individual skills and behaviors and applying them effectively in the real world. This is a particularly difficult transition for the head injured individual. These homelike residential centers provide a structured approach and specially trained staff. While primarily using the community to develop and practice daily living skills, many provide specific training classes and groups to improve basic cognitive and social skills.

Respite Care Programs.   Families frequently provide personal care assistance and around-the-clock supervision to severely disabled family members. Respite care is designed to help preserve the family caretakers by giving them short term relief from these responsibilities. The developmental disability (DD) care system has offered this service routinely for up to 2 weeks yearly for its patients. Some head injury care centers have only recently offered this service, and it has been selectively available based upon bed availability, medical and other specialized patient needs, and funding availability.

SUMMARY

In the past 20 years the scope of the problem of rehabilitating those suffering the effects of traumatic head injury and their families has become much clearer. Much has been learned about the nature and treatment of residual deficits, disabilities, and handicaps. Useful treatment approaches and techniques have been identified.

It has also become clearer that no single facility can provide for all short- and long-term needs. Nonmedical facilities such as community colleges, charitable organizations, and religious groups have valuable roles to play. Most effective use of these resources depends on development of a true system of care, which presently does not exist. To create a system of care in a community requires incentives. Additionally new organizational relationships, including cooperative and collaborative ventures, will be required. Each demands a degree of sharing and cooperation that may be new and anxiety-provoking to the organizations involved.

The development of a system of care can have both positive and negative effects. Patient empowerment and functional independence could be compromised by learned reliance on a protective system of services that fuels a "future improvement" orientation. Families and their communities, while presented with a more complete and coordinated array of services, may need to spend more money on these services. Against these potential negatives rests the real possibility of a more uniform and improved level of patient and family independence that decreases long-term social support costs. A systems approach to development of independence and reduction of misery is long overdue.

REFERENCES

1. Bush, G, Spivak, MP and Spivak, ML: Testimony of the National Head Injury Foundation to the Senate

Appropriations Subcommittee on Labor Health and Human Services, Education and Related Agencies

Relative to FY 1987 Appropriations for Programs Authorized by the Rehabilitation Act of 1973. As Amended May 9, 1986.

2. Cervelli, L and Berrol, S: Description of a model care system. In Berrol, S et al (eds): Head Injury Rehabilitation Project Final Report. NIHR Grant #13-P-59156/9, San Jose, CA, Santa Clara Valley Medical Center, 1982, p iv.
3. Cole, JR, Cope, DN and Cervelli, L: Rehabilitation of the severely brain injured patient: A community-based, low-cost community model. Arch Phys Med Rehabil 66:38, 1985.
4. Hackler, E and Tobis, JS: Reintegration into the community. In Rosenthal, M et al (eds): Rehabilitation of the Head Injured Adult. FA Davis, Philadelphia, 1983, p 429.
5. Smith, RK: Prevocational programming in the rehabilitation of the head injured patient. Phys Ther 63:84, 1983.
6. Eames, P and Wood, R: Rehabilitation after severe brain injury: A follow-up study of a behavior modification approach. J Neurol Neurosurg Psychiatry 48:613, 1985.
7. Mackworth, N, Mackworth, J and Cope, DN: Towards an interpretation of head injury recovery trends. In Berrol, S et al (eds): Head Injury Rehabilitation Project Final Report. NIHR Grant #13-P-59156/9. San Jose, CA, Santa Clara Valley Medical Center, 1982, p viii.
8. National Head Injury Foundation, Office of Special Education and Rehabilitative Services, Rehabilitation Services Administration, Office of Special Education Programs, National Institute of Handicapped Research, Council of State Administrators of Vocational Rehabilitation, and National Association of State Directors of Special Education: Cooperative Agreement (A Memorandum of Understanding), 1985.
9. Office of Health Systems Management, Division of Health Care Standards and Surveillance: Head Injury in New York—A Report to the Governor and the Legislature. New York State Department of Health, 1986.
10. Anderson, DW and McLaurin, RL (eds): Report on the National Head and Spinal Cord Injury Survey. National Institute of Neurological and Communicative Disorders and Stroke. J Neurosurg (Suppl) 53:1, 1980.
11. Miller, JD: Early Evaluation and Management. In Rosenthal, M et al (eds): Rehabilitation of the Head Injured Adult. FA Davis, Philadelphia, 1983, p 37.
12. Rinehart, MA: Considerations for functional training in adults after head injury. Phys Ther 63:33, 1983.
13. Berrol, S et al (eds): Head Injury Rehabilitation Research Project Final Report. Grant No. RSA 13-P-59156/9-03. San Jose, CA, Santa Clara Valley Medical Center, 1982.

14. Benton, A: Behavioral consequences of closed head injury. In Central Nervous System Trauma Research Status Report. National Institute of Neurological and Communicable Disorders and Stroke, 1979, p 84.
15. Lezak, MD: Living with the characterologically-altered brain injured patient. J Clin Psychiatry 39:592, 1978.
16. National Council on the Handicapped: Toward Independence—An Assessment of Federal Laws and Programs Affecting Persons with Disabilities—With Legislative Recommendations. US Government Printing Office, Washington, DC, 1986.
17. Taylor, H, Kagay, MR and Leichenko, S: The ICD Survey of Disabled Americans: Bringing Disabled Americans Into the Mainstream. Lou Harris and Associates, New York, 1986.
18. Magrab, P and Elder, T (eds): Planning for Services to Handicapped Persons. Brookes, Baltimore, 1979.
19. Ackoff, R: The systems revolution. In Lockett, M and Spear, R (eds): Organizations as Systems. Open University Press, Milton Keynes, England, 1980, p 26.
20. Rubin, I, Plovnick, M and Fry, R: Initiating planned change in health care systems. J Appl Behav Sci 10:107, 1974.
21. Kelley, M: The opportunity in rehabilitation, growing need offers exceptional opportunities for long term care facilities. Contemp Long-Term Care 10:38, 1987.
22. Starr, P: The coming of the corporation. In The Social Transformation of American Medicine: The Rise of a Sovereign Profession and The Making of a Vast Industry. Basic Books, New York, 1982, p 420.
23. Tarlov, A: Shattuck Lecture—The increasing supply of physicians, the changing structure of the health service system, and the future practice of medicine. N Engl J Med 308:1235, 1983.
24. Loughran, EL: Networking, coordination, cooperation and collaboration: Different skills for different purposes. Commun Educ J 9:28, 1982.
25. Reed, H: Typical Partnership Problems. Presented at conference Collaborations and Linkages sponsored by University of Massachusetts School of Education and Center for Community Development, Northampton, MA, 1986.
26. Schuartz, SR, Goldman, HH and Churgin, S: Case management for the chronically mentally ill: Models and dimensions. Hosp Commun Psychiatry 33:1006, 1982.
27. Voorhes, PA: Identification of the mental health needs and services being provided to the physically disabled in Santa Clara County, CA. Department of Physical Medicine and Rehabilitation, Santa Clara Valley Medical Center, 1982, unpublished data.

Chapter 32

Educational Strategies

DOUGLAS E. HARRINGTON, Ph.D.

STATEMENT OF THE PROBLEM

The incidence of head injury by age groupings indicates that there is a disproportionately high rate of injury in adolescents and young adults.[1] The estimated cumulative risk for brain injury in children through the age of 15 is 4.0 percent in boys and 2.5 percent in girls.[2] Because of age- and health-related factors combined with the neuroplasticity of the younger, developing brain, survival rates are estimated to be much higher for the younger age groups.[2] However, the previously held notion that children sustaining serious brain injuries are relatively impervious to cognitive, behavioral, and motor consequences is being forcefully challenged.[3, 4] Even in cases with children sustaining so-called mild head injuries, there are reports of personality changes, irritability, school learning problems, headaches, and memory and attention deficits.[5]

These studies suggest that education for brain injured individuals, after their acute medical care and rehabilitation has been completed, is an inevitability. The highest incidence of head injury victims by age grouping falls within the years when education remains either a compensatory requirement or a viable, realistic, and age-appropriate option.

Yet, in spite of this inevitability, the educational process for individuals with neurologically based learning and behavioral disturbances remains confusing and controversial. The American Psychiatric Association classifies brain damaged conditions as "organic brain syndromes." Neurologists have introduced the term "neurobehavioral disorders." The educational system, however, has not created an analogous descriptive term for brain injury. In fact, PL 94-142, the National Education Act guaranteeing a free and appropriate education for all individuals with disabilities, does not include a specific category for brain-related disorders.

HISTORIC OVERVIEW

In spite of the current lack of recognition of traumatic brain injury within the educational field, the concept of neurologic disorders is not new to educators. The origin of clinical reports on acquired brain dysfunction in childhood can be traced back to the early 1920s.[6, 7]

At the same time, Orton[8] was writing about "word blindness" in school-aged children. He postulated a relationship between brain functioning and specific types of reading disability because of similarity between children with reading disorders and brain damaged adults with left cerebral lesions. In the 1930s, a paper outlined a childhood behavioral syndrome referred to as "organic driveness."[9] In the 1940s, a major contribution to the field was made by Strauss and Lehtinen[10] in outlining the psychopathology and education of brain injured children. A contributing factor to the confusion and controversy within this literature was its primary association with children suffering from "minimal brain dysfunction." Unfortunately, a large proportion of these "brain damaged children" were given the diagnosis

476

based on a pattern of behavior rather than from any known pathologic alteration of brain tissue.[11] Consequently, those children with a well-defined pathologic lesion either by history or evaluation were grouped with those children without such documented lesions. The ultimate result appears to have been a lack of acceptance by the education field of the concept of brain damage and any specialized pedagogy directed toward serving these students.

During the 1950s and 1960s researchers such as Kephart, Frostig, Kirk, Cruickshank, and Myklebust kept the notion of neurology and education alive. However, during this time, there was a greater emphasis placed upon the behavioral science of learning through the operant conditioning and behavior modification literature. The interest was on what was happening outside the cranium, not inside. Then in the late 1960s and early 1970s with the emergence of brain imaging techniques allowing medical science to look inside the active brain, the pendulum began swinging back in the direction of the neurosciences. In 1978, the annual Yearbook of the Society for the Study of Education devoted its entire contents to information on education and the brain.[12] More recently, researchers such as Hewett, Satz, Gaddes, Hynd, Rourke, and Hartlage have contributed numerous articles and studies on the relevance of studying the brain as it relates to education. In fact, Cruickshank[13] has proposed the idea of a new type of educator—the neuroeducator—who would be responsible for guiding the education field in the synthesis of neuroscience research and literature with the fundamentals of learning and pedagogy.

Recently, there has been growing literature on educating the student with traumatic brain injury.[14–19] In California, the legislature has recently adopted Title V Regulations (a document that regulates special education services for the disabled in the California Community College system), which includes a specific category for brain injured students.

GOVERNMENT MANDATE
PL 94-142

The purpose of the federal education legislation (PL 94-142) originally passed in 1975 and then revised in 1981 is (1) to ensure that all handicapped children have available to them a free appropriate public education which includes special education and related services to meet their unique needs; (2) to ensure that the rights of handicapped children and their parents are protected; (3) to assist states and localities to provide for the education of all handicapped children; and (4) to assess and ensure the effectiveness of efforts to educate those children.

In PL 94-142, the term "handicapped children" is defined as those children who, when evaluated, are found to have handicaps which in order to benefit from education require specially designed instruction or require related services including transportation, speech pathology/audiology, psychologic services, physical and occupational therapy, recreation, early identification and assessment of disabilities, medical services for diagnostic or evaluation purposes, school health services, social work services, and/or parent counseling and training. Special handicapping categories listed in the regulations include mentally retarded, hard of hearing, deaf, speech impaired, visually handicapped, seriously emotionally disturbed, orthopedically impaired, other health impaired, deaf-blind, multihandicapped, or specific learning disabilities. As mentioned earlier, a category for students who have sustained traumatic brain injury is not included—that is, unless concomitant to the brain injury is one or more of the handicaps listed, such as vision and/or hearing loss.

In reviewing the specific definitions of each handicapping condition, there are some categories under which the student with traumatic brain injury may be identified. These categories include mental retardation, orthopedic impairment, other health impairment, specific learning disability, and speech impairment. However, more often than not, a student with traumatic brain injury does not "fit" into one of these classifications. The reason is that each category leaves out the primary deficit areas usually associated with post-traumatic head injury, specifically cognitive and behavioral disturbances. These disturbances meet the intention of the law by being handicaps that adversely effect a student's ability to benefit from education without specially designed instruction or related services. However, without a specific category identifying and defining these handicaps, educators remain unaware and underprepared to provide service to the student with brain injury.

Section 504

Section 504 of the Rehabilitation Act of 1973 ensures that all disabled students will have access to postsecondary education when appropriate. Section 504 provides protection for disabled adults in areas of admissions, curriculum, and physical accessibility. The Association on Handicapped Student Service Programs in Postsecondary Education is one of the national organizations working for appropriate education opportunities for disabled adults. In California, primarily through the efforts of the California Association of Postsecondary Educators for the Disabled, a specific diagnostic category has been adopted within disabled student service guidelines for students with acquired brain injury. In addition, the Chancellor's Office of the California Community Colleges has developed a consortium of professionals which has recently published a handbook outlining educational services appropriate for students with acquired brain injuries in the California community college system.[18]

NHIF/OSERS Agreement

In 1985, a Cooperative Agency Agreement[20] was adopted and signed by the National Head Injury Foundation (NHIF) and the Office of Special Education and Rehabilitative Services (OSERS), Council of State Administrators of Vocational Rehabilitation (CSAVR), and the National Association of State Directors of Special Education (NASDSE). The purpose of the agreement was to provide an outline for the parties to work together to promote the delivery of improved and expanded research, education, and rehabilitation services for the head injured population.

Included in the goals of the agreement directly relevant to education were (1) to recognize traumatic brain injury (TBI) as a specific disability, (2) to increase knowledge about TBI to educators, (3) to expand and stimulate an array of innovative services and strategies in education to this population, and (4) to expand scientific knowledge through research and development. To further implement the agreement between the national level agencies, state and local special education agencies are encouraged to create and/or review and renew their own appropriate agreements specifying how they will structure local cooperation and planning to better service this population.

THE DILEMMA OF RETURNING TO SCHOOL AFTER TBI

Case 1. John was a healthy, energetic, and high-achieving 16-year-old high school student. He was planning to take the scholastic aptitude test (SAT) in his junior year with his sights set on one of the major state universities, which his older brother had attended.

In early summer at the end of his sophomore year, the patient was involved in a serious motor vehicle accident in which he sustained a severe closed head injury with right frontal-temporal brain contusions. He was comatose for 2 weeks and experienced a post-traumatic confusional state for an additional 3 to 4 weeks. Once he was stabilized medically and orthopedically, he was transferred to the acute medical rehabilitation unit. He approached his rehabilitation care with the same positive outlook and fervor that he had used throughout his life up to the time of the accident. Remarkably, John was able to be discharged from the hospital to outpatient treatment after 8 weeks of acute rehabilitation. His therapists and doctors all commented on how "miraculous" his recovery had been. In spite of the seriousness of his acute injuries, everyone was feeling optimistic and encouraged about his long-term prognosis.

Once he was placed in an outpatient therapy program, the fall semester had started and his school district provided a home teacher in the afternoon in order to keep up with his studies. The home teacher was not familiar with students with traumatic brain injury. The home teacher was able to tutor him in English and government for the next 3 months. She attempted to review with him his algebra book from the previous semester, but John was having difficulty with some of the basic concepts. By the second semester everyone felt he was ready to return to school. However, the home teacher was concerned about his math work and referred John to the school psychologist for evaluation. The psychologist was backlogged with testing referrals and was not able to schedule John until 4 weeks into the semester. However, with the speech pathologist's evaluation from the hospital, the psychologist was able to schedule John into two 30-minute sessions per week with the speech therapist at school.

John enrolled in a full six-period day with a few modifications including the speech therapy, an office aide job, and a sixth-period individualized gym class to work on reconditioning.

By the second week of the semester, John began expressing concern to his parents. They, too, were becoming concerned because for the first time they were getting calls from the attendance office that John was regularly tardy to his classes. By the fourth week, the school psychologist had completed his evaluation and scheduled a meeting with his parents. He had what he thought was good news. John's measured IQ score still fell at the high end of the average range; although there was some difficulty noted with the timed motor and visual spatial tasks. In the achievement areas, he was still above grade level in his written language score and sight vocabulary. He was now 2 years below grade level in his math achievement but close enough to his expected performance that it was not considered a severe discrepancy. The psychologist painted a very optimistic picture to John's parents considering the seriousness of his acute injuries. No specific recommendations were made other than continuing with the speech therapy. When the parents brought up a concern about John's attendance problem, the psychologist explained that that was something typical of students after returning from a long absence to school and that it should improve in a few weeks. His parents left the meeting feeling confused and worried.

By the end of the first quarter, John was failing his algebra class. His math teacher recommended that he drop the class and because of his awareness of John's accident decided not to penalize him, by giving him a withdrawal rather than an "F." John was beginning to feel very discouraged. His English teacher had called his parents and said that in discussions in the classroom on the literature that was assigned, it appeared that John was not comprehending the assignments. The Government teacher had sent in a discipline slip to John's counselor because on one occasion in class when dis-

cussing Middle Eastern affairs, John stood up and blurted out an obscenity. John's parents noticed that the phone had essentially stopped ringing in his room. His girlfriend came over to see him now less frequently. John was spending Friday and Saturday nights at home, whereas before his accident, he would rarely spend a weekend night at home. Things were drastically different, yet John essentially looked the same. His parents began to admit that even though John was physically the same, his behavior was much more childlike and irresponsible.

This case example illustrates some of the difficulties encountered by students returning to school. After traumatic brain injury, the medical field can perform miracles in saving lives and returning individuals to what appear to be normal physical specimens. However, residual cognitive and behavioral deficits can be quite subtle but devastating. Many times, these deficits are not recognized and assistance is not provided.

John was experiencing cognitive and behavioral problems influencing his educational program. Even after individual evaluation by the school psychologist, however, these problems were not identified. He was not found to be eligible for special education resources, except for speech therapy. His academic program was too demanding and his teachers were not made aware of his difficulties. Rather than discouraging John, his teachers tended to overlook problems and to make excuses for his behavior. They tended to "pass him along" even though he was nowhere near the caliber of student he was before. Even the medical and rehabilitation professionals were not much help because they tended to be so optimistic and positive about John's recovery that unrealistic expectations were created on everyone's part.

The dilemma of returning to school after a traumatic brain injury is that life is just not the same. Expectations and future plans need to be re-evaluated and modified. Cognitive and behavioral difficulties are not well identified, and appropriate special education resources are generally not well established. Although acute rehabilitation can provide substantial assistance in maximizing spontaneous recovery from the injury, it is the long-term reintegration of the individual into a successful educational program working toward a future that is the real challenge for this population.

INDIVIDUALIZED EDUCATION PROGRAM

It is mandated in PL 94-142 that every handicapped student is entitled to a written statement that is developed and implemented to appropriately address the needs of that student in special education. Meetings are to be scheduled at least annually for the purpose of developing, reviewing, and revising a handicapped student's individualized education program (IEP). Each meeting to review the IEP must have in attendance a representative or administrator of the school program other than the student's teacher, one or both of the student's parents (or guardian), the student (when appropriate), and any other individual at the discretion of the parent or agency. If a student has been evaluated for special education for the first time, the school shall ensure that a member of the evaluation team participates in the meeting or that someone is present who is knowledgeable about the evaluation results. In addition, the school is to take steps to ensure that the parents are an integral part of the meeting.

The IEP for each student must include

☐ A statement of the student's present educational performance level
☐ A statement of annual goals, including short-term instructional objectives
☐ A statement of the specific special education and related services to be provided and the extent to which the student will participate in regular education services
☐ The projected dates for initiation of services and anticipated duration of services
☐ Appropriate objective criteria and evaluation procedures which are to be reviewed at least annually to determine whether short-term objectives are being achieved

The purpose of the IEP is to provide a framework from which to understand a handicapped student's current performance level, needs based upon that performance level, goals directed toward meeting the needs, and the types of services necessary to realistically attempt to reach the goals. It is a vehicle provided to all parents and handicapped students which allows educational services to be directed toward the handicapping condition. It is also a method of monitoring, reviewing, and revising the education program if the disability is not being appropriately addressed. The IEP process can provide parents and students with TBI with a method that can assist the transition and ultimate success in returning to school.

ASSESSMENT

Assessment of the student with TBI is extremely complex. The reasons for the complexity include

☐ The complicated and multiple problems that can occur when the brain is traumatized.
☐ Brain injuries are never the same: even when the location of the injury is similar, the manifestations from individual to individual can be very different.
☐ Recovery from brain injury is dependent on many factors including age, developmental stage, intensity of medical intervention, medications, location of damage, time since accident, preaccident student traits, familial support, socioeconomic status, and postaccident adaptive success.
☐ There are very few tests that have been developed and standardized specifically for the brain injured, especially within the education field.
☐ Very few personnel in education have any background or experience in evaluating neurologically based conditions.

Yet, in spite of its complexity, an adequate assessment is critical to the development and implementation of an appropriate educational plan. In fact, the assessment phase of an IEP proposal is the most critical in being able to develop reasonable goals and objectives for the student and in ultimately deciding what types of educational services are necessary.

The ingredients for adequately assessing a student with traumatic head injury include

☐ The educator's awareness of each student's educational ability and performance before the injury
☐ The educator's awareness of the six most typical areas in which a student's educational performance can be impacted by a

traumatic brain injury (i.e., cognitive, behavioral/psychosocial, emotional/personality, communication, academic, and psychomotor)

☐ The educator's knowledge that each of the areas in which performance can be negatively influenced falls somewhere on the continuum from mild to severe

☐ The educator's knowledge of assessment strategies within each of the six areas

☐ The educator's understanding of brain-behavior-learning relationships

Because of the complex nature of assessment after traumatic brain injury, it is recommended that the educational evaluation be completed by a multidisciplinary team of professionals found within the education field and that this team interact and interchange information so that data that cross interdisciplinary lines can be understood by all those involved. The following specialist categories should be typically included

☐ Special education teacher
☐ School psychologist
☐ Speech/language specialist
☐ School social worker/counselor
☐ School nurse
☐ Adaptive physical education specialist
☐ School administrator

When appropriate, additional consultation and evaluation may be requested from the following disciplines: physical therapists, occupational therapists, vocational rehabilitation specialists, neuropsychologists, neurologists, physiatrists, orthopedic specialists, and psychiatrists.

It is cautioned that professionals involved in the assessment process must have specific expertise in the administration and interpretation of the tests or procedures utilized.

It also must be recognized that assessment of the brain injured student may require adaptation of typical assessment procedures provided to other students. The choice of procedures must take into consideration the student's postaccident status. For example, the length of time, complexity, type of direction, type of response, provision for practice, and pacing of the material may all need to be modified to maximize the appropriateness of the assessment. Suggested adaptation procedures include

☐ Modifying the method of student response, such as allowing for pointing, gesturing, underlining, and so forth

☐ Modifying the length, complexity, or modality of test directions

☐ Giving multiple choice or examples

☐ Enlarging print or decreasing the amount of print on a given page

☐ Giving opportunity for timed and untimed responses

☐ Testing the limits to understand the student's maximum performance level

☐ Providing delimiting factors (e.g., stress, speed, noise) that may highlight the student's limitations in performance

☐ Providing assessment in a variety of settings (e.g., 1:1, small versus large, quiet versus noisy)

☐ Considering motoric or sensory deficits

☐ Considering medications, time of day, and fatigue factors

☐ Allowing for serial behavioral observations over time

If procedures are adapted, consideration must also be given to the standardization of the assessment tools. One must be careful in drawing conclusions of a standardized nature when standardized procedures are not followed.

Although each student's performance will be different, there are certain general characteristics which need to be observed in nearly all evaluations. In testing situations, as well as eventually in the classroom, close observation of the following characteristics needs to occur and be considered:

☐ Level of attention span, distractibility, and orientation to time, place, and task

☐ Adaptability, i.e., adjustment to changes in content, format, or routine

☐ Perseveration, i.e., tendency to repeat certain words, phrases, or actions

☐ Tolerance to stress, such as time, noise, or frustration

☐ Fatigue, i.e., the student's mental and physical stamina

☐ Passive-aggressiveness, i.e., resistance to complete tasks, work refusals, belligerence

☐ Factors related to emotional adjustment including anxiety, depression, fear of failure, frustration-tolerance

☐ Tendency to become tangential or circumstantial in activity

☐ Degree to which external structure, cueing, and prompting is required

☐ Tendency to distort, confuse, or misperceive facts

☐ Processing time, delayed response or slowed performance

☐ Degree of confusion or comprehension

☐ Degree to which new information interferes with recent learning

☐ Lack of consistency in performance over time

☐ Utilization of compensatory strategies

With the aforementioned information in mind, assessment is suggested in the following areas: (1) preinjury traits and abilities, (2) medical history/description of injury, (3) cognitive abilities, (4) behavioral/psychosocial performance level, (5) communication/speech skills, (6) academic performance level, (7) emotional/personality status, and (8) psychomotor/physical status.

Preinjury Traits/Abilities

It is very important to always consider the student's preinjury status and abilities. It is generally believed that the student with above-average intellectual, academic, and social abilities has the best prognosis for long-term recovery and adaptability. It is also believed that if a student has an academic or behavioral difficulty before the injury, then this difficulty will likely remain (or worsen) after the injury. Therefore, preinjury factors can help provide insight into a student's eventual performance profile.

Assessment of preinjury factors can be obtained through a variety of procedures. The school administrator or counselor can review the cumulative school record for achievement scores, report cards, and behavioral referrals. The parents can be interviewed by the counselor or social worker to review school history and to help identify preinjury strengths, habits, interests, and hobbies. If the student has been evaluated for special education in the past, prior test results and IEPs can be considered. Preinjury health records can also be reviewed by the school nurse to consider prior medications or medical conditions that may be complicated by the current injury.

The purpose of the preinjury records review is to develop a profile of strengths and weaknesses that the student displayed prior to injury. This can assist with understanding how the student's status has been affected by the injury, which can assist the school, family, and student in developing realistic plans for the future. In addition, because of the nature of learning problems typically found after brain injury, often preinjury experiences and abilities can be utilized in planning more successful postinjury activities.

Medical History/Description of Injury

The medical history is very critical in understanding a student's postinjury status. There are three critical factors to consider: (1) length and depth of coma, (2) length of post-traumatic amnesia, and (3) type and location of brain damage. The quality and length of a coma, as well as the post-traumatic amnesia period, are generally prognostic indicators of long-term outcome. (For full description of acute medical assessment, see Chapters 3 and 4.) The type and location of injury is important in order to distinguish a localized, focal injury from a more global, diffuse one. In addition, different neurobehavioral conditions can exist depending upon the neuroanatomic region(s) involved. In addition, the student's current medical status, including medications and possible further medical plans or complications (e.g., seizures, surgeries), needs to be closely monitored and considered.

The school nurse, speech/language specialist, and/or school psychologist may be the best education personnel involved in this process. However, typically these professionals are not routinely trained in the neurosciences as part of their background. Consequently, specialized inservice and training should be established, or a specialized professional such as a neuroeducator and/or outside consultation needs to be provided.

Cognitive Abilities

Cognition is the mechanics of the thinking process involved in the perception, acquisition, organization, and utilization of information. (See Chapters 12, 22, and 27 for an extensive review of the fields of cognitive assessment, training, and rehabilitation.) Since a primary goal of the education field is to convey and increase knowledge in the students it serves, understanding how cognitive functions are affected after brain injury is critical.

Within the educational field, the most typical assessment procedure of cognitive function is an individualized intelligence (IQ) test administered by a school psychologist. However, IQ testing may be an inadequate measure of functional behavior after a brain injury. A student with a sensory or severe motor impairment will not be capable of performing validly on a standardized IQ test. On the other hand, a student may score well on measured intelligence but applied, so-called executive, performance may be severely impaired. In order to develop a clearer and more detailed description of a student's cognitive profile, it is recommended that in addition to general intelligence, assessment should be broken down into a variety of cognitive performance areas:

☐ Arousal/alertness
☐ Orientation (person, place, time, activity)
☐ Perceptual skills (visual, auditory, tactile)
☐ Sustained attention/concentration
☐ Speed of processing
☐ Learning and memory·
☐ Spatial analysis (shape, size, dimension)
☐ Conceptual functions (reasoning, categorizing, sequencing)
☐ Executive functions (planning, problem solving, flexibility of thinking, detouring)
☐ Generalization of learned skills

Cognitive assessment needs to be completed by individuals with a background in learning theory, developmental psychology, and neuropsychology. The school psychologist with a background in neuropsychology is probably the best-trained educator for this task. In addition, assistance from the speech/language specialist and special education teacher may be appropriate. The special education teacher can be particularly helpful in identifying learning strengths and

strategies as they relate to the school curriculum while the speech/language specialist can assist with understanding how cognitive impairments will influence communication skills. Assistance may also be obtained from outside consultants such as occupational therapists and neuropsychologists.

Behavioral/Psychosocial Performance Level

The behavioral aspects of psychosocial skills can be the most difficult to understand and manage in the long-term readjustment after traumatic brain injury.[21] These skills are typically evaluated with either adaptive behavioral/developmental scales or descriptive behavior-rating scales. Unfortunately, there are very few of these types of scales that have been specifically developed or standardized for students with brain injuries. The parent and the rehabilitation personnel can be helpful in explaining how the student's behavior has been since the brain injury. However, it must be understood that there are certain phases, or levels, of recovery that all patients with TBI typically progress through, which are more reflective of their recovery phase than long-term behavioral outcomes.[22] Also, preaccident behavioral and social functions need to be evaluated and are generally accepted as predictors of possible behavioral patterns after the brain injury.

Psychosocial behavioral disturbances that must be considered include

☐ withdrawal
☐ perseveration
☐ low frustration tolerance
☐ irritability/restlessness
☐ disinhibition
☐ impulsivity
☐ fatuousness
☐ egocentricity
☐ lack of awareness/acceptance of disabilities
☐ lack of initiation
☐ lack of follow-through
☐ poor goal directed behavior
☐ poor generalization
☐ fatigue
☐ poor personal hygiene

The personnel involved in the assessment of these areas may include the school psychologist, school social worker, and school counselor.

Communication/Speech Skills

Students with brain injuries often display a wide range of communication disorders. The severity and type is often dependent upon cause, location, and type of injury, as well as preaccident status and developmental stage. Speech may be impacted by slowness, poor articulation and motor planning, or word finding difficulties. Communication deficits may involve the receptive and expressive aspects of written or oral communication, or may involve the student's internal mediation of language. There is no single test battery with norms which has been established specifically for students with traumatic brain injury. Consequently, communication skills assessment requires utilization of tests evaluating a variety of deficits, including aphasia and apraxia. Typically, the evaluation should include assessment in the following areas: (1) audiology, (2) receptive language, (3) expressive language, (4) pragmatics, and (5) motor speech dysfunction.

Academic Performance Level

Students with TBI often present with gaps in academic learning. One must evaluate lost skills, understand previously acquired skills that simply need refreshing or review, and take into consideration cognitive deficits and limitations and how they will affect the acquisition of new skills. Initially, it is always important to obtain information about the student's prior level of academic performance. Standardized achievement testing can be used to measure current performance levels; however, it is important to understand that standardized scores may not reflect how a student will actually perform in class. Cognitive factors like memory, organization, comprehension, speed of thinking, and fatigue can all have a negative impact on a student's performance even though he or she may be "reading at grade level." Most importantly, observational diagnostic teaching methods can be used to help determine learning styles, strategies, and deficits. In the case of high school

students, evaluation of graduation credits is needed to better determine the length of time and pacing of academic classes toward ultimate obtainment of a diploma. An academic assessment should include basic reading (i.e., decoding), reading rate, reading comprehension, spelling, handwriting, written composition, mathematical calculation and reasoning, consumer mathematics, and study skills.

The special education teacher, with assistance from the speech/language specialist and the school psychologist, is the ideal professional to assess this area.

Emotional/Personality Status

Emotional and personality problems are typically quite complicated following TBI. The source of these problems comes from three primary areas: (1) preexisting difficulties that may remain or have become exacerbated after the injury, (2) organically based neurobehavioral disturbances, and (3) reactive, adjustment problems in coping with the circumstances following the injury.[23] There may be many types of problems, including depression, anxiety, emotional lability, apathy, giddiness, antisocial traits, aggression/anger, poor reality testing, confabulation, dependency, excessive orderliness, suspiciousness, and lack of empathy.

Tests of personality and emotional adjustment have generally not been standardized on a TBI population. What may be interpreted as "hypochondriacal" on a test of personality may be an entirely appropriate behavior pattern for a brain injured person. These types of tests are usually administered and interpreted by trained psychologists, although some counselors may have had appropriate training on certain instruments. Close observation of behavioral performance and self or family report may be the most valid measurement of performance in these areas.

Psychomotor/Physical Status

The student with TBI may also suffer from a variety of physical impairments, which may result from damage to the central nervous system or from injury to other body systems from the same accident, such as peripheral nerve or musculoskeletal problems. An assessment of a student's physical status can be an integral part of educational programming, depending on how the physical problems can be remediated through adaptive physical education programs and how the problems may affect other school-related behaviors such as mobility, coordination, and strength. Areas to be considered in psychomotor assessment include fine motor coordination, gross motor coordination, balance, motor planning, kinesthetic awareness, laterality and directionality, spatial orientation and awareness, strength, and stamina. In addition, a student's ability to participate in a game, team sport, or recreation program will also influence adjustment in other areas including emotional and social functioning.

The psychomotor assessment can typically be completed by an adaptive physical education specialist. In some cases, consultation by a physical therapist, occupational therapist, or physiatrist can assist with evaluation.

PLACEMENT

Once the assessment of the student has been completed and the IEP has developed goals and objectives related to the needs identified in the assessment, the student should be appropriately placed within the kindergarten through 12th (K–12) grade educational system. Unfortunately, placement decisions are not always easy or clear-cut. If students have never received special education assistance in the past, they may feel resentful about the extra help. Since students also typically have good recollection of prior skills and abilities, they may continually try to compare their current abilities with premorbid ones. In this way, placing students in services or classes with other handicapped students may be interpreted as a sign of failure. Also, most education personnel are generally underprepared and inexperienced in instructing a student with TBI, so the chances of placing the student with experienced professionals is rather limited.

A range of service can be provided: from regular education classes with minimal modification to specially designed residential centers far from the mainstream of prior education experience. However, the educational institution is mandated to insure that placement and implementation of services occurs within the "least restrictive environment." The term "least restrictive" means that education will occur in an appropriate environment in which the child is educated to the maximum extent with children who are not handicapped, and that removal from regular education will only occur when the nature or severity of the handicap is such that education within regular classes cannot be achieved satisfactorily.

Typically, the range of alternatives within the K–12 system includes

□ Regular education with modification
□ Regular education with designated instructional (ancillary) services such as speech/language, health, psychology/counseling, occupational or physical therapy, physical education, contracting/behavior modification, and study skills/tutorial services
□ Regular education with resource program (partial day) assistance
□ Special day program (self-contained, full-day class)
□ Nonpublic private special school
□ Residential school

In addition, special education may be provided in home instruction or hospital instruction services.

There are several qualities unique to TBI students which must be considered in placement alternatives. First of all, because of the recovery process from brain injury, the student's performance over time will be highly variable. Consequently, a review of the student's progress may need to occur more frequently than for other handicapping conditions. The student's rate of change typically will tend to be faster during the 12–18 month postinjury period, but recovery can continue over much longer intervals of time. Also, recovery and progress will be dependent upon age, maturation, and developmental factors. Recovery after brain injury does not typically mean returning to preinjury status. Rather, the recovery is usually a lifelong process in which return of functioning is discussed in relative terms, such as percentage of recovery compared with preinjury status.

In placement, one needs to consider each student's needs. Some students may benefit from being placed in very similar circumstances to their previous education program in order to take advantage of familiarity in routines and surroundings. Other students may be too traumatized in returning to their previous environments and may be better off getting a new start someplace else.

The most important quality of any student's placement, even in the least restrictive environment, is structure. Students with a brain injury function best when they are provided organized, structured, and clearly stated instructional services within a consistent routine with minimal disruptions. High-school-age students may not be capable of assuming independent responsibility for their educational program as they did before. They may need assistance in getting from class to class, organizing their notebook, planning their assignments, and recognizing problems when they arise.

Placement alternatives must also be as flexible as possible. Students may re-enter school at any time depending upon when they are released by their physician. Students may require speeded or slowed curriculum, as well as repetition, review, or modification of curriculum. Graduation requirements may need to be modified or waived. Some students may be able to function only within certain time periods of the day, or for only limited lengths of time. Other students may have to work around outside medical and therapy appointments. Many times a decision must be made in the curriculum between the importance of teaching a specific content or teaching a process by which further information can be obtained. For example, is it more important for a student to take a required class, such as World History, or an ancillary service, such as memory compensation with a speech/language specialist? Being flexible within the school schedule and placement to satisfactorily meet the student's needs can be one of the most challenging areas of postinjury education.

POSTSECONDARY EDUCATIONAL PLACEMENT ALTERNATIVES

The guidelines for IEP's, assessment, and placement alternatives are not as clearly defined in postsecondary situations as they are in the K–12 system. PL 94-142 is mandated as a right of students and their families while the student remains in the K–12 system. Technically, students may remain in this system until they obtain a high school diploma or until they reach their 22nd birthday. However, many times older adolescent and young adult students (e.g., 18- to 21-year-olds) are not interested in returning to high school alternatives. In addition, many students may sustain their injuries while enrolled in college or other postsecondary educational programs and want to return to the same or similar environments.[24]

There are various options to consider outside of the K–12 educational system, including adult education, trade schools, community colleges, and 4-year colleges and universities. However, the key to success in any of these postsecondary alternatives is the awareness of the institution of the unique learning needs of the TBI students and the willingness to accommodate resources to meet these needs.

One such institution, the California Community Colleges, has made a substantial commitment toward integrating these students within their system. In 1985, the Chancellor's Office of the California Community Colleges conducted a survey of the 106 campuses within its system. Of the 51,000 students with disabilities enrolled, 2500 were found to have acquired traumatic brain injuries. A consortium of community college leaders was brought together from the fields of medicine, speech pathology, adaptive physical education, psychology, learning disabilities, counseling, and administration. The consortium developed a handbook[18] identifying resources within the system which could be drawn together to service the needs of the students with TBI. Personnel within the system include speech/language specialists, counselors and psychologists, learning disabilities specialists, adaptive physical education specialists, physical disability specialists, allied health professionals, adaptive computer technologists, paraprofessional tutors and aides, mainstream faculty, and administrators. The handbook outlines how these personnel can be utilized in screening and admission procedures, assessment, curriculum, IEP development and implementation, and computer-assisted technology. The handbook also provides an overview of the nature of acquired brain injury and basic neuroanatomy written with the educator in mind. It also contains a unique student profile matrix that provides a conceptual framework in which the complex needs of these students can be understood.

Within the California Community Colleges system, there is a range of available resources varying from campus to campus. Generally, these resources can be described in five program examples: (1) limited services, (2) learning disability programs, (3) self-contained off-campus programs, (4) full-spectrum on-campus resources, and (5) full-spectrum campuses with available off-campus self-contained centers.

Campuses with limited services have available counseling through disabled student services offices. The counselor can help the student select classes within the college curriculum based upon the student's abilities and interests. These courses can provide an evaluation of the viability of a student returning to a college-based curriculum, and of how much assistance is truly needed. In the beginning, courses may be taken on an "auditing" basis so as not to jeopardize credits or academic standing. Typically, these campuses also offer physical conditioning and recreation through adaptive physical education classes. Also, enabling services such as advance registration, accessible parking, note takers, test facilitators, readers, tutors, and interpreters can be provided.

Many campuses offer learning disability programs which are already servicing adult learning-disabled students. Although the student with TBI is different from the learning-disabled adult, many similarities exist that allow for mixing of resources to both disabled groups. Learning disability programs generally offer in-depth psychoeducational assessments, tutorial services in basic skills, mainstream classes, remedial education classes, and specialized classes for improvement in such areas as study skills, communication skills, or career guidance. In addition, they provide the previously discussed service such as adaptive physical education, transition-to-mainstream classes, and enabling services.

Several campuses offer off-campus specialized centers specifically designed to the needs of students with brain injuries. These self-contained centers may range from ones that focus on young adults with TBI to those that focus on a population of older adults recovering from strokes. Because of the self-contained nature of these programs, the environment can be engineered to intensify services in the areas of cognitive retraining, psychosocial retraining, and behavior management. Students who may not be successful on a regular campus because of the degree of their cognitive or behavioral deficits may be managed well within a self-contained center.

Several campuses offer a full spectrum of uniquely designed services for students with brain injuries, while at the same time provide maximum integration within regular on-campus activities. The uniquely designed classes typically include cognitive retraining, speech and language training, psychosocial skills training, computer-assisted and -adapted technology, vocational preparation and job placement, skills training on community transition, and even family education on brain injury. These campuses typically have community college personnel trained or experienced in brain injury rehabilitation methods along with their special education background. These campuses usually also provide services available in other programs including adaptive physical education, mainstream transition, and enabling services. Some may offer specialized off-campus centers and, thus, offer a full range of resources from the most intensive to the least restrictive.

The California Community Colleges system has taken a state and national leadership role in the development of uniquely specialized resources within an educational context for the TBI population; however, there are many questions and concerns that require further study. A primary concern revolves around the issue of funding. These programs and resources are quite expensive, yet education dollars remain rather limited. Many people question the appropriateness of college institutions providing remedial education resources. There are many unanswered questions about curriculum, assessment procedures, and the degree of professional training required of personnel who teach TBI students. Even recognizing which student is appropriate for the community college and which student may not be appropriate is not easily accomplished at present. Considerable research and development is needed and must be supported by educational institutions.

INTERVENTION

Ultimately, once assessment, goal-setting, and placement have been accomplished, the implementation of services begins. Educational intervention entails consideration of many of the unique qualities and learning patterns of traumatically brain injured students. Methods of service will require modification from student to student. Each lesson plan and instructional method should consider the specialized cognitive, behavioral, and physical needs of each student.

Teaching Strategies

Wittrock[25] reviews some of the literature in cognitive science and neuropsychology as it relates to education and knowledge acquisition. Special teaching strategies she proposes include (1) remediation of attentional problems through verbal mediation strategies, extrinsic reward paradigms, insertion of questions within the lesson to direct attention and information processing, and utilization of novel/discrepant instruction; (2) enhancing memory by providing semantic meaning to rote data or by utilizing mental imagery; (3) improving comprehension and retention by regularly summarizing information as it is being taught; (4) improving learning by analyzing the student's learning style across two major paradigms—verbal-analytic learning using propositional and sequential analyses versus spatial-holistic learning using imagery and appositional synthesis—and then matching the learning style with the teacher instructional style; (5) facilitating information processing through the use of metacognitive (i.e., cognitive self-monitoring) strategies. These suggested pedagogic strategies are applicable to all teaching situations. However, they have particular relevance to teaching those with TBI, since these students have definitive cognitive and neuropsychologic impairments.

The educator should make every effort to understand how each student's cognitive, behavioral, and physical impairments affect his or her ability to benefit from the instructional program. Consideration should be given as to how these deficits can be remediated and how these deficits can be circumvented through compensatory strategies. These suggested pedagogic strategies apply to all teaching situations; however, they have particular relevance to teaching TBI students.

Compensatory Instructional Strategies

Whether the instruction is being provided in the regular classroom or in a specialized training center, there are certain cognitive and behavioral characteristics that require compensatory strategies. These methods can be categorized according to the specific problem that is being compensated for:

1. Deficits in attention/concentration
   a. Provide allowance for rest periods
   b. Classrooms should minimize distractions
   c. Attention should be continually monitored and refocused
   d. Instructions should be short and concise
   e. Assignments must be relevant, novel, and stimulating
   f. Time of day, medications, and fatigue factors should be closely monitored
2. Deficits in memory (typically short-term, new learning problems)
   a. Repetition
   b. Overlearning
   c. Memory compensation tools (e.g., notetaking, tape recording)
   d. Utilize mental imagery techniques
   e. Learning should be relevant and meaningful
   f. Teach memory mnemonics
   g. Attempt to anchor learning to previous experience
3. Deficits in sensory perceptual skills
   a. Multisensory, multimodality instruction
   b. Accommodate to student's perceptual strengths
   c. Modify the environment to accommodate needs (e.g., close seating, placement of material in appropriate visual fields)
4. Deficits in speech/communication
   a. Provide assistive devices such as notetakers, tape recorders, communication boards

b. Utilize paraphrasing, verbal repetition, and summarizing

c. Provide cueing, prompting, and role playing

d. Utilize concrete, concise verbal instruction

e. Utilize video and audio recordings

f. Allow nonverbal communication such as gesturing, signing, pantomime

5. Deficits in higher reasoning and problem-solving skills

a. Provide a highly structured environment

b. Utilize well-defined goals and objectives

c. Provide ongoing feedback

d. Provide frequent planning and scheduling meetings

e. Provide frequent summarizing of data

f. Provide assistance with prioritizing and sequencing

g. Provide assistance with alternative solutions

h. Allow time for slower processing/discourage impulsive responding

i. Highly reinforce any self-monitoring or self-correcting behaviors

6. Deficits in physical functioning

a. Students should have complete accessibility

b. Assistive devices such as wheelchairs and print enlargers should be provided

c. Accommodation for speed of performance should consider physical disability

Interfacing With Medical/Rehabilitation Services

Before a student returns to school, and as part of the assessment process, it is strongly recommended to obtain all acute and medical rehabilitation records. This information will assist in analyzing the severity and type of brain injury sustained and highlight any important ongoing medical and rehabilitation issues. It is very important to identify the attending physician who will continue to follow the student on an outpatient basis. Any medical problems or questions can be directed to the physician by the school nurse. The effects of medications and their impact on the student's education perfor-

mance should be understood. Often, members of the medical rehabilitation team may be available to the school to provide inservice training or specific consultation on a particular student.

Cognitive Re-education

The field of cognitive rehabilitation is a rapidly expanding area of treatment where the focus is on training or improving thinking and acquisition skills.[26, 27] In the education field, there has been considerable discussion of the efficacy and value of cognitive teaching strategies.[28–30] However, in only limited cases has this technology been applied to the education of students with TBI.

Harrington and Levandowski[31] reviewed the value of a cognitive re-education program using standardized neuropsychologic testing as an outcome measure. These authors were able to show statistically significant gains made by students in a program specifically designed to enhance cognitive performance in a population of traumatically brain injured students. The program is a community college–based education service for young adults with acquired brain injuries. The students attend a full-time education program for approximately 18 to 24 months, which provides cognitive re-education, psychosocial training, and vocational preparation. The cognitive education aspect of the program uses an instructional hierarchy so that students progress through sequential modules of instruction from the basic to the complex:

Module 1— Attention/Concentration
Module 2— Perceptual Processing
Module 3— Organizational Processing
Module 4— Higher Reasoning/Problem Solving

All students must progress through each module, but the pace and speed with which students move through the modules is dependent on individual needs. Although no control group was provided to verify that improvements were made because of experience in the program, the program does indicate the value of such a service for traumatically brain injured in an educational setting.

Psychosocial/Behavioral Training

Psychosocial and behavioral functioning have clearly been identified as the most problematic long-term rehabilitation issues after traumatic brain injury.[21, 32–35] It is the psychosocial and behavioral problems which will likely be the greatest obstacles to successful educational re-entry. Consequently, it is imperative to develop adequate plans to deal with these problems within the school environment. These problems may range from the very subtle to the very extreme. Specific strategies which can be provided within an educational context include: one-to-one counseling and guidance, small-group therapy programs, peer support groups, rap groups, social skills training groups, guidance and communication classes, and education or parent groups for family members. In addition, behavioral contracting, contingency management, timeout, video feedback, role playing, and peer pressure can be effective school-based strategies. Consultation with an outside psychotherapist or behavioral psychologist familiar with head injury problems can be beneficial, as can consultation with a neurologist or neuropsychiatrist regarding beneficial medications.

There are certain suggestions that can be employed to enhance student awareness of personality or behavioral issues. For example, before gains can be made in behavioral areas, the student needs to recognize his or her own strengths and weaknesses. Therefore, provision of constructive feedback in a concrete manner, such as using graphs and charts to document progress, can help each student's awareness.

In addition, whenever there are behavioral problems, it is very important to analyze the environmental factors that may be contributing to the difficulties. Some tasks may be too frustrating or beyond the student's physical or cognitive limitations. The environment has to remain consistent and regular, with few changes in routine. Many times behavioral problems can be easily redirected when confronted in a supportive but firm manner. Students must recognize the educator as a trustworthy, fair, and consistent authority figure. They often are looking for guidance from significant others because their self-evaluation and guidance system are confused and uncertain.

Coping strategies for management of anger, frustration, depression, social isolation, and fear of failure (anxiety) can be provided. Didactic and therapeutic strategies for stress managment can be offered. These students also have to redevelop a sense of control over their lives. Often students feel paranoid or impotent as a consequence of suffering a traumatic experience. They need to develop a sense of personal competency and self-direction.

Many students also become very egocentric in their perception of the world. Their ability to remain empathetic toward others becomes quite restricted. Exploring personal values and how these students view themselves in relation to others can be helpful. Recognizing the feelings of others and identifying alternative perspectives on problems can also facilitate growth. Social skills training can be done in the classroom or as part of an individual or group counseling program.

Communication/Speech

Traumatic brain injury can result in a wide range of communication problems. Such problems require the direct care of a speech and language specialist. However, these problems can interfere with all aspects of the student's education. Therefore, it is imperative for the speech/language specialist to communicate with all personnel involved with the student. The primary areas of deficit were outlined in the earlier information on assessment. The intervention can be a one-to-one therapy session, small-group session, classroom special program, and/or consultation with other educational personnel.

Physical Education

As previously reviewed in the assessment information, an individual with TBI may suffer a variety of physical impairments. A psychomotor adaptive physical education program can help enhance performance in problem areas as well as promote psychosocial skills, self-concept, and appropriate recreation skills. Psychomotor programs can be one-to-one, self-directed with supervision, group exercise classes, or team sports. Activities can be divided into three major categories: (1) individualized therapeutic activities, (2) activities that parallel existing or regular physical education classes, and (3) activities directed toward leisure time and recreation.

Whatever physical education plan is developed, medical clearance for the activity by the attending physician is essential. In addition, consultation from a physical therapist familiar with head injury is strongly recommended in order to avoid contraindicated activities for a given person's physical problems.

Mobility Training/Orientation

Often after a brain injury, the patient remains in a state of spatial disorientation or confusion. This confusion can lead to difficulties with navigation, following directions, or identifying locations. In addition, motor impairments such as hemiplegia and sensory impairments such as blindness or visual field loss may impede a student's ability to traverse the environment. Assistance must be provided to help these students be better oriented to the environment and have full physical accessibility. Suggestions include (1) minimizing changes in classes or degree of independent mobility, especially in the early transition back to school; (2) providing a peer buddy system until students are independent on campus; (3) allowing extra time between classes for going from one place to another; (4) providing orientation maps that students always carry with them; (5) providing instruction in what to do if lost; and (6) helping students become better oriented in the community. In the most extreme cases, some students may unknowingly leave the grounds and have difficulty finding their way back to campus. These students obviously need a very structured and controlled environmental program.

Parent/Family Support

Finally, it is imperative that the school recognize that rehabilitation and recovery from the effects of TBI involves the entire family. It is important to include the family members in all aspects of the educational process and to ensure that the rights of the student and family are enforced and re-

spected. One of the greatest strengths of the IEP is its guarantee of involvement of the family in the student's education program. Family members are to be integral parts of the IEP team and must give consent for all decisions relative to the IEP. Suggested activities to involve the parents in the program include:

1. Always follow the rule of informed consent when it comes to evaluation, identification, and placement decisions.

2. Have special parent conferences to review progress at every grading period.

3. Provide parent education and communication workshops.

4. Provide parent and family support groups within the local school or by referring the families to support agencies in the community.

5. Have close liaison with the social service departments at each rehabilitation program that serves the traumatically brain injured.

6. Have available referrals to family counselors, therapists, and psychologists who specialize in working with persons with TBI.

SUMMARY

The chapter has provided an overview of traumatic brain injury as it applies to the field of education. Neurologically based disorders of learning and behavior have substantial historic roots. However, at present, there is considerable controversy and lack of recognition regarding the learning and behavioral problems of students with TBI in our schools. Epidemiologic studies are revealing a rapidly growing population of students with acquired traumatic brain injuries returning to school. Recent government mandates and growing professional and public awareness are beginning to resolve the controversy and recognize this growing population.

The process of individualized education programs, federally defined in Public Law 94-142, can provide a vehicle so that students with TBI may return to a meaningful educational experience. Currently very few education personnel receive specialized training or experience in working with such students. Specialized educational strategies in the areas of assessment, placement, and intervention are reviewed in this chapter. Educators need to recognize that specialized training is necessary in order to effectively meet the unique cognitive, behavioral, emotional, and physical needs of these students.

REFERENCES

1. Annegers, JF et al: The incidence, causes, and secular trends of head trauma in Olmstead County, Minnesota. Neurology 30:912, 1980.
2. Rivara, FP and Mueller, BA: The epidemiology and prevention of pediatric head injury. J Head Trauma Rehabil 1:4, 7, 1986.
3. Rutter, M, Chadwick, O and Shaffer, D: Head injury. In Rutter, M (ed): Developmental Neuropsychiatry. Guilford Press, New York, 1983.
4. Ewing-Cobbs, L, Fletcher, JM and Levin, HS: Neuropsychological sequelae following pediatric head injury. In Ylvisaker, M (ed): Head Injury Rehabilitation: Children and Adolescents. College-Hill Press, San Diego, 1985.
5. Boll, TJ: Minor head injury in children—out of sight but not out of mind. J Clin Child Psychol 12:1, 1983.
6. Ebaugh, FG: Neuropsychiatric sequelae of acute epidemic encephalitis in children. Am J Dis Child 25:89, 1923.
7. Strecker, E and Ebaugh, F: Neuropsychiatric sequelae of cerebral trauma in children. Arch Neurol Psychiatry 12:443, 1924.
8. Orton, S: Word-blindness in school children. Arch Neurol Psychiatry 14:581, 1925.
9. Kahn, E and Cohen, LH: Organic driveness. N Engl J Med 210:748, 1934.
10. Strauss, AA and Lehtinen, V: Psychopathology and Education of the Brain-Injured Child, Vol 1. Grune & Stratton, New York, 1947.
11. Birch, HG: The problems of "brain damage" in children. In Birch, HG (ed): Brain Damage in Children: The Biological and Social Aspects. Williams & Wilkins, Baltimore, 1964.
12. Chall, JS and Mirsky, AF: Education and the Brain. Seventy-Seventh Yearbook of the National Society for the Study of Education, Part II. The University of Chicago Press, Chicago, 1978.
13. Cruickshank, WM: A new perspective in teacher education: The neuroeducator. J Learn Disabil 14:6, 1981.
14. Savage, RC and Carter, RC: Re-entry: The head injured student returns to school. Cogn Rehabil 3:2, 1984.
15. Cohen, SB et al: Educational programming for head injured students. In Ylvisaker, M (ed): Head Injury Rehabilitation: Children and Adolescents. College-Hill Press, San Diego, 1985.
16. Savage, RC and Pollack, I (eds): An Educator's Manual: What Educators Need to Know About Students with Traumatic Brain Injury. National Head Injury Foundation, Framingham, MA, 1985.
17. Rosen, CD and Gerring, JP: Head Trauma: Educational Reintegration. College-Hill Press, San Diego, 1986.
18. Cook, J et al: The ABI Handbook: Serving Students with Acquired Brain Injury in Higher Education. California Community Colleges, Sacramento, 1987.
19. Light, R et al: An evaluation of a neuropsychologically based re-education project for the head injured child. J Head Trauma Rehabil 2:1, 1987.
20. National Head Injury Foundation: Cooperative Agency Agreement. Framingham, MA, 1985.
21. Brooks, N (ed): Closed Head Injury: Psychological, Social and Family Consequences. Oxford University Press, Oxford, 1984.
22. Malkmus, D, Booth, B and Doyle, M: Models and strategies in cognitive rehabilitation. In Rehabilitation of the Head Injured Adult: Comprehensive Cognitive Management. Rancho Los Amigos Hospital, Downey, CA, 1980.
23. Rosenthal, M: Behavioral sequelae. In Rosenthal, M et al (eds): Rehabilitation of the Head Injured Adult. FA Davis, Philadelphia, 1983.
24. Hall, DE and DePompei, R: Implications for the head-injured reentering higher education. Cogn Rehabil 3:4, 1986.
25. Wittrock, MC: Education and recent neuropsychological and cognitive research. In Benson, DF and Zaidel, E (eds): The Dual Brain: Hemispheric Specialization in Humans. Guilford Press, New York, 1985.
26. Adamovich, B, Henderson, JA and Auerbach, S: Cognitive Rehabilitation of Closed Head Injured Patients: A Dynamic Approach. College-Hill Press, San Diego, 1985.
27. Trexler, LE (ed): Cognitive Rehabilitation. Plenum Press, New York, 1982.
28. Sternberg, RJ: Intelligence Applied: Understanding and Increasing Your Intellectual Skills. Harcourt, Brace, Jovanovich, San Diego, 1986.
29. Feuerstein, R: Instrumental Enrichment: An Intervention Program for Cognitive Modifiability. University Park Press, Baltimore, 1980.
30. Nickerson, RS, Perkins, DN and Smith, EE: The Teaching of Thinking. Lawrence Erlbaum Associates, Hillsdale, NJ, 1985.
31. Harrington, DE and Levandowski, DH: Efficacy of an educationally-based cognitive retraining programme for traumatically head-injured as measured by LNNB pre- and post-tests. Brain Injury 1:1, 65, 1987.
32. Lezak, MD: Living with the characterologically altered brain injured patient. J Clin Psychiatry 39:592, 1978.
33. Oddy, M, Humprey, M and Uttley, D: Subjective impairment and social recovery after closed head injury. J Neurol Neurosurg Psychiatry 41:611, 1978.
34. Levin, HS, Benton, AL and Grossman, RG: Neurobehavioral Consequences of Closed Head Injury. Oxford University Press, Oxford, 1982.
35. Prigatano, GP: Neuropsychological Rehabilitation After Brain Injury. Johns Hopkins University Press, Baltimore, 1985.

Chapter 33

Returning to Work After Traumatic Head Injury

JOY V. COOK, M.A.

"When can I go back to work?" is probably the question most frequently asked of rehabilitation specialists working with survivors of traumatic head injuries. Return to work remains the leading indicator of recovery after a brain injury, and it is what survivors strive for most, often to the neglect of quality of life issues such as personal relationships, family life, and leisure activities.[1] A review of the current literature, however, does not present an encouraging picture of this group's work potential.

As the field awaits adequate outcome studies, reviewing the current literature suggests return to gainful employment with traditional rehabilitation from 12 percent[2] to 100 percent.[3] For example, in a recent study Ben-Yishay and coworkers described a holistic approach to return to work, including occupational trials following an intensive remedial/preparatory program (cognitive, interpersonal, and vocational components), as effective in helping 84 percent of the patients to resume productive work, 63 percent of them in competitive employment.[4] In a text on neuropsychologic rehabilitation, Prigatano and associates reported that 60 to 65 percent of patients are able to obtain and 50 percent to maintain competitive employment after a highly structured approach centered on social behavioral change.[5] These findings, along with those of other studies,[4] can be confusing, however, as they are based on programs with patients having deficits from various etiologies, diverse evaluation procedures, inconsistent definitions for success, and, most importantly, a paucity of long-term follow-up studies.

Limiting the discussion of the vocational potential of this population to job acquisition, however, ignores the significant problem surrounding job retention. Rehabilitation counselors in the field report that 75 percent of head injured workers will lose their jobs in the first 90 days, about half of them quitting with complaints of reduced satisfaction with their jobs or of work that is beneath their abilities.[6] In a study of 44 young adults 2 years after their accidents, researchers report that many of those who returned to their former jobs found they could no longer cope with their previous responsibilities. Adjustments had to be made, often by trial and error, to accommodate their altered abilities. Others were in new but unsuitable jobs and they, like those who were still not employed, presumably needed to make further adjustments in order to retain their jobs.[7]

Employer terminations equal those of voluntary resignations, and are usually accompanied by reports of unsuitable work behaviors and inability to integrate into the work routine. Employers often complain about brain injury survivors' irregular punctuality and attendance, their interpersonal problems with coworkers, and the inability to manage their personal lives along with their work.

Although what has been presented depicts a rather distressing picture of the vocational potential of survivors of traumatic brain injury, there is in these studies good evidence that progress is being made in the development of viable rehabilitative approaches that enhance the potential for returning a significant percentage of this population to work. Prospects are brighter for these people than ever before.

LIMITATIONS AFFECTING VOCATIONAL POTENTIAL

Conservative estimates indicate 7.5 million Americans sustain traumatic head injuries annually.[8]* Seventeen percent of these injuries will be severe enough to be considered major, and the remaining 83 percent of this population, even after having achieved "total physical recovery," may exhibit problems that preclude their abilities to resume premorbid lifestyles. This is a young population; nearly 30 percent of the victims are between the ages of 17 and 44, with the potential for a long work life ahead of them.[8] The problems caused by the brain injury are not isolated to one function or body part but may cause any combination of cognitive, speech/communication, psychosocial/emotional/coping, and/or physical impairments. A more detailed look at how these major problems can affect a survivor's potential for vocational rehabilitation is outlined below.

Cognitive limitations[9] affect the functions necessary for effective thinking and, therefore, job performance. The following are seven areas for consideration when appraising the effects of traumatic head injury on cognitive processes:

1. Attention/concentration—sustaining mental concentration to complete job tasks
2. Perceptual processing—perceiving information in one or more sensory modalities
3. Orientation—orienting to time, place, people, and events

4. Memory—storing, retaining, and retrieving old and new information
5. Organization—ordering and maintaining order in reception, synthesis, and expression of thoughts
6. Problem solving and executive functioning—setting goals, initiating action, monitoring implementation, flexibility working toward desired outcomes, recognizing task completion
7. Generalization—applying or transferring learned skills to other situations

Speech/Communication limitations[9] can cause minimal to severe breakdowns in the communication process, thus influencing the individual's effectiveness in work situations. The following are four areas for consideration when appraising the effects of traumatic head injury on communication processes:

1. Receptive language—comprehending vocabulary and utterances of varying complexity, length, and rate; having a well-organized semantic system for higher-level language processes (abstractions, concept formation, verbal reasoning, problem solving); speed of processing information
2. Expressive language—word finding, organizing thoughts, and expressing thoughts clearly in varied, demanding, and stressful situations
3. Pragmatics—adhering to the rules of conversation including interrupting/turn-taking, appropriate conversational topics, vocabulary, and physical distances
4. Motor speech—articulating; exhibiting voice quality, rate, and pitch within normal limits

Psychosocial limitations[9] are probably the leading causes of work failure. They may be organically based, direct results of the microscopic destruction of neural tissue found in closed head injury, or functionally based adjustment reactions to the victim's feelings of hopelessness and helplessness in trying to cope with the new and poorly understood disability. The following is further clarification of these two areas for consideration when appraising the effects of traumatic head injury on psychosocial behaviors:

---

*By definition, head injuries include trauma to the head which is *not* associated with brain injury. Over 6 million of all head injuries (1976) were of this type.

Organic Behavior Disorders. These neuropsychological problems are related to the severity and loci of the brain lesions and may manifest themselves in loss of impulse control, perseveration, obsessive-compulsive behaviors, emotional lability, reduced frustration tolerance, disinhibition, poor social judgment, fatuousness, egocentricity, lack of initiative, and/or social viscosity. Evidence of microscopic tissue damage which may lead to such disorders has been documented even in cases of whiplash and mild head injury.[10, 11]

Functional Behavior Disorders. Coping and adjustment are cognitive functions, disruption of which can be manifested in affective disorders such as anger, fear, depression, anxiety, irritability, mistrust, and denial. The severity of these disorders may be unrelated to the severity and locus of the injury. It has been estimated that 65 percent of victims of severe traumatic head injury develop significant psychiatric disabilities which further retard recovery to their premorbid levels of functioning.[12] This estimate has been substantiated in numerous studies. Rimel reported that psychologic responses to an injury are a significant factor in the long-term disability of patients with minor head injury.[13] Rimel and colleagues,[14] in another study of the moderately impaired, and Levin and associates,[15] reporting on severely impaired patients, arrived at similar conclusions after long-term follow-ups that the patients' psychologic responses to their injuries were substantial impediments to recovery.

Physical limitations[9] can diminish the capacity to do physical labor or complete a workday. The following are four areas for consideration when appraising the effects of traumatic head injury on physical abilities:

1. Post-traumatic epilepsy—electrical disruptions in brain activity; frequency and severity of the seizures and even the antiseizure medication can restrict day-to-day work and leisure activities[16]
2. Motor limitations—a range of problems from fine and gross motor control to weakness and paralysis
3. Sensory limitations—diminished or lost vision, hearing, smell, touch, and taste
4. Physical stamina limitations—endurance insufficient for work requirements

PROGNOSTIC INDICATORS

As there is no consistent predictor of job readiness, and as patients may exhibit a range of problems and of different levels of severity, vocational specialists face substantial challenges in guiding the preparation and return of these individuals to work. There are multiple premorbid and post-traumatic conditions that can be considered when attempting to estimate vocational potential. These prognostic indicators have been indicated as significant in current research:

☐ **Type of brain injury:** Diffuse injuries cause combinations of different types of problems at varying levels of severity, while localized injuries may result in an isolated disability to one specific brain area and behavioral function.[9]

☐ **Severity of brain injury:** Severe head injury is defined by a score of 8 or less on the Glasgow Coma Scale at acute hospital discharge;[17] good recovery is associated with briefer periods of coma;[15] diagnosis of focal lesions by CT scan and intracranial surgery suggests at least moderate head injury,[14] with subdural hematoma being the most common diagnosis.[18]

☐ **Post-traumatic amnesia (PTA):** With PTA lasting 24 hours or more, 20 to 30 percent of survivors will require less taxing employment than they performed premorbidly; 10 percent will be unemployable.[19]

☐ **Age:** The decreasing rate of return to work after age 40 may be due to victims' diminished ability to adapt and/or employers' reluctance to support victims with relatively short work lives.[20, 21]

☐ **Physically handicapping conditions:** Depending on the job, preinjury physical disability can be an obvious impediment to employment.

☐ **History of previous neurologic insults, premorbid alcoholism, drug abuse, and psychiatric problems:** The cumulative effects of multiple brain injuries and pre-existing personality disorders are clear predictors of failure to return to work;[22, 23] it is reasonable to assume that those who exhibited premorbid adjustment problems will find it harder to overcome their disabilities of any kind.[1]

☐ **Supportive families, significant**

others, employers: Understanding and encouraging advocates provide support, reinforce and help generalize learned behaviors, and are more willing to adapt to new levels of competence.

☐ **Intelligence, education, socioeconomic group, and work history:** Preinjury occupational status and social factors are positively related to outcome.[1, 24–26] It has been suggested that people who were in professional positions premorbidly will have more resources to buffer the effects of the brain injury and that their employers will be more indulgent and cooperative.[13, 20, 25, 26]

☐ **Specific disabilities:** For example, post-traumatic epilepsy can preclude the ability to return to some professions.[16]

☐ **Local economic conditions:** It will be more difficult to find employers willing to accommodate to the needs of disabled employees in economically depressed geographic areas.

☐ **Jobs requiring speed, efficiency, and safety:** Employers in industrial settings will have additional requirements that may pose significant barriers to new and returning employees seeking these jobs.[27]

Now that we have explored the characteristics of brain injury that affect vocational potential, we turn to an explanation of appropriate and effective rehabilitation.

VOCATIONAL REHABILITATION

A model vocational rehabilitation program will have these components:

☐ An interdisciplinary team approach
☐ Flexible evaluation procedures
☐ Behaviorally based training/education
☐ Job placement
☐ Long-term follow-up

The Interdisciplinary Team

It has been documented in the literature that an interdisciplinary approach to rehabilitation dramatically enhances the ability of patients with brain injuries to meet their vocational goals.[26] With the varied and complex needs of individuals with traumatic head injury, the investment in the team approach is not only logical but vital to assessment and training/education.

The interdisciplinary team works in an integrated fashion: sharing information, coordinating treatment plans, ensuring consistency in priorities and approaches. The team may consist of allied health professionals, neuropsychologists, vocational counselors, physicians, work evaluators, private and state vocational rehabilitation counselors, educators, job trainers, significant others, the prospective employer, and the head injured patient.

Interdisciplinary team meetings are appropriate settings to which to invite significant others to share their thoughts and feelings and learn together about the patient. "Family education is a hallmark of an effective vocational rehabilitation program."[28] These meetings are opportunities to enhance patient/family/team communication, and to develop realistic, well-structured expectations for short- and long-term goals. To the extent possible, patients' families can be enlisted to help reinforce and generalize the things that are learned at the meetings.

Evaluation Procedures

THE CASE HISTORY

The evaluation begins with the acquisition of historic information: a patient's medical status, premorbid lifestyle and behaviors, education and work history, and current levels of functioning based on interdisciplinary team reports. A comparison and analysis of this information will provide invaluable insights as to what job types might be contraindicated for medical reasons, level of premorbid functioning compared with present functioning, and capability of returning to previous jobs. If a new vocation is indicated, premorbid interests and hobbies can provide a base from which to investigate and plan.

Vocational specialists can begin gathering information on the preinjury work history while the patient is still in a coma. "Diagnostically interviewing" former employers and coworkers, obtaining detailed job information, and identifying work values, primary reinforcers, and the importance of work in the patient's premorbid life reveals information that can be useful to the rehabilitation team, and the information gleaned from these interviews can be used in later work evaluation and job training.[29]

FLEXIBLE EVALUATION PROCEDURES

Due to the multiplicity of deficits evident in individuals with brain injury, the tasks and roles of vocational specialists and evaluators are very complex.[6] The findings of the interdisciplinary team's assessments should be corroborated by and integrated with the results of vocational assessments to obtain an overall picture of work potential, and to provide focus for programming and planning.

The head injured individual's employability is affected by continually evolving factors. Physical, cognitive, and behavioral changes occur steadily and dramatically during the first 6 to 12 months after injury. Vocational evaluations should be delayed until this period of spontaneous recovery has passed and functional stability is maintained.

Vocational evaluation of the individual with traumatic head injury is a different process from that used with other disabled populations. Effective vocational evaluation requires individualized planning, flexible and varied procedures in actual/realistic job situations, and repeated evaluations over time and under varying conditions.[28]

A comprehensive evaluation will include formal and informal measurements of the following areas pertinent to work:

□ **Attention and concentration**—selective attention
□ **Executive functioning**—goal-setting and task completion
□ **Interpersonal behavior**—communication and social judgment
□ **Problem solving and judgment**—mental flexibility and understanding cause-effect relationships
□ **Memory**—potential for learning new information
□ **Orientation**—grasp on time and place
□ **Perception**—auditory and visual perceptual skills
□ **Organization**—higher-level thinking: analysis, classification, sequencing, screening the relevant from the irrelevant
□ **Gross and fine motor skills**—functioning, potential, and adaptations

□ **Premorbid abilities and interests**—personality, education, and occupation prior to brain injury
□ **Endurance**—sustained performance without excessive fatigue or loss of concentration

Other factors for consideration[9] are

□ **Self-concept**—ability to realistically appraise skills and to match them with realistic vocational choices
□ **Adaptability to job requirements**—ability to follow directions, work under supervision, move from task to task, work under stress, be punctual, and meet specific job requirements
□ **Personal appearance**—self-care and appropriate dress
□ **Mobility in the community**—community transportation resources and ability to get around in the community

EVALUATION TOOLS

As it has been established that the range and type of limitations that may be exhibited by individuals with brain injuries are unique, it stands to reason that there may be inherent problems in using traditional vocational assessments to measure the impact of the deficits attributed to the brain injury. Vocational competency issues are confounded by inconsistencies in performance; by the need for longer periods of time to complete the procedures; and by anger directed at the evaluator, inward, or at the family.[30]

Formal psychometric assessments may be administered by a variety of allied health professionals such as educators, psychologists, and speech/language pathologists to measure academic abilities, interests, personality traits, speech and language functions, and the like.

The nature of the clinical distraction-free environment during assessment may mask underlying problems, however. Such assessments may provide misleading information, and their results should be substantiated by observation, over time, under stress, and in varying environmental conditions. For example, performance on a reading test in a quiet setting will not give a true indication of a patient's ability to read at the same level of comprehension with distraction and varying demands of text length and complexity. The patient's performance on isolated items may not be a valid measurement of his or her skill level in a subject, particularly with the complications of fatigue and stress. Levels of performance may be dependent on patients' abilities to reference previous learning and poor short-term memory will affect new learning. By its nature, the structure imposed by the test environment simply does not offer realistic perspectives on the effects of executive skills on independent functioning.

Vocational assessment relies on tools that resemble the real work task as closely as possible. Some commonly used vocational assessment tools include job-based work samples and job site observations. For head injured clients, the need for realistic work samples is particularly critical, the ideal work sample being on the job site, at the precise work station, and with the exact tools and materials to be used.[28]

Work samples may be employed selectively and can be useful in evaluating former skills or identifying new ones.[31] A creative work evaluator may mix and match several systems, effectively varying time, instructions, and methods of administration. In tests that are designed to be sequentially more difficult, continuing to test beyond "ceilings" may reveal islands of abilities that may have been overlooked through strict adherence to the administration instructions.[28]

While vocational evaluators depend exclusively on normative data for their other clients, when evaluating individuals with brain injuries, such comparisons may be misleading.[29] Based on the client's performance on an isolated work sample, there may not be adequate evidence to predict sufficient selective attention to perform in the presence of distraction. Does the client have the physical and mental endurance to perform the task at the same rate for a regular shift? With interruptions does the client exhibit ample executive skills to reinitiate the task and follow through to completion?

Even when work behaviors are sufficient for the job, communication and psychosocial issues may interfere with the client's ability to retain it. Subtle language disturbances, such as standing too close or touching when conversing, and more obvious behavioral problems, may affect interaction with coworkers. It is important to have sufficient opportunity to observe disinhibition and reactive behaviors.

When physical limitations prevent an individual from performing a particular work sample, adaptations can be made so that the sample can still be used. If performance on a particular work sample requiring two hands is impossible due to a nonfunctioning hand, judgments about the individual's ability to perform two-handed tasks may not be valid. With modifications the work sample may be performed with one hand. This kind of ingenuity and creativity, frequently necessary with head injured clients, complicates the evaluation process and increases the time required to complete the evaluation, but the results are truly representative of the client's abilities.[30]

INFORMAL TESTS

Another way to assess vocational abilities of clients with brain injuries is to use evaluator-developed job simulations. While formal evaluations test single skills, the informal types obtain information on functional abilities. They provide assessments of learning potential/memory for unfamiliar tasks. Observation can provide increased understanding of a client's thinking process relative to problem solving, organization, planning, and follow-through to job completion. Even more important, it provides an opportunity for an assessment of compensatory skills. Such creativity and individualization may be required to evaluate work potential for each client with a head injury adequately.

Once more, the team approach is essential when using a variety of methods to determine the vocational potential of this population. A synchronized and well-integrated team can make valuable and specific recommendations for remediation, training, and job restructuring based on a client's thought process, ability to compensate, and identified strengths and weaknesses.

The following table of assessment procedures is based on the Vocational Assessment Procedures Analysis prepared by the New York State Head Injury Association Vocational Rehabilitation Task Force.[29] These instruments are not necessarily recommendations, and are provided for informational purposes.

VOCATIONAL ASSESSMENT PROCEDURE ANALYSIS

Category	Available Procedures	Comments
Work Performance: manual and finger dexterity, eye-hand and bimanual coordination, following instructions, color discrimination, speed of production	Normed, manual psychometric tests, i.e., Crawford Small Parts Dexterity Test (CS-PDT),[32] Hand Tool Dexterity Test,[33] Purdue Pegboard Test[34]	Low predictability since so trait-specific; good comparison over successive administrations, norms invalid for brain injured
	Normed aptitude tests, i.e., Bennet Mechanical Comprehension Test (BMCT),[35] Flannigan Industrial Tests (FIT),[36] Minnesota Clerical Test (MCT),[37] General Aptitude Test Battery (GATB),[38] Office Skills Tests[39]	Standardized, often written instructions and strict normative data; may be useful to measure abstract knowledge in specific areas. Record changes when not using normative procedures and data
	Commercially available trait factor work samples, i.e., JEVS Work Samples: In-Depth Vocational Assessment for Special Needs Groups,[40] Vocational Information and Evaluation Work Samples (VIEWS),[41] VALPAR Component Work Sample Series[42]	Realistic tasks to determine specific information, i.e., speed, attention to detail, coordination. Helpful in exploring modifications to work sites. Can be too abstract for some patients. Norms and standards unusable. Record changes when not using normative procedures and data
	Commercially available job samples, i.e., Singer Vocation Evaluation System,[43] Comprehensive Occupational Assessment and Training Systems (COATS),[44] Tower System[45]	Realistic outcome/product/tasks for career exploration. Tasks can be broken down and modified. Awkward audiovisual instructions. Norms and standards unusable. Record changes when not using normative procedures and data
	On-the-job assessment	Most useful overall assessment when patient is job ready and/or support, i.e., job coach, is available
Cognitive Factors: memory, speed of processing, perception, judgment and problem solving, language processing and expression, academics	Psychometric tests used by various disciplines	Good baseline data, administered over time can demonstrate change
Work Behaviors: attention, adherence to rules authority, response to criticism, work tolerance	Psychometric scales, i.e., Social and Prevocational Information Battery-T (SPIB-T),[46] Street Survival Skills Questionnaire,[47] Traumatically Head Injured Assessment Scale,[48] self-reports, significant other reports	Validity dependent on subjective information; use several sources of information. Scales offer useful behavioral categories for observations
	Situational observations, i.e., on-the-job, psychosocial interaction	Use specific observational techniques, i.e., interval recordings, timed and random samplings, narratives. Can be compared with similar samplings of competitive workers. Helpful during team staffings

VOCATIONAL ASSESSMENT PROCEDURE ANALYSIS
(Continued)

Category	Available Procedures	Comments
Physical Abilities: standing, walking, sitting, bending, lifting, stooping	Standardized range of motion, strength, tolerance tools used by various disciplines	Sufficient for baseline data and comparisons over time; but not sufficient for determinations of actual work performance
	Situational observations i.e., on-the-job, during assessment	Be specific in use of indicators of time, weight, distance, and so on
Interests/Temperaments: expressed, assessed, observed	Picture-interest survey, i.e., Wide Range Interest-Opinion Test (WRIOT),[49] Geist Picture Interest Inventory,[50] Reading Free Vocational Interest Inventory (R-FVII)[51]	Carefully monitor administration to reduce misinterpretation. Divide longer tests into several administrations. Some are limited to specific occupations. Highly variable information supplied by each
	Written interest surveys, i.e., Strong-Campbell Interest Inventory (SCII),[52] California Occupational Preference Survey (COPS),[53] Kuder Occupational Interest Survey, Form DD (KOIS),[54] Premorbid Worker Trait Questionnaire[55]	Depend on reading ability, or read to client. May have interpretive information. Some require computer scoring
	Informal discussions with patient and significant others	May be best method of identifying interests
	Tours, job trials, and situational assessments	Best when structured and combined with counseling. Can be effective for unrealistic clients

Behaviorally Based Training/Education

A training and education program for individuals with head injuries should be based on the following:

An In-depth Interdisciplinary Vocational Evaluation With Consideration for Premorbid Job Characteristics and Interests. The results of the vocational evaluation and associated information will provide the necessary information for the rehabilitation specialist to determine the client's readiness for vocational training.

Exploration of Vocational Choices; A Job Match Between Interests and Skills. Based on premorbid and present interests, work experiences, residual strengths and limitations, vocations can be explored.

Realistic Appraisal of the Magnitude of the Discrepancy Between the Vocational Goal, Abilities, Limitations, and Effectiveness of Compensatory Strate-

gies. The rehabilitation specialist examines the feasibility of achieving the vocational goal based on client's performance in work trials. If the goal is determined to be unrealistic, a modified goal will be identified.

Even unrealistic expectations expressed by clients or families can have positive implications. They may motivate for clients to comply with medical/therapeutic regimens. In other cases, they may not be unrealistic at all but may be goals that require significantly more time and effort than usual to attain.[28]

In cases when clients have unrealistic job expectations the following guidelines are suggested:[28]

☐ Client is responsible for gathering job information from multiple sources.
☐ Client interviews and observes key worker contacts.
☐ Client participates in work trials.
☐ Counselor does not hinder counseling

relationships by direct confrontation; instead uses families, counseling group members, video recordings, and so on.

This technique can provide the time for cognitive and emotional adjustment before a client actually tries a job at which he or she is not likely to be successful.

On-going Counseling to Confront Problems, Deal With Stressors and Reinforce Client's Skills and Assets. A career counselor is calm, consistent, positive, and sensitive to the need for time for psychologic and emotional adjustment. Early in the counseling relationship, specific goals, relevant cues, and positive reinforcements are established.[28]

A Prescriptive Behaviorally Based Training Plan that Maximizes Cognitive, Physical, and Behavioral Abilities, and Compensatory Techniques and Adaptations. Training is centered on a specific job, at a specific place of employment, with a specific piece of equipment. Each job will be test analyzed, or broken down into a sequence of "do-able" steps. Positive and meaningful reinforcements are identified and built into the process. The job may need to be fitted to the person, rather than the person fitted to the job. Attention should be paid to job modification, job restructuring, or job engineering to adapt the tasks to the client's abilities.[28] The emphasis of the training/education program will be on the maximization of cognitive strengths, development and reinforcement of compensatory skills, and use of adaptations. Learning styles will determine teaching strategies.

Alignment of Family/Employer Acceptance and Support. The attitudes, support, and involvement of the client and family will directly affect the plan's success. Families may have to deal with changes in attitudes regarding positions of lesser status. Employers will need information and guidance in formulating realistic expectations; a client's work may not be up to usual productivity levels. Vocational specialists and job coaches should be available for problem solving, support, and reinforcement for both the client and the employer.

Work Trials

Work or occupational trials are nonpaying work experiences designed to provide real-ity orientation and feedback regarding work habits and behaviors, as well as job performance. Work habits are related not only to the physical and cognitive demands of a given assignment but also to an attitude and a sense of one's public presentation. Work behaviors include attendance, interpersonal skills, ability to understand and follow instructions, anticipatory behavior, selective attention, concentration, and executive skills. Stamina, body mechanics, dexterity, and personal grooming are also relevant. Work trials can last from 3 months to a year, or longer if instructional strategies continue to produce desirable changes in work habits and behaviors.

In a rehabilitation hospital setting, such as the one at New York University, work situations are designated within the medical complex in offices, shops, libraries, and so forth. Vocational counselors from the head trauma program serve as personal counselors, tutors, and supervisors. Work competency, productivity, and interpersonal skills are rated by both the vocational counselor and the actual job supervisor. Each patient's work abilities are compared with those of competitively hired employees doing the same jobs. Comparable competitive performance for a minimum of 6 weeks is considered competence. Some patients may be shifted from one job to another until work reliability is established.[4]

Job Placement

A recommendation for the appropriate type of job setting will be possible as the client progresses in the work trial, and observations are made about work habits, work behaviors, and job performance. Employment may be attempted on a part-time basis to examine the generalization of desirable work traits and physical/mental stamina.

Inventories are available that may help to identify vocational levels of the clients.[48, 55, 56] These inventories rate work habits (i.e., punctuality, attendance, psychosocial behaviors). The information gleaned from these inventories can be used to determine the level of assistance and employment, competitive or avocational, that will be appropriate for each individual.

An empathetic and supportive employer may be sought from a list of previous employers, family members, friends, or community-affirmative business people. Here again, the rehabilitation specialist may have to devise a creative plan to recruit and enlist the right employer for the right job for the client.

There are also alternatives to work that can provide meaningful life activity for those clients for whom competitive employment is not a realistic choice. The Avocational Activities Inventory[57] can be helpful in the selection of such appropriate activities based on interest and ability. The support of the family is again critical in successful avocational placement. The interdisciplinary team is invaluable in providing and/or recommending long-term support for families.

The Departments of Vocational Rehabilitation

The Departments of Vocational Rehabilitation are state- and federally funded agencies, products of the Rehabilitation Act of 1973, Section 504. The mission of these agencies is to help individuals with disabilities enter or return to work and live more independently.

Vocational rehabilitation counselors prepare individualized written rehabilitation plans (IWRP) for each client. These plans may include one or more of the following services:[6]

- [ ] Cognitive rehabilitation
- [ ] Behavioral management
- [ ] Psychosocial rehabilitation
- [ ] Physical therapy
- [ ] Occupational therapy
- [ ] Speech and language therapy
- [ ] Neuropsychology
- [ ] Counseling services
- [ ] Recreational therapy
- [ ] Vocational services

Eligibility for services is based on a reasonable expectation of getting and retaining a job following rehabilitation services. An applicant is interviewed and scheduled for medical and other examinations. The resulting information is reviewed to learn the type and extent of the disability, and how much work an applicant can perform. If it is determined that the applicant is eligible he or she is accepted as a vocational rehabilita-

tion client. Examinations, counseling, training, and vocational services are provided free of cost. Medical care and special equipment may be billed on a sliding scale according to income.

Appropriate requests for services are those directly related to vocational concerns. Care should be taken to enroll clients with head injuries for vocational rehabilitation services only when medical and functional stability has been achieved. The client must be alert, oriented, out of post-traumatic amnesia, able to understand what has happened, and prepared to participate actively in vocational planning.[6]

Because clients with head injuries present a wider range of cognitive, social, physical, and self-care issues than do clients with other disabilities, vocational counselors may need more information to understand the implications for successful vocational rehabilitation for this client group. For example, brain injured clients may require longer training programs than clients with other disabilities. The 60-day follow-up rule used with other groups may not allow sufficient time to determine job retention for this group.

To address these issues, and to inform vocational rehabilitation counselors of the implications of serving patients with brain injury, the State Departments of Rehabilitation in California and Colorado have implemented informative workshops for their counselors. During preliminary workshops, guest speakers provide general information on cognitive and psychosocial issues. During other workshops, difficult cases may be dealt with in a group problem-solving process. These two states have also developed codes to identify brain injured clients, to document numbers served, and to follow their long-term vocational progress.

Replication of these counselor training programs with state-developed Memos of Understanding or Cooperative Agreements, sponsored by the National Head Injury Foundation, will further this population's ability to access the services and benefits of the Departments of Vocational Rehabilitation.

Employment Models

There are two employment models that hold potential for minimizing the job retention dilemma previously mentioned in this chapter: transitional and supported employment.

Transitional employment is funded, time-limited job site training that is a necessary step for the client hoping to gain paid employment, who needs to adjust to a job in a regular work setting.

Supported employment is a funded, ongoing intensive service model that enables clients to gain and maintain paid employment in a regular work setting. This model funds placement, training, and follow-up for the client's work life. It has the advantage of being able to fit the job to the client, not the client to the job.[28]

Job coaches are professional staff personnel provided in either of the two employment models. Their responsibilities include training/education specific to the job, modification of work behaviors, travel training, family counseling, and agency coordination. They are skilled at communicating with employers and coworkers to achieve conflict and problem resolution. They understand job analysis, and train clients on the job site daily. After training has concluded, it is their ongoing responsibility to contact employers and make follow-up observations regularly. They are recalled when job requirements change and clients need to develop new skills.

Based on the job retention record of individuals with head injuries, the supported employment model seems a viable solution to otherwise rather bleak employment prospects for this population. It is a promise of support for the client's work life. Because of this commitment, there are ethical considerations for funding programs using this model. The humanitarian and financial benefits, quality of life issues, wage-earning potential, and tax revenues need to be weighed against the cost of supported employment.

It is hoped that future Vocational Rehabilitation Act amendments will provide definitions and state funding for supported work employment programs for survivors of head injuries. Regardless of the level of federal funding, vocational specialists will need to be creative in identifying fiscal resources for their clients. One creative supported employment specialist has developed a self-support plan using a Supplemental Security Income work incentive program to fund supported employment for his clients.[58]

CONCLUSION

With continuing advances in medical interventions, victims of brain injury will have correspondingly improved chances for survival. Treating the growing numbers of survivors will pose continuous challenges to rehabilitation professionals, but it is encouraging to know that during the last few years methodologies have emerged that demonstrate potential for improving the vocational prospects of this group.

The prominence and tireless lobbying efforts of the National Head Injury Foundation are responsible for securing national attention for the head injured and for the need for rehabilitation research. The National Institute on Disability and Rehabilitation Research has been responsive to the Foundation's efforts, and has made head injury a top priority for research funding.

It will be the ongoing support of national and private endowments that will yield new methodologies, evaluation tools, and standardized measurements for success and long-term follow-up studies. From this research will emerge demonstration projects that will document the vocational potential of brain injured individuals with appropriate interventions and resources. The numbers of accessible community-based programs will grow as their cost and therapeutic effectiveness are documented. With increasing evidence of long-term job retention, more and more permanent funding will be directed to supported work programs. Training programs will develop to prepare professional and paraprofessional vocational specialists to staff these projects.

Care must be taken, however, to ensure that we do not neglect life quality issues in our search for vocational strategies. By definition, quality of life encompasses the subjective qualitative aspects of recovery such as physical, emotional, and material well-being; interpersonal relationships; social, community, and civic activities; personal development and fulfillment; and recreation. Although "material well-being" can come from gainful employment, it is important that this well-being not come at the expense of "sociopersonal aspects of existence." Somehow, as we search for vocational solutions for our clients, we must also be committed to discovering new paths that will lead them to improved life satisfaction and wellness.[59]

REFERENCES

1. Humphrey, M and Oddy, M: Return to work after head injury: A review of post-war studies. Injury 12:107, 1980.
2. Thomsen, IV: Late outcome of very severe blunt head trauma: 10–15 year second follow-up. J Neurol Neurosurg Psychiatry 47:260, 1984.
3. Wrightson, R and Gronwall, D: Time off work and symptoms after minor head injury. Injury 12:445, 1980.
4. Ben-Yishay, Y et al: Relationship between employability and vocational outcome after intensive holistic cognitive rehabilitation. J Head Trauma Rehabil 2:35, 1987.
5. Prigatano, GP et al: Neuropsychological Rehabilitation after Brain Injury. Johns Hopkins University Press, Baltimore, 1985, 131.
6. The Silent Epidemic: Rehabilitation of people with Traumatic Brain Injury. Rehab Brief. National Institute of Handicapped Research, Washington, DC, 1986.
7. Weddell, R, Oddy, M and Jenkins, D: Social adjustment after rehabilitation: A two year follow-up of patients with severe head injury. Psychol Med 10:243, 1980.
8. Caveness, W: Incidence of cranio-cerebral trauma in the United States with trends from 1970 to 1975. Adv Neurol 22:1, 1979.
9. Cook, J et al: ABI handbook: Serving students with acquired brain injury in higher education. California Community College Chancellor's Office, Disabled Students Programs and Services, 1987.
10. Omaya, AK, Faas, F and Yarnell, PR: Whiplash injury and brain damage: An experimental study. JAMA 204:285, 1968.
11. Omaya, AK and Gennarelli, TA: Cerebral concussion and traumatic unconsciousness: Correlation of experimental and clinical observations on blunt head injuries. Brain 97:633, 1974.
12. Bruckner, FE and Randle, APH: Return to work after severe head injuries. Rheumatol Phys Med 2:344, 1972.
13. Rimel, RW et al: Disability caused by minor head injury. Neurosurgery 9:221, 1981.
14. Rimel, RW et al: Moderate head injury: Completing the clinical spectrum of brain trauma. Neurosurgery 11:344, 1982.
15. Levin, HS et al: Long-term neuropsychological outcome of closed head injury. J Neurosurg 50:412, 1979.
16. Dikmen, S and Morgan, S: Neuropsychological factors related to employability and occupational status in persons with epilepsy. J Nerv Ment Dis 168:236, 1980.
17. Teasdale, G and Jennett, B: Assessment of coma and impaired consciousness: A practical guide. Lancet 2:81, 1974.
18. Gennarelli, TA et al: Influence of the type of intracranial lesion on outcome from severe head injury: A multicenter study using a new classification system. J Neurosurg 56:26, 1982.
19. Brown, JC: Late recovery from head injury: Case report and review. Psychol Med 5:239, 1975.
20. Heiskanen, O and Sipponen, P: Prognosis of severe brain injury. Acta Neurol Scand 46:343, 1970.
21. Gilchrist, E and Wilkinson, DM: Some factors determining prognosis in young people with severe head injuries. Arch Neurol 36:355, 1979.
22. Lishman, WA: The psychiatric sequelae of head injury: A review. Psychol Med 3:304, 1973.
23. Gjone, R et al: Rehabilitation in severe head injuries. Scand J Rehabil Med 4:2, 1972.
24. Bond, MR and Brooks, DN: Understanding the process of recovery as a basis for the investigation of rehabilitation for the brain injured. Scand J Rehabil Med 8:127, 1976.
25. Rusk, HA, Block, JM and Lowman, EW: Rehabilitation of the brain-injured patient. In Walker, AE et al (eds): Late Effects of Head Injury. Charles C Thomas, Springfield, IL, 1969, p 327.
26. Najenson, T et al: Rehabilitation after severe head injury. Scand J Rehabil Med 6:5, 1974.
27. Crawford, D: Rehabilitation after severe head injury: The role of the employer. Injury 1:169, 1969.
28. McMahon, B: Vocational programs and approaches that work. In Burns, PG, Kay, T and Pieper, B: A Survey of the Vocational Service System as It Relates to Head Injury Survivors and Their Vocational Needs. New York State Head Injury Association, Albany, 1986, p 131.
29. Burns, PG, Kay, T and Pieper, B: A Survey of the Vocational Service System as It Relates to Head Injury Survivors and Their Vocational Needs. New York State Head Injury Association, Albany, 1986.
30. Musante, SE: Issues relevant to the vocational evaluation of the traumatically head injured client. Vocational Evaluation and Work Adjustment Bulletin, Spring:45, 1983.
31. Jellinek, HM and Harvey, RF: Vocational educational services in a medical rehabilitation facility: Outcomes in spinal cord and brain injured patients. Arch Phys Med Rehabil 63:87, 1982.
32. Crawford, J: Crawford Small Parts Dexterity Test (CSPDT). The Psychological Corporation, a subsidiary of Harcourt Brace Jovanovich, Cleveland, OH, 1956.
33. Bennett, GK: Hand Tool Dexterity Test. The Psychological Corporation, a subsidiary of Harcourt Brace Jovanovich, Cleveland, OH, 1965.
34. Purdue Pegboard Test, Science Research Associates, Chicago, 1968.
35. Bennett, GK et al: Bennett Mechanical Comprehension Test (BMCT). The Psychological Corporation, a subsidiary of Harcourt Brace Jovanovich, Cleveland, OH, 1970.
36. Flanagan, JC: Flanagan Industrial Tests (FIT). Science Research Associates, Chicago, 1970.
37. Andrews, DM, Peterson, DG and Longstaff, HP: Minnesota Clerical Test (MCT). The Psychological Corporation, a subsidiary of Harcourt Brace Jovanovich, Cleveland, OH, 1979.
38. General Aptitude Test Battery (GATB). United States Department of Labor, Division of Tests, Employment and Training Administration, Washington, DC, 1970.
39. Office Skills Tests. Science Research Associates, Chicago, 1977.
40. J.E.V.S. Work Samples: In-Depth Vocational Assessment for Special Needs Groups. Vocational Research Institute—J.E.V.S., Philadelphia, 1976.
41. Vocational Information and Evaluation Work Sam-

ples (VIEWS). Vocational Research Institute—J.E.V.S., Philadelphia, 1977.

42. VALPAR Component Work Sample Series. Valpar International, Tucson, AZ, 1985.

43. Singer Vocational Evaluation System. New Concepts, Morris, IL, 1988.

44. Comprehensive Occupational Assessment and Training Systems (COATS). Prep, Inc., Trenton, NJ, 1980.

45. TOWER System. International Center for the Disabled. New York, 1967.

46. Halpern, A et al: Social and Prevocational Information Battery—T (SPIB-T). CTB/McGraw-Hill, Monterey, CA, 1979.

47. Street Survival Skills Questionnaire, McCarron-Dial Systems, Dallas, 1980.

48. Traumatically Head Injured Student Assessment Scale. Coastline College, Costa Mesa, CA, 1986.

49. Jastak, JF and Jastak, S: Wide Range Interest Opinion Test (WRIOT). Jastak Associates, Wilmington, DE, 1979.

50. Geist, H: Geist Picture Interest Inventory. Western Psychological Services, Los Angeles, 1971.

51. Becker, RL: Reading Free Vocational Interest Inventory (RFVII). Elbern Publications, Columbus, OH, 1981.

52. Strong, EK and Campbell, DP: Strong-Campbell Interest Inventory (SCII). Consulting Psychologists Press, Palo Alto, CA, 1981.

53. Knapp, RR, Grant, B and Demos, GD: California Preference Survey (COPS). Educational and Industrial Testing Service (EDITS), San Diego, 1971.

54. Kuder, F: Kuder Occupational Interest Survey, Form DD, (KOIS). Science Research Associates, (SRA), Chicago, 1970.

55. Premorbid Worker Trait Questionnaire. Coastline College, Costa Mesa, CA, 1986.

56. Crewe, NM and Athelstan, GT: Functional assessment in vocational rehabilitation: A systematic approach to diagnosis and goal setting. Arch Phys Med Rehabil 62:299, 1981.

57. Overs, RP, Taylor, S and Adkins, C: Avocational counseling manual: A complete guide to leisure guidance. Haewkins and Associates, Washington, DC, 1977.

58. Nielson, GB: Unpublished material, 1978.

59. Klonoff, PS, Snow, WG and Costa, LD: Quality of life in patients 2 to 4 years after closed head injury. Neurosurgery 19:735, 1986.

Chapter 34

Medicolegal Aspects of Head Injury

KENNETH I. KOLPAN, J.D.

Persons who incur head injury will necessarily face legal problems as a result of their injury. The nature of the injury with its resultant treatment, as well as the cause of the injury (often a motor vehicle accident), leads to involvement in the legal system. Legal rights of the head injured and concomitant responsibilities of health care providers occupy an important role in the treatment of the head injured patient from acute stages through subacute rehabilitation and the posthospital rehabilitation stage. Early medical treatment for head injuries involves emergency treatment of person(s) who will be unable to give consent for treatment; other medical treatment is long range, raising legal issues of insurance coverage. Finally, many head injuries are the result of motor vehicle accidents, sports injuries, or trauma caused by a responsible third party. The responsible party is sued in what is known as personal injury litigation. Each of these areas—medical treatment, insurance coverage, and personal injury compensation—is affected by the law.

This chapter discusses three areas in which legal issues are likely to emerge. The topics are discussed according to a medical chronology—acute care, rehabilitation, and long-term planning—though the legal concerns do not neatly fit into any time sequence. Nor does each person with a head injury face every legal problem discussed subsequently; however, these are the most common legal problems when a head injury occurs. The following discussion uses statutes and legal cases for illustrative purposes only and is not a substitute for seeking competent legal advice.

TREATMENT

As soon as medical personnel provide emergency treatment to a person with a head injury, the law is involved with the issue of informed consent. Because persons with head injury are unable to respond to medical personnel as a result of their injury, *informed consent* is dealt with in a common sense fashion. The law finds that the injured party implicitly gives his or her consent to provide the necessary medical treatment. *Implied consent* allows medical treatment to be rendered without the provider fearing liability (i.e., committing an unlawful battery) for giving treatment without a patient's authorization.

For implied consent to apply, the injured party must require emergency treatment to save life or limb and the treatment rendered must be so limited. Once the emergency treatment is no longer required, the doctrine of implied consent does not govern.

Absent in an emergency, actual informed consent for medical treatment must be obtained before the treatment is rendered. This principle recognizes that each individual person has a constitutional right to privacy and self-determination. At the same time, the law provides that medical personnel are at substantial risk if they treat a person without authority. If the head injured person is competent, consent is obtained from the patient as long as he or she is 18 years of age or older. If the head injured person is deemed incompetent by a court of law, informed consent must be obtained from the patient's legally authorized representative. An example follows:

Case 1. Mr. W is a 45-year-old man with chronic organic brain syndrome due to a traumatic accident years ago. The injury resulted in physical disabilities and cognitive impairments. Mr W. also has difficulty controlling his behavior. He is at a substantial risk of harm to himself as he consistently gets up from his wheelchair, but he does not have sufficient balance to maintain ambulation.

During his hospitalization, Mr. W had a suprapubic catheter placed. Subsequently Mr. W developed problems with the catheter as it became twisted or clogged. He could identify his need to urinate but was unable to do so. His treating physician recommended removal of the catheter and dilatation of the narrowed urethra. Although considered a simple procedure, the surgery was not without risks. The patient was at risk from the anesthesia and possible infection. Permission for the recommended surgery was needed.

Mr. W was unable to assent to the procedure because he could not understand nor remember for but a moment any of the information about the proposed surgery. Unmarried and without family, the patient had no representative who might be authorized to make the consent decision. The treating physician was unable to arrange for the operation unless he could obtain consent from someone authorized to speak on Mr. W's behalf.

This case went to the local probate court for resolution. This is an example of a guardian being required to represent the needs of a head injured patient. A *guardianship* proceeding requires that a physician (not any other professional) opine that the patient is either mentally ill or retarded. (Some states vary on this first requirement.) Since head injuries do not necessarily fit in either category, doctors all too often describe a patient as mentally ill, though the patient is not thought of in that context.

The second point required in a guardianship proceeding is that the patient is unable to care for himself as a result of impaired thinking.

A third criteria must be met: that Mr. W's impairment prevents him from appreciating the consequences of his decision relative to the offered medical treatment.

In seeking the court's determination relative to incompetence and authorization for the medical procedure, a proposed treatment plan had to be submitted. After the court had found Mr. W sufficiently impaired as to render him incompetent to decide his own course of medical treatment, the court reviewed the risks and benefits of the treatment, the patient's prognosis with or without treatment, and the nature of surgery. A person was appointed as Mr. W's guardian with specific authorization to consent to customary and usual medical treatment.

Before the court allowed the guardian to assent to the proposed surgery, Mr. W's wishes had to be accounted for. The guardian was to decide the treatment issue according to Mr. W's wishes were he able to express them now. This is the "substituted judgment" principle; it replaces the long-followed paternalistic approach of courts toward incompetents.

A *guardian ad litem* (an investigator) was appointed to ascertain the patient's wishes. The *guardian ad litem* met with Mr. W and the medical staff. She found Mr. W to be incompetent and a danger to himself. Further, she weighed the risks of the proposed surgery with its benefits and recommended that the guardian assent to the procedure. The court agreed.

The appointing of a guardian with authority to consent to customary and usual medical treatment is essential to the ongoing treatment of the head injured. Previously, appointed guardians in some states do not automatically have authority to consent to medical treatment and must return to the court for such authorization. Even where guardians have authorization to consent to medical treatment, it may not extend to psychotropic medication. Health care providers should be aware of this point.

When a patient requires psychotropic medication, the procedure involved is more detailed to protect both the rights of the head injured and the potential liabilities of the provider. The rest of Mr. W's case addresses this point.

Mr. W's injury caused him to have behavior problems. The medical staff recommended psychotropic medication (as opposed to state institutionalization) as reasonable means of managing his behavior. Though the psychotropic medication is not as invasive as surgery, the known side effects of the medication such as tardive dyskinesia are substantial. Mr. W's treatment plan included the antipsychotic medication, Mellaril, which, according to his treating physician, was used to control his aggressive symptoms. It was stated that the medication was not treating the underlying brain injury but rather the patient's outbursts. The court reviewed the treatment plan involving psychotropic medication before it would approve it.

The above procedure in Mr. W's case evolves from the case of ·Rogers v Okin,[1] which states that antipsychotic medication cannot be administered to a patient, absent an emergency against the patient's will unless a judge, using a substitute judgment standard, determines that the patient would have consented to the administration of antipsychotic medication. The court required a treatment plan that must include

1. Patient's express preferences even while incompetent
2. Religious convictions of the incompetent person (as it affects treatment)
3. Impact on the head injured person's family
4. Probability of side effects from the proposed medical treatment
5. Prognosis without the proposed treatment
6. Prognosis with the proposed treatment

The treating doctor is then asked to write a treatment plan covering each of these six factors. A judge reviews each and makes a substituted judgment decision whether or not the patient would assent to the proposed antipsychotic medication.

The court reviewed and approved the plan for Mr. W. Court involvement did not end; periodic reviews were to be submitted to the court.

By virtue of the Rogers case,[1] the incompetent's right to choose his or her own medical treatment is preserved even though the individual is unable to fully understand the treatment. At the same time, the health care provider is protected because a court order has set out the parameters of the treatment. Though somewhat cumbersome, the court does offer necessary protection to all involved. In an emergency, antipsychotic medication may be provided to an unwilling patient as long as other specific requirements are followed and the justification for not seeking court involvement does not go beyond the described emergency.

Issues of informed consent are not limited to the acute emergency phase of treating the head injured. As the head injured continue to survive for longer periods of time in institutions, hospitals, rehabilitation facilities, and nursing homes, courts are extending their involvement in treatment of these patients in order to protect the rights of those unable to speak for themselves. In 1976, Karen Quinlan, a patient in a persistent vegetative state, was being maintained on a ventilator.[2] Questions arose regarding removal of the ventilator. A guardian, appointed by the court, sought permission to withdraw the ventilator. The court allowed removal of the ventilator since the life-prolonging ventilation (not life-saving treatment) was not invasive and the underlying condition was itself not treatable. Ms. Quinlan died some 9 years after the ventilator was removed.

The Quinlan case opened the door for legal challenges to other treatment modalities given to persons with head injury, e.g., nutrition and hydration. In Re: Claire Conroy,[3] guidelines for withholding sustenance were established. The case, however, dealt only with an incompetent, institutionalized elderly person with severe mental and physical disabilities who had a limited life expectancy of less than a year. Conroy does not apply to the head injured population or to head injury facilities. Nevertheless, the court's discussion of withdrawing sustenance is worth noting.

A lower court in New Jersey had approved withdrawal of hydration for Ms. Conroy, though it was tantamount to allowing her to die.[4] A higher New Jersey court limited the extent of the Conroy decision since Conroy was not brain dead, comatose, or in a vegetative state. Though medical evidence was inconclusive as to whether she experienced pain, there was no reasonable possibility of her returning to a "cognitive" life—that is, awareness of her environment. The court limited its decision to the following set of circumstances: elderly persons residing in nursing homes who are likely to die within 1 year despite receiving treatment. In those circumstances, sustenance could be withdrawn.[5]

The Conroy decision reaffirms a person's right to determine treatment even if it results in the person's death. The court emphasized that withdrawing sustenance is not suicide because it is not a self-inflicted wound that causes death, rather the underlying disease is the cause of death.

The *Conroy* court used a balancing test to come to its decision. On one hand the court reviewed the patient's right of self-determination and on the other hand the state's countervailing interests in preserving life, protecting innocent third parties, and upholding the integrity of the medical profession. The court declared that life sustaining treatment could be withheld or withdrawn from an incompetent patient if that particular patient would have refused the treatment under the circumstances involved.

The *Conroy* case is important to rehabilitation specialists who treat the head injured because it is a reminder that a person's mental condition (incompetence) does not change the person's basic right to determine his or her own course of medical treatment even if the medical treatment, such as hydration and nutrition, is life sustaining. This legal principle was most recently advanced in a case that did involve a patient with a head injury.[6]

Paul Brophy suffered a ruptured aneurysm located at the apex of the basilar artery. As a result, he was in a persistent vegetative state. A gastrostomy tube had been placed 7 months after his injury to provide for nutrition and hydration. Brophy's wife was appointed his guardian, and she asked the court's permission to withdraw or clamp his feeding tube. A lower probate court refused her request.

The court was well aware of the number of persons affected by its decision. In a footnote, the court cited the President's Commission Report stating that the causes and places of death in the United States have changed dramatically over the years. It is now estimated that institutional settings account for 80 percent of the deaths that occur.[6] The primary cause of death is progressive illness rather than acute causes. Providers watched this case closely since the institution where Brophy resided refused to remove or clamp the G tube as requested by the guardian's wife.

The *Brophy* court stated that Brophy was not terminally ill (unlike *Conroy*) and that he could live on for several years although he had a shortened life expectancy due to nonaggressive therapies making him susceptible to secondary complications. (See later discussion of life expectancy of a person with a head injury.) The court recognized that the G tube itself was not painful but found that death by dehydration was pain-

ful. With this factual context set, the court decided that the G tube could be removed and the facility would not be compelled to remove it. The facility was ordered to assist in the transfer of Brophy to a facility that would carry out the court's order (p. 441).[6]

The Massachusetts Court followed the "substituted judgment approach." It analyzed Brophy's expressed preferences, his religious convictions, the impact of the decision on his family, the probable side effects of the proposed treatment, and his prognosis both with and without treatment. Unlike many cases involving young head injured persons, Brophy had expressed his preferences for nontreatment were he to be in a persistent vegetative state. His religious convictions and the impact on his family were equally clear. His preferences were supported by his family. The court focused its attention on Brophy's wishes making his constitutional right of privacy paramount. The fact that Brophy was comatose in no way lessened his constitutional guarantee against invasion of his privacy through unwanted medical treatment (pp. 427–436).[6] His incompetence did not affect his legal right to choose medical treatment; it only changed the manner by which his choice was implemented. The court directed Brophy's wife (his guardian) to carry out his wishes (pp. 441–442).[6]

The *Brophy* case does not mean that treatment can be withdrawn or withheld in all circumstances involving seriously head injured persons. Each case calls for a balancing of the individual's right of self-determination and the state's interest in the preservation of life. The court focused on the patient's desires and not on the type of treatment involved, even though the nature of the treatment is considered. Emphasis on the type of treatment—extraordinary or ordinary—detracts from the issue, which is the patient's preferences. This is true whether the treatment is to be withheld or withdrawn (pp. 437–438).[6] In conclusion, the *Brophy* decision upholds an individual's right to choose or refuse medical treatment regardless of his or her physical or mental condition.

DECISION MAKING

When patients lose their ability to make treatment decisions, they may also lose the ability to make other personal decisions such as signing contracts, conducting business, and spending money. Like medical treatment decisions, the personal decisions are carried out by the head injured person unless that person becomes incompetent. If a court adjudicates a patient to be unable to appreciate other personal decisions, someone must be appointed the lawful representative. It is not sufficient that a spouse, friend, or health care provider take over these responsibilities. The better course of action is the court appointing a person legally responsible to assume the personal decision making. The court procedure ensures that an appropriate person will be named, his authority clearly delineated, and his decisions accounted for. Most courts require periodic accounting to the court and make the appointment subject to removal for acts of bad faith or fraudulence. Different jurisdictions provide different titles: guardians of the property, conservator, trustee, receiver; but the effect is to guard the incompetent person and his or her assets while providing protection to the person legally authorized to make decisions on behalf of the incompetent head injured individual.

Since head injuries require extensive medical treatment, payment for medical services is crucial. When conflicts arise, legal consultation follows.

INSURANCE COVERAGE

Head injury patients who require lengthy hospitalization, rehabilitation care, and outpatient therapies may pay for their treatment through their health care insurance. Because of the limitations, either monetary ceiling or contractual definitions, health care insurance is often a major obstacle to obtaining optimal rehabilitation treatment. If a person has a medical insurance plan, the coverage is more often for acute hospitalization up to some limit and for rehabilitation care to a lesser limit. The gap between available health care insurance and optimal rehabilitation is a cause for pursuing personal injury litigation, but compensation from such litigation is usually years away while insurance coverage for the required treatment is needed immediately. To the disappointment of families of head injured and some institutions, available health insurance is usually inadequate to cover required treatment for head injuries. An example follows:

Case 2. A man who had suffered a head injury had been in a skilled nursing facility for several years. He had made progress in the head injury program. The facility had provided periodic evaluations to the governmental insurance payor. As the patient's progress waned, the insurer sent notice to the facility that it would no longer pay for the services rendered, and gave the facility 30 days to make arrangements for the patient's transfer. With limited resources, the family's choice was to transfer the head injured person to a facility that would accept governmental payments (Medicaid or Medicare) at a lower per diem, but that type of facility did not provide the unique treatment found in this head injury facility.

This case is not unusual. The insurer claimed that its contract did not provide for custodial "care" in a skilled nursing facility. Their contract defined "custodial care" to be care without the capability of progress or improvement. The fact that the patient was in a head injury facility that was licensed as a skilled nursing facility only reinforced the insurer's perception that the facility was providing custodial care. The facility sought legal advice on how to proceed. Discussion with staff and administration revealed that the patient was involved in many therapies aimed at improving his physical and mental condition. Progress, albeit slow, was continuing. When medical records were reviewed, the records failed to document the patient's progress, though he responded to respiratory therapy, speech therapy, and sensory stimulation program in measurable ways. The facility appealed the insurer's decision to the company's internal review board. After reading the current reports, documented progress, the planned objectives, goals, and actual changes in the patient's condition, the review board reversed its earlier decision and paid for the patient's continued care at the head injury facility.

This example shows that insurers, like laypeople, are unfamiliar with head injury programs. Providers have an obligation to educate payors (private or government) about the efficacy, purpose, and results of these relatively new programs. Treatment reports must carefully document the patient's recovery and rehabilitation, even when progress is slow and difficult to measure. Insurers are concerned about expansion of their contracts into areas that appear to be costly. Though this is a legitimate concern, a head injury program that does fall within the health insurance contract obligates the insurer to provide payment for the head injury program as long as it is well documented. This is true whether the payor is a private carrier or a governmental program. This issue does not arise when the family has sufficient private resources or the injured person has received personal injury compensation from a responsible party. When money comes from a private source or a liability suit, the injured person has the freedom to choose the location and nature of treatment and is not limited by contractual provisions. This is the reason why personal injury litigation is a viable alternative to financing needed rehabilitation care.

PERSONAL INJURY COMPENSATION LITIGATION

Traumatic head injuries are often a result of a motor vehicle accident, sports injury, or a defective product. Under many of these circumstances, another person or entity may be liable for the injury to the patient. A personal injury lawsuit seeks a judicial determination that a party (defendant) was negligent, caused the injury, and should compensate the injured party. If the defendant has insurance, payment to the injured party comes from the liability insurance carrier when the matter is settled or ends in judgment for the injured party. Once payment is received, it is unrestricted and can be used by the injured party for appropriate medical treatment. Before personal injury litigation reaches that point, there are numerous legal hurdles that must be overcome.

If the head injured person is going to sue for compensation, there are time limits within which legal proceedings must be commenced (Statute of Limitations). Limits may vary according to the jurisdiction (e.g., 2 or 3 years) and to the defendant involved in the type of legal action (e.g., medical malpractice). If a person fails to file within the requisite time period, the suit is forever barred. Some time limitations may be tolled due to the injured person's age (minority), incapacity (incompetence), or because the

jurisdiction follows the "rule of discovery."

The latter rule states that the Statute of Limitations starts to run when the injured person "discovers or reasonably should have discovered" the injury. States that follow this rule recognize that some injuries are not readily discoverable and that these time limitations to file suit should not begin until that injury is or should have been discovered. The rule balances the defendant's interest in not being forever at risk for a lawsuit and the injured party's right to sue for injuries that are discovered late. A case example follows:

> **Case 3.** A mason was hit on the head by $4 \times 4 \times 8$ inch timber. He was told he had a bad concussion. Twenty-four hours later he was listless and became depressed. He was examined by two different neurologists but no neurologic symptoms were noted. At a clinic, he was diagnosed as being anxious and depressed. He entered psychotherapy. The psychiatrist said his symptoms were related to his accident and described him as having "compensation neurosis." Nearly 2 years after the accident, he was diagnosed as having chronic, mild, organic symptoms associated with brain trauma. Nearly 3 years after the accident, his attorney received a report from a forensic psychiatrist relative to his injury. Some 4½ years after the accident, the mason filed a lawsuit even though there was a 3-year Statute of Limitations. The jurisdiction did follow the "rule of discovery."

The question raised by this illustration is: When did the Statute of Limitations begin to run: when the mason was injured or nearly 3 years later when the mason states he was first informed of his medical condition? If the mason's reasoning is accepted, then his lawsuit will go forward. Otherwise, it is barred by the 3-year Statute of Limitations.

In the case of *Gore v O'Connell's Sons*,[7] the court stated that the Statute of Limitations generally runs from the time of injury. Only when the condition is inherently unknowable, such as in a latent disease (asbestosis), does the rule of discovery apply. Because the mason had sought out medical treatment and his doctors had related his medical condition to the trauma, the medical condition was not inherently unknowable even in retrospect. When a condition becomes manifest, such as the symptoms the mason had, the Statute of Limitations is not tolled. Unfortunately for the mason and other persons who have head injuries, if they develop problems related to trauma and fail to identify them within the time allotted under the Statute of Limitations, they may have lost an opportunity for personal injury compensation. Early identification and legal action may be advisable. However, once a lawsuit is instituted, early resolution of the lawsuit may be ill-advised.

In a case involving a 15-year-old boy injured in an automobile accident,[8] early resolution of his lawsuit was detrimental. Suit had been brought against the driver for negligence within the 3-year Statute of Limitations. The suit resulted in a jury verdict for the head injured boy. Less than 3 months after the jury verdict, the boy suffered symptoms of seizures for the first time. Medical evidence was submitted to the trial judge months after the jury verdict that the seizures were a direct result of the automobile accident. Medical testimony established that the seizure could not have been discovered during the time between the automobile accident and the jury verdict even with appropriate medical care being given during that time.

The injured boy's seizures were real and causally related to his automobile accident but the jury did not consider it in awarding compensation to him. This case was reopened under local rules permitting a new trial where there is "newly discovered evidence" which was not available to the injured party during the jury trial and such evidence would have affected the ultimate jury decision (e.g., the amount of damages would have been more).[9]

Though this lawsuit was reopened, cases that settle can rarely be opened when undiscovered medical problems arise which are causally related to the incident involved in a lawsuit. This is troublesome because 90 percent of personal injury cases, including those involving head injuries, settle without a trial. Issues of fraud or incompetence may be sufficient basis to challenge a settlement. When a person's unknown medical condition manifests itself after the settlement, the injured person is without recourse. To protect against this situation, attorneys representing the head injured person must be aware of the late consequences of head injuries such as behavioral problems, seizures, and dementia. Similarly, juries and opposing counsel must be made aware of these late sequelae. Experts familiar with these medical complications are an important part in the representation of a head injured person.

EXPERT TESTIMONY

Since most people do not understand the nature of head injury, how it occurs, and its consequences, expert testimony is the best way to convince opposing counsel, insurers, and jurors about head injury. For example, expert evidence about CT findings, x-ray films, EEG, whether abnormal or not, must be explained to the unknowing; otherwise, incorrect decisions regarding compensation will be made. Basic medical evidence about anatomy and how a head injury occurs even without outward signs must be explained. The significance of negative findings on CT and skull x-ray films and EEGs must also be provided. Otherwise, head injured persons, especially those with so called "minor or moderate" injury, will not receive just compensation. A recent court case demonstrates.

Case 4. A 26-year-old who suffered a head injury from a 400-pound garage door being pulled down on her head was subsequently examined at a hospital where x-ray and CT films and EEG results were all within normal limits. She continued to have substantial impairments in cognition, memory, and concentration which were all documented in neuropsychologic testing. An expert neurologist was called to testify as to the seriousness of her injury notwithstanding the normal findings. His explanation is found in Table 34–1.

The apparent absence of objective evidence of injury is a major impediment in establishing that a head injury has occurred. Attorneys need this documentation to effectively represent their clients. The neuropsychologist is the key. Before a neuropsychologist can present his or her findings in a courtroom, it must be established that the training and education received by the neuropsychologist is adequate to allow him or her to render an opinion regarding brain injury. Further, the neuropsychologist must explain the nature of the tests, the norms involved, the reliability, the validity, and the purposes of the individual subtests. Since the impairments documented in neuropsychologic testing such as memory, concen-

Table 34–1. TRANSCRIPT OF TESTIMONY

Q Are you aware of any medical reason why a person with a head injury would have a normal CAT Scan?

A The CAT Scan gives us a snapshot, a photograph of the anatomy of the brain as if someone had taken a brain out and were able to slice it and then look at each individual piece. But the significant injuries that are done to people who have head injuries are not as a result of large hemorrhages or strokes but rather they are done on a microscopic level because the individual cells and the connections from one cell to another are actually torn. The tearing is done on such a microscopic level that the CAT Scan may not be able to tell us that this injury has occurred but rather we see in the patient in examining them (sic) an insult and, knowing the laboratory research that has been done on the nature of the head injury, we can then infer that the damage that has been done is the result of what is called a shearing effect or a tearing of the fibers that travel from one cell to another, and these are too small to be seen on the CAT Scan.

THE COURT. And if a person had a head injury, could they [sic] have a normal EEG and still have brain damage?

THE WITNESS. The reason is that the EEG again is a very gross test. It records the electrical activity from the brain but takes in very large territories and the test is done by placing wires on the skull and recording the electrical activity produced by the brain. Unfortunately, the test only tests the upper outer two-thirds of the brain because we can't get to the undersurface and it only records information approximately one inch deep into the brain. And so any damage that is done deeper than one inch or on the undersurface will not show up on the EEG. Also, there is a requirement of a fairly significant injury to the brain to reduce the amount of electrical activity both in how rapidly electricity is produced and also in the degree or the voltage from the electricity that the brain produces. So you can have a fairly significant injury without change in the EEG just as you can have very significant abnormality in a person's ability to function after birth injuries, such as [sic] retarded people may have absolutely normal EEG's and normal CAT Scans and yet their ability to function in life may be very much less in quality and degree than a person who isn't retarded.

Q Doctor, can persons with head injury have a normal skull film Xray as well?

A Certainly.

Q Why is that?

A In order to produce a skull fracture, you often deal with a different force than you do with the problem inside the brain. We are talking about two different consistencies. The skull can take up a great deal of force without breaking whereas the brain is loose inside the skull. The brain has an ability to shift slightly within the skull so that when the head is struck, the brain may shift inside. And the inner surface of the skull is not completely smooth so that there are some irregular areas that can produce an abrasion of the brain. Also, the brain moves inside the skull the way a person moves inside a car when the brakes are applied in a very hard manner. We move forward when the brakes are applied. When the skull is struck and stops, the brain will continue to move forward. The movement is not always just straight forward but there is a twisting motion because pressure is applied to the brain when it strikes the inside of the skull and, as far as the pressure waves are concerned, there is only one way for that pressure wave to move and that is down toward the center of the brain. And if the head hasn't been struck absolutely straight, there is a bit of a twist or torque that occurs to the brain so that there is an impact injury of actually hitting of the brain inside the skull and also a twisting injury that occurs.

From Transcript.[10]

tration, and attention are difficult to otherwise demonstrate in a courtroom (the head injured person appears better than he is because it is an orderly setting), the objective findings on neuropsychologic testing are essential evidence in personal injury litigation. A jury can understand the quantifications under each subtest and, hopefully, appreciate the significance of the patient's test scores from the norm. A piece of demonstrative evidence may be helpful (Table 34–2).

As the neuropsychologist testifies about the test scores, each test is described, the norm is emphasized and the significance of the patient's score in terms of the norm is explained. In this way, the jury can see and hear objective evidence that quantifies the incurred brain injury.

With sufficient background, foundation,

Table 34–2. SAMPLE: SUMMARY OF NEUROPSYCHOLOGIC FUNCTIONS/BRAIN IMPAIRMENT (HALSTEAD-REITAN SERIES)—EXHIBIT 8

Test	Halstead-Reitan Battery Suggested Cut-offs for Brain Damage	Score
Category	51 or more errors	77 errors
Seashore rhythm	25 or less correct	17 correct
Speech-sounds perception	8 or more errors	34 errors
Finger-tapping	50 or less taps per 10 second interval	19 taps (RH) 16.4 taps (LH)
Trail-making		
Part A	40 or more seconds	81 seconds
Part B	91 seconds or more	270 seconds
	No. tests administered in this section: 5	
	No. tests suggesting brain damage: 5	
Aphasia screening	No suggested cut-offs	4 errors (2 in repeating multisyllabic words, 1 in subtraction calculation, and 1 in copying cube)

From Transcript.[10]

and training the neuropsychologist may offer an opinion regarding the cause (e.g., of the accident) of the head injury. Some jurisdictions, however, do not allow a neuropsychologist to render an opinion regarding causation and prognosis related to brain injury;[11] other jurisdictions are more willing.[12]

If the neuropsychologist is a trained vocational rehabilitation specialist, he or she could proffer an opinion regarding the person's present and future employability. If not, an expert in vocational rehabilitation should testify to assist the jury in its decision related to the head injured person's ability to return to work.

An important expert in the head injured person's case is a person who is familiar with long-term planning for the head injured. A psychiatrist, neurologist, neuropsychologist, or rehabilitation counselor may all provide the specifics of such long-term planning (including lifelong institutional care, if that is appropriate). The long-range plan must then be quantified in dollar terms and the present cost of such a plan projected over the person's expected lifetime. An economist will provide this testimony.

Not only the extent, frequency, and cost of the itemized treatments but also the duration of the treatment influence the ultimate cost of long-term care for the head injured person. Obviously, if a head injured person's life expectancy is reduced it will dramatically affect the extent of the long-term treatment. Life expectancy tables provide guidance; they provide the number of years a person will continue to live, according to a statistical pool and for the general population. Estimating a life expectancy of a person in a coma or with serious head injury may become an arguable point that is not easily resolved by using the usual life expectancy tables. Each side of a lawsuit contests whether the head injury is a life-threatening situation affecting life expectancy or, as long as a person is medically stable and receives medical treatment, the injury has no effect on life expectancy. The latter point posits that head injury itself is not life threatening and that secondary complications, if appropriately treated, will not affect a head injured person's life expectancy.

Persons who provide long-term treatment to the head injured (including those in coma) will be asked to testify about life expectancy of the patient in question and to document the same. Existing life expectancy tables and previous research on this population may be unreliable, as they do not include head injured patients who receive aggressive trauma care and rehabilitation treatment.

Added to compensation for a person's lost employment and cost of long-term care is payment for pain and suffering and loss of enjoyment of life. Head injured persons must endure through their lifetime a recognition but not reconciliation that their present condition is unlike that of their former self. It is difficult to assess pain and suffering, and more so when the person is in a prolonged coma. In a recent New Jersey case, a patient who was in coma for 6 years sued a local county for causing an automobile accident.[13] Each attorney had an expert who assumed diametrically opposed opinions concerning her ability to appreciate pain. A "Day in the Life" videotape showed the person in daily activities including therapy. The film was to be shown to the jury. During the film, the patient smiled after a compliment from one of her medical staff. Defense counsel, after reviewing the tape, felt the jury would interpret the patient's smile as evidence that the patient did respond to her environment as the plaintiff's expert opined. The plaintiff's expert was ready to testify that her repeated grimacing during physical therapy was further evidence that she responded to environmental stimuli.

Finally, the plaintiff's neurologist was expected to testify that he replicated the patient's grimaces during his neurologic examination. This case was settled, in part, because the videotape presentation provided graphic evidence supporting plaintiff's contentions regarding her pain and suffering.

SETTLEMENTS

Personal injury suits usually end with a settlement. A settlement can be made in one lump sum or over a period of time (e.g., structured settlement). Each method has its advantages and drawbacks. A lump sum is a certain amount that can be invested and, hopefully, preserved over a person's lifetime. The lump sum, not the investment, is nontaxable. When a substantial sum of money is involved, some families may be ill-equipped to manage the money and thus it may not last through the time it is needed.

A structured settlement addresses this last point by providing periodic payments, some of which may be guaranteed for a number of years (and is paid to the person's estate when he or she dies). The remaining portions of payments are made over the person's lifetime. Under current law, the periodic payments are nontaxable. The payments usually provide for a cost of living and are periodic lump sum payments. Structured settlements are inflexible, give the head injury person no control over the monies, and depend on the insurance company's solvency and any other underlined guarantors.

Each case is different. The settlement must be appropriate in light of the facts of the case, the needs of the injured party, and the abilities of the person handling the finances.

CONCLUSION

The head injured confront lifelong problems in obtaining medically appropriate treatment and payment for the care. Legal principles often determine whether a head injured patient will receive needed treatment. Providers and families of the head injured individual, through understanding of their legal responsibilities and rights, will be better able to provide and obtain maximum rehabilitation treatment.

REFERENCES

1. Roberts v Commission of the Department of Mental Health.
2. In re Karen Ann Quinlan, 70 NJ 10 (1976).
3. In the Matter of Claire Conroy, 98 NJ 321 (1985).
4. In the Matter of Claire Conroy, 190 NJ Super. 453 (1983).
5. In the Matter of Claire Conroy, 190 NJ Super. 321 (1985).
6. Brophy v New England Sinai Hospital, Inc, 398 Mass 417 (1986).
7. Tanya Gore et al v Daniel O'Connell's Sons, Inc, 17 Mass App Ct 645 (1984).
8. David A VanAlstyne v Richard Whalen, 15 Mass App Ct 340 (1983), 20 Mass App Ct 239 (1985).
9. Mass R Civ P No 60(b)(2).
10. Transcript, Susan Berberian v K-Mart Corporation, Norfolk County, Mass Civil Action Number 137202 (February 5, 1986).
11. GIW Southern Valve Company v Robert C. Smith, 471 So 2d81 (Fla App 2 Dist 1985).
12. Simon v Simon, 385 Mass 91, 106 (1982); Lavasco v Parkhurst Marine Ry Co, 322 Mass 64 (1947).
13. Sharon Feller et al v County of Bergen, Superior Court of New Jersey, Law Division, Bergen County Docket No L-065644-83.

Section V
Conclusion

MITCHELL ROSENTHAL, Ph.D.

In the last six years, since publication of the 1st edition of this text, an expansion in rehabilitation practices and types of programs serving the head injured patient has been seen. Efforts to rehabilitate head injured patients have moved beyond the medically oriented acute rehabilitation sphere into long-term postacute service delivery programs such as day treatment, independent living, residential treatment, supported employment, educational reintegration, and the like. Therapeutic intervention techniques have developed a firmer basis which can be traced to a better understanding of the recovery process and of which therapeutic interventions are likely to produce long-term functional gains. In this section, a comprehensive overview of major therapeutic techniques is presented which, it is hoped, will guide both the novice and the experienced clinician to understand the optimal methods of treating physical and neurobehavioral dysfunction after traumatic brain injury.

Treatment of the motor dysfunctions resulting from head injury is often overshadowed by the need to manage the overwhelming cognitive and behavioral sequelae. Despite a relatively good recovery in motor function in a significant proportion of the brain injured population, it is important to recognize that many severely brain injured individuals experience a variety of motor dysfunctions which are an important factor in the total recovery picture. Rinehart highlights the fundamental principles that need to be considered in developing a treatment plan for motor and sensorimotor dysfunction. The author notes the inter-relationship between motor dysfunction and cognitive impairments and the need to consider the latter in the context of any motor treatment program.

Zoltan reviews the major categories of visual-perceptual and perceptual-motor deficits following traumatic brain injury. These deficits, if left untreated, have a great impact on performance of basic daily living tasks, vocational performance, and the capacity to drive an automobile. A rationale for the application of specific therapeutic techniques (i.e., neurodevelopmental, sensory-integrative, transfer of training, and functional) is articulated and related to specific types of deficits, corresponding sites of lesions and clinical manifestations.

Swallowing disorders have become a greater focus for rehabilitation treatment during the past few years. Adamovich presents a discussion of the major types of swallowing disorders, methods of diagnosis, and treatment. Though speech/language pathologists have become the major treators of swallowing disorders in many rehabilitation centers, the author argues for an interdisciplinary approach with specific roles for the occupational therapist, rehabilitation nurse, physician, respiratory therapist, physical therapist, and dietitian.

Cognitive rehabilitation—a commonly used, but ill-defined term—has become the rubric under which most efforts at rehabilitating cognitive disabilities have fallen. Several chapters in this section address cognitive rehabilitation techniques. McNeny and Dise describe the process of reality orientation training, which has become a fundamental practice in the treatment of the low-

516

level brain injured patient and the patient who emerges from coma and is confused and agitated. The casual observer may deem these procedures simple and common sensical, yet many clinicians often fail to implement these procedures in a sound, consistent manner. Though well-controlled studies have not yet been performed to document the effectiveness of reality orientation, seasoned brain injury clinicians will likely attest to its value as an integral part of the early rehabilitation process.

For the cognitive therapist, whether identified as a speech/language pathologist, occupational therapist, neuropsychologist, or special educator, methods of remediating or compensating for cognitive disabilities such as problem-solving, memory, and organizational skills have become better articulated. Adamovich presents a detailed illustration of specific cognitive rehabilitation procedures as applied to the brain injured adult. She notes that cognition and communication should not be artificially separated and that all communication disorders following brain injury are interrelated to fundamental cognitive disorders. Treatment of communication disorders has expanded to include a focus on the provision of sophisticated augmentative communication devices, which can greatly enhance the communicative capacities of the brain injured adult.

Ben-Yishay and Prigatano present their formulation of the current state of the art of cognitive or neuropsychologic rehabilitation practice. They present an effective argument for a holistic model that is supported by their own extensive research data. The results of their research provide clear evidence that cognitive disabilities are generally not remediated or restored to baseline levels. Instead, their work supports the notion that many brain injured adults, given an intensive cognitive rehabilitation program, can learn effective compensatory strategies which can lead to higher levels of social adaptability and a greater likelihood of return to work and satisfying interpersonal relationships.

As Bond and others have previously noted, the most troubling long-term sequelae of head injury for the relatives are the behavioral and interpersonal deficits. When the first edition of this text was published, behavioral intervention strategies were only sporadically and ineffectively employed in the treatment of head injured patients. Since that time, behavioral methods have become an important part of the treatment of the acute and postacute brain injured patient. Eames, Haffey, and Cope present a conceptual model for employing behavioral and pharmacologic intervention techniques with head injured individuals. All therapists working with these patients, regardless of discipline, would be well-served by reading the indications, contraindications, and side-effects of such treatments. Too often, behavioral and pharmacologic interventions are viewed as "quick fixes" and often, due to this inadequate preconception, result in failures.

Previous research that has documented the long-term burden of head injury on the relatives, as well as the emergence of national organizations such as the NHIF in the United States and Headway in Great Britain, has led clinicians to focus more rehabilitation efforts on the family. Muir, Rosenthal, and Diehl have provided an overview of the variety of family intervention strategies currently in practice. Family education is now provided extensively and in multiple formats—brochures, books, videos, and educational and support groups. The emergence of families as case managers for their relatives has caused the rehabilitation team to include them in every phase of the rehabilitation effort—from the intensive care unit to the day treatment center. Yet, the authors emphasize the need for better evaluation procedures and systematic research to understand how rehabilitation efforts affect family function and overall outcome.

For many, the ultimate criterion for successful rehabilitation after head injury is return to school or to work. Because of the pervasive residual neurobehavioral sequelae, this goal may be very difficult to accomplish. Fortunately, the educational and vocational systems have recently awakened to the plight of the brain injured. Harrington describes the history of integrating children with special needs into the educational system and clearly demonstrates how the needs of the brain injured are uniquely different from other populations. He addresses ways in which special education approaches need to be used at an elementary and secondary school level. Since many brain injured persons are of college age or are in college at the time of injury, it is also important for college educators to be aware of the problems of the brain injured and to find effective ways of meeting their needs. He provides some guidelines and recommendations for postsecondary reintegration for those brain injured who are capable of entering the system, through either community colleges or traditional 4-year colleges.

The majority of young brain injured persons face years of social isolation and economic hardship if they are unable to enter the workplace. Cook offers a perspective on the special vocational needs of the brain injured. She articulates some of the difficulties inherent in traditional vocational assessment procedures and newer methods of vocational assessment and training. The "supported employment" model, in which a brain injured person is placed in an employment setting and provided with a full-time job coach, is one that has been the focus of considerable state and federal support in the past few years and has led to the proliferation of specialized programs for the brain injured. In the next few years, one would hope that research will demonstrate the viability and cost-effectiveness of this model.

Lack of adequate recreational pursuits for the brain injured person is increasingly viewed as a major obstacle toward successful rehabilitation of these individuals. Fortunately, rehabilitation programs have come to view therapeutic recreation as a mandatory, rather than an optional, part of their treatment programs despite the lack of third-party reimbursement for these services. Berger and Regalski present a staged model for the provision of therapeutic recreation services, based on the Rancho Los Amigos Levels of Cognitive Functioning Scale. From this schema, it can be clearly seen how therapeutic recreation can be used to foster improved cognitive function, social skill development, and self-esteem. For the many head injured patients who may be forever unable to return to work or school, an ability to effectively use leisure time may be the only safeguard against social isolation, major depression, and family dysfunction.

Effective rehabilitation care of the brain injured requires not only sophistication in medical and therapeutic intervention, but also an understanding of the complex medicolegal issues so often involved in long-term management. Kolpan reviews the many medicolegal issues facing the brain injured person which so many therapists are only vaguely familiar with: issues regarding competency, guardianship, rights to withdraw nutrition, liability litigation, obtaining disability benefits, expert testimony, medical documentation, and so forth. To adequately serve our patients and families, physicians, psychologists, and therapists must become conversant with these issues and assist families who are confronted by these many perplexing medicolegal concerns.

The notion of community reintegration and systems of care is addressed by Cervelli. Our understanding of the long-term recovery of the brain injured patient has led to a realization that rehabilitation must continue in some form for many years after the initial neurologic injury. As Cervelli points out, the acute medical model is not well suited to provide the longitudinal care needed by so many who sustain brain injury. The role of the case manager has become crucial in providing the linkage between the various elements of the care system, which are not well coordinated. However, case managers are not yet a standard part of the rehabilitation effort and, in many cases, represent the needs of a third party (i.e., insurance company, employer), rather than the patient or family. As the system of care becomes more diverse and differentiated with the advent of day treatment, residential care, respite care, coma treatment, and lifelong residences, effective community reintegration efforts become paramount to maintain the gains achieved by heroic medical efforts and skilled acute rehabilitation programs.

Thus, this section illustrates the ways in which rehabilitation efforts have become more sophisticated in the past few years. It is reasonable to say that more brain injured patients are receiving intensive rehabilitation for longer periods of time in more diverse settings than ever before. Yet, our research efforts have lagged behind advances in clinical practice. The burden of proof remains for rehabilitation researchers to demonstrate the cost-effectiveness of these new, intensive, often expensive treatments and the improvements in ultimate functional outcome so desperately sought after by survivors of head injury and their families.

REHABILITATION OF THE CHILD WITH TRAUMATIC BRAIN INJURY

Ernest R. Griffith, M.D., Editor

Chapter 35

Scope of the Problem—Early Assessment and Management

DEREK A. BRUCE, M.B.Ch.B

After the first few weeks of life, trauma becomes the major cause of death throughout infancy and childhood. Estimates of the current annual rates for head trauma in children vary from 12,000 total head injuries per 100,000 children to 230 cases requiring hospitalization per 100,000 children.[1-5] Although almost all children may sustain minor injuries to the head that never come to medical attention, approximately 10 percent of children can be expected to sustain some significant trauma. The most common injuries are scalp lacerations and contusions, with only a small proportion (as low as 2 percent) of the injuries being severe enough to warrant hospitalization or produce brain damage. The cause of the trauma varies depending on the source of the data. The most frequent cause of trauma, however, is a fall, with the most frequent cause of fatality being a motor vehicle accident. The distribution of injury by age also varies depending on the origin of the statistics; most importantly, the cause of severe trauma varies markedly with age and may be an important prognostic indicator. Two to five million children sustain some degree of head trauma each year. The frequency is greater in children from birth to age 5 than in those aged 5 to 14. Every year approximately 200,000, or 3 to 4 percent, are hospitalized, and there are approximately 5000 deaths annually as a result of head trauma. Thus, the mortality rate from head trauma has been estimated as high as 10 per 100,000 children per year.

Of even greater social and economical significance are the number of children left with neurologic, intellectual, or psychiatric difficulties that were precipitated or aggravated by the head injury. It seems likely that up to 50 percent of children who recover consciousness after severe head trauma (comas lasting more than 6 hours) will have some intellectual or psychiatric problem that can be identified in the first 1 to 2 years post-trauma. The impact of these abnormalities on the child's life experience and future progress is not known.

Age is the major determinant of the type of trauma that children are exposed to. The incidence of brain trauma during birth is unknown. Essentially all children delivered vaginally will have evidence of scalp trauma—caput succedaneum. However, the incidence of intracranial trauma is small. At Children's Hospital of Philadelphia (CHOP), we saw 25 neonatal head injuries in 5 years, with a total head injury admission rate of about 250 children per year. The majority of the newborn injuries are mild; however, cephalohematomas, skull fractures, intraparenchymal hemorrhage, and subdural and epidural hematomas do occur.

The lesions are usually the result of focal stress—for instance, forceps or slow deformation during delivery. Thus, diffuse damage from trauma is rare. Nonetheless, our experience has not been encouraging, with 10 percent dying and 30 percent having poor development. The major cause of the severe injuries was mid or high forceps application, injuries that could and should have been avoided.

Through the first year of life, the infant is exposed to trauma from falling, from adult abuse, and from motor vehicle accidents. Motor vehicle trauma is usually sustained as a result of being a passenger in a car. With the introduction of good car restraint seats for children, and their enforced use, such injuries will be decreased but not eliminated. As much as 90 percent of the mortality may be prevented by use of good car restraints.

The commonest mechanism of injury of the child is a fall.[6] In the first 6 to 9 months, this is usually the result of custodian carelessness. The child is dropped or rolls from the bed or changing table. The degree of trauma is dependent on the height of the fall and the surface upon which the child falls. Such falls commonly produce skull fractures, which are usually linear and often extensive. These minor falls rarely produce unconsciousness or intracranial injury, despite dramatic looking fractures. Such injuries are often associated with delayed subgaleal hematomas, occurring 3 to 7 days after trauma, which are self-resolving. Major self-induced injury is very uncommon, but falls down steps while in a walker, or out of an unguarded window can result in severe brain injury. These injuries also are avoidable with simple precautions.

In our experience at CHOP, 80 percent of head injury deaths in the first 2 years of life are the result of custodian-induced trauma. As noted, it is rare for an infant to sustain sufficient trauma to produce unconsciousness as a result of the accidental injuries of childhood.[7] This is probably due to a number of factors, including skull elasticity and the lack of the upright position. It is extremely difficult to induce traumatic unconsciousness in animals other than primates, in part because of the alignment of the brainstem with the cerebral hemispheres and peduncles. Thus, when an unconscious child is seen and the history is either nonexistent or is that of minor trauma, the veracity of these statements is suspect, and custodian induced trauma is the presumed cause.

These children suffer long delays prior to initiating the appropriate care because

1. Seeking medical care is usually delayed in the hope the child will recover.

2. On arrival at the hospital, there is usually no history of severe trauma—or often of any trauma at all—and thus time is spent seeking a cause for the coma (e.g. infection).

3. There is a reluctance on the part of the medical staff to accept that the injury is as severe as it actually is in these small children.

The outcome in this group of children is very poor; 7 to 30 percent die; 30 to 50 percent are left with significant cognitive, intellectual, or neurologic deficits; and 30 percent have a chance for normal development. The only solution to this problem is prevention. It is a mistake to imagine that this sort of trauma occurs only to underprivileged children. Child abuse is a ubiquitous cross-societal occurrence and will continue until children are seen as independent people and not the property of their parents or custodians. Occurrence rates are difficult to estimate, but approximately 1500 children die as a result of child abuse per year, almost a third of all other head injury deaths.

Falls are the most frequent cause of childhood head trauma (42 percent).[1, 6, 8, 9] Falls occur at all ages. Most of these are accidental but could be avoided with better safety measures and parent and child education. However, the skull is presumably designed to sustain trauma, and since human beings are exploratory beasts, the childhood environment must not be made too restrictive. The majority of head trauma does not produce permanent alterations in the child's functional state.[10]

Once the child is able to venture farther from the restricted environment of home and parental supervision, injuries by motor vehicles take first place in producing major trauma. The majority of these injuries involve the child as a pedestrian, but some series report up to 40 percent occur to children as passengers in vehicles.[11] Pedestrian injuries tend to occur in the 5- to 10-year age group, most frequently between 2 and 4 P.M. when school is let out. The alterations in speed limit will have little effect on the incidence of these injuries, but prevention through parent and child education can be expected to have a significant effect. Bicycles become an important factor in accidental trauma to children beginning in the latter part of the first decade and proceeding into the early part of the second decade.

While trauma is sustained as a result of sporting and recreational activities, the actual number of severe injuries to the head and neck is very small.[12] This is an area where proper coaching and identification of the student athlete as a person, rather than as an object, to obtain gain for the school or team, would certainly cut down the incidence of major CNS trauma. The major injuries are sustained in contact sports (e.g., football, rugby) and in horseback riding. The improvements in training and equipment have significantly reduced the number of fatal injuries in high school football.[13, 14] More than half the serious head and spine injuries occur during nonorganized recreational activities. The increased use of off-the-road vehicles by children has produced a large number of injuries that are not prevented by wearing helmets and in certain areas of the country represents a serious new head injury problem.

A consistent finding in all series is that male children sustain head injuries twice as frequently as do their female counterparts. While many accepted myths may be quoted to account for this, a good study to identify why this is so would be of great potential importance. An understanding of the reasons why the incidence is higher in boys could decrease childhood head injury by approximately 30 percent.

PATHOPHYSIOLOGY

Most severe head trauma is the result of acceleration/deceleration forces applied to the brain, with or without impact to the skull. Our understanding of some of the pathology associated with this type of injury has increased over the last 5 years and has led to some redefinition of head injury pathology. To evaluate the trauma, we consider the clinical history and associate that with the dynamic living pathology as demonstrated by the computed tomography (CT) or magnetic resonance imaging (MRI) scan. Since the introduction of this methodology, the pathology is no longer limited to autopsy descriptions. The first useful clinical offshoot of this is the division of head injuries into focal versus diffuse injury.

Usually, focal injury results from impact trauma and is associated with a skull fracture or brain contusion. Diffuse injury is a result of sheering stresses set up from the acceleration/deceleration profile. The latter results in injury that may be invisible on the CT or MRI scan, yet results in unconsciousness that may be prolonged. At least part of this diffuse injury is diffuse axonal damage. The white matter is exposed to a variety of forces which result in stretching or distortion of the axons and myelin sheaths. The least definable degree of this type of injury may be clinical concussion, the most severe, prolonged unconsciousness resulting ultimately in the vegetative stage.

There is transient physiologic disruption of function, which is reversible. Myelin sheath disruption occurs with underlying disturbance of axonal transport, identified as retraction balls. If the damage is mainly to the myelin sheath, this is also probably reversible. Finally, there is total axonal disruption, which is probably irreversible.[15] Thus, recovery will depend on the relative degree of each type of injury the brain has sustained. This type of injury can occur anywhere in the central nervous system (CNS) but is most prominent in the corpus callosum, internal capsule, and regions of the superior cerebellar peduncles. Primary brainstem injury occurs, but it is rare that there is only brainstem injury; usually associated diffuse injury to the white matter of the hemispheres is also present. The importance of this is that even a child with "brainstem injury" is potentially salvageable and is at risk for the progression of all the pathophysiologic changes that can lead to secondary damage (Fig. 35–1). The term "brainstem injury" has little clinical or pathologic value and is best abandoned in favor of the more accurate term, "diffuse injury."

The concept of secondary injury versus primary injury is not new and has been discussed earlier. At present, we have no specific therapy for the direct mechanical effects of trauma to the brain. There are a series of pathologic events, triggered by the injury, that are progressive. Prevention

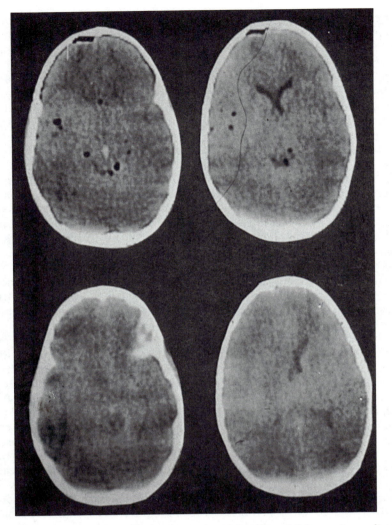

Figure 35–1. A 4-year-old child struck by an automobile. The child was immediately comatose (GCS = 4) with fixed, dilated pupils. *Top,* initial scan showed air in the subarachnoid space and a periaqueductal hemorrhage. This could be dismissed as "brainstem injury." *Bottom,* 24 hours later, however, the ICP was markedly elevated, and a repeat CT scan now shows severe brain swelling, absence of cistern, ventricular compression, and a right-to-left shift of the lateral ventricles, thus emphasizing that "diffuse injury" is more appropriate than "brainstem injury."

of these is the goal of both early and late therapy. These events are hypoxemia, hypercarbia, hypotension, and intracranial hypertension. These may be all early accompaniments of the head injury, since apnea, bradycardia, and intracranial hypertension often occur concomitant with the injury. The same events may occur later as a result of expanding intracranial mass, systemic shock secondary to other injuries, diffuse brain swelling, or prolonged hypoventilation secondary to airway obstruction as a result of the comatose state. The avoidance of the secondary injury will limit the degree of brain damage to that sustained around the period of the injury itself and, therefore, is likely to modify the outcome.

The common pathology of damage from these secondary events is ischemia. This may be global, when associated with severe intracranial hypertension or shock, or focal due to herniation syndromes (subfalcine, transalar, transtentorial, or through the foramen magnum). The brain can be diffusely swollen due to an increase in blood volume (brain swelling), an increase in brain water content (brain edema), or a combination of *both*. The detrimental results of the swelling are the production of intracranial hypertension, herniation, and ischemia. Brain swelling is a common finding on CT scans in children with severe head trauma (Fig. 35–2).[16] The most frequent cause appears to be congestion (increased cerebral blood volume [CBV]), often accompanied by an increase in cerebral blood flow (CBF).[16, 17]

It appears that at an early stage, in the first 12 to 24 hours, the cerebral metabolism of oxygen may also be increased, even in the presence of coma.[18] There is evidence in experimental models to suggest that this increased metabolic activity may be focal in the basal ganglia, rather than diffuse throughout the cortex. This does not appear to be the result of seizure activity.

On the CT scan, two forms of early brain swelling are identified. In one, the brain parenchyma appears normal or even slightly increased in density on the CT. This is hyperemic congestion and appears to carry with it a good prognosis. The second is that of diffuse low intensity of the supratentorial brain. This latter is usually the after-effect of ischemia, or is a manifestation of severely elevated intracranial pressure with very low or absent cerebral blood flow to the cortex. This is nearly always associated with death. Occasionally patients survive with severe neocortical destruction. Cerebral edema, which appears as areas of focal low density on CT scan, is rarely seen in the first 24 hours, except around intracerebral hematomas. Early areas of low density on CT suggesting focal ischemia do not seem to be associated with a worsened prognosis.

The pathophysiology associated with pediatric head injury is dynamic and changes from day to day and sometimes from hour to hour. Elevated intracranial pressure (ICP) is initially produced by the traumatic event. If the ICP remains severely elevated, the child usually dies prior to arrival at the hospital. With short paramedic response times and rapid evacuation, on-site intubation, and resuscitation, an increasing number of children who would have died at the roadside are now likely to reach the hospital with functioning cardiovascular systems. Some of

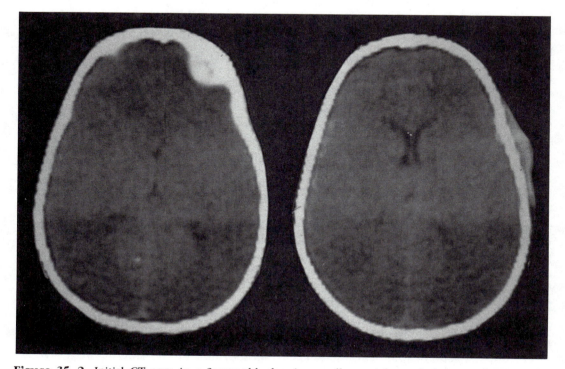

Figure 35–2. Initial CT scan in a 3-year-old, showing small ventricles and absence of CSF in the peri-mesencephalic and pineal region cisterns: diffuse brain swelling.

these patients will have equal intracranial and arterial pressures and be brain dead.

To identify this situation at the earliest time, intracranial pressure monitoring in the emergency room can be helpful. Elevated ICP in the early stages of head injury is most frequently due to vasodilatation and, in many cases, cerebral hyperemia. This results from traumatic insult to the blood vessels, plus the combination of hypoxia and hypercarbia. Control of the ICP at this time is best achieved by hyperventilation to $Paco_2$ between 20 and 25 torr, controlling blood pressure within the normal range, supplying adequate Po_2 to maintain a Pao_2 of 80 to 100 torr, and avoiding interference with cerebral venous return by keeping the head and neck in midline. Elevation of the head 20 to 30 degrees can also be helpful in decreasing intracranial venous pressure, provided that the systemic arterial pressure is adequate.

Another cause of elevated ICP is the presence of an intracranial mass lesion. Such a lesion must be identified as early as possible by CT scan and, if surgically significant, should be removed. Elevated intracranial pressure later in the course of the head injury is more likely due to true cerebral edema (increase in water content) or may be associated with alterations in serum osmolality as a result of the syndrome of inappropriate antidiuretic hormone secretion. Finally, increases in intracranial pressure that occur 7 to 10 days after trauma may be the result of secondary hydrocephalus. Each of these causes of intracranial hypertension has its own specific therapy.

EARLY ASSESSMENT

Birth Trauma

Since the forces the skull and brain experience during delivery are usually static, there is an association between the appearance of the child's head after birth and the degree of suspected cerebral trauma. High and mid forceps applications have, in our experience, been the major causes of serious brain injury during delivery. They have been responsible for depressed skull fractures, subdural and epidural hematomas, intracerebral hematomas, and hemorrhagic contusions. The common "ping-pong" depressed skull fracture, which is unassociated with overlying scalp trauma, is almost certainly the result of pressure of the pelvic bony prominences on the skull and not of obstetrical intervention.

For children suffering severe intrapartum trauma, the initial Apgar score is usually low and frequently the 5-minute Apgar is also low. Focal neurologic deficits are uncommon, but scalp and facial bruising and frank evidence of forcep marks, or scalp lacerations, are common. Seizures occurring in the first 24 hours after a traumatic delivery are often associated with the presence of an intracranial hematoma and are an indication for a CT scan, if hypoglycemia and hypocalcemia are not present. Decreasing level of consciousness is difficult to evaluate at this age, but the presence of a full or bulging fontanelle, split sutures, or increasing head size are all important parameters.

Similarly, the occurrence of intermittent apnea or bradycardia should suggest the possibility of cerebral injury, if delivery has been traumatic. Even quite extensive cortical damage cannot be identified by the neurologic examination at this age, and a guarded prognosis is necessary for these children because signs of spasticity may not occur for at least 6 months. The mortality rate from head injuries sustained during birth is low, but the long-term cognitive dysfunctions may be as high as 30 percent.

First Year of Life

The later in the first year of life the injury occurs, the easier is the neurologic evaluation. The use of the Glasgow Coma Score (GCS) is not valuable for children under 1 year old. Speech is obviously not yet present, but in this age group replacement of speech by crying can be done effectively. If the child cries spontaneously, then a full four points are given for speech. If there is no crying, then one point is given with no effort to grade in between. Eye opening early in the first year of life only occurs for short periods through the day, even in quite normal babies; therefore, its significance is difficult to evaluate. Infants with severe head injury may exhibit rhythmic eye opening which may appear quite purposeful, and yet they may still be suffering from severely elevated ICP, decreased cerebral blood flow, and irreversible brain injury.

Infants with documented evidence of no

cerebral blood flow have been seen to exhibit repetitive arm and leg movements that look like bicycling activity and that can readily be mistaken for purposeful and spontaneous motor activity. It is easy for the physician to be fooled by such motor activity, especially if this is associated with rhythmic eye opening. Based on these clinical findings, there is often delay in tracheal intubation and in obtaining a CT scan until further obvious and usually fatal deterioration occurs.

A vital part of the early examination in this group of children is funduscopic examination to look for retinal hemorrhages. These rarely occur from accidental injury and are the hallmark of a shaking impact injury.[7] They are usually associated with significant secondary brain damage due to hypoxia, hypercarbia, and elevated intracranial pressure and should always be taken as a sign of potentially severe brain trauma. There is a common misbelief that small babies are protected from changes in intracranial pressure because of the presence of the fontanelle and open sutures. In fact, the presence of an open fontanelle is no protection against elevated ICP. The ICP can equal the blood pressure just as easily in an infant as it can in a child with closed sutures.

The fontanelle cannot be accurately used to estimate the ICP. The best that can be achieved by feeling the fontanelle is to state (1) that the ICP is elevated and (2) that the fontanelle appears more tense or less tense than it did at some time in the past. The need for early aggressive management to prevent or control elevated ICP is just as important in the infant as in the older child, and when brain injury is suspected, early intubation, hyperventilation, and CT are prerequisites of treatment. If the brain appears swollen, the intracranial pressure should be monitored. Brain swelling in these little children can progress rapidly, within a few hours, to produce massively elevated ICP and no cerebral blood flood.

In children over 1 year of age, the GCS is fairly applicable. Until age 2 to 2½, speech cannot be graded, but crying does not occur in coma. Therefore, we give a score of four if there is any crying and one if there is not. The remainder of the scoring system, eye opening, and motor responses are applicable in the acute stages of injury. As accurate a history as possible of the presence or absence of spontaneous ventilation and the muscle tone at the scene of the accident will help to identify the children (1) who have suffered acute cervicomedullary injury, and (2) who are at risk for having had significant amounts of cerebral anoxia or ischemia. The occurrence of early apnea is associated with a poor prognosis and may be the only indicator of cervicomedullary junction damage in the unconscious intubated child.

The history of the mechanism of injury is important:

1. To estimate the forces involved
2. To suggest the likely presence of other injuries—either spinal or abdominal
3. To define the likely presence of focal or diffuse cerebral injury, including a mass lesion

Children struck by automobiles are likely to sustain a diffuse injury without focal mass lesions. Children who fall off their bicycles are more likely to sustain focal epidural hematomas than diffuse injury.

Seizures are fairly common after head trauma in childhood. Seizures occur in about 3 to 5 percent of reported head traumas. In children, more than half of the seizures will be associated with severe head trauma, and more than half of the early seizures will occur within the first 24 hours.[19-22] It is vital to establish whether a seizure has occurred or not. It is common that children are transferred from one hospital to another following trauma. Often the reason for the transfer is an acute change in consciousness. In up to half of these cases, this may be the result of a seizure that was either atypical, or simply not seen by the medical attendants.

The response to such a clinical deterioration will be different if a seizure is the suspected cause. Frequently, the acute changes result in the insertion of an endotracheal tube in association with the giving of Pentothal (Abbott) and a muscle-paralyzing agent. It then becomes impossible for the receiving hospital to evaluate the true extent of the underlying cerebral injury, as judged by the level of consciousness. Frequently, the CT scan is either normal or shows mild swelling. These children then may receive intracranial pressure monitoring because of concern that the change in state was the result of elevated ICP. Thus, there is a potential for them to receive much more therapy than is really required. Certainly it is better to err on the side of overtreatment in this situation than to permit secondary damage to occur as the result of elevated ICP; however, good observation of the patient and an effort to elicit a history of any potential seizure will prevent this over-response in the majority of cases.

All children who sustain traumatic injury must be assumed to have multiple trauma until proven otherwise. Cerebral injury does not produce hypotension unless there is a cervicomedullary disruption and this should be apparent from the general examination: flaccidity and apnea. A careful but rapid, general physical examination is required in every child. The most frequent accompanying trauma is abdominal injury followed by long bone injury. Accompanying chest injury can also produce acute deterioration as a result of hemothorax or pneumothorax. The general dictum that head trauma is more properly considered to be craniospinal trauma does not apply to the child. The history of the injury is extremely important. In a suspected shaken impacted child, or in a less than one year old who is an unrestrained passenger in a car, cervicomedullary injury is common, but x-ray films are usually negative. In the older child, the history will help the physician to decide on the risk of associated spinal injury. It must be realized that up to 40 percent of spinal cord injuries in children are accompanied by normal x-ray films.[23] The frequency of injury to the spine is 50 or more times less than that of injury to the head. Thus, the practice of taking routine lateral cervical spine x-ray films is of very questionable value. Certainly urgent resuscitation and intubation should not be delayed for the purpose of obtaining such cervical spine x-ray films.

MANAGEMENT

The management of the child with severe head trauma is not materially different from that of the adult and is designed to prevent secondary damage. The standard ABC's of resuscitation are followed: clearing the *airway* manually to remove secretions and debris; establishing good air movement in and out of the lungs *(breathing)*; and ensuring an adequate *circulation*. Once the airway is open, the children will usually spontaneously hyperventilate. If there is any evidence of hypoventilation, then bag and mask hyperventilation should be commenced. Gentle posterior pressure on the cricoid cartilage closes the esophagus, thus preventing air from entering and distending the stomach, a maneuver that also prevents aspiration of gastric contents. This simple maneuver should be performed during intubation. Following this, a rapid general physical examination is performed to evaluate the neurologic system: both cranial and spinal systems, the chest, the abdomen, and the extremities. In children, it is rare for shock to be due to head injury.

As soon as the basic resuscitation is under way, intravenous (IV) access is required. Ideally, this is achieved with as large an IV catheter as possible. In small children, a cutdown or femoral IV line may be the only option. At the time of IV line insertion, blood is drawn and sent for complete blood count (CBC), type and cross-match, electrolytes, blood urea nitrogen (BUN), glucose, and clotting studies. Blood gases, ideally arterial, are obtained as early as possible during resuscitation to evaluate oxygen, CO_2, and acid-base status. In small children, the use of the Doppler blood pressure system, with an appropriate-sized cuff, may be necessary to obtain satisfactory recordings. If shock is present, resuscitation should employ a mixture of crystalloid and colloid, with blood being given as soon as possible, depending on how easily the hypotension can be controlled. If hypotension cannot be reversed and adequate blood pressure maintained, the use of the MAST suit may be helpful in maintaining an adequate blood pressure long enough to get the child to the operating room.

The timing of insertion of an endotracheal tube will depend on the patient's clinical state. A child who is in a coma, has ineffectual ventilation with poor or absent airway reflexes, or is apneic requires immediate intubation. If adequate ventilation can be readily achieved, either with bag and mask or by the patient, then intubation can be performed in a more organized fashion. Ideally, intubation is performed after hyperventilation with 100 percent O_2, and nondepolarizing muscle relaxant is given, followed by sodium pentothal.

As noted earlier, pressure on the cricoid cartilage will prevent regurgitation and aspiration of gastric contents. Once the endotracheal tube is in place, a chest x-ray film is obtained to ensure correct placement. This is often a good moment to obtain other x-ray films (e.g., of the long bones and abdomen). Patients who may require intubation are those with a GCS score below 8 and those with obvious airway obstruction or shock. It is usual to pass a nasogastric tube to decompress the stomach, and all children with acute head trauma should be assumed to have a full stomach. When there is extensive nasal and facial trauma, there is often damage to the cranial base in the cribriform region, and passing a nasogastric tube can result in the tube entering the cranial cavity. In these latter circumstances, an oral gastric tube is much safer once the airway has been secured. In general, in the unconscious patient, it is better to pass the nasogastric tube after intubation has been accomplished. This is certainly true if the cough or gag reflexes are impaired.

The use of ICP monitoring during the resuscitation and emergency phases of therapy is controversial. I believe that the criteria for ICP monitoring should be (1) GCS of 5 or less, and (2) the presence of shock plus GCS below 8. During the period of fluctuating blood pressure that occurs with resuscitation and efforts to control shock, the brain is at major risk as a result of episodic rises in ICP with each rise in blood pressure. Not only will this produce intermittent brain ischemia when the blood pressure drops and the ICP rises, but these repeated waves of elevated ICP can abolish cerebral vascular pressure autoregulation. The only way to know what is occurring in the intracranial space during resuscitation is to measure the ICP.

The other advantage of inserting an ICP monitor in the emergency room is that during the second period of risk, which occurs between leaving the resuscition area and reaching either the operating room or the ICU, an objective measure of the ICP is available. This is a period when secondary injury is likely to occur as a result of being unable to monitor CO_2, arterial pressure, or ICP. To minimize this risk, we use portable monitoring of ICP, arterial pressure, and pulse oximetry during the transport. While undergoing CT, the patient's end tidal CO_2 is monitored. Thus, the possibility of a secondary injury occurring during this period of movement is minimized. Reasons for ICP monitoring later, after stabilization, are a CT scan that shows significant focal mass effect and shift, progressive neurologic deterioration, or postoperatively, after the removal of a mass lesion, if brain swelling is present.

SPECIAL STUDIES

The single best investigation for visualization of acute traumatic brain injury is the CT scan. This should be obtained in all unconscious children as soon as possible after stabilization and should also be obtained in all children showing disturbed consciousness or with focal neurologic deficits (Fig. 35–3). An uninjected CT scan is usually all that is required in the emergency setting. There is mild concern that a CT scan obtained too early after trauma may miss the later development of a hematoma. This is rare in children, but any deterioration in the neurologic exam, or unexpected increase in ICP, should be reason enough to repeat a CT scan immediately. The timing of routine follow-up CT scans will depend upon the clinical state of the patient, the findings on the initial CT scan, and any other non-neurologic injuries that are present. In general, we like to repeat the CT scan at about 5 days prior to removing the ICP monitor, and again at 10 days to 2 weeks. Further follow-up studies are performed at a month and then yearly. Follow-up CT scans are usually done with and without contrast media.

The MRI scan has not yet become a valuable tool in the first hours after trauma. In the early stages, acute bleeding may be invisible. Also, the problems of obtaining an MRI scan with all the resuscitation equipment attached to the child are significant. After a few days, however, these problems lessen and the MRI scan demonstrates small subdurals and areas of cerebral contusion more readily than does the CT scan (Fig. 35–4).[24] It is not clear whether diffuse axonal injury will be better appreciated on the MRI scan than on the CT scan. Later follow-up studies suggest a good correlation between changes in the MRI scan and neurocognitive outcome. This has not been our experience at CHOP in a limited number of children. It does appear that the best early study is still the CT scan, but that for follow-up the MRI scan may prove more sensitive

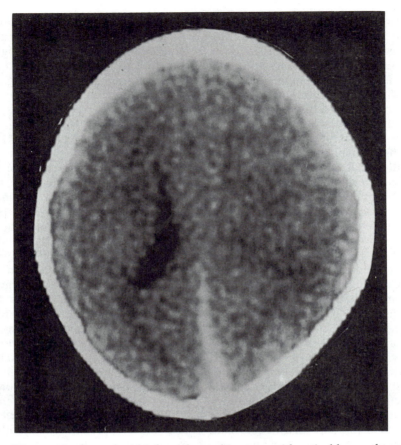

Figure 35–3. CT scan of a 4-month-old infant admitted in coma with retinal hemorrhages and no history of trauma. CT scan shows the typical interhemispheric subdural seen with the shaking impact type of injury.

to measure the degree of underlying brain injury.

Angiography is rarely performed if CT scanning is available. In the absence of a CT scan, however, angiography will demonstrate the presence and degree of any mass lesion. It is preferable to perform angiography than to do no study at all to identify a potentially treatable surgical mass lesion. Angiography is still occasionally required, in addition to CT scan, to evaluate arterial injury or arterial spasm following head trauma.

MANAGEMENT OF ELEVATED ICP

The early control of the ICP by hyperventilation has been discussed. If, despite moderate hyperventilation, the ICP remains above 20 to 25 torr, then increased hyperventilation to a CO_2 at least 20 torr is recommended. Early in the course of resuscitation, an ICP over 40 torr despite pentothal, muscle paralysis, endotracheal intubation, and hyperventilation is almost invariably fatal, unless a surgically treatable mass lesion is present.[25, 26] When such an ICP is found, a CT scan must be obtained as quickly as possible. The contents of the intracranial space are limited to blood volume, brain volume, CSF volume, and the presence of any other mass (e.g., a hematoma). The ability to manipulate these various intracranial contents is also limited. Thus, when considering therapy for elevated ICP, the most likely cause of the elevated intracranial pressure has to be considered. The CT scan will demonstrate which component is responsible for the elevated ICP.

Recovery from the surgical removal of the

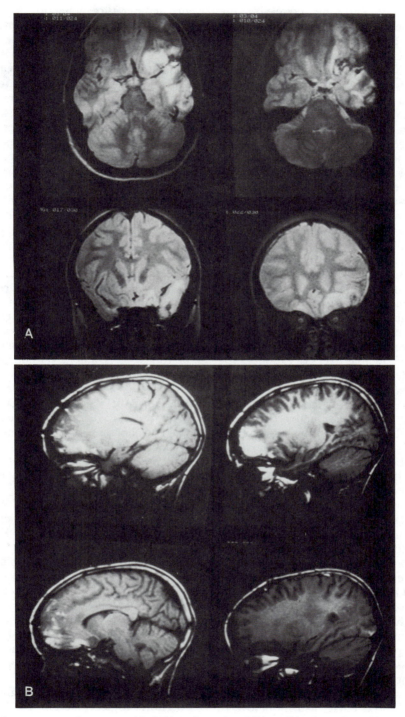

Figure 35–4. MRI scan of a 7-year-old child, 3 days after falling off his bicycle. GCS was never below 10. *A,* Axial and coronal MRI shows basal frontal and left temporal contusions with underlying edema of the white matter. *B,* Sagittal cuts show the multifocal frontal contusions.

mass lesion is dependent upon the level of neurologic function at the time of surgery. The worse the neurologic condition, the worse the outcome. Thus, mass lesions, although relatively uncommon in children (20 to 30 percent) must be identified and, if surgically significant, removed as soon as possible. This is one method of ICP control. As discussed earlier, about 50 percent of children who are unconscious after head injury appear to have increased cerebral blood flow, cerebral hyperemia, and congestion. If this is a correct delineation of the pathophysiology, then the major factor producing the elevated ICP is vasodilatation and increased cerebral blood volume (CBV).[27] This is best controlled by hyperventilation, which has its effects directly on the cerebral blood vessels producing vasoconstriction, a decrease in blood flow, and a decrease in blood volume.

If hyperventilation fails to control the ICP in the first 24 to 48 hours after trauma, then there are other ways to decrease cerebral blood flow, blood volume, and metabolism. Obviously, one does not want to decrease blood flow below that necessary to meet the metabolic demands of the tissue. Sedative drugs (e.g., sodium pentothal or pentobarbital) decrease cerebral metabolic needs and by chemical autoregulation decrease cerebral blood flow and blood volume. Thus, these agents can be helpful in controlling the ICP in the early stages. There is no evidence that these drugs have any "protective" effects and they should be used only when ICP and arterial pressure are being monitored. Other sedative agents (e.g., Etomidate) have been used to control ICP, and the mechanisms are probably similar. The addition of large amounts of these agents can result in decreased peripheral resistance and hypotension. If very large quantities are given, there may be direct effects on cardiac function; thus, additional monitoring of central venous pressure or cardiac output and pulmonary artery and capillary wedge pressures may become necessary. The amount of these drugs to be used should be just enough to control the ICP within the desired range, usually below 20 torr, and not to shoot for a specific blood level or EEG effect.[28, 29]

Hypothermia decreases cerebral metabolism and cerebral blood flow and, therefore, is of potential value in controlling intracranial pressure that is due primarily to increased blood volume. In children who are receiving barbiturates to control ICP, the core temperature generally drifts down to 34°C because the barbiturates interfere with central mechanisms for heat control and produce peripheral vasodilatation. This moderate hypothermia is probably beneficial. Therapeutic hypothermia to levels of 30 to 31°C can be used (below this level there is a markedly increased risk of cardiac arrhythmia). The use of deeper hypothermia, in addition to barbiturates, has been discouraged because of an apparent increase in pulmonary complications, especially severe pneumonias. These complications were seen most frequently in children with Reye's syndrome who were being treated with barbiturates to control intracranial pressure.[30] Such severe pneumonias are rarely seen in similarly treated head injury patients and it is possible that Reye's syndrome predisposed these children to such problems. Nonetheless, there is currently a reluctance to use a combination of deep hypothermia below 34°C degrees and the barbiturates. The use of hypothermia alone, to 30 to 31°C, is still a potentially valuable therapy when other methods of ICP control have failed.

Removal of CSF is an effective way to lower the ICP. This will be most effective when an increase in CSF volume is causing the increased ICP. In children with severe head injuries, the amount of CSF, as estimated by CSF cisternal volume and ventricular volume on CT, is reduced (see Fig. 35–2). Thus, while an increase in CSF volume is rarely the prime factor producing the increased ICP, the removal of CSF from the ventricles will still lower the ICP. Unfortunately, when the CSF volume is limited, this is not a very useful therapy since the drainage system will become dysfunctional as the ventricles collapse and no more CSF is available. CSF may only be withdrawn with safety from the ventricular system and not by lumbar puncture. CSF production continues despite moderate increases in ICP, and theoretically, decreasing CSF production would be helpful in controlling ICP. Chemical efforts to decrease CSF production have not been effective in the treatment of elevated ICP that accompanies head trauma. Diamox is rarely used, but Lasix and ethacrynic acid are used, both of which may have some effect on CSF production.

The final factor that can produce elevated

ICP is an increase in brain volume due to edema (increased water content). Edema, except around intracerebral hematomas, is rarely found in the early stages after head injury. The edema that is being treated is extracellular white matter edema (vasogenic edema).[31] The presence of intracellular astrocytic edema has been described in experimental head injury, but its importance in clinical head injury has yet to be established. Vasogenic edema is formed by disruption of the blood brain barrier and the flow of plasma filtrate into the extracellular spaces of the brain. The driving force for the fluid flow is the capillary pressure, minus the plasma oncotic pressure, and this is balanced by brain tissue pressure and extracellular brain oncotic pressure. Thus, the higher the blood pressure, the greater the rate of edema formation. Theoretically, lowering the arterial pressure would be a valuable way to decrease edema formation rate. Unfortunately, this is dangerous if the ICP is elevated.

Lowering the systemic arterial pressure (SAP) will effectively lower the cerebral perfusion pressure (CPP) (CPP = SAP − ICP) and, thus, lead to a potential decrease in cerebral blood flow (CBF). Even if pressure autoregulation is present, the drop in CPP will lead to vasodilatation to maintain CBF, and the increase in CBV may offset any improvement in ICP that might have been achieved by limiting edema formation. Keeping the blood pressure around the normal for age is the safest management in preventing either too high or too low arterial pressures. When the ICP is elevated, lowering the SAP should not be used as a means to lower ICP. Corticosteroids are effective in improving the function of the leaky blood brain barrier in tumors, but there is no evidence that they play a similar role in trauma. There are no studies that show any significant benefit in ICP control or outcome from the use of steroids. In children, there are no studies that show any detrimental effects for steroid usage and, thus, whether or not steroids are used in the treatment of head injuries, is an individual decision for the physician managing that particular child. The current trend is that fewer centers are using corticosteroids as part of management.

The established treatment of cerebral edema is the use of hyperosmotic agents (e.g., urea, mannitol, glycerol). These are believed to withdraw fluid from the brain (probably the normal brain) across the osmotic gradient created from blood to brain. Osmotic agents will decrease the ICP even in the absence of brain edema, and the exact mechanism remains unclear. The rapid infusion of these hypertonic solutions will increase the serum osmolality from 5 to 15 milliosmoles. This sudden increase in osmotic load also produces cerebral vasodilatation and transient increases in cerebral blood flow. This is why osmotic agents are not recommended in the early treatment of children with severe head injuries. If they are to be used, the child should be hyperventilated to lower the blood flow and prevent the potential increase in blood flow, blood volume, and ICP that could occur. Rapid infusions of these solutions can raise the arterial pressure, which can also be deleterious by raising intracranial pressure.

The greatest benefit from osmotic agents is likely to occur 24 to 48 hours after the head injury, at which time cerebral edema is often present and the hyperemia is usually controlled. If the ICP cannot be controlled in the first 24 hours by a combination of hyperventilation, head-up position, barbiturates, and CSF drainage, then osmotic agents have to be used even though the effect may be small. Tubular diuretics (e.g., furosemide and ethacrynic acid) cannot be relied on to effectively decrease the ICP, unless fluid overload is present.

PROGNOSTIC FACTORS

Age and Mechanism of Injury

In most studies of outcome after head injury, patients younger than 15 to 18 years of age have a better outcome for the same level of coma. However, there is also the suggestion that children less than 5 years of age have a worse outcome than those over 5. How much of the improved outcome in childhood is a factor of the mechanism of underlying injury and the extent of primary damage and how much is a function of the plasticity and recoverability of the younger brain remains unclear. Measures of depth of coma do not reflect the absolute degree of primary injury or of diffuse axonal injury. It might be expected that the loading forces to the brain would have a good correlation with the final outcome. Children are rarely involved in very high–speed accidents, suggesting that the loading forces to the child's brain are, indeed, less than those for the average adult injury. I am unaware of any study that has compared outcome in adults and children who have been exposed to similar forces (e.g., automobile passengers). Would there still be a difference in recovery? Certainly the mechanism of trauma has an effect on expected survival. Child abuse appears to carry with it a much poorer prognosis for the same initial neurologic examination than do pedestrian injuries. This may be one reason why outcome in the child under age 5 appears to be so bad. At CHOP, 80 percent of deaths in children under 2 years of age are due to abuse by an adult custodian, although child abuse accounts for approximately 20 percent of the trauma admissions. There is also a very high mortality for unrestrained infants as automobile passengers, and this appears to be related, specifically, to cervicomedullary trauma. Although good studies are still unavailable, extensive clinical experience suggests that the mechanisms of injury have a significant effect on both mortality rate and degree of recovery.

Glasgow Coma Scale

Except in the first year of life, the GCS appears to be a reliable indicator of early brain injury. For each GCS value, the outcome is better for children than for adults, but the trends are similar. The highest mortality and morbidity are with GCS scores of 3. In children, unlike adults, a GCS score of 4 is associated with significant recovery rates. Perhaps the largest difference is in children with GCS scores of 5 and above, in whom expected mortality rates are very low and expected good recovery rates very high.

Brain CT Scan

The value of the initial CT scan has not been well studied. In our experience, there are findings on the initial scan that correlate with the final prognosis. The findings of small hemorrhages in the corpus callosum, thalamus, or mid-brain, which have been suggested to be the CT scan hallmarks of se-

vere diffuse axonal injury, are associated with higher mortality and more severe morbidity than any other CT pattern. Diffuse swelling with decreased ventricular size and compressed cisterns is associated with a good prognosis, if the brain density is normal or increased. In situations when the supratentorial brain is of low density, with loss of the gray-white interface, severe brain ischemia is present and the incidence of death is close to 100 percent. Any survivors have been left with severe brain injury. The only exception is the very young infant, in the first few weeks to months of life, in whom the brain density can be difficult to interpret. This pattern of diffuse low density, sometimes with normal density of the basal ganglia, is usually associated with severely elevated ICP, close to the systemic arterial pressure levels, and is a sign of minimal cerebral perfusion. While global decrease in brain density carries with it an extremely grave prognosis, focal areas of low density inferring focal ischemia are not associated with a worsened outcome.

Intracranial Pressure

In general, the higher the ICP, the higher the mortality rate.[25, 32–34] However, there does not appear to be a good correlation between the quality of survival and elevated ICP (Table 35–1). The majority of early deaths appear to be related to intracranial hypertension, and improvements in outcome are related to the early control of the intracranial pressure. Thus, although ICP is an important parameter, it may be a reflection of the degree of injury as much as a cause of secondary injury. Those patients who have significant diffuse axonal damage may have a very poor functional recovery despite never having elevated ICP.

Location of Treatment

It is unclear whether the location of treatment of the head injury influences the outcome or not. For adult head injuries, it has been demonstrated that the more hospitals the patient visits on route to the final place of treatment, the higher the mortality rates. It is thus important to get the pediatric patient to a hospital capable of managing pedi-

Table 35–1. LEVEL OF ICP RELATED TO NEUROLOGIC OUTCOME IN 41 SEVERELY HEAD INJURED CHILDREN [26]

ICP	Good Recovery Moderate Disability	Severely Disabled/ Vegetative	Dead
20 torr	75%	8.0%	17.0%
21–40 torr	87%	6.5%	6.5%
+41 torr	50%	6.0%	44.0%

atric problems at the earliest possible time. Better results in general are reported from children centers than from adult trauma centers.[11, 26, 35, 36] Although the reports from Sick Children's Hospital in Toronto show mortality rates similar to those from adult centers, the number of patients with GCS scores of 3 or 4 is considerably higher than in most other series.[35] It is difficult to avoid the fact that the best results come from units dedicated to the care of children, suggesting that the direction toward centralized pediatric care for severe trauma is a sensible and logical one.

Functional and Behavioral Effects

Minor head injuries in children, those not associated with loss of consciousness, do not appear to produce significant physical morbidity. Only 7 percent are likely to have complaints of headache by 1 month and other indices of physical health are normal.[37, 38] However, there is a high incidence of alterations in play and daily activities (25 percent). Parents report significant increase in school absenteeism over the first month. The rates of these disturbances are approximately twice the population norms. In addition, disturbances of mood and affect are seen: the pediatric post-traumatic syndrome.[39] The lack of physical morbidity makes it unlikely that the behavioral changes are a result of cerebral injury. There appears to be a very direct relationship between the functional disturbance and intrafamilial stress and anxiety.[37, 38] The incidence of behavioral difficulties or frank psychiatric problems following more severe head injuries is also about 25 percent.[40–42] It is interesting that here, too, there appears to be a relationship to family anxiety and stress,[41] and it is still unclear whether these disturbances are the result of the psychologic and stress reactions of the child and family or are directly related to neurocircuitry damage from the trauma. The similarity between the mild and severe injuries in this particular area suggests that there is not a direct relationship between severity of trauma and behavioral response, whereas in the areas of neurologic function and cognitive ability such a relationship does appear to exist.

Length of Coma and Outcome

Even brief unconsciousness in teenagers and children can be followed by memory deficits, trouble concentrating, and headaches.[43, 44] With loss of consciousness for a few minutes, rapid recovery of memory function occurs over days up to 1 month.[43, 45] The greater the length of coma, the greater the incidence and degree of memory disturbance.[46] Following even prolonged coma, there is usually significant neurologic recovery in children. The chronic vegetative state occurs in 2 percent or less of children who suffer severe head injury.[11, 26, 47] Of all children who survive with GCS scores of 8 or less, 90 percent can be expected to recover to a moderately disabled state or better within 3 years.[11, 26, 40, 48–50] A coma lasting more than 3 months seems to be the cut-off point for this expected recovery. The degree of neurologic recovery appears also to be related to the locus of injury but, more importantly, to the GCS score on admission. Twenty percent of children with a GCS score of 5 to 7 and 50 percent of those with GCS scores of 3 and 4 can be expected to have permanent neurologic deficits.[26] In children with a mean duration of coma of 6 weeks, only 10 percent had a normal neurologic examination, yet

70 percent were functioning independently or with minimal help.[49] Thus, diffuse injuries that leave neurologic deficits seemed to be coped with quite well. The major exception appears to be that of residual ataxia.

Cognitive disturbances appear to be a more serious sequela of severe head trauma than are neurologic disturbances. Coma of only 3 days' duration has been reported to produce a drop in overall IQ.[51] Yet, coma of up to 2 weeks duration has been recorded to be consistent with a normal rate of learning in more than 90 percent of children.[52] Coma up to 3 months has been associated with a return to scholastic function but often with some special help in up to 70 percent of children.[26] Performance aspects of IQ appear to be the most affected.[40] Of note, is that younger children appear to have greater intellectual sequelae than do older children and teenagers.[42, 46, 53] What is most surprising is not that a significant number of children have a severely impaired cognition after severe head injury[42] but that so many make a good recovery. It is increasingly clear that the limitations on intellectual recovery and future life performance after severe head injury are the result of complex interactions between neurological, intellectual, and behavioral alterations, some of which are clearly related to the severity of the trauma as measured by the GCS and the length of coma and some of which are not. Future studies in the area may be more beneficially directed to the study of the children who recover and function well after severe trauma rather than those who do poorly. What is it that permits a good functional recovery in the face of residual brain damage?

MORTALITY

The mortality rate for children sustaining severe head trauma is lower than for older age groups.[25, 54–57] Pagni and coworkers reported 61 percent mortality rate in adults compared with 32 percent for individuals under 19 years old.[58] Overall mortality rates for severe head injury in children vary from 9 to 38 percent,[11, 26, 33, 34, 48, 59, 60] and the risk of death correlates with the GCS. Current studies suggest that 15 to 25 percent overall mortality rates for children with GCS scores of 8 or less are currently possible. The mor-

Table 35–2. OUTCOME FOLLOWING PEDIATRIC HEAD TRAUMA*

Investigators	Glasgow Coma Score	
	3–4	5–7
Bruce et al[26]	28%	0%
Humphreys et al[35]	73%	20%
Walker et al[11]	74%	8%
Berger et al[36]	50%	24%

*Mortality rate in percentages as related to depth of coma.

tality for those with GCS scores of 5 or above varies from 0 to 20 percent (Table 35–2).[11, 26, 35, 36] For those with GCS scores of 3 or 4, the mortality rate ranges from 28 to 75 percent.[11, 26, 35, 36] Children with GCS scores of 4 have mortality rates ranging from 17 to 75 percent, with most recent series being 10 to 15 percent in the absence of multiple trauma. Children in flaccid coma with GCS scores of 3 have mortality rates from 50 to 100 percent. When spontaneous ventilation is preserved, recovery to a moderately disabled state may occur in up to 40 percent of those with flaccid coma. For all groups of children with severe head injuries, the presence of multiple trauma and shock essentially doubles the expected mortality rate. Early deaths seem to be due to intracranial hypertension, and up to 50 percent of all head injury deaths may, in fact, occur prior to hospitalization. In some reported series the mortality rate for children 5 years old or younger is higher and cognitive dysfunction appears to be greater than in those more than 5 years old.[42, 54, 61] This may be less a function of age than of the type of trauma the children are exposed to. By far the most common cause of major trauma and mortality in a child under age 2 appears to be child abuse. Hospital deaths at all ages are primarily the result of the head injury (80 percent) and only 20 percent appear to die from secondary complications.

SUMMARY AND CONCLUSIONS

Head injury in children is a serious public health problem. There is little evidence to suggest that minor head injuries or moderate head injuries produce significant permanent brain damage, but they may have significant effects on daily function, many of which may be related to intrafamilial anxiety and stress. Even after less serious injuries, family support and counseling, as well as medical care for the child, become very important. The reintroduction to school should be well planned, and whatever ancillary support is needed should be organized early to minimize stress. The outcome from severe head injuries depends on the severity of the injury. The lower the GCS score and the longer the duration of coma, the greater the risk of permanent neurologic and cognitive damage. Behavioral and functional changes, though less clearly related to the severity of trauma, are very important in determining the final functional capacity. Our

understanding of the primary and secondary pathophysiology that occurs after head trauma in children has improved markedly over the last few years. This has resulted in improved early care, both at the accident site and in the intensive care unit, and has resulted in improved survival rates. The long-term functional effects and their causes are not clearly clarified. If rehabilitation is to be fully effective, it has to be comprehensive and as noted previously, the study of those who do well may be of greater benefit than of those who do poorly. Finally, recent evidence suggests that there may be an increased vulnerability in small children younger than 5 years old to residual permanent brain dysfunction following severe mechanical trauma.

REFERENCES

1. Annegers, JF: The Epidemiology of Head Trauma in Children. In Shapiro, K (ed): Pediatric Head Trauma. Futura Publishing Co, Mount Kisco, NY, 1983, p 1.
2. Anderson, DW and McLaurin, RL: The National Head and Spinal Cord Injury Survey. J Neurosurg Suppl 53:S-1, 1980.
3. Accident Facts. National Safety Council, Chicago, 1982.
4. Annual Summary for the United States 1979: Monthly Vital Statistics Report. DHHS Vol 28, No 28, No 13. Nov 13, 1980.
5. Vital Statistics of the United States. Government Printing Office, Washington, DC, 1981.
6. Hendricks, EB, Harwood-Nash, DCF and Hudson, AR: Head injuries in children, a survey of 4465 consecutive cases at the hospital for sick children, Toronto, Canada. Clin Neurosurg 11:46, 1964.
7. Billmire, RE and Myers, PA: Serious head injury in infants: Accident and abuse. Pediatrics 75:340, 1985.
8. Zimmerman, RA et al: Computed tomography of craniocerebral injury in the abused child. Radiology 130:687, 1979.
9. Annegers, JF et al: The incidence, causes and secular trends of head trauma in Olmstead County, Minnesota, 1935–1974. Neurology 30:912, 1980.
10. Casey, R, Ludwig, S and McCormick, MC: Morbidity following minor head trauma in children. Pediatrics 78:497, 1986.
11. Walker, ML, Storrs, BB and Mayer, T: Factors affecting outcome in the pediatric patient with multiple trauma concepts. Pediatr Neurosurg 4:243, 1983.
12. Bruce, DA, Schut, L and Sutton, LN: Brain and cervical spinal injuries occurring during organized sports activities in children or adolescents. Clin Sports Med 1:495, 1982.
13. Torg, JS: Athletic Injuries to the Head, Face, and Neck. Lea and Febiger, Philadelphia, 1982.
14. Torg, J et al: National football head and neck registry: 14 year report on cervical quadriplegia. JAMA 197:369, 1984.
15. Gennarelli, TA et al: Diffuse axonal injury and traumatic coma in the primate. Ann Neurol 12:564, 1982.
16. Bruce, DA et al: Diffuse cerebral swelling following head injuries in children: The syndrome of "malignant brain edema." J Neurosurg 54:170, 1981.
17. Ito, V et al: Brain swelling and brain edema in acute head injury. Acta Neurochir (Wien) 79:120, 1986.
18. Swedlow, D et al: Cerebral blood flow AJDO₂ and CMRO₂ in comatose children. In Go, KG and Baethmann, A (eds): Brain Edema. Plenum Press, New York, 1984, p 365.
19. Annegers, JF et al: Seizures after head trauma. A population study. Neurology 30:683, 1980.
20. Kollevold, T: Immediate and early cerebral seizures after head injuries. Part I. J Oslo City Hosp 26:99, 1976.
21. Hendricks, EB and Morris, L: Post traumatic epilepsy in children. J Trauma 8:547, 1968.
22. Jennett, B: Epilepsy After Non-Missile Head Injuries. 2nd Edition. Wm Heinemann, Medical, London, 1975.
23. Pang, D and Wilberger, JE Jr: Spinal cord injury without radiographic abnormalities in children. J Neurosurg 57:114, 1982.
24. Jenkins, A: MRI scan after head trauma. Lancet 2:445, 1986.
25. Bruce, DA et al: Outcome following severe head injury in children. J Neurosurg 48:679, 1978.
26. Bruce, DA et al: Pathophysiology, treatment and outcome following severe head injury in children. Child Brain 5:174, 1979.
27. Zimmerman, RA et al: Computed tomography of pediatric head trauma: Acute general cerebral swelling. Radiology 126:403, 1978b.
28. Bruce, DA et al: The effectiveness of iatrogenic barbiturate coma in controlling increased ICP in

61 children. In Shulman, K et al (eds): Intracranial pressure. Springer-Verlag, Berlin, 1980, p 630.

29. Raphaely, R et al: Management of severe pediatric head trauma. Pediatr Clin North Am 27:715, 1980.

30. Frewein, T et al: Outcome in severe Reye's syndrome with early pentobarbital coma and hypothermia. J Pediatr 100:663, 1982.

31. Bruce, DA: Management of cerebral edema. Pediatr Rev 4:217, 1983.

32. Miller, JD et al: Significance of intracranial hypertension in severe head injury. J Neurosurg 47:503, 1977.,

33. Gobiet, W et al: Treatment of acute cerebral edema with high dose of dexamethasone. In Beks, JWF, Bosch, DA and Brock, M (eds): Intracranial Pressure. Springer-Verlag, New York, 1976, p 231.

34. Shapiro, K and Marmarou, A: Clinical application of the Pressure—Volume index in treatment of pediatric head injuries. J Neurosurg 56:819, 1982.

35. Humphreys, RP et al: Severe head injuries in children: Concepts. Pediatr Neurosurg 4:230, 1983.

36. Berger, MS, Edwards, MSB and Bartkauski, HM: Outcome from severe head injury in children and adolescents. J Neurosurg 62:194, 1985.

37. Casey, R, Ludwig, S and McCormick, MC: Morbidity following minor head trauma in children. Pediatrics 78:497, 1986.

38. Casey, R, Ludwig, S and McCormick, MC: Minor head trauma in children: An intervention to decrease functional morbidity. Pediatrics 80:159, 1987.

39. Black, P et al: The post traumatic syndrome in children. In Walker, AE, Caveness, WF and Critchley, M (eds): The Late Effects of Head Injury. Charles C Thomas, Springfield, IL, 1969, p 142.

40. Flach, J and Malmros R: A long term follow up study of children with severe head injury. Scand J Rehabil Med 4:9, 1972.

41. Klonoff, H, Law, MD and Clark, C: Head injuries in children: A prospective five year follow up. J Neurol Neurosurg Psychiatry 40:1211, 1977.

42. Brink, JD et al: Recovery of motor and intellectual function in children sustaining severe head injuries. Dev Med Child Neurol 12:565, 1970.

43. Gronwall, D and Wrightson, P: Delayed recovery of intellectual function after minor injury. Lancet 2:605, 1974.

44. Gronwall, D and Wrightson, P: Cumulative effect of concussion. Lancet 2:995, 1975.

45. Levin, HS and Eisenberg, HM: Neuropsychological impairment after closed head injury in children and adolescents. J Pediatr Psychol 4:389, 1979.

46. Levin, HS and Eisenberg, HM: Neuropsychological outcome of closed head injury in children and adolescents. Child Brain 5:281, 1979.

47. Tomei, G et al: Features of the clinical evolution following the acute stage in severe traumatic coma in childhood. A study of 45 cases of the so-called Apallic syndrome. Mod Probl Pediatr 18:280, 1977.

48. Carlsson, CA, Von Essen, C and Lofgren, J: Factors affecting the clinical course of patients with severe head injury. Parts 1 and 2. J Neurosurg 29:242, 1968.

49. Brink, JD, Imbus, C and Woo-Sam, J: Physical recovery after severe closed head trauma in children and adolescents. J Pediatr 97:721, 1980.

50. Stover, SL and Zeiger, HF Jr: Head injury in children and teenagers: Functional recovery correlated with the duration of coma. Arch Phys Med Rehabil 57:201, 1976.

51. Shaffer, D, Chadwich, O and Rutter, H: Psychiatric outcome of localized head injury in children in outcome of severe damage to the central nervous system. CIBA Foundation Symposium, 34, Elsevier, New York, 1975, p 191.

52. Heiskanen, O and Kaste, M: Late prognosis of severe brain injury in children. Dev Med Child Neurol 16:11, 1979.

53. Lange-Cisack, H et al: Prognosis of brain injuries in young children (one until five years of age). Neuropaediatrae 10:105, 1979.

54. Jennett, B et al: Severe head injuries in three countries. J Neurol Neurosurg Psychiatry 40:291, 1977.

55. Akerlund, E: The late prognosis in severe head injuries. Acta Chir Scand 117:275, 1959.

56. Cedermartk, J: Uber Verlauf, Symptomatologie und Prognose Kaniozerebraler Verletzungen. Acta Chir Scand (Suppl 75):86, 1942.

57. Marshall, LF and Bowers, SA: Outcome prediction in severe head injury. In Wilkins, RH and Rengechary, SS (eds): Neurosurgery. McGraw-Hill, New York, 1985, p 1606.

58. Pagni, CA et al: Severe traumatic coma in infancy and childhood. J Neurosurg Sci 19:120, 1975.

59. Becker, D et al: The outcome from severe head injury with early diagnosis and intensive management. J Neurosurg 47:491, 1977.

60. Gruskiewicz, J, Doran, Y and Peyser, E: Recovery from severe craniocerebral injury and brain stem lesions in childhood. Surg Neurol 1:197, 1973.

61. Raimondi, AJ and Hirachauer, J: Head injury in the infant and toddler: Lance Scoring and Outcome Scale. In Villani, R et al (eds): Advances in Neurotraumatology. Excerpta Medica, Amsterdam, Congress Series 612, 1983, p 99.

Chapter 36

Specific Problems Associated With Pediatric Head Injury*

KENNETH M. JAFFE, M.D.
JOYCE D. BRINK, M.D.
ROSS M. HAYS, M.D.
ANNA J.L. CHORAZY, M.D.

Each year an estimated one million children in the United States sustain closed head injuries.[1] Over 150,000 of these children are admitted to hospitals where they are surviving in increasing numbers due to improvements in before hospital care, medical transport, and intensive medical-surgical management.[2, 3] The improved survival rate and physical outcome in moderately and severely brain injured children, as compared with adults, has led to the prevailing contention that children are spared the seriously disabling effects of head injury. This notion is contrary to the available evidence. It has resulted in an overestimate of the capabilities of head injured children who, because of the increased likelihood of achieving independence in motor function and activities of daily living, are underserved by the health care and educational systems.

What are the specific problems that follow childhood closed head injury? With broad categorization, they can be divided into those of a neuropsychologic nature and those of a more physical or medical-surgical realm. This chapter reviews these multifac-

eted, complex, and often inter-related problems. To responsibly serve this population, health care professionals and educators must first understand the consequences of head injury and their far-reaching implications. Many of these problems are reintroduced in Chapter 37, which emphasizes methods of assessment.

NEUROPSYCHOLOGIC SEQUELAE

Behavioral and Psychiatric Effects

The association of adverse behavioral change and closed head injury has been well documented since 1936 when Blau described the "post-traumatic psychopathic personality."[4] The occurrence of behavioral sequelae after pediatric brain injury is now well established. However, considerable disagreement persists regarding the nature of disordered behavior and its precise etiology. The following case study depicts the early behavioral abnormalities that may result from head trauma, even during the course of a good physical recovery.

*This work was supported in part by grant R49 CCR002299-01: Outcome of Closed Head Injury in Childhood from the Centers for Disease Control.

Case 1. While on her bicycle, a 10-year-old girl rode off an embankment, striking her unprotected head on a cement driveway 10 feet below. When first examined after the injury she was moving her extremities purposely but not responding to voice. Her Glasgow Coma Scale (GCS) score was 10. She was intubated in the field and transported by helicopter to a tertiary care center. The initial cranial CT scan was normal. Her acute care included intracranial pressure monitoring for 5 days. A cranial CT scan at 24 hours after admission showed diffuse cerebral edema and bilateral frontal subdural effusions without mid-line shift. Mannitol was used intermittently to maintain intracranial pressure within normal limits. Four days after injury she was inconsistently responding to some simple commands and demonstrating purposeful movements of her extremities (GCS = 15). On the fifth day, she was increasingly agitated. Her speech was incoherent and she attempted to strike or bite staff members working with her.

She was transferred to a rehabilitation center closer to her home 2 weeks after injury. At the time of admission, she continued to demonstrate unprovoked aggressive behavior with attacks of hitting, kicking, and biting during any attempt at physical examination. She was confused and disoriented to time and place. Her short-term memory was impaired and she was unable to describe why she was hospitalized. She could walk but showed poor judgment and safety awareness. There were no focal neurologic findings. She fought any type of physical restraint and her behavior became aggressive when any tasks were requested of her. She also became violent when questions were asked that she could not successfully answer. She repeatedly said, "I hate you and I want to go home." When asked where she was, she often said, "School." Chloral hydrate, administered as sedation prior to an EEG, exacerbated her screaming and striking out, necessitating cancellation of the procedure. To prevent self-injury, she slept on a mattress on the floor.

One parent remained with her at all times during the first week in the rehabilitation center. By the end of this week she was calmer, and her attention span improved to 15 to 20 minutes. Physical restraints were avoided. In order to reduce agitation, she was permitted to walk as much as desired with staff or family members. Shaping of behavior was accomplished through positive reinforcement. Television watching and stickers were awarded for cooperation and specific tasks completed. By the second week (4 weeks postinjury), she could answer questions more appropriately, had fewer episodes of agitation, and was orientated to person, time, and place. In expressive and receptive language she scored at the 12th grade level.

At the end of the second week, a day pass was allowed and during the following week, an overnight pass. While at home she had no outbursts of aggressive behavior. Her ability to focus on tasks steadily improved. Cognitive assessments 6 weeks after injury and prior to discharge from the rehabilitation center showed her to be functioning at a high-average range of intelligence. Her full-scale IQ was 111, with a verbal score of 115, and a performance score of 104. Achievement test scores were in the high-normal range.

Behavioral sequelae may be divided into two categories: those that are manifest during the course of acute recovery (as presented in the illustrative case history) and are more likely to be transient and predictable, and those documented in long-term follow-up studies which are considered to be more permanent. The former is described by Divack and coworkers as occurring in three stages.[5] The *early stage* is marked by agitation, regression, and impaired information processing. This early syndrome of "cerebral irritation" has been well described by Jennett as a stage of restless, disorganized behavior before full consciousness and orientation are regained.[6] It may persist for many days or weeks. The agitation and irrational behavior, characterized by random and frequently nonpurposeful motor activity and verbal outcries, is not responsive to sedation. Pharmacologic intervention with tranquilizers may actually aggravate the symptoms by further clouding the sensorium of a disoriented child. Theoretically, tranquilizers can also interfere with recovery after head injury.[7]

Another early behavioral abnormality following head injury is much less common. Todorow describes an abnormal psychologic response consisting of a "feigned death" state or "sleeping beauty syndrome," mimicking an "organic coma vigil."[8] Motionless and apathetic, the child appears to be escaping a traumatic and frightening situation by not responding to any environmental stimuli. It is difficult to determine in the early course, whether the total lack of response is organic or psychoreactive.

A *middle stage* includes intolerance of stimulation such as touch and noise. Denial or underestimation of deficits frequently results in decreased patient compliance and increased demands on staff and family to control behavior. The *final stage* results from the adverse wedding of subtle cognitive deficits and increasing awareness of impairment. This frustrating combination produces loss of self-esteem, depression, anger, and risk-taking behavior.

Aspects of long-term behavioral disturbance attributed to traumatic brain injury in children include attentional deficit, overactivity and restlessness, aggressiveness, destructiveness, tantrums, impulsivity, and socially disinhibited behavior. There is diversity of opinion regarding the etiology of this altered psychologic functioning. Blau initially postulated that brain injury alone resulted in dramatically altered behavior.[4] There is support for this theory based on associations of the severity of behavior with location of the brain injury, age at onset, and duration of coma. However, studies are inconsistent in reporting these associations. More recently, attention has been focused on the child's reaction to acquired cognitive deficits as a source of stress and behavioral change. A third factor is the recognition of increased incidence of premorbid psychologic problems in the pediatric head injured population. It is likely that all three factors contribute to the psychiatric and behavioral sequelae of brain injury.

Klonoff and Low investigated age at injury and found little difference in behavioral outcome comparing younger children (less than 9 years old) with older children.[9] Conversely, in another study Brink and associates did find significant differences based on age.[10] Younger children (less than 10 years old) displayed hyperactivity, decreased attention, loss of impulse control, and increased aggression, whereas older children displayed more affective disorders and impaired judgment. Hjern and Nylander reported an increase in behavioral disturbances in children with persistent neurologic deficits after head injury.[11] Similarly, an increase in chronic behavioral disorders correlated positively with secondary complications of injury (e.g., cardiac arrest and respiratory failure) in the long-term follow-up studies by Flach and Malmos.[12] The location of brain injury may also be associated with severity of behavioral change. Naughton reports greater psychologic problems with brainstem lesions than in hemispheric injury.[13] The severity of behavior disturbance was also directly correlated with duration of coma in a retrospective study by Shaffer and colleagues.[14]

The psychiatric sequelae of head injury in children are complex. Patients can exhibit exacerbation of premorbid difficulties as well as develop new deficits. Rutter has postulated that the disinhibited behavior changes noted after traumatic brain injury may be unique to patients suffering head injury.[15] By prospectively studying children who suffered head injury, experienced posttraumatic amnesia of greater than 7 days, and had documented absence of premorbid psychologic morbidity, he identified a new behavioral symptom complex which occurred after injury in a significant number of patients. A combination of behaviors resembling organic frontal lobe syndrome includes euphoria, lack of judgment, disinhibition, childish behavior, and apathy.[16] This interplay of deficits — especially poor judgment, childish behavior, and disinhibition — exposes pediatric head injury patients to the dangers of abuse and exploitation.

The stress created by awareness of acquired cognitive deficits in the recovery phase persists over time and is a likely contributor to psychosocial dysfunction. Fuld and Fisher attributed the majority of personality change after brain injury to this "secondary stress of impaired perceptual and cognitive abilities."[17] The family experiences the stress as well. This was noted by Klonoff and Low, who found increased anxiety, apprehension, and overprotectiveness in parents of brain injured children as well as significant denial and caution in the children.[9] The combination resulted in "deterioration of home functioning" in 15 percent of families by 2 years postinjury.

The effect of traumatic brain injury on the family has been more objectively studied by Brooks and McKinlay.[18] Using a questionnaire including bipolar adjectives, relatives reported the extent and nature of personality change after traumatic brain injury. There was a positive correlation between the relatives' perception of the severity of personality change and the duration of post-traumatic amnesia. Specific negative changes were noted in two general areas: difficulty in impulse and behavioral control on one end of the spectrum and increasing aspontaneity of behavior (listlessness, poor motivation) on the other. The former group of behavior disorders was perceived as a greater burden to the family. The relatives' perception of personality changes as a burden to the family was positively correlated with increasing time postinjury. The same patients were perceived as a relatively "greater burden" at 12 months after injury than at 3 months, despite increasing gains in motor and cognitive recovery. The implications are that distance in time from traumatic brain injury influences general recovery positively. However, the severe impact on the family is often delayed until recovery has plateaued and efforts at community reintegration have begun.

Pre-existing behavioral disturbance was less appreciated in earlier studies. Later Jennett and coworkers reported that the majority of children with psychiatric sequelae after head injury were maladjusted prior to their accident.[19] More specifically, Black and associates found that a third of children with closed head injury had pre-existing behavioral disturbances.[20] Twenty percent of these affected children demonstrated new behavior disorders after brain injury. Premorbid personality factors may be *causally* related to the head injury, but the nature of sequelae may be more related to the type of injury itself.

There is a clear over-representation of children with premorbid personality problems in the traumatically brain injured population. There is also an apparent increase in disordered families. The implications for rehabilitation of the brain injured child are evident. Disorganized family situations and poor parenting expose children to an increased risk of head injury. These families also have less resources to expend in coping with the long term management of a disabled child. It has been recommended by Brooks[18] and others that the best results can be achieved with a twofold approach: modification of patient behavior in the recovery period and early anticipatory guidance, education, and psychoemotional support for the family and other caregivers.

Language

The prognosis for recovery of communication skills after pediatric brain injury is good. In long-term studies, recovery of functional language with rehabilitation has been reported to be as high as 92 pecent.[21] Of these, one quarter have some detectable language deficit. There is, however, a strong suspicion that, when carefully evaluated, all significantly head injured patients will demonstrate at least some short-term, subtle language disturbance.[22]

The factors that are often helpful in predicting general outcome in pediatric closed head injury do not strongly correlate with recovery of language. Long-term follow-up studies suggest that age at injury has some predictive value and that infants have an overall poorer outcome.[2] There appears to be an inverse relationship between age at the time of acquired brain damage (traumatic and nontraumatic) and the degree of language recovery, with the best language outcome in children sustaining brain injury under 1 year of age.[23, 24] Age at the time of traumatic brain injury may also affect the type of language disturbance. Adolescents more frequently acquire dysarthrias and deficits in written language whereas younger children have been reported to have a higher incidence of verbal apraxia.[25] Duration of coma, a significant predictor of general outcome,[2, 10] is less useful in establishing the prognosis for recovery of speech.[22]

Children display nonaphasic or motor-speech disorders less often than true aphasia. Dysarthria, described by Sarno as a spectrum from mild articulatory imprecision of consonant groups to completely unintelligible speech, is clinically similar in children and adults.[22] It affects one third of those with acquired language dysfunction. In addition to difficulty with articulation, children demonstrate hypernasality, phonatory weakness, monopitch, and slow rate of speech. Long-term studies suggest that mutism is more frequently seen in children than adults.[26, 27]

The most common category of language disorder in pediatric traumatic brain injury is expressive aphasia. True agrammatism, seen in congenital language dysfunction and characterized by poor verbal repetition, is less often associated with traumatic brain injury.[25] The areas of difficulty most frequently encountered are in confrontation naming and word retrieval. The ability to organize expressive language is frequently affected and has important implications for academic functioning. Functional receptive communication appears to be impaired less often. Studies using gross measures of receptive language skills to compare children one year after traumatic brain injury to matched controls have demonstrated little difference in auditory comprehension.[28] Those children with gross receptive deficits, however, tend to have poorer language recovery overall. This group of more seriously impaired patients is a subset of the larger group who demonstrate subtle receptive deficits in school.

It has been demonstrated in adult patients with brain injury that all will have at least some subtle deficit when carefully evaluated.[22] This is significant in view of the fact that the majority of the patients appear to have full recovery of normal conversation. An analogous situation exists in children. Although routine testing may not demonstrate subtle acquired language difficulty, the challenge of the classroom frequently does. Long-term studies to describe the natural history of language dysfunction over time are presently unavailable. Educational studies report that after brain injury, 70 percent of children demonstrate a functional drop in comprehension of spoken language and 90 percent show decreased reading comprehension when stressed by increasing workload despite normal scores on the Wechsler Intelligence Scale for Children–Revised (WISC-R).[26] Longitudinal studies of academic performance indicate that subtle deficits in language acquisition exert an increasingly greater influence as the demands and expectations of the school curriculum increase with age.[26] Carefully organized language evaluation by clinicians familiar with brain injury may accurately characterize subtle deficits so that the academic program may incorporate constructive strategies to help compensate for such language difficulty.

Language disturbance after brain injury is inextricably linked to the other areas of cognitive functioning including attention, memory, perception, new learning, reasoning, problem solving, and judgment. The developing child confronts tasks especially in the areas of acquisition of social skills and academic achievement that will be greatly affected by even subtle receptive language dysfunction. Although the outcome for recovery of functional language is good, careful attention must be directed toward identification and remediation of remaining subtle deficits in order to successfully reintegrate the brain injured child into his or her environment.

Intellectual Ability

Following head injury, the majority of children and adolescents will recover gross and fine motor skills and physical independence. Intellectual impairments, however, result in more serious long-term disability. Levin and coworkers have published data comparing intellectual recovery in children and adolescents matched for the severity of their brain injury, based on the Glasgow Coma Scale (GCS).[29] Table 36–1 summarizes the Wechsler Verbal and Performance IQ scores at least 6 months after injury.

The important findings are that young children with severe injuries (GSC less than or equal to 8) showed significantly lower intellectual quotients at follow-up than adolescents. Verbal and Performance IQ scores below 80 were found in 33 percent and 40 percent of the children, respectively, whereas no adolescent had an IQ score below 80. This abnormal intellectual capacity was related significantly to impairments of memory. Brink and associates reviewed 52 severely brain injured patients (age range two to 18 years at injury) whose duration of coma was at least 1 week (median duration 4 weeks).[10] Children under 10 years old showed significantly lower IQ scores than those who were older. Only one third of the entire study population had full scale IQ scores greater than 85 at follow-up 1 to 7 years after injury.

These studies point out that the immature brain does not appear to have a selective advantage in the recovery of higher cognitive functions after a traumatic injury as had been previously thought. Intellectual outcome does, however, appear to be directly related to the severity of the injury in both children and adolescents.[10, 28] The duration

Table 36-1. LONG-TERM INTELLECTUAL RECOVERY

	GCS ≤8		GCS >8	
	Median	Range	Median	Range
Children	(n = 15)		(n = 9)	
Verbal IQ	90	50–137	91	81–113
Performance IQ	87	45–118	100	82–118
Adolescents	(n = 14)		(n = 7)	
Verbal IQ	98	83–128	93	80–130
Performance IQ	105	80–117	114	91–120

From Levin, HS et al.,[29] with permission.

of coma rather than the initial GCS score has the strongest correlation to long term outcome and intellectual function.[29] Chadwick and colleagues established a strong "dose-response" relationship between the duration of post-traumatic amnesia (PTA) and intellectual impairment.[30] No long-term or permanent intellectual deficiency was found in children whose PTA was less than 2 weeks. However, 6 of the 10 children with a PTA of more than 3 weeks showed persistent intellectual compromise. Levin and Eisenberg found that only patients with coma greater than 24 hours had significant decreases in IQ at 6 to 18 months after injury.[28]

Improvement in intellectual functioning can continue during the first year after injury and into the second.[10, 30] Klonoff and coworkers documented such improvement for as long as 5 years after injury.[21] Researchers have found a dissociation between scores on the Verbal and Performance subtests of the WISC-R postinjury.[30] Performance IQ deficits are both more severe and persistent as compared to verbal IQ deficits. With time this early discrepancy between performance and verbal IQ lessens. The recovery pattern of performance IQ is depicted in Figure 36–1. Poor performance IQ reflects impairments in speeded performance, motor dexterity, and problem solving following head injury. Verbal subtests demand retrieval and use of overlearned material, which appears to be better preserved.

In summary, the main points related to intellectual functioning following head injury in children are as follows:

1. Young children have relatively lower IQs than adolescents with similar severity of injury.
2. There is a direct relationship between

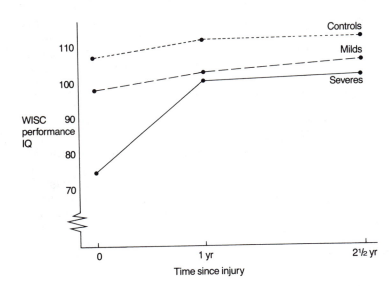

Figure 36–1. Recovery of performance IQ after head injury. (From Chadwick, O, et al.,[30] with permission.)

the severity of brain injury, as measured by duration of coma, and long term intellectual impairment.

3. Performance IQ, at least initially, is more affected than verbal IQ.

4. Improvement in intellectual function can occur for many years after injury.

Memory Disturbances

Memory deficits are common in the child and adolescent recovering from head trauma. Impairment of long-term storage and retrieval of information was observed in nearly half of 64 patients (age range 6 to 18 years) studied by Levin and Eisenberg.[31] The two tests used included the selective reminding procedure requiring recall of 12 common words, and a continuous recognition memory task that used line drawings of familiar things. Performance was directly related to the severity of the acute neurologic injury as measured by GCS and duration of coma. Focal lesions involving the left temporal lobe were associated with particularly severe impairments of verbal memory and learning. The findings in a different 1-year follow-up study using the same tasks are illustrated in Figure 36–2.[29]

Once again, long-term retrieval varied according to the severity of injury but not according to age. Severely injured adolescents demonstrated recovery of verbal memory, but still performed at follow-up at an impaired level when compared to adolescents with lesser degrees of injury. Although improvement in intellectual function occurs with time, memory deficits appear to be more persistent.

Other Neuropsychologic Deficits

Other deficits of neuropsychologic function seen following head trauma are in visual-motor and visual-spatial skills such as copying of geometric figures, construction of three-dimensional block designs, and discrimination of faces. These tasks appeared to be more impaired than verbal skills. Levin and Eisenberg found that visual-spatial impairment was present in one third of children after closed head injury.[28] Retardation of motor speed and proficiency is another

common finding. Speed involving eye/hand coordination is especially sensitive to the effects of brain injury.[30]

Scholastic Achievement

Cognitive and behavioral impairments following closed head injury often lead to compromised academic performance. When Klonoff and coworkers reviewed educational progress among head injured children, they found 24 percent of the total had failed a grade or were in remedial classrooms (Table 36–2).[21] Among the older children, 13 percent had repeated failures or were no longer in school. Among 33 survivors of severe brain injury, Mahoney and colleagues found only 29 percent were in regular schools and free of behavioral and neurologic problems.[2] In Brink's series of children with prolonged coma, only 8 of 34 children were attending regular school.[10] Despite the importance of academic ability to a child's overall adaptive functioning, there is a paucity of data on post-traumatic academic problems.

Shaffer and associates[32] studied 88 school age children under the age of 12 years who had a history of unilateral compound depressed skull fracture, dural tear, and underlying cortical damage noted at surgery. Reading ability was assessed 2 years after injury when all of the children were attending school. Fifty-five percent had scores at least 1 year below their chronologic age and 33 percent were at least 2 years below age level. At greatest risk for reading delays were those children injured before the age of 8 years who had a period of unconsciousness greater than 3 days. Reading deficiency was thought to be due to their decrease in general intelligence. Arithmetic scores are also affected after head injury and reduced relative to both pre-traumatic and post-traumatic reading scores. This is the case even for children with normal intelligence.

Factors influencing school performance after head trauma also include memory, visual-spatial ability, motor proficiency, attention, and behavioral control. Because the underpinnings of academic success are so complex, it is not surprising that school failure occurs even in the face of normal intelligence and achievement test scores. Jacobson and coworkers[33] summarized some of

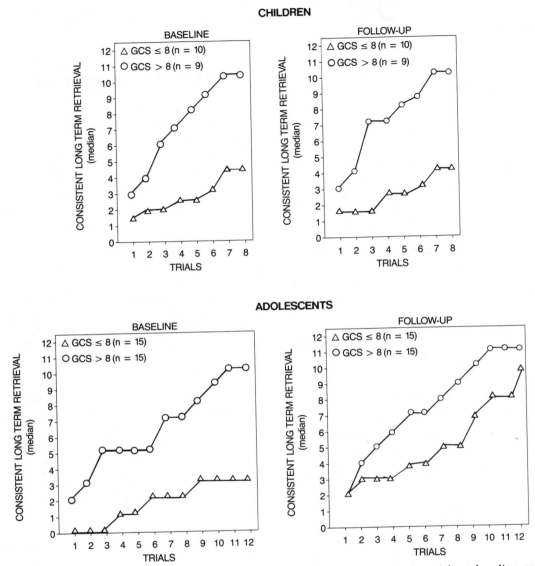

Figure 36–2. Consistent long-term retrieval for children and adolescents by trials at baseline and follow-up (GCS = Glasgow Coma Scale). (From Levin, HS, et al.,[29] with permission.)

Table 36–2. EDUCATIONAL PROGRESS 5 YEARS AFTER HEAD INJURY

	Younger (<9 years old)	Older (≥9 years old)	Total
Normal	58 (74.3%)	26 (66.7%)	84 (71.8%)
Failed grade/still in normal stream	12 (15.4%)	7 (17.9%)	19 (16.2%)
Special/remedial classes	8 (10.3%)	1 (2.6%)	9 (7.7%)
Successive failures/no longer in school		5 (12.8%)	5 (4.3%)

From Klonoff, H et al.,[4] with permission.

the common problems of adolescents returning to school following head trauma. These include impairments in abstract thinking, ability to organize work, reading comprehension, generalizing information, making judgments, and predicting consequences—all of which can have an impact on scholastic achievement.

MEDICAL AND SURGICAL PROBLEMS

Closed head injury in children is associated with both medical and surgical complications. Many of these present during the early days following injury, whereas others do not become evident for months. Almost any organ system can be affected, depending on the severity and mechanism of the injury and subsequent treatment. Familiarity with the constellation of problems that can potentially complicate recovery leads to early recognition, prompt treatment, and reduced morbidity.

Nutrition and Feeding

The presence of malnutrition on medical, surgical, and rehabilitation units[34-38] bespeaks the need for aggressive nutritional support for hospitalized patients. Hypermetabolism following trauma in adults has been well documented and may result in reduced circulating protein to depleted muscle and fat reserves.[39-42] Although there are no published reports from metabolic studies of children with head injury, many metabolic studies have been performed on children who are critically ill, have been severely burned, are on renal dialysis, or are receiving total parenteral nutrition. A similarity between outcome status of adult patients with severe head injury and those with burns of the body surface has been observed. Both demonstrate hypertension, tachycardia, hyperthermia, and wasting of the body mass with seemingly adequate nutrition. The hyperadrenergic state of patients with burns, sepsis, and systemic trauma requires increased nutritional support due to hypermetabolism and a hyperdynamic cardiovascular state in which there is increased delivery of oxygen to the tissues.[40] The child with traumatic brain injury

is at particular risk for compromised nutrition. Even without associated abdominal injury, intestinal stasis is common for days after head trauma. Limited calories are initially provided through peripheral intravenous alimentation. Following the return of intestinal motility, isotonic enteral feedings are introduced. Major abdominal injuries or prolonged ileus necessitate the institution of enteral hyperalimentation.

The presence of abnormal oropharyngeal muscle tone, sensation, movement disorders, and pathologic reflexes can result in feeding and swallowing disorders.[43] Oropharyngeal dysfunction, as well as gastroesophageal reflux, can be a cause of aspiration. A detailed nutritional and a multidisciplinary feeding/swallowing evaluation will help formulate recommendations about appropriate consistency, texture, and temperature of food, positioning requirements, method of food delivery (oral versus tube), and oral feeding techniques (see Chapter 37).

Malnutrition and aspiration are not the only issues related to feeding. Later during recovery, caloric intake exceeding metabolic requirements can lead to obesity, especially but not only for the child with compromised independent mobility. Hypothalamic injury may also result in true hyperphagia.[44] Early detection of this problem can be achieved through careful monitoring and reporting of dietary habits and semiweekly weighings.

Gastrointestinal Tract

Gastrointestinal bleeding, as common in children after head injury as in adults, can be due to gastric acid hypersecretion, reflux esophagitis, stress peptic ulceration, or mucosal damage from nasogastric tube feedings.[45-50] Monitoring the stool for occult blood should be a routine nursing practice. Pancreatitis, which is associated with increased intracranial pressure, must be included in the differential diagnosis of abdominal pain following head injury.[51]

Respiratory System

There are many ways in which children differ from adults in respiratory function. The smaller size of a young child's airway has clear implications for airway management. Infants have a more rapid respiratory rate and heart rate than older children and adults. Children's resting oxygen consumption per unit of body weight is twice that of adults. Furthermore, children in distress are more likely to increase the rate than the depth of respiration. Children fatigue more easily with labored breathing than do adults, and reach a point of respiratory insufficiency more quickly.[52] Small children have enlarged lymphoid tissue (tonsils and adenoids) which, when infected, can produce swelling and increased secretion that can occlude the airway and cause obstruction, especially when compounded by neuromuscular swallowing dysfunction.

Following head injury, many children undergo endotracheal intubation at the scene, during transport, or upon admission to the hospital. The risk for developing laryngotracheal stenosis or granuloma formation increases with the duration of endotracheal intubation and the amount of trauma inflicted during initial tube placement. Long-term risk of pediatric tracheostomy is well documented in the literature.[52] Subglottic stenosis, tracheal granulomas, fused vocal cords, and paralysis and the loss of phasic adduction of the cords due to prolonged decreased ventilatory resistance have all been documented as problems for tracheostomy decanulation in children.

Hypertension

Systemic hypertension is a frequent finding in brain injured children, occuring in 20 percent of patients under 18 years of age with severe injury.[53] Although usually resolving spontaneously, hypertension may persist for months, and require medication.[54] It appears to be secondary to a hyperadrenergic state[55] associated with increased intracranial pressure and a poor neurologic outcome.[46, 47, 56, 57] Hypertension and tachycardia may be an expression of a generalized autonomic mass reaction to severe injury of the hypothalamic area and its connections. While mild hypertension can be safely monitored, sustained elevations in blood pressures should not automatically be attributed to the head injury. Other treatable causes should be investigated. If the degree of hypertension is felt to represent

a significant health risk, antihypertensive medication can be administered. The continuing need for such pharmacologic management should be periodically reassessed. The possibility of cognitive and affective pharmacologic side effects must be weighed against the desired benefits.[58]

Fever and Infection

The unique problems of assessing fever in children, most familiar to pediatricians, should be kept in mind. Fever may represent an insignificant viral illness or a life-threatening central nervous system infection. It is most frequently associated with viral or bacterial infections, especially of the ears and upper respiratory tract.[59] Sinusitis must be suspected in any child with fever who has undergone nasotracheal intubation.[61] Lower airway causes of fever include pneumonia, bronchitis, aspiration, and atelectasis. With a basilar or compound skull fracture or penetrating brain injury, the risk of bacterial meningitis[61] or brain abcess is enhanced. Indwelling Foley catheters and urinary stasis from incomplete bladder emptying may produce urinary tract infections. Central and peripheral intravascular lines predispose patients to bacteremia and should be discontinued when they are no longer needed.[62, 63] Fever represents a medical emergency in children who have undergone splenectomy due to blunt abdominal trauma and splenic laceration. Because of the risk of fulminant bacteremia, antibiotics should be administered after multiple cultures of body fluids have been obtained. Prior to discharge from the hospital, the asplenic child should be properly immunized and the patient and family informed of the risks and management of the postsplenectomy state.[64]

Hypothalamic injury can be responsible for a so-called fever of central origin. Before this diagnosis is accepted, all sources of infection must be vigorously and carefully excluded. The same approach should be followed before making the diagnosis of drug-induced fever.

Parasitic and fungal infections are rare but should be kept in mind. Furthermore, any inflammatory process may cause fever.[65] Severe spasticity may be a cause of low-grade fever.

Endocrine Disorders

Diverse clinical presentations of endocrine dysfunction of the pituitary-hypothalamic area can occur as a result of head injury in children. Dysfunction can be transient or permanent, partial or complete.[66–72]

During the first week or two after injury, posterior pituitary hyperfunction is reflected by the usually self-limited syndrome of inappropriate secretion of antidiuretic hormone (SIADH).[73, 74] Insufficiency of antidiuretic hormone secretion, central diabetes insipidus (DI), found by Roberts in 3.5 percent of severely brain injured children, may be transient or permanent.[44, 75]

Anterior pituitary reserve should be carefully evaluated in the presence of diabetes insipidus because hypopituitarism, growth impairment, and isosexual precocious puberty have been reported following moderate to severe head injury.[70, 76–79] Growth hormone deficiency is clinically significant only in children in whom it may result in short stature (if severe) or delayed onset of growth (if mild). Although pituitary hormone deficiencies are more commonly reported following head injury than is precocious puberty, the latter can occur as a result of accelerated maturation of the hypothalamic pituitary axis.[80–82] Long-term follow-up should include observation for the signs and symptoms of these conditions. Unexplainable vague symptoms of poor growth (height and weight), malaise, anorexia, persistent low reading of temperature, pulse or blood pressure, sexual immaturity, and laboratory findings of hyponatremia and hypoglycemia should trigger suspicion and further evaluation.[70]

Dermatologic Conditions

In many centers, steroids are still routinely employed in the acute management of closed head injury. The steroid-induced acne that results will resolve spontaneously with discontinuation of the medication. Treatment may, however, be necessary and does not differ from that of nonsteroid-induced acne.

Decubitus ulcers, although preventable, are not uncommon in the head injured child who remains at bedrest for an extended period of time. Predisposing factors include poor hygiene, incontinence, compromised nutrition, spasticity, casting, and positioning problems. The cornerstone of treatment remains strict pressure relief complemented by proper nutritional support, local wound care including debridement of necrotic tissue, and antibiotic treatment of significant wound infections.

Musculoskeletal Disorders

FRACTURES AND DISLOCATIONS

Since the majority of pediatric and adolescent head trauma is due to motor vehicle accidents, there is a high incidence of extracranial injuries, particularly of the skeleton.[83–86] The most serious orthopedic problems are spine and extremity fractures and dislocations. These may be difficult to initially diagnose in the comatose patient. As alertness improves, all musculoskeletal complaints deserve careful evaluation in order to detect occult injury. In the series reported by Hoffer and colleagues, 38 percent of severe head injured patients sustained fractures.[85] These injuries are summarized in Table 36–3.

Fractures of the femur occurred most frequently, followed by fractures of the clavicle, forearm and wrist, tibia, and humerus. Six of 112 patients under 18 years of age had cervical spine fractures. Because spinal as well as pelvic fractures can be easily

Table 36–3. FRACTURE AND DISLOCATION ASSOCIATED WITH CLOSED HEAD INJURY

Fractures and Dislocations	69 Fractures in 43 Patients
Femur	21
Tibia	9
Ankle and foot	3
Pelvis	2
Lumbar spine	1
Clavicle	15
Shoulder dislocation	1
Humerus	6
Elbow dislocation	1
Forearm and wrist	10
Cervical spine fractures	6
Quadriplegia	5

From Hoffer, M et al.,[85] with permission.

overlooked, radiologic examination of the cervical spine and pelvis is indicated in the unconscious, head injured child with multiple trauma.

Orthopedic management of fractures and joint injuries attempts to achieve reduction during initial care. Because of complex care requirements, as well as agitation and combativeness that are frequently associated with head injury, open reduction and internal fixation have become the standard of care for many fractures.[87–89]

Heterotopic Ossification

Heterotopic ossification is a process in which new bone is formed in tissues which do not usually ossify. When mature, it has the same x-ray pattern as normal bone. Histologically, it is identical to bone found in other parts of the body.

The complication of heterotopic ossification occurs less frequently in children than in adults, and less frequently after head injury than spinal cord injury. Its cause is unknown. In two series of 112 and 139 head injured children, 6 (5 percent) and 21 (15 percent) developed this condition, respectively.[85, 90] Usually the heterotopic ossification is focal and involves the hip, thigh, shoulder, and elbow.

The clinical signs of heterotopic ossification include a decrease in range of motion (in spite of an active therapy program), pain, redness, and swelling in the involved area. It may be confused with cellulitis, septic arthritis, thrombophlebitis, or fracture. Occurring anywhere from 2 to 12 months after the head injury, there is usually no prior history of injury to the involved extremity.

Because of the risk of joint ankylosis, passive range-of-motion exercises, carried to the point of joint resistance, should be continued in its presence. For adults, forceful joint manipulation, under general anesthesia, of joints affected by heterotopic ossification has been advocated by Garland and coworkers.[91] During childhood this procedure must be done with extreme caution because of possible damage to epiphyseal growth plates. Surgical excision should only be considered when the restriction in joint range of motion interferes with functional gain and rehabilitation or care needs. In 20

affected joints reported by Brink and Hoffer, only two underwent surgical excision.[92] This was performed after ossification had matured and there was no reported recurrence following surgery. Treatment with diphosphonates, although recommended for adults, has not been studied in children. The low incidence of heterotopic ossification in children and reports of rachitic-like bony changes following the pediatric use of etidronate disodium appear to be relative contraindications to its prophylactic application, especially in prepubertal children.[93] The recent study by Mital and coworkers suggests that salicylate therapy (60 mg/kg of body weight/day) may prevent the progression of ectopic ossification.[90] This observation awaits further investigation.

Immobilization Hypercalcemia

Immobilization of children, regardless of the cause, may result in immobilization hypercalcemia.[94–97] Clinical symptoms may include vague lethargy, alteration of mood, gastrointestinal distress, nausea, or anorexia. Urolithiasis is usually a *late* manifestation, but may appear early.

Scoliosis

Scoliosis can occur in patients with residual spasticity following head injury. In a series of 221 patients, scoliosis of greater than 30 degrees was observed in 19 (9 percent).[98] Children should be watched carefully for this complication, especially as they go through the accelerated growth of puberty.

Leg Length Discrepancy

During long-term follow-up for head injury, three patients in a series of 112 were found to have leg length discrepancy unrelated to fractures.[85] All three were hemiplegic, ambulatory, and 6 years of age or younger at the time of initial injury. The hemiplegic side was shortened (tibia and femur) by 2 to 5 cm when compared with the nonaffected side. The child who has onset of hemiplegia at a young age should be monitored for this complication. Leg length equalization procedures may be necessary, depending on the magnitude of the discrepancy.

Neurologic/Neurosurgical Disorders

MOTOR

Spasticity with or without ataxia is the most common motor deficit following severe head injury in children. It is found in 40 to 77 percent in reported series.[56, 98, 99] Spastic hemiparesis or hemiplegia is noted most frequently, with upper extremity impairment resulting in the greatest disability when the dominant hand is involved. The loss of fine motor hand function may be further complicated by parietal lobe damage and disturbance of discriminative sensory functions on the opposite side of the body. Sensory extinction or inattention can result in neglect of the upper extremity, even when there is potentially useful motor function. During childhood, spasticity may increase for the first 6 months after injury with a peak usually reached at 2 to 3 months.

The next most frequent motor disorder following pediatric head injury is ataxia, found more commonly in children than adults. When ataxia occurs in combination with spasticity, it is usually more pronounced in the less spastic extremities. This particular combination of motor deficits has been reported in 20 to 39 percent of pediatric and adolescent patients with severe head trauma.[56, 99] Ataxia alone is less common. Severe ataxia can be very disabling, interfering with basic skills such as feeding and ambulation. It is also associated with dysarthria and impaired speech intelligibility. In children, ataxia has been observed to improve over 2 to 3 years in contrast with the more limited recovery potential from this impairment in adults. Table 36–4 summarizes the motor deficits of 344 head injured adolescents at 1 year follow-up.

Other motor disorders including dyskinesias occur only rarely.[44] The management of motor disabilities is discussed elsewhere in this book (see Chapters 10, 23, and 38).

Table 36–4. RESIDUAL MOTOR DEFICITS

	N	%
Spasticity	119	38
Ataxia	25	8
Spasticity and ataxia	124	39
"Soft" signs	10	3
"Normal"*	31	10
Spinal cord injury	4	1
Peripheral nerve injury	4	1

*"Normal" indicates normal neurologic examination. From Brink, JD et al.,[53] with permission.

SPINAL CORD INJURY

The combination of head injury and spinal cord injury occurred in 1 percent of a large series of pediatric head injury patients.[56] The early diagnosis of this condition in a comatose patient can be easily overlooked. Cervical spine films should be routine in assessing the comatose child injured in a motor vehicle accident or in a fall from a height.[100] The level of spinal cord injury is most commonly cervical but can be thoracic or lumbar. The diagnosis should be suspected if there is abnormal anal sphincter tone, a differential response to pain in the upper versus the lower extremities, or a flaccid symmetrical paraparesis or paraplegia. In young children, spinal cord injury commonly occurs without confirmatory radiologic evidence of vertebral disruption, compounding the diagnostic difficulty.[101] Somatosensory evoked potentials may be a useful diagnostic aid, especially with incomplete spinal cord injury.[102] The diagnosis of incomplete spinal cord lesions may not be made definitively until the patient regains consciousness and a more detailed sensory and motor examination can be performed.

PERIPHERAL NEUROLOGIC INJURY

As with spinal cord damage, peripheral nerve injury is uncommon. It must be considered, however, when a flaccid paralysis or weakness of an extremity persists in a patient who otherwise is improving. A fractured clavicle should alert the clinician to the most common site of lower motor neuron injury, the brachial plexus. Peroneal and radial nerve injury occur less frequently but may be associated with long bone fractures.[56] Pelvic fractures can result in damage to the lumbosacral plexus or pelvic nerve, resulting in a monoparesis or neurogenic bladder.[103, 104] The diagnosis of peripheral neurologic injury can be confirmed by electromyography and nerve conduction studies.

SKULL FRACTURES

During the first 2 to 3 years of life, dural tears beneath a skull fracture predispose children to herniation of brain or fluid-filled subarachnoid tissue, resulting in the development of a "growing" (enlarging) skull fracture.[105, 106] In this age group, fracture lines should be carefully palpated for fluid collections and plain skull radiographs should be obtained periodically. Delay in the diagnosis can result in neurologic compromise.

Fractures involving the base of the skull are not always detected radiologically.[83, 107] Careful clinical inspection of the cranium will lead to the detection of the pathognomonic signs of basilar skull fractures. Fractures of the anterior cranial fossa are associated with periorbital hematoma (raccoon's eyes) and cerebral spinal fluid rhinorrhea, whereas fractures of the middle cranial fossa, with mastoid hematoma (Battle's sign) and cerebral spinal fluid or bloody otorrhea. Intracranial air, cerebral spinal fluid leakage, and a predisposition to meningitis occur as a result of dural tearing and fistula formation. Central nervous system infection can develop, however, without clinical or radiologic evidence of a basilar skull fracture.[107]

Fractures of the temporal bone are important because of its proximity to structures of critical importance.[108] Most temporal bone fractures (70 to 80 percent) are of the longitudinal type, resulting in damage to the tympanic membrane and structures of the middle ear (hemorrhage, ossicular chain disruption) (Fig. 36–3).[109] The resultant hearing deficit (see further on) usually resolves spontaneously but if not requires tympanotomy.[110] The post-traumatic perineural edema of the seventh cranial nerve following a longitudinal fracture results in a delayed, spontaneously resolving facial weakness or paralysis.[111]

Transverse fractures of the temporal bone are responsible for the remaining 20 to 30 percent of basilar skull fractures (Fig. 36–

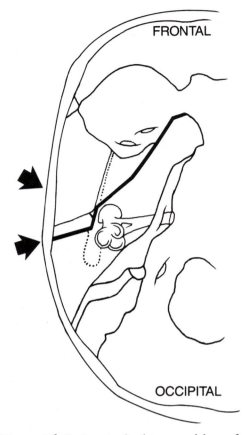

Figure 36–3. Longitudinal temporal bone fracture *(heavy line)*. The causative blow *(arrows)* is struck from a lateral direction on the temporal or parietal area of the skull. (From Goodwin, WJ,[108] with permission.)

4).[110] The vestibular apparatus, cochlear, and facial nerve are most frequently damaged, accounting for vertigo, a permanent and total sensory neural hearing deficit, and immediate onset of facial paralysis, respectively.

POST-TRAUMATIC HYDROCEPHALUS

Ventriculomegaly is a frequent finding after head injury.[112] Most often it is due to cerebral atrophy (hydrocephalus ex vacuo), a loss in the mass of cerebral white matter due to diffuse axonal injury. The ensuing reciprocal increase in the volume of the ventricular system may be found as early as 2 weeks after injury. In adults its presence is related to the severity of the injury as well as the quality of recovery.[113]

Post-traumatic communicating hydro-

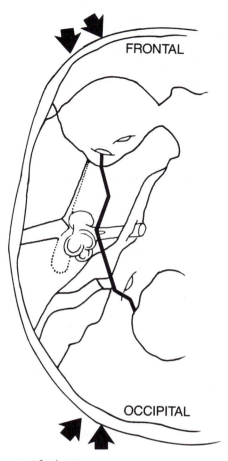

Figure 36–4. Transverse temporal bone fracture *(heavy line)*. The causative blow *(arrows)* is struck from an anterior or posterior direction. (From Goodwin, WJ,[108] with permission.)

cephalus, the other cause of ventricular enlargement, is unusual even among patients with severe head injury.[114] The interference with cerebrospinal fluid flow, presumably due to subarachnoid hemorrhage, leads to progressive dementia, impaired consciousness, ataxia, failure to improve, or behavioral and cognitive changes. Most often it occurs within the first year after trauma. When cerebrospinal fluid pressure is elevated, clinical improvement usually follows shunting. Subdural cerebrospinal collections or hygromas need only be treated if associated with clinical findings.

AUDITORY AND VESTIBULAR DISORDERS

Vestibular and cochlear dysfunction, including sensorineural hearing loss, posi-

tional vertigo (rare in children), and spontaneous and positional nystagmus, may be a complication of head injury.[111, 115–117]

Most instances of conductive hearing deficits following head injury are due to the hemotympanum associated with longitudinal fractures of the temporal bone and perforation of the tympanic membrane.[110] Both conditions usually improve spontaneously. Permanent tympanic membrane perforation is rare. Conductive losses can also be due to injuries of the ossicular chain which may be successfully managed many weeks after the initial trauma.[111] Cochlear concussion is generally responsible for the sensorineural hearing deficit after head injury. The ensuing high frequency hearing disturbance is characteristically above the critical speech range. Improvement in traumatic sensorineural hearing deficit occurs more frequently in children than adults.[110] Depending on the severity and type of hearing loss, amplification may be warranted. Transverse fractures of the temporal bone are usually associated with total and permanent sensorineural deficits.[110, 118]

As many as 40 percent of children immediately after trauma will have sensory and peripheral vestibular disturbances. In 6 months only half as many will be affected.[117] Unlike for adults, the persistence of dizziness is unusual. A thorough otologic assessment must be performed on any child with vestibular or auditory disorders (see Chapter 37).

VISUAL DISTURBANCES

A variety of visual disturbances may be caused by damage to the visual pathways or the cranial nerves innervating the extraocular muscles.[119–121] Visual impairments may result from either penetrating wounds around the eye or blunt cranial trauma that affects the visual pathways and the visual cortex. Blunt trauma as a cause of retinal detachment is highest in the first three decades of life.[122, 123]

Optic nerve injury may be due to stretching, tearing, contusion, or vascular compromise.[123] This usually occurs in the fixed canalicular portion of the second cranial nerve's course and results in monocular blindness, impaired acuity, or a field defect. Lesions of the optic tracts or radiations result in homonymous field defects. In contrast to cortical blindness, which is usually transitory, complete recovery is the exception with any of these aforementioned conditions.[124]

Traumatic injury to the oculomotor, trochlear, or abducens nerves can result in diplopia. Because of the high incidence of spontaneous resolution, surgical intervention for traumatic ophthalmoplegia should be delayed during the first year after injury.[125] Functional improvement will usually result from alternate eye patching under the guidance of an ophthalmologist.

Amblyopia is a concern in any child younger than 8 years of age. During this early period of life, visual deprivation or a misalignment of the eyes may produce suppression of the deviating eye and loss of visual acuity. Young children with traumatic third cranial nerve palsies have an inability to accommodate. If the child has a developmental hypermetropic refractive error and an accompanying inability to accommodate, profound amblyopia may result if not properly assessed and treated.

POST-TRAUMATIC SEIZURES
AND EPILEPSY

Early post-traumatic seizures are those that occur within the first week after head injury. During childhood, they are more common than in the adult years and also more likely to occur after a minor head injury.[126, 127] Children under age 3 account for most of this increased incidence, with 75 to 85 percent of early seizures occurring within the first 24 hours of injury.[126] This is in contrast to adults, in whom half of all post-traumatic seizures occur more than 24 hours after injury.

Early post-traumatic seizures, predominantly focal and focal becoming generalized,[126, 128, 129] can, if prolonged and recurrent, increase cerebral edema and intracranial pressure. Because of this, Kennedy and Freeman advocate the short-term administration of anticonvulsants following an early seizure *only* if focal neurologic findings and/or focal brain damage (intracranial hematoma, cerebral laceration) are found.[130] Their recommendation does not stem from any convincing evidence that early seizures predispose to late post-traumatic epilepsy, defined as two or more seizures that occur more than 1 week after head injury.

Late post-traumatic epilepsy occurs more in adults than in children. The overall incidence in nonbiased pediatric populations is between 1.5 and 2.0 percent.[127, 128, 131] Even in a prospectively studied population of severely injured children, the incidence of epilepsy was only 2.3 percent.[132] Most late epilepsy occurs within 12 months of head injury and the peak onset is within 3 months.[130] Just under half of all late seizures have focal features, of which approximately 50 percent are temporal lobe epilepsy.[130] Almost three quarters of all late seizures become generalized.[127]

A recent critical review advocates that long-term prophylactic treatment of late post-traumatic epilepsy in childhood not be undertaken.[130] This recommendation appears warranted in view of the presently available data: the economic cost and morbidity of anticonvulsants are significant;[133, 134] the risk of head injured children developing late epilepsy is low; and prospective studies have failed to demonstrate the effectiveness of such prophylactic therapy.

SUMMARY

The neuropsychologic consequences of head injury have a profound influence on a child's ability to function at home, in the community, and most importantly at school. The educational setting demands the acquisition of new knowledge and maximally taxes cognitive, linguistic, visual-motor, and behavioral skills. A child's ability to successfully function in the protected hospital setting after awakening from coma is not a reliable predictor of future successful adaptive functioning. The population of head injured children should be targeted for support, anticipatory guidance, and careful evaluation and follow-up so that their reintegration into school, peer group, and family can occur smoothly.

The medical and surgical problems that are associated with head injury can range from the trivial to the profound. Knowledge of these potential problems can lead to the prevention of many and the early detection of most. The triad of prevention, early detection, and prompt treatment can mean the difference between reduced morbidity or the compounding of long-term disability.

REFERENCES

1. Spivack, MP: Advocacy and legislative action for head-injured children and their families. J Head Trauma Rehabil 1:41, 1986.
2. Mahoney, WJ et al: Long-term outcome of children with severe head trauma and prolonged coma. Pediatrics 71:756, 1983.
3. Bruce, DA et al: Outcome following severe head injuries in children. Neurosurgery 48:679, 1978.
4. Blau, A: Mental changes following head trauma in children. Arch Neurol Psychiatry 35:723, 1936.
5. Divack, JA et al: Behavior Management. In Ylvisaker, M (ed): Head Injury Rehabilitation: Children and Adolescents. College Hill Press, San Diego, 1985, p 347.
6. Jennett, B: Head injuries in children. Dev Med Child Neurol 14:137, 1972.
7. Feeney, DM et al: Amphetamine, haloperidol, and experience interact to affect rate of recovery after motor cortex injury. Science 217:855, 1982.
8. Todorow, S: Recovery of children after severe head injury. Psychoreactive superimpositions. Scand J Rehabil Med 7:93, 1975.
9. Klonoff, H and Low, MD: Disordered brain function in young children and adolescents: Neuropsychological and electroencephalographic correlates. In Reitan, RM and Davison, LA (eds): Clinical Neuropsychology: Current Status and Application. John Wiley & Sons, New York, 1974.
10. Brink, JD et al: Recovery of motor and intellectual function in children sustaining severe head injuries. Dev Med Child Neurol 12:565, 1970.
11. Hjern, B and Nylander, I: Late prognosis of severe head injury in childhood. Acta Paediatr Scand (Suppl)152:113, 1964.
12. Flach, J and Malmos, R: A long-term follow-up study of children with severe head injury. Scand J Rehabil Med 4:9, 1972.
13. Naughton, JAL: The effects of severe head injuries in children. Psychological aspects. Proceedings of an International Symposium on Head Injuries. Churchill-Livingstone, Edinburgh, 1971, p 106.
14. Shaffer, D et al: Psychiatric outcome of localized head injury in children. In Outcome of Severe Damage to the Central Nervous System. Ciba Foundation Symposium 34, Elsevier, Excerpta Medica, Amsterdam, North-Holland, 1975.
15. Rutter, M: Psychological sequelae of brain damage in children. Am J Psychiatry 138:12, 1981.
16. Gerring, JP: Psychiatric sequelae of severe closed head injury. Pediatr Rev 8:115, 1986.
17. Fuld, RA and Fisher, P: Recovery of intellectual ability after closed head injury. Dev Med Child Neurol, 19:495, 1977.
18. Brooks, DN and McKinlay W: Personality and behavioural change after severe blunt head injury — a relative's view. J Neurol Neurosurg Psychiatry 46:336, 1983.
19. Jennett, B et al: Predicting outcome in individual patients with head injury. Lancet 1:1031, 1976.
20. Black, P et al: The head injured child: Time course of recovery, with implications for rehabilitation. Proceedings of an International Symposium on Head Injuries. Churchill-Livingstone, Edinburgh, 1971, p 131.
21. Klonoff, H et al: Head injuries in children: A prospective five year follow-up. J Neurol Neurosurg Psychiatry 40:1211, 1977.
22. Sarno, MT: The nature of verbal impairment after closed head injury. J Nerv Ment Dis 168:685, 1980.
23. Woods, BT and Carey, S: Language deficits after apparent clinical recovery from childhood aphasia. Ann Neurol 6:404, 1979.
24. Teuber, HL: The brain and human behavior. In Held, R, Leibowitz, HW and Teuber, HL (eds): Perception. Springer-Verlag, Heidelberg, 1978, p 893.
25. Alajouanine, T and Lhermitte, F: Acquired aphasia in children. Brain 88:653, 1980.
26. Ylvisaker, MA: Language and communication disorders following pediatric head injury. J Head Trauma Rehabil 1 (4):48, 1986.
27. Levin, HS et al: Mutism after closed head injury. Arch Neurol 40:601, 1983.
28. Levin, HS and Eisenberg, EM: Neuropsychological outcome of closed head injury in children and adolescents. Child Brain 5:281, 1979.
29. Levin, HS et al: Memory and intellectual ability after head injury in children and adolescents. Neurosurgery 11:668, 1982.
30. Chadwick, O et al: A prospective study of children with head injuries. II. Cognitive sequelae. Psychol Med J 11:49, 1981.
31. Levin, HS and Eisenberg, HM: Neuropsychological impairment after closed head injury in children and adolescents. J Pediatr Psychol 4:389, 1979.
32. Shaffer, D et al: Head injury and later reading disability. J Am Child Psychiat 19:592, 1980.
33. Jacobson, MS et al: Followup of adolescent trauma victims: A new model of care. Pediatrics 77:236, 1986.
34. Mize, CA et al: Undernutrition of pediatric inpatients: Repeated nutrition status evaluation. Nutr Supp Serv 4:27, 1984.
35. Pollack, WM et al: Malnutrition in critically ill infants and children. J Parent Ent Nutr 6:20, 1982.
36. Newmark, SR et al: Nutritional assessment in a rehabilitation unit. Arch Phys Med Rehabil 62:279, 1981.
37. Parsons, HG et al: The nutritional status of hospitalized children. Am J Clin Nutr 33:1140, 1980.
38. Merritt, RJ and Suskind, RM: Nutritional survey of hospitalized pediatric patients. Am J Clin Nutr 32:1320, 1979.
39. Clifton, GL, Robertson, CS and Choi, SC: Assessment of nutritional requirements of head injured patients. J Neurosurg 64:895, 1986.
40. Clifton, GL and Robertson, CS: The metabolic response to severe head injury. In Miner, ME and Wagner, KA (eds): Neurotrauma: Treatment, Rehabilitation, and Related Issues. Butterworths, Boston, 1986, p 73.
41. Deutschman, CS et al: Physiological and metabolic response to isolated closed-head injury. J Neurosurg 64:89, 1986.
42. Young, B et al: Metabolic and nutritional sequelae in the non-steroid treated head injury patient. Neurosurgery 17:784, 1985.
43. Ylvisaker, M and Logemann, J: Therapy for feeding and swallowing disorders following head in-

jury. In Ylvisaker, M (ed): Head Injury Rehabilitation: Children and Adolescents. College Hill Press, San Diego, 1985, p 195.

44. Roberts, AH: Severe Accidental Head Injury: An Assessment of Long-Term Prognosis. Unwin Brothers, Ltd, Surrey, England, 1979.

45. Curci, MR et al: Peptic ulcer disease in childhood reexamined. J Pediatr Surg 11:329, 1976.

46. Lloyd, CW et al: Pharmacokinetics and pharmacodynamics of cimetidine and metabolites in critically ill children. J Pediatr 107:295, 1985.

47. Kamada, T et al: Gastrointestinal bleeding following head injury: A clinical study of 433 cases. J Trauma 17:44, 1977.

48. Norton, L, Greer, J and Eiseman, B: Gastric secretory response to head injury. Arch Surg 101:200, 1970.

49. Norton, L et al: Gastric secretory response to head injury. Arch Surg 101:200, 1970.

50. Watts, C and Clark, K: Gastric acidity in the comatose patient. J Neurosurg 30:107, 1969.

51. Eichelberger, MR et al: Acute pancreatitis and increased intracranial pressure. J Pediatr Surg 16:562, 1981.

52. Myers, EN, Stool, SE and Johnson, JT: Tracheotomy. Churchill-Livingstone, New York, 1985.

53. Brink, JD, Imbus, C and Woo-sam, J: Physical recovery after severe closed head trauma in children and adolescents. J Pediatr 97:721, 1980.

54. Pang, D: Pathophysiologic correlates of neurobehavioral syndromes following closed head injury. In Ylvisaker, M (ed): Head Injury Rehabilitation: Children and Adolescents. College-Hill Press, San Diego, 1985, p 3.

55. Clifton, GL et al: Cardiovascular response to severe head injury. J Neurosurg 59:447, 1983.

56. Brink, JD et al: Physical recovery after severe closed head trauma in children and adolescents. J Pediatrics 97:721, 1980.

57. Kanter, RK et al: Association of arterial hypertension with poor outcome in children with acute brain injury. Clin Pediatr 24:320, 1985.

58. Solomon, S et al: Impairment of memory function by antihypertensive medication. Arch Gen Psychiatry 40:1109, 1983.

59. Wright, PF et al: Patterns of illness in the highly febrile young child: Epidemiologic clinical and laboratory correlates. Pediatrics 67:694, 1981.

60. Smith, AL: Personal communication, 1987.

61. Hirschmann, JV: Bacterial meningitis following closed cranial trauma. In Sande, MA, Smith, AL and Root, RK (eds): Bacterial Meningitis. Churchill-Livingstone, New York, 1985, p 95.

62. Morgan, BC: Complications from intravascular catheters. Am J Dis Child 138:425, 1984.

63. Stamm, WE: Prevention of infections: Infection related to medical devices. Ann Int Med 89:764, 1978.

64. American Academy of Pediatrics: Report of the Committee on Infectious Diseases, ed 2. American Academy of Pediatrics, Elk Grove Village, IL, 1986.

65. Kluger, MJ: Fever. Pediatrics 66:720, 1980.

66. Brown, DR and McMillan, JM: Posttraumatic anterior hypopituitarism-revisited: The role of TRH provocative release prolactin in the confirmation of anterior pituitary damage. Pediatrics 59:948, 1977.

67. Doczi, T et al: Syndrome of inappropriate secretion of antidiuretic hormone (SIADH) after head injury. Neurosurgery 10:685, 1982.

68. King, LR et al: Pituitary hormone response to head injury. Neurosurgery 9:229, 1981.

69. Klachko, DM et al: Traumatic hypopituitarism occurring before puberty: Survival 35 years untreated. J Clin Endocrinol 28:1768, 1968.

70. Klingbeil, GEG and Cline, P: Anterior hypopituitarism: A consequence of head injury. Arch Phys Med Rehabil 66:44, 1985.

71. Ratcliffe, PJ et al: Late onset post-traumatic hypothalamic hypothermia. J Neurol Neurosurg Psychiatry 46:72, 1983.

72. Valenta, LJ and DeFeo, DR: Post-traumatic hypopituitarism due to a hypothalamic lesion. Am J Med 68:614, 1980.

73. Robinson, AG: Disorders of antidiuretic hormone secretion. Clin Endocrinol Metab 14:55, 1985.

74. Born, JD et al: Syndrome of inappropriate secretion of antidiuretic hormone after severe head injury. Surg Neurol 23:383, 1985.

75. Hadani, M et al: Unusual delayed onset of diabetes insipidus following closed head trauma. J Neurosurg 63:456, 1985.

76. Barreca, T et al: Evaluation of anterior pituitary function in patients with posttraumatic diabetes insipidus. J Clin Endocrinol Metab 51:1279, 1980.

77. Shaul, PW et al: Precocious puberty following severe head trauma. Am J Dis Child 139:467, 1985.

78. Miller, WL et al: Child abuse as a cause of posttraumatic hypopituitarism. N Engl J Med 302:724, 1980.

79. Paxson, CL and Brown, DR: Post-traumatic anterior hypopituitarism. Pediatrics 57:893, 1976.

80. Shaul, PW, Towbin, RB and Chernausek, SD: Precocious puberty following severe head trauma. Am J Dis Child 139:467, 1985.

81. Costigan, DC et al: The "empty sella" in childhood. Clin Pediatr 23:437, 1983.

82. McKiernan, J: Precocious puberty and non-accidental injury. Br Med J 14:1059, 1978.

83. Hendrick, EB et al: Head injuries in children: A survey of 4465 consecutive cases at the Hospital for Sick Children, Toronto, Canada. Clin Neurosurg 11:46, 1964.

84. Irving, MH and Irving, PM: Associated injuries in head injured patients. J Trauma 7:500, 1967.

85. Hoffer, M et al: Orthopedic management of brain injured children. J Bone Joint Surg 53A:567, 1971.

86. Gillogly, SD et al: Orthopaedic problems in head-injured children and adolescents (abstr). Proc Am Acad Orthop Surg 1986, 70A.

87. Bellamy, R and Brower, T: Management of skeletal trauma in the patient with head injury. J Trauma 14:1021, 1974.

88. Fry, K et al: Femoral shaft fractures in brain-injured children. J Trauma 16:371, 1976.

89. Ziv, I and Rang, M: Treatment of femoral fracture in the child with head injury. J Bone Joint Surg 65-B:276, 1983.

90. Mital, MA et al: Ectopic bone formation in children and adolescents with head injuries: Its management. J Pediatr Orthop 7:83, 1987.

91. Garland, ED et al: Forceful joint manipulation in head-injured adults with heterotopic ossification. Clin Orthop 169:133, 1982.

92. Brink, J and Hoffer, M: Rehabilitation of brain injured children. Orthop Clin North Am 9:451, 1978.

93. Rogers, JG et al: Use and complications of high-dose disodium etidronate therapy in fibrodysplasia ossificans progressiva. J Pediatr 91:1011, 1977.

94. Tori, JA and Hill, LL: Hypercalcemia in children with spinal cord injury. Arch Phys Med Rehabil 59:443, 1978.

95. Cristofaro, RL, and Brink, JD: Hypercalcemia of immobilization in neurologically injured children: A prospective study. Orthopedics 2:485, 1979.

96. Van Zuiden, L et al: Immobilization hypercalcemia. Can J Surg 25:646, 1982.

97. Chan, GM et al: Bone mineral status in childhood accidental fractures. Am J Dis Child 138:569, 1984.

98. Hoffer, M and Brink, J: Orthopedic management of acquired cerebral spasticity in childhood. Clin Orthop 110:244, 1975.

99. Costoff, H et al: Survivors of severe traumatic brain injury in childhood — late residual disabilitiy. Scand J Rehabil Med (Suppl) 12:10, 1985.

100. Bruce, D: Clinical care of the severely head injured child. In Shapiro, K (ed): Pediatric Head Trauma. Futura Publishing, Mount Kisco, New York, 1983, p 27.

101. Pang, D and Wilberger, JE: Spinal cord injury without radiographic abnormalities in children. J Neurosurg 57:114, 1982.

102. Mizrahi, EM and Dorfman, L: Sensory evoked potentials: Clinical application in pediatrics. Pediatrics 97:1, 1980.

103. Reichard, SA et al: Pelvic fractures in children — Review of 120 patients with a new look at general management. J Pediatr Surg 15:727, 1980.

104. Looser, KG and Crombie, HD: Pelvic fracture: An anatomic guide to severity of injury. Am J Surg 132:638, 1976.

105. Sekhar, LN and Scarff, TB: Pseudogrowth in skull fractures of childhood. Neurosurgery 6:285, 1980.

106. Rothman, L et al: The spectrum of growing skull fracture in children. Pediatrics 57:26, 1976.

107. Jennett, B and Teasdale, G: Management of Head injuries. FA Davis, Philadelphia, 1981.

108. Goodwin, WJ: Temporal bone fractures. Otolaryngol Clin North Am 16:651, 1983.

109. Nelson, JR: Neuro-otologic aspects of head injury. Adv Neurol 22:107, 1979.

110. Vartiainen, E: Auditory and Vestibular Disorders Following Head Injury in Children. University of Kuopio Publications, Kuopio, Finland. 1983.

111. Healy, GB: Hearing loss and vertigo secondary to head injury. N Engl J Med 306:1029, 1982.

112. Kishore, PRS et al: Posttraumatic hydrocephalus in patients with severe head injury. Neuroradiology 16:261, 1978.

113. Van Dongen, KJ and Braakman, R: Late computed tomography in survivors of severe head injury. Neurosurgery 7:14, 1980.

114. Cardoso, ER and Galbraith, S: Posttraumatic hydrocephalus — a retrospective review. Surg Neurol 23:261, 1985.

115. Browning, GG, Swan, IRC and Gatehouse, S: Hearing loss in minor head injury. Arch Otolaryngol 108:474, 1982.

116. Vartiainen, E, Karjalainen, S and Karja, J: Auditory disorders following head injury in children. Acta Otolaryngol (Stockh)99:529, 1985.

117. Vartiainen, E, Karjalainen, S and Karja, J: Vestibular disorders following head injury in children. Int J Pediatr Otorhinolaryngol 9:135, 1985.

118. Shapiro, RS: Temporal bone fractures in children. Otolaryngol Head Neck Surg 87:323, 1979.

119. Anderson, DP and Ford, RM: Visual abnormalities after severe head injuries. Can J Surg 23:163, 1980.

120. Crompton, MR: Visual lesions in closed head injury. Brain 93:785, 1970.

121. Smith, JL: Some neuro-ophthalmological aspects of head trauma. Clin Neurosurg 12:181, 1964.

122. Assaf, AA: Traumatic retinal detachment. J Trauma 25:1085, 1985.

123. Anderson, RL, Panje, WR and Gross, CE: Optic nerve blindness following blunt forehead trauma. Ophthalmology 89:445, 1982.

124. Griffith, JF and Dodge, PR: Transient blindness following head injury in children. N Engl J Med 278:648, 1968.

125. Mealey, J: Skull fractures. In McLaurin, R (ed): Pediatric Neurosurgery, Surgery of the Developing Nervous System. Section of Pediatric Neurosurgery of the AANS. Grune & Stratton, New York, 1982, p 289.

126. Salazar, AM et al: Epilepsy after penetrating head injury. I. Clinical correlates: A report of the Vietnam head injury study. Neurology 35:1406, 1985.

127. Annegers, JF et al: Seizures after head trauma: A population study. Neurology 30:683, 1980.

128. Raimondi, AJ and Hirschauer, J: Head injury in the infant and toddler. Child Brain 11:12, 1984.

129. DeSantis, A et al: Early post traumatic seizures in adults: Study of 84 cases. J Neurosurg Sci 207, 1979.

130. Kennedy, CR and Freeman, JM: Post traumatic seizures and post traumatic epilepsy in children. J Head Trauma Rehabil 1:66, 1986.

131. Hendrick, EB and Harris, L: Post traumatic epilepsy in children. J Trauma 8:547, 1968.

132. McQueen, JK et al: Low risk of late post-traumatic seizures following severe head injury: Implications for clinical trials of prophylaxis. J Neurol Neurosurg Psychiatry 46:899, 1983.

133. Reynolds, EH: Chronic antiepileptic toxicity: A review. Epilepsia 16:319, 1975.

134. Vining, EPG et al: Effects of phenobarbital and sodium valproate on neuropsychological function and behavior. Ann Neurol 14:360, 1983.

Chapter 37

Rehabilitative Assessment Following Head Injury in Children

MARK YLVISAKER, Ph.D.
ANNA J. L. CHORAZY, M.D.
SALLY B. COHEN, M.Ed.
JOYCE P. MASTRILLI, O.T.R./L.
CINDY BLACK MOLITOR, P.T., M.S.
JAMES NELSON, Ph.D.
SHIRLEY F. SZEKERES, Ph.D.
ANNE S. VALKO, M.D.
KENNETH M. JAFFE, M.D.

After severe head injury, the scope of problems requiring thorough assessment can be very broad. In addition, traditional methods of assessment often require modification or flexibility in interpretation as a result of the particular combinations of cognitive, psychosocial, and motor problems that in many cases distinguish head injured children from those whose impairments are congenital. The interaction of normal developmental phenomena with the consequences of traumatic brain injury further complicates the assessment. A complete discussion of assessment of children with head injuries would, therefore, be an ambitious undertaking indeed. Our goal in this chapter is to highlight those aspects of cognitive, sensorimotor, and medical assessment that have a strongly pediatric focus and that relate in important ways to practical management decisions within a rehabilitation setting. Throughout the chapter, we emphasize the need for rehabilitation professionals to integrate their assessments, to focus on issues of functional significance, and to consistently relate assessment findings to normal development.

COGNITIVE ASSESSMENT

Cognitive and related psychosocial deficits tend to be more common than motor deficits in head injured children as a group (see Chapter 36), although within this group, individual children's profiles can vary dramatically. Furthermore, cognitive deficits, even if mild, can have a profound effect on the life of a developing child. The community that a child re-enters includes school, with its attendant demands on cognitive and behavioral integrity. Since the pretraumatic knowledge base of a child is less well developed than that of a head injured adult, reduced learning efficiency may have a more significant long-term effect on a child than on a comparably injured adult.

The cognitive profiles of head injured

children often differ from those of children who are developmentally delayed or who have congenital learning disabilities.[1] Therefore, thorough assessment, coupled with an interpretation of the assessment results that is based on an understanding of head injury sequelae, may be necessary to secure special services for head injured children. The importance of careful cognitive assessment is further underscored by the fact that closed head injury typically results in brain damage (e.g., microscopic shearing lesions) that is not detected by standard neuroradiologic procedures or neurologic assessment and that may not result in readily observable changes in the child's overall functioning.[2]

Given the scope of the term "cognitive" (i.e., all mental processes and systems involved in acquiring and using knowledge), several rehabilitation professions have a legitimate interest in assessing cognitive functioning. These include psychology/neuropsychology, special education, occupational therapy, and speech-language pathology. In a rehabilitation facility, this shared interest in cognitive assessment easily leads to overtesting. From the perspective of a single discipline, however, *under*assessment is a possible result, since rehabilitation professionals often lack a shared vocabulary and conceptual framework with which to communicate assessment results and their implications to one another. Consequently, an integrated picture of the child's cognitive functioning may not emerge despite a large amount of testing. In addition, several aspects of cognitive functioning that are particularly important in the rehabilitation of head injured children are not addressed by standardized tests. Therefore, our focus in this section of the chapter is on *integrated* cognitive assessment within a rehabilitation setting for the purpose of planning, evaluating, and modifying cognitive rehabilitation programs and treatment.

Goals of Assessment

Decisions regarding the selection of assessment instruments or procedures, the timing of assessment, and even who should perform the assessment vary with the goal of assessment. Assessment of a head injured child may be for purposes of determining the presence or absence of brain damage, classifying the child under pre-established diagnostic categories, formulating a prognosis, establishing eligibility for educational or rehabilitation services, placing a child in an educational setting, or establishing where in a curriculum to begin instruction. It may also be used to prepare for legal testimony, describe outcomes in a group of head injured children, evaluate the effectiveness of intervention, or plan cognitive rehabilitation or special education programs and modify intervention in an ongoing way.

Each purpose places its own set of constraints on the assessment and inappropriate or incomplete information may be the result when an assessment tool designed to serve one purpose (e.g., diagnosing brain damage) is used to serve another purpose (e.g., planning treatment). Diagnosing brain damage or making inferences from behavior (including test results) to central nervous system (CNS) status requires that there be firm evidence supporting such inferences—i.e., established correlations between certain types of test results and patterns of CNS functioning *for head injured children.* Research in this area is insufficient to support confident inferences of this sort for young children.[3, 4] Using brain-behavior relationships validated with adults is inappropriate in light of the unique organization of cognitive behavior in children at various stages of cognitive development and the presumed differences between children and adults in the CNS activity underlying these differences in cognitive organization. Consequently, the focus of cognitive assessment of children is more properly on behavioral variables and the inter-relationships among these variables than on presumed relations between behavior and CNS status. Furthermore, diagnosis of brain damage is typically not at issue in the case of children whose head injury is severe enough to require a period of rehabilitation.

Establishing eligibility for services or programs requires the use of assessment instruments that are acceptable to those individuals or agencies responsible for making decisions regarding eligibility. However, since the cognitive profile of a head injured child with a residual learning impairment may be quite different from that generally expected of a child whose learning impairment is congenital (e.g., a head injured child with a learning impairment *may* lack the significant discrepancy between verbal and performance IQ that is often associated with learning disabled children), tests used to establish eligibility must be interpreted in light of what is known about outcome following severe head injury. School administrators and others responsible for placement decisions must be shown that *flexibility* in eligibility criteria for head injured children is often necessary to ensure appropriate programs for them.

Classification or diagnosis and prognosis require the use of tests that are validated in relation to the questions being asked by the assessment. Few cognitive assessment instruments have been validated for use with head injured children. In particular, none of the tests of cognitive or academic functioning has yet been shown to be a good predictor of school learning in the long term post-injury. The questions that need to be answered in order to fine-tune cognitive rehabilitation, however, do not necessarily require the use of standardized tests. It is to this topic—assessment for planning rehabilitation—that we now turn.

Rehabilitation-Relevant Assessment

The objectives of cognitive assessment that is administered for purposes of planning and refining cognitive rehabilitation are:

☐ To identify an individual child's pattern of strengths and weaknesses within the broad domain of cognitive functioning, so that weaknesses are not neglected and so that strengths are exploited in the remediation of or compensation for deficits

☐ To identify which among the strengths and weaknesses have the most powerful functional implications in the child's real world

☐ To set goals and specific objectives for cognitive rehabilitation; to modify these as often as is warranted by changes in the child's functioning or by his or her response to treatment

☐ To obtain baseline levels in all areas of treatment and to measure progress

☐ To determine which type of intervention is most effective in promoting functional cognitive improvement (e.g., component process training vs. compensatory strategy training)

☐ To identify, for each child, effective styles of learning and thinking so that therapy and classroom instruction can be customized for that child

☐ To identify what task, environmental, interpersonal, and motivational variables have the greatest effect on adaptive cognitive functioning and on learning

Meeting these objectives requires the integration of formal testing, informal assessment (including interviews of family members, teachers, nursing staff, and others), and, most importantly, diagnostic therapy or prescriptive teaching that is designed to answer questions that remain unanswered by the formal cognitive assessment.

ROLE OF FORMAL ASSESSMENT

Standardized tests of cognitive, cognitive-communicative, cognitive-perceptual, and academic functioning provide *levels* of functioning in a variety of cognitive and cognitively based areas that aid therapists and classroom teachers in selecting tasks at the appropriate level of difficulty in given areas. In addition, these tests provide an overall profile of strengths, weaknesses, and patterns of performance, and contribute to explanations of impaired performance. Well-chosen tests may reveal subtle problems that are not obvious in daily functioning but that could have significant implications in a demanding classroom or social setting. In some cases, formal test results can serve as baseline scores for measuring progress in therapy; this, however, is true only if the test measures those skills that are the explicit targets of treatment. Table 37–1 includes brief descriptions of several tests and test batteries that are commonly used by psychologists, special educators, speech-language pathologists, or occupational therapists in the assessment of head injured children's cognitive abilities.

Frequently, formal tests yield results that are inaccurate or incomplete in relation to the child's habitual cognitive functioning in the classroom or other demanding settings.[62] Conditions of formal assessment may, by their very nature, compensate to

Table 37–1. SELECTED TESTS OF COGNITIVE, COGNITIVE-PERCEPTUAL, COGNITIVE-LANGUAGE, AND ACADEMIC FUNCTIONING IN CHILDREN

Wechsler Intelligence Scale for Children–Revised (WISC-R)

Age range: 6–16 years

Content areas: wide range of intellectual functions

Comments: yields verbal IQ, performance IQ, and full-scale IQ, plus scaled scores on 12 subtests; although not validated specifically for use with head injured children, has been widely used to measure global intelligence, and to assess mental retardation, organic brain damage, learning disabilities, and mental disease; some evidence that the WISC-R is sensitive to brain damage in children;[5, 6] widely used in outcome studies of head injured children; found by Chadwick and colleagues[7] to be as sensitive to brain damage following head injury in children as more specific neuropsychologic measures; adequate performance on the WISC-R may not, however, predict a normal rate of academic learning following head injury;[8, 9] verbal-performance splits cannot be given the same neuropsychologic interpretation in children as in adults;[10, 11] not considered an acceptable basis for drawing inferences about lateralization and localization of brain lesions in children.[10]

Kaufman Assessment Battery for Children[12]

Age range: 2–6 to 12–16

Content areas: sequential processing ability; simultaneous processing ability; achievement

Comments: attempts to reduce the emphasis on language in the measurement of intellectual ability; attempts to separate assessment of native ability from measures of acquired knowledge; useful in the psychoeducational evaluation of learning disabilities and educational planning; used in several studies of mentally retarded and learning disabled children,[13, 14] but not head injured children; limited validation for use with brain injured children

Luria-Nebraska Neuropsychological Battery—Children's Revision[15]

Age range: 8–12 years

Content areas: 11 summary scales: motor, rhythm, tactile, visual, receptive speech, expressive speech, writing, reading, arithmetic, memory, intellectual processes

Comments: does not purport to measure all of the neuropsychologic skills in children and is questionable in its use with head injured children since its weak areas include memory skills, especially delayed or long-term memory, and complex integrative skills;[16] controversy as to whether or not Luria's theories have been successfully translated into standardized test procedures;[17–19] results have been found to complement those of the WISC-R.[6]

Halstead-Reitan Neuropsychological Battery

Age range: Reitan-Indiana tests: 5–8 years;[20] Halstead-Reitan tests: 9–14 years[21]

Content areas: includes the WISC-R and measures of academic achievement in addition to specialized neuropsychologic measures, and assesses a broad range of neuropsychologic functions

Comments: in addition to level of performance, is said to identify deficits of pathognomonic significance and differential patterns of ability, and to yield comparisons of the two sides of the body,[22] has been used in long-term follow-up studies of head injured children;[8] for older children has been shown to be fairly good at differentiating brain damaged from normal children,[23–25] but has not been shown to predict specific real-life behavioral correlates;[26] for younger children lacks specific age norms and has not been thoroughly validated.[27]

McCarthy Scales of Children's Abilities[28]

Age range: 2½ to 8½ years

Content areas: verbal ability, short-term memory, numerical ability, perceptual performance, motor coordination, lateral dominance

Comments: yields a general cognitive index; tasks are more game-like than many tests (useful for capturing attention of head injured children); good standardization and reliability; respectable correlations with academic achievement; successful differentiation between children with and without learning problems; weak areas include social comprehension, judgment, and verbal abstract reasoning.[29]

Assessment in Infancy[30]

Age range: birth to 24 months

Content areas: sensorimotor cognitive development

Comments: standardized on a small and unrepresentative sample; not norm-referenced; excellent breakdown of sensorimotor skills within a Piagetian framework.

Assessment of Children's Language Comprehension[31]

Age range: 3–6 years

Content areas: comprehension of spoken language as related to length and complexity of the message

Table 37–1. *(Continued)*

Comments: yields information related to the number of language elements that can be processed in one clause or active declarative sentence; measures functional working memory span for meaningful linguistic input; provides important information about young children's processing abilities similar to that provided by the Token Test for older children and adults

Clinical Evaluation of Language Functions[32]
Age range: grades K–12
Content areas: language functioning in the following areas: phonology, syntax, semantics, memory, word finding, and retrieval grouped under processing subtests, production subtests, and supplementary subtests
Comments: means and standard deviations available for each subtest and the entire battery; suggests formats for analyzing error responses and for extension testing to explore variables which seem to be primary in contributing to a child's error responses; includes useful exploration of naming and word retrieval abilities, often impaired following head injury

Illinois Test of Psycholinguistic Abilities[33]
Age range: 2–10 years
Content areas: several psycholinguistic abilities, grouped by channel (e.g., auditory versus visual input and motor versus vocal output), process (e.g., reception, expression), and level of organizing (automatic versus representational)
Comments: yields standard scores as well as age scores for each subtest; intended to delineate specific abilities and disabilities relevant to planning treatment; although not currently as widely used as in the recent past, does yield useful information about head injured child's organizational abilities; verbal expression subtest can yield information about information retrieval (time, effort, and fluency), knowledge of objects, and perception of features

The Word Test[34]
Age range: 7–12 years
Content areas: several aspects of semantic knowledge (associations, synonyms, semantic absurdities, antonyms, definitions, multiple definitions)
Comments: yields standard scores for each subtest; useful exploration of a child's ability to organize and express critical semantic knowledge

Neurosensory Center Comprehensive Examination for Aphasia[35]
(pediatric norms in Gaddes and Crocket)[36]
Age range:
Content areas: wide range of verbal skills
Comments: not widely used in clinical language evaluations of children, but has been used by Levin and colleagues in outcome studies of head injured children;[37, 38] word fluency subtest is a clinically useful indicator in older head injured children and adolescents

Test of Visual Perceptual Skills (Nonmotor)[39]
Age range: 4–12 years
Content areas: visual discrimination, visual memory, visual-spatial relationships, visual form constancy, visual sequential memory, visual figure-ground, visual closure
Comments: yields standard scores as well as age scores for each subtest; requires good attentional abilities; useful in delineating visual-perceptual strengths and weaknesses

Motor-Free Visual Perception Test[40]
Age range: 4–9 years
Content areas: spatial relationships, visual discrimination, figure-ground relationships, visual memory, visual closure
Comments: yields means and standard deviations as well as age scores for the entire battery; requires good attention and impulse control

Developmental Test of Visual-Motor Integration[41]
Age range: 4–14 years
Content areas: visual-motor skills involved in copying geometric forms (simple to complex)
Comments: yields standard scores and percentiles; can be administered individually or to a group; has been used in studies of brain injured, educably retarded, partially sighted, and developmentally delayed children; useful component of the assessment of organizational abilities in head injured children; requires the ability to write and to follow directions

Test of Visual-Motor Skills[42]
Age range: 2–13 years
Content areas: visual-motor skills involved in copying forms
Comments: can be administered individually or to a group; limited use in research; results depressed by problems with attention/concentration, impulse control, or direction following

Table 37–1. (*Continued*)

Learning Accomplishment Profile: Diagnostic Edition, Revised (LAP-D)[43]
Age range: 6 to 72 months
Content areas: physical, psychomotor, cognitive, and language functions
Comments: yields only developmental ages; standard scores not available; norms based on a limited number of children; assessment based on task analysis which facilitates diagnostic prescriptive teaching; useful as a criterion-based measure to evaluate programming; provides a useful breakdown of cognitive skills that are basic to learning; can provide information on basic processing and thought organizational abilities for older head injured children. The *Learning Accomplishment Profile* (*LAP*)[44] provides additional criterion-referenced information for establishing educational objectives. The *Early Learning Accomplishment Profile for Developmentally Young Children* (Early LAP)[45] includes a more refined breakdown of milestones and educational objectives for young handicapped children, birth through 36 months.

The Developmental Resource (Vol 1)[46]
Age range: birth to 6 years
Content areas: sensorimotor/cognitive development; gross and fine motor development; self-help skills
Comments: provides an excellent breakdown of skills for infants and very young children; items are useful in probing cognitive abilities in areas such as perception, organization, problem solving

Revised Pre-Reading Screening Procedures[47]
Age range: entering grade 1
Content areas: integrative processing abilities (auditory, visual, kinesthetic, language) needed for academic subjects in first grade
Comments: group administration; facilitates development of multisensory educational programs; complex oral directions are difficult for head injured students; can be used to monitor on-task behavior, overload, flexibility, task organization, and expressive organization

Slingerland Screening Tests for Identifying Children With Specific Language Disability[48, 49]
Age range: grades 1–6 (supplemented by the *Specific Language Disability Test*[50] *for grades 6–8*)
Content areas: variety of processing abilities related to language, reading, and fine motor tasks
Comments: yields only rough cut-off scores suggestive of a learning disability; results indicate areas of processing strength and weakness relevant to remedial programming; useful for evaluating organizational and integrative abilities and timed performance; test directions can be complex and difficult for head injured students

Peabody Individual Achievement Test[51]
Age range: grades 1.5–12.
Content areas: reading, spelling, mathematics, and general information
Comments: yields grade equivalent scores and percentile ranks; standardized on large samples of children in mainstream education; pointing response makes test useful for children with motor speech or fine motor impairments; minimizes memory requirements; limited amounts of reading material benefit students with overload problems

Woodcock Reading Mastery Series[52]
Age range: grades K–12
Content areas: letter identification, sight vocabulary, word attack, word comprehension, and passage comprehension
Comments: yields grade level scores and percentile ranks; standardized on large samples of children in mainstream education; requires oral responses; passage comprehension (silent reading) requires retrieval abilities

Diagnostic Reading Scales[53]
Age range: grades 1–8
Content areas: sight vocabulary; oral and silent reading comprehension; listening comprehension
Comments: yields grade scores; standardized on a large sample of children in mainstream education; includes phonics and word analysis tests; recall required for open-ended questions

Group Diagnostic Reading Aptitude and Achievement Tests—Intermediate Form[54]
Age range: grades 3–9
Content areas: reading comprehension, written spelling, math computation, copying, integrative visual-motor, visual-sequencing, and auditory-sequencing tasks
Comments: Paragraph comprehension (silent reading) subtest includes written questions, the option of referring back to the paragraph (thereby reducing memory demands), and a printed multiple choice response format

Woodock-Johnson Psychoeducational Battery: Tests of Cognitive Ability, Tests of Academic Achievement, Tests of Interest Level[55]

Table 37–1. *(Continued)*

Age range: grades 1–12 (standardized on subjects age 3–80+)
Content areas: many areas of cognitive functioning (verbal and nonverbal) academic achievement, and interest with psychological, educational, and vocational implications
Comments: yields grade, percentile, and age scores; cluster scores and part scores also available; evaluation of reasoning skills (e.g., concept formation and analysis-synthesis subtests) and of new learning skills (visual-auditory learning subtest) is very useful for head injured students; can be used to monitor performance from preschool through adulthood; can compare achievement and aptitude against the same population

Detroit Tests of Learning Aptitude[56] (DTLA-2)
Age range: 6–17 years
Content areas: variety of intellectual abilities in linguistic, cognitive, attentional, and motoric domains
Comments: revised form of the original DTLA; improved statistical foundation, including standard scores for each age; useful for determining strengths and weaknesses among an individual's intellectual abilities; can help to identify students needing special education placement; useful assessment of attention/concentration, short and long-term memory, expressive organization, nonverbal reasoning, and problem solving; directions may be wordy

Key Math Diagnostic Arithmetic Test[57]
Age range: grades K–9
Content areas: variety of processing abilities in academic areas related to mathematics
Comments: yields grade equivalent scores; provides criterion-referenced information for instructional programming; combines mathematics and language skills; requires integrative abilities; useful assessment of organizational and problem-solving abilities in head injured students

Gates-McKillop Reading Tests[58]
Age range: grades 1–12
Content areas: word-calling/decoding abilities; vocabulary knowledge; oral spelling
Comments: yields grade norms and ratings of skills; norm population not described; reading comprehension *not* evaluated; oral spelling scores useful for students with visual or fine-motor impairments.

Inventory of Basic Skills[59]
Age range: grades K–6
Content areas: wide variety of cognitive and academic skills
Comments: criterion referenced; provides supplementary information that is useful for defining instructional objectives for individual students and for measuring performance in specific areas; *Comprehensive Inventory of Basic Skills[60]* (grades K–9) and *Inventory of Essential Skills[61]* (secondary classrooms) provide additional criterion-referenced assessment materials that are useful in developing instructional programs

some degree for deficits that are common following head injury. These unintended compensations include the following:

☐ The controlled and distraction-free testing environment may compensate for attentional impairments

☐ The use of short tasks and relatively brief testing sessions may compensate for reduced endurance, persistence, and attention span

☐ The use of very clear test instructions and examples may compensate for weak task orientation and impaired flexibility in shifting from one type of task to another

☐ The use of highly structured tasks and clear instructions may compensate for a general lack of initiation and spontaneous problem solving

☐ Test items that do not include real-life *amounts* of information to be processed or *rate* of delivery may compensate for weak integration of information and generally reduced efficiency of information processing

☐ The use of tests that do not require the storage and retrieval of information from day to day (or longer periods) may compensate for learning impairments

☐ Tests that measure *pretraumatically* acquired knowledge or skills may generate false optimism with regard to new learning

☐ The encouraging interaction style of a

skilled examiner may compensate for the child's inability to cope with interpersonal stress or the perception of demands

Following head injury, performance often varies with the setting, the familiarity and interest level of a task, and the people in the environment. Exploration of variables such as these requires going beyond strictly formal assessment.

In addition to the possible sources of inflated results listed here, formal tests generally lack procedures for eliciting and describing the strategies that a patient spontaneously uses to accomplish a task, or for measuring the effects of various suggested strategic procedures on performance of a task. These issues are important in planning therapy or special education.

ROLE OF INFORMAL ASSESSMENT

Given the variability in functioning from setting to setting and from task to task that is common in head injured children, observing the child in a variety of settings, and obtaining information from family members, nursing staff, and teachers are essential components of the assessment. This is particularly true of children whose responsiveness is limited, who remain somewhat confused, or who continue to have significant processing impairments. Family members may see the child's optimal functioning in a familiar environment with familiar activities. In addition, family members often have occasion to observe and document impaired functioning in areas that are difficult to measure formally (e.g., practical problem solving, orientation to established routines, initiation and inhibition, appropriateness of social interaction, safety and social judgment, endurance, and persistence).

It is useful to give observation forms to parents (and to nursing staff in the case of inpatients) so that they can systematically collect information on selected aspects of cognitive functioning, for example: (1) how attention and concentration vary with factors such as time of day, type of activity, familiarity of the activity, person, level of distractions in the environment, instructions, and incentives; (2) at what level of complexity performance of activities of daily living (ADLs) breaks down; (3) how many tri-

als the child needs in order to learn new routines or routes; (4) how much and what type of cueing the child needs to accomplish routine tasks; (5) how the child responds to stress, including requests to hurry, tasks that are demanding, and a busy environment; (6) how spontaneous and effective the child is in social interaction and practical problem solving.

Including parents (or nursing staff) in the assessment of these aspects of cognitive functioning also contributes to their education in the effects of head injury and helps them to feel part of the rehabilitation team. This lays the foundation for their important role in treatment.

Exploring Cognitive Functioning: Hypothesis Testing and Diagnostic Therapy

Many questions are not answered until treatment or classroom instruction is begun. These include questions about the child's learning rate and style, factors that influence learning (including environment, types of tasks, behavior management systems, and compensatory strategies), relative contributions of various cognitive impairments to functional problems, and the effectiveness of alternative types of intervention. Treatment, especially in the initial stages, includes a series of experiments designed to define the child's cognitive problems as precisely as possible and to isolate the most effective approach to rehabilitation.

The appendix to this chapter presents a set of probes that are useful in answering these questions. The probes are listed in a conceptual framework that includes general categories of cognitive processes and systems and important assessment questions within each category. The cognitive framework defined by the categories and questions is not intended to suggest a model of cognitive functioning or a theory of cognition. Rather, the framework is designed to *organize* descriptions of cognitive functioning, to promote *complete* descriptions, to *integrate* assessment findings from a number of professionals who might not otherwise speak a mutually understandable language, and to focus attention on the *functional* dimensions of cognitive weakness. The general categories of cognition that we use are

1. **Component Processes:** attentional processes, perceptual processes, memory/learning processes, organizing processes, reasoning/problem-solving processes

2. **Component Systems:** working memory, long-term memory (knowledge base), executive system, and response system

3. **Functional-Integrative Performance:** including the performance variables efficiency, scope, manner, and level

Elsewhere, we have discussed these categories in some detail.[63]

The use of *questions* in the table is designed to promote active *detective work* or *hypothesis testing* on the part of all professionals who work with head injured children. The hallmark of a competent evaluator, given the goal of rehabilitation planning, is knowing what questions to ask and various ways to answer those questions. Rehabilitation-relevant assessment in this sense is ongoing as long as the child continues to receive rehabilitation or special education services.

The assessment probes listed in the appendix were organized by individuals representing the rehabilitation professions most intimately interested in cognitive rehabilitation: neuropsychology, special education, speech-language pathology, and occupational therapy. Because the focus is cognition, the grouping of tasks may not be familiar to some clinicians. Speech-language pathologists, for example, will find probes related to language functioning spread throughout the table. This is appropriate, given the goal of isolating and describing those skills and deficits that have a cognitive basis.

The probes themselves are simply illustrations of tasks (or in some cases interview questions) that are useful in answering important assessment questions. In some cases, we have included formal tests as appropriate probes. Tests such as the Stanford-Binet Intelligence Scale[64] include tasks that are extremely useful for probing cognitive functioning. In most cases, however, the probes are tasks that are not standardized or norm referenced and hence can be modified as needed to answer specific questions about the functioning of an individual child. However, because of the absence of standardization and of normative information, it is essential that clinicians *not* use these tasks to document the existence of a problem or to diagnose a specific cognitive disorder or type of brain damage. This is not the purpose of these probes. Even in using the probes appropriately—as tools in the investigative work that is needed to fine-tune treatment and to assess in functional terms the effects of treatment—it is important for clinicians and teachers to have a thorough understanding of normal cognitive development and a sensitivity to the normal variability in performance of tasks that are used to probe the cognitive functioning of a brain damaged child. In probing organizing processes, for example, we recommend having the child explain a favorite game to a person who knows nothing about the game. This is a demanding yet practical organizational task and often reveals very good or very weak organizational abilities. However, normally developing children and adolescents often give superficial or poorly organized descriptions of games. Therefore, results must be interpreted cautiously. Often, only relatively extreme results of probes—positive or negative—have interpretable significance. The practical value of probe tasks, as well as tests, is largely a function of the amount and variety of experience that the clinician has with the task with normally developing as well as handicapped children.

The cognitive processes and systems outlined in the appendix constitute a broad operational definition of cognitive functioning. Nevertheless, descriptions of a child's component processes and systems may not, taken together, yield an accurate or complete description of the child's performance of demanding functional tasks (that require the efficient integration of many processes and systems) in unstructured settings. Observation of functional-integrative behavior in natural contexts is both the beginning and the end of cognitive assessment. Assessment *begins* with such observations because exploration of component processes and systems is largely for purposes of discovering why performance of functional-integrative behavior in real-life contexts is less effective than it should be. Assessment *ends* with such observations because the effectiveness of cognitive intervention must ultimately be measured against real-life criteria.

We have found it important to track four broad dimensions of functional-integrative behavior that cut across cognitive processes and systems.

1. **Efficiency** (including the *amount* of work accomplished and *time* required, holding quality constant). Efficiency can be probed in a number of ways, for instance, holding all else constant, by systematically increasing the *amount* of information to be processed (or work to be accomplished) and observing the rate of decline in performance; or by systematically increasing the *rate* at which information must be processed (e.g., compare timed versus untimed performance) and observing the rate of decline in performance. Input and output channels can be systematically varied.

2. **Scope.** Scope of performance includes the variety of settings in which effective functional performance can be maintained. Probes involve comparing the child's performance of functional-integrative tasks in simple and structured settings with performance in complex and unstructured settings; one-on-one versus group; familiar versus unfamiliar settings; with familiar people versus strangers. Generalization of newly learned skills should be carefully tracked from the context of learning to other functional settings.

3. **Level.** Determine at what levels (academic level, language level, general developmental level) the child can maintain functional performance.

4. **Manner.** Manner refers to the characteristic way in which the child performs a task. Probes involve observing the child and noting characteristics of behavior along the following dimensions: impulsive versus reflective; rigid versus flexible; dependent (needing cues) versus independent; passive versus active; and egocentric versus nonegocentric.

Each probe in the appendix is classified as being relevant to the early childhood (roughly ages 2 to 5 years), middle childhood (roughly ages 6 to 11 years), and/or adolescent (roughly ages 12 to 18 years) phase of development. Many aspects of cog-

nitive development exist on a continuum and cannot readily be divided into stages.[65] An individual child's cognitive development is dynamic and is influenced by a large number of factors. Nevertheless, the overall differences in functioning among preschoolers, grade school–age children, and older children are well recognized in research and also in educational systems and practices. Table 37–2 describes key aspects of cognitive development at each of the three age ranges. These global bench marks of cognitive development can serve as guides to the selection or construction of probe tasks and to the interpretation of results. Thus, for example, verbal probes appropriate for school-age children or adolescents can often be turned into preschool probes by using real objects and by framing the task in a context that is action based and meaningful for the young child. It must be remembered, however, that there is a wide range of performance in each of the age groupings and that the level of a child's cognitive behavior may vary with the task, depending on the child's familiarity, task-specific knowledge, motivation, and other factors. Furthermore, many children who have the potential to function at a given cognitive level fail to do so for environmental reasons. Flavell,[66] Kail,[67] and Siegler[65] all present very useful general descriptions of cognitive development.

Introduction of Formal Assessment in the Sequence of Recovery

Assessment of cognitive functioning based on structured observation and probes begins when the child is admitted to the rehabilitation facility or unit, regardless of the level of cognitive functioning. Behavioral checklists or guided observation forms are useful for nurses and stimulation team members to track responsiveness and changes early in recovery.

As the child becomes more alert but remains significantly confused, the administration of selected tests or portions of tests may be indicated, but only if (1) the degree of confusion would not completely invalidate results of the test and (2) the results would have implications for how the patient

**Table 37–2. IMPORTANT ASPECTS OF COGNITIVE
DEVELOPMENT**

Attention/Perception

E: Attentional focus is on surface information, salient features, or the present state of the event; inspection is incomplete; gaze is interrupted by salient features and selected features are searched repeatedly

M: Child can perceive a growing number of features of objects and events; focus is on relevant information, not necessarily salient perceptual attribute; can take alternative perspectives; growing control over attentional and perceptual processes

A: Increasingly, attention is directed to whatever features the task demands; scanning is systematic; attentional and perceptual processes can be self-regulated according to the individual's long-term goals

Memory/Learning

E: Performance is largely a function of the situation; motives and activity play a major role in recall; memory in a practical activity is superior even to memory in play; limited and slow search for target information; strategies rarely used in memory tasks, occasionally in "real" situations (e.g., paying special attention to objects that they will have to gather for an activity); limited ability to assess own recall readiness and to focus learning efforts on only that information that is not already known

M: Performance is less a function of the situation; will maintain a search of memory and searching is faster; uses strategies such as rehearsal; begins to use a study strategy, given external cues

A: Can use retrieval strategies and maintain extended search of memory; can use study strategies effectively (e.g., elaboration; topic sentences in note taking); may modify material during rehearsal to enhance recall; deliberately eliminates trivial information in order to focus on essential information; differentiates known from unknown information and concentrates on the latter in studying

Organization

E: Preference for "familiar event" or episodic organizational schemes rather than those based on hierarchical semantic categories

M: Hierarchical semantic organization (e.g., superordinate categories) becomes well established; recalls well organized text better than poorly organized text, but cannot identify the cause of the improved recall or actively reorganize a text to improve recall

A: Can impose organization on random text; can reorganize text; is aware that improved organization enhances recall

Reasoning

E: One-to-one correspondence and number conservation develop, but child relies on counting rather than observation and understanding of the transformation made; limited understanding of cause and effect, may rely on contiguity to determine cause

M: Growing facility with operations on numbers; steadily improving measuring skills; can perform mental operations such as rotating images and can represent transformations that have been made; problem solving progresses from simple trial and error to concrete experimentation

A: Thinks hypothetically—can consider relations between possible events; can solve problems in a hypotheticodeductive manner (i.e., project consequences of possible solutions and accept or reject the solution on the basis of those projections); understands abstract concepts; can reason deductively, using rules of logical reasoning, regardless of the truth of the statements involved

Working Memory

E: Limited functional "space" in working memory which limits the possibility of rehearsal

M: Memory span of about 6 units; makes possible more rehearsal

A: Working memory of 7($+/-2$) units; functional capacity greatly enhanced by active organizational abilities ("chunking")

Knowledge Base

The knowledge base grows steadily throughout childhood with consequent improvements in the ability to organize information, process quickly, interpret accurately, and solve problems efficiently

Executive System

E: Early developments in executive system include seeking aid and asking questions, inhibiting impulses in response to instruction (e.g., during "quiet time"), planning activities (e.g., bringing coat, hat, and mittens before asking to go outside), and using different communicative styles with different types of communication partner; the preschool child has little metacognitive awareness of cognitive processes, but begins to understand mental terms such as "know," "understand," "remember," "forget," and so on; the limited development of the executive system is evidenced by impulsivity, disinhibition, egocentrism, here-and-now orientation, and low frustration tolerance

M: Growing metacognitive awareness; can suggest ways to remember more effectively, including internal mnemonics; understands the effects of delay on memory; growing decentration; can take alterna-

Table 37–2. *(Continued)*

tive perspectives; steadily growing behavioral self-control and inhibition; growing ability to set long-term goals and work toward them
    A: With some encouragement and guidance, can reflect on own behavior, thinking, learning style, etc.; can recognize and compensate for cognitive weaknesses; can deliberate about long-term goals and formulate complex plans for achieving goals; can monitor and evaluate own cognitive performance

E = early childhood (roughly 2–5 years)
M = middle childhood (roughly 6–11 years)
A = adolescence (roughly 12–18 years)

is treated. The Peabody Picture Vocabulary Test,[68] for example, is easy to administer, does not place a significant demand on the child's processing abilities, and yields information about receptive language that makes a difference in how the rehabilitation team interacts with the patient.

Administration of a comprehensive formal assessment should not occur until the following conditions are met:

1. The child's ability to follow directions and remain appropriately oriented to a task is not so compromised that interpretation of results is impossible
2. The child's attention span is adequate for valid administration of selected tests (at least 20 minutes)
3. The child is not in a stage of rapid recovery

If a comprehensive assessment is administered during a period of rapid cognitive recovery, the results will lack rehabilitation implications. During this period, brief screening instruments and informal probes can be used to identify the patient's strengths and weaknesses for purposes of planning treatment.

Interpreting Test Results

Head injured children often have pockets of intact abilities that easily lead to mistaken inferences about their anticipated success in a demanding classroom or social situation. For example, reading (decoding) skills may be relatively intact despite significant difficulty with reading comprehension; or comprehension at the sentence or short paragraph level may be adequate despite an inability to integrate and comprehend the amount of information presented in stan-

dard reading assignments that are several pages long.[69, 70] Similarly, computational skills may be adequate despite an inability to apply those skills in the context of word problems or other functional mathematics activities. A child may be well oriented and exhibit good safety and social judgment in a sheltered hospital, school, or home setting but be quite unsafe under conditions that are unfamiliar or stressful.

The ways in which the conditions of formal testing may compensate for commonly observed cognitive problems in head injured children may result in optimal performance on testing that is far superior to habitual performance in a demanding classroom. On the other hand, it is possible that a head injured student will perform surprisingly well in the classroom, given the familiarity of the setting and materials relative to the unfamiliar setting and tasks of formal assessment. Therefore, in making judgments about academic placement and needed intervention, there is no substitute for diagnostic therapy and prescriptive teaching, with careful monitoring of the child's response to instruction in a natural setting.

Predicting long-term outcome and academic success is equally difficult. To date, no studies of head injured children have documented the predictive validity of early psychologic, educational, or related measures in relation to long-term outcome—academic progress or vocational adjustment. In many cases, head injured children have a premorbid history of learning difficulties or behavioral problems. The complex interaction of these phenomena with normal developmental problems and traumatic brain damage renders prediction especially hazardous. Our own experience[9] as well as that of others[8] indicates that normal or even above average IQ scores often accompany a below average rate and level of learning (based on academic achievement tests).

These considerations necessitate a careful and appropriately qualified interpretation of test results for family members and for school personnel who lack experience with head injuries in children. Test results, particularly IQ scores and grade levels, can have a powerful impact on family members and on patients themselves. It is the obligation of professionals to clarify for family members the often confusing scatter of abilities that typically accompanies traumatic brain injury and to support the need for special services to strengthen weak areas of functioning while at the same time modulating the report and recommendations to fit the family member's own stage of response to the injury.

Special Considerations in the Assessment of Preschoolers

A set of interesting problems is encountered in the assessment of cognitive functioning in children in the 2-to-5-year range. First, the absence of reliable pretraumatic levels of functioning renders it particularly difficult to establish which aspects of the child's current functioning, if any, are a result of the injury. Careful interviewing of parents and examination of whatever preschool records may be available are helpful in establishing possible effects of the injury and in exploring the child's rate and efficiency of new learning.

Second, the wide variability in *normal* development in this age range[3] contributes to the difficulty in identifying effects of the injury and in predicting long-term outcome. Psychologic and related language testing of preschoolers is known to be of questionable predictive validity· even for normally developing children. Because of the variability in normal development, the wide variety of behaviors that are considered normal for preschoolers and the lack of follow-up studies of children injured in the preschool years, it is often difficult to convince parents to accept the need for intervention or careful monitoring of the child's development.

Our experience suggests that preschoolers, like older children, often evidence problems in the areas of attentional control, language processing related to the amount or complexity of information to be processed or to the rate of its delivery, organizational skills, and rate of new learning. These problems, if subtle, may have no functional consequences until the child faces the learning demands of a classroom. For these reasons, preschoolers should be carefully monitored through the early grade school years even if their functioning appears to be within normal limits. Particularly careful monitoring should occur when the child begins formal education to rule out the need for special education or other supportive services.

The most important component of diagnostic assessment of very young children who appear to have experienced nearly complete recovery involves teaching them information, rule-governed activities (e.g., games), or vocabulary that can be assumed to be new for the child, and systematically documenting the child's rate and manner of learning. Diagnostic treatment should also include representational play and social interaction with gradually increasing cognitive and social stress—to detect possible deficits of organization, planning, problem solving, and retrieval that might not be evident in normal interaction or in testing.

SENSORIMOTOR ASSESSMENT

The key to assessment of head injured children for planning functional gross and fine motor rehabilitation is thorough developmental assessment that focuses on the quality of movement and sensorimotor organization. Because developmental changes occur through the interplay of sensory and motor systems,[71, 72] it is not possible to neatly separate those systems in assessment. The extent of control over movement, the quality of those movements, and how the control is modified and augmented through therapeutic intervention form the foundation for the development of mature functional abilities following head injury.

Developmental assessment identifies the components of movement,[73] which are prerequisites for acquiring those functional skills (e.g., dressing, walking, self-feeding) that serve as the goals of rehabilitation. The use of a developmental framework allows clinicians to focus on the primary problems that interfere with further development, thereby providing a starting point for treatment and a systematic ordering of treatment objectives. Targeting and thoroughly developing the underlying components of movement patterns ultimately enables the child to use those components in a *variety* of functional activities and as a base for further development. In addition to identifying impaired components of movement, assessment establishes the necessary baselines against which to measure progress.

In contrast to the developmental sensorimotor impairments of a child with prenatal or perinatal neurologic insult, head injured children experience a sudden disorganization of a previously intact sensorimotor system and the disruption of functional abilities that were to some degree established before the injury. Since the process of reacquisition of previously acquired abilities differs from that of acquiring new skills, assessment must take into account pretraumatic development as well as post-traumatic skills and deficits. There may also be scattered sparing of functions following diffuse brain damage, further distinguishing the assessment and treatment of head injured children from that of children delayed from birth.

The child's age at the time of injury and at the time of assessment influences motor assessment in several ways. Children's bones are malleable and respond differently to stress than do those of adults.[74] If the child is in a period of rapid growth, tight muscles can become further shortened, abnormal muscle activity can change the shape of growing bones, and decreased weight-bearing can inhibit growth. Furthermore, growth both changes the child's center of gravity,[75] which can exaggerate balance problems, and increases the effort required to move against gravity, which can exaggerate abnormal patterns of movement.

Each phase of childhood entails a unique focus in assessment. Children who are injured in infancy lack a foundation of previously acquired motor skills. Therefore, their assessment and treatment closely resemble those of children with congenital neurologic disorders. The preschool years are a time of refinement of gross and fine motor skills. Consequently, the focus following head injury is not merely on reacquiring lost skills, but also on further re-

finement. Assessment of school-age children must highlight functional academic skills (e.g., writing) and equipment or adaptations needed for academic success. Adolescents, similar to adults in motor functioning, are in a phase of social self-consciousness that necessitates a focus in assessment on identifying ways to achieve maximum independence with a minimum of stigma or self-perceived "differentness." Motor assessment must also include a careful evaluation of the family's ability and willingness to be an integral member of the treatment team and of their training needs. Finally, for many severely injured children, adaptive equipment (e.g., adaptive seating, power mobility, communication aids, environmental controls) may have a powerful impact on functional abilities and therefore requires careful evaluation.[76]

Assessment Parameters

Functional motor control and the quality of motor performance are based on sensorimotor components that must be individually analyzed for their effect on motor control. This assessment is based largely on careful observation of the patient during functional activities and therapeutic handling. Parameters to be evaluated are

- ☐ Range of motion
- ☐ Muscle tone
- ☐ Muscle strength
- ☐ Reflexes
- ☐ Sensation (including visual, auditory, tactile, and vestibular sensation, proprioception, and kinesthesia)
- ☐ Posture
- ☐ Postural reflex mechanisms (righting, equilibrium, and protective reactions)
- ☐ Motor planning (praxis)

Each of these parameters will be discussed separately, although their separation is to some degree artificial. Following assessment of each area, their integration into functional abilities is evaluated and the impact of each on motor control is analyzed. Assessment of functional abilities occurs in the areas of gross motor skills (e.g., walking, transferring), fine motor skills (e.g., manipulating materials, writing), and activities of daily living (e.g., dressing, grooming).

RANGE OF MOTION

Assessing the motor system includes determining the range of joints as well as soft tissue (e.g., hamstring length and isolated hip and knee range). Trunk mobility should be assessed in flexion, extension, and rotation. Limitations in range of motion may be due to soft tissue contractures, spasticity, capsular adhesions, fractures with internal fixation, or heterotopic ossification. Range of motion measures provide baselines for treatment and indicate positioning, splinting, or casting requirements.[77] In addition, assessing range of motion enables clinicians to observe tonal influences in resistance to completing the range and to determine the effect of range of motion on limitations of active movement.

Clinicians should use only slow, gentle movements in assessing range of motion, particularly if muscle tone is high. Movement synergies (e.g., scapulohumeral rhythm) are considered during this assessment, as is the effect of position on range of motion. Care must be taken if there is suspicion of fractures, bone decalcification, or heterotopic ossification. Interpretation of results should not be based on adult norms, since children's joint ranges vary relative to adult standards due to developmental biomechanical factors.[78]

MUSCLE TONE

Normal muscle tone (slight continuous contraction of a muscle) is necessary to maintain posture and enable movement against gravity.[79] Abnormal muscle tone limits movement potential or leads to abnormal movement patterns. High tone limits active movement, may reduce passive range of motion, and may lead to contractures; low tone inadequately supports movement against gravity; fluctuating tone reduces stability and gradation of movements needed for control.

Assessment of muscle tone includes (1) observing the effects of position changes and movement on tone; (2) feeling the muscle at rest and during movement, comparing tone throughout the body; and (3) treating the child to determine the effects of therapeutic handling on tone. Throughout this assessment, it is essential to evaluate the effects of abnormal tone on active movement.

Since muscle tone in head injured children can vary significantly with the level of arousal, agitation, lability, or medication, it is important to make several observations. It is also valuable to acquire detailed information regarding pretraumatic status, including photographs or videos of the child, if available, since there is some variability in muscle tone among normally developing children.

REFLEXES

Following severe head injury, developmentally primitive reflexes may reemerge as a result of neural disinhibition.[80] These include the symmetrical and asymmetrical tonic neck reflexes, the tonic labrynthine reflex, positive support reflex, Babinski's reflex, Galant's reflex, startle reflex, flexor withdrawal reflex, grasp reflex (plantar and palmar), and stepping reflex. Assessment should focus on the influence of primitive reflexes on tone and movement rather than on the reflex in isolation.[79] This enables therapists to plan positioning and treatment to decrease the effects of the reflexes and thus to allow mature patterns of movement to emerge. Interpretation of reflex testing in head injured *infants* must be guided by the normal developmental timetable for the integration of specific reflexes.

MUSCLE STRENGTH

Manual testing of muscle strength has several limitations with head injured children. The testing procedure is not applicable to infants or children with major cognitive limitations, norms are not available for all age ranges, and grading of strength is difficult with young children. Following head injury, strength may be reduced as a result of prolonged inactivity or orthopedic injury. Standard procedures for testing muscle strength can be found in Kendall and McCreary.[81]

SENSATION

In addition to visual and auditory assessment (discussed later in this chapter), it is important to assess vestibular functioning and tactile sensation, proprioception, and kinesthesia.[82]

Vestibular Sensation. Clinical observation that focuses on vestibular functioning and its effects on sensorimotor skills yields information useful for positioning and treatment. Because of the frequently lowered seizure threshold following head injury, tests of postrotary nystagmus[83] are not advised. The following observations should be included in the assessment of the vestibular system: body orientation in space; the child's response to movement; postural reactions, including righting (with and without vision occluded), equilibrium, and protective responses; postural background movements; and oculomotor control, including the presence or absence of nystagmus.

Tactile Sensation. The response to tactile stimulation as well as tactile discrimination should be assessed, if possible.[79] Very young or cognitively impaired children can be evaluated by methodically and incrementally introducing a stimulus (e.g., deep touch, pressure, pain, or temperature) and observing the child's response. Discriminating touch (e.g., 1–2 point, sharp/dull, stereognosis) can be assessed with higher functioning children.

Proprioception/Kinesthesia. Proprioception (the awareness of joint position) and kinesthesia (the awareness of joint movement) are both important in the assessment of posture and movement, and are closely linked to vestibular function. In the case of patients with the necessary cognitive and motor skills, proprioception and kinesthesia can be assessed by having these individuals copy the position or movement of one limb with the opposite limb (vision occluded). In other cases, assessment of proprioception and kinesthesia can be based on observations like the following: Does the patient seem aware of his or her posture and maintain it? Does the patient correct his or her posture only when given visual feedback? Does he or she neglect a limb or side of the body (e.g., allow an arm to dangle in the spokes of the wheelchair)? Does the patient need to visually monitor fine movements? Does the patient have difficulty placing a limb when it is out of his or her visual field (e.g., placing a foot while walking)?

POSTURE

Assessment of posture presupposes an understanding of normal posture, which is maintained by means of vestibular, tactile,

proprioceptive, and visual feedback. Pediatric assessment additionally presupposes a knowledge of developmental norms, including developmental differences in bone structure and the biomechanics of postural adjustments. For example, the use of abdominal muscles and the position of the pelvis during maintenance of posture is quite different in toddlers versus young school-age children versus adolescents.[84] An adult-like gait pattern is not achieved until age 7.[85, 86]

Tools for assessing posture include the use of a plumb line and a postural grid. More subjective, but functionally useful, methods include careful observation of the child's alignment, possible asymmetries, trunk and head position, and base of support. Since posture is of primary importance as a stable base from which to move, it is critical to observe postural adjustments during movement or when the child is passively moved. It is also important to determine whether the child's posture is maintained automatically or deliberately. This is accomplished by comparing posture when the child is attending to a task and when he or she is attending to posture only.

POSTURAL REFLEX MECHANISMS

Balance is maintained by means of postural reflex mechanisms.[80] Assessment of these responses in head injured children assumes an understanding of their acquisition in normal development.[73] The responses should be assessed through transitions to all applicable developmental positions: prone, supine, quadruped, sitting, kneeling, and standing. Assessment is based on careful observation of the child's responses and postural realignment following displacement of either the child or the surface. These responses are elicited by tactile, proprioceptive, vestibular, and visual stimulation.

There are two postural reflex mechanisms to be assessed:

1. **Righting Reactions:** These responses support the maintenance of posture and alignment when the body's center of gravity is displaced within the base of support. Righting reactions serve to maintain head and trunk orientation in relation to gravity, to the surface, and to each other. Righting responses are generally in straight planes of movement.

2. **Equilibrium Reactions:** These responses support the maintenance of posture when the body's center of gravity is displaced outside the base of support. Equilibrium reactions serve to recover a stable base and to prevent falling. Responses include diagonal and rotary movements and involve the extremities as well as the head and trunk. In addition, *protective responses* should be assessed. These responses, which include protective extension of the upper extremities and protective stepping of the lower extremities, enable individuals to catch themselves when righting and equilibrium reactions are insufficient to maintain balance.[87]

MOTOR PLANNING (PRAXIS)

Motor planning, or praxis, is the purposeful and goal-directed, yet automatic, initiation and performance of an efficient and effective sequence of movements. Adequate motor planning entails the ability to conceptualize, organize, and execute a sequence of unfamiliar actions.[88] Assessment of motor planning is based on careful observation of movement transitions (e.g., moving from lying to sitting) and on a comparison of performance between familiar and unfamiliar tasks. Motor planning may also be assessed with the *Southern California Sensory Integration Test.*[89]

The results of an isolated test must, however, be interpreted cautiously. Judgments of a child's motor planning skill must be related to more general cognitive skills, including attention, organization, initiation, and memory.

Functional Integration

Following assessment of these sensorimotor components, their integration within functional motor activities is assessed. The goals of assessment are to determine the influence of abnormal muscle tone, reflexes, or sensation on active movement and to describe the quality of that movement or the way in which it is performed, rather than merely noting that a motor skill has been acquired. This involves observation of the child in a large number of motor activities, as well as settings, that are developmentally appropriate and important for that child. In the case of each observation, it is essential to determine *how* the child performs the activity (the quality of skills), the speed and coordination of performance, and the specific reason for difficulty if normal functioning is not observed. If, for example, a child is unable to stand to transfer, it is important to know if the cause is limited range of motion, hypertonicity or hypotonicity, or impaired motor control. Finally, it is necessary to determine if performance of functional activities exacerbates abnormal tone or motor patterns.

Gross Motor Abilities. With the aforementioned considerations in mind, the following questions should be answered: Can the child move away from mid-line and retain his or her balance? Can the patient lose control of center of gravity and regain it? Can the patient move in and out of positions? Can he or she take weight on arms and legs? Can the patient stabilize proximally with a decreasing base of support? What transitional movements are present: Can the patient roll in both directions? Move to sitting over both sides of the body? Assume all fours? Move to kneeling and up to standing? Move from sitting to standing? How does the patient move around the environment? Can he or she creep? Crawl? Walk? Does the patient require assistance or devices for walking? Do orthotic devices, if present, correct or mask a problem? Can the child transfer to and from bed? Wheelchair (or adapted tricycle)? Toilet seat? Shower chair? Bathtub? What equipment is needed to promote more effective and independent gross motor activity?

Fine Motor Abilities. The following questions should be answered: Is the child's reach graded and directed? Can he or she cross mid-line? Is the patient's grasp graded and functional for handling a variety of shapes and sizes of objects? Does he or she demonstrate isolated finger control in activities such as pointing, finger plays, or typing? Can the patient manually manipulate objects and accurately release them? Are speed and coordination adequate for tasks like writing, buttoning, and bouncing and catching a ball? Is bilateral coordination adequate during symmetrical and reciprocal activities such as unscrewing a toothpaste lid or scissoring? What is the child's hand dominance (pretrauma and post-trauma)? Is there spontaneous use of the nondominant hand as an assist? Since functional fine motor skills are closely related to both visual perceptual and cognitive abilities, exploration of fine motor functioning should include the detective work described in the cognitive assessment section of this chapter. Reduced writing speed, for example, may be the result of motor incoordination, impaired visual, perceptual or visual-motor functioning, fluctuating attention, confusion regarding the task, or impaired academic skills.

Activities of Daily Living. The following questions should be answered: Can the child self-feed, dress, groom, and toilet? Is the child as independent and safe in the community as is appropriate for age and background? Can he or she cook and prepare meals (if age-appropriate)? Is the patient as independent and effective in play or other leisure activities as is appropriate for age and background? Coley[90] presents a developmental sequence of self-care skills and their developmental prerequisites.

Since the performance of activities of daily living is the cognitively and socially based application of available motor skills, each activity should be analyzed in terms of several variables.

1. **Motoric Considerations:** Does the child have adequate control, balance, strength, and endurance for the task?

2. **Attention:** Are attention span and selective attention adequate for the task? Should the environment be free of distractions?

3. **Perception:** Are figure-ground mechanisms adequate for the child to find an item in a store or pick out socks from a drawer? Can he or she identify the front and back of a shirt?

4. **Memory:** Does the child remember how to do an activity such as tying shoes? Can the child retain instructions? Does he or she need cueing for each step?

5. **Organization:** Can the child sequence the steps of a task such as dressing? Can he assemble the materials necessary for a task such as making a sandwich?

6. **Problem Solving/Judgment:** If problems arise or the circumstances are not familiar, can the child act effectively? Is he or she safe unsupervised in a kitchen or on a playground?

7. **Initiation:** Does the child engage in appropriate ADLs without prompting or cueing?

8. **Efficiency:** Can the child complete tasks in a reasonable amount of time? At what level of complexity can he or she work?

Formal and Informal Assessment

For the most part, the assessment procedures just discussed are informal, that is, not part of a standardized test or battery of tests. There are several reasons for this emphasis on informal procedures. Most standardized tests of motor development rely on motor milestones. An assessment that is relevant to planning a program of rehabilitation, in contrast, must identify, through careful analysis that is not part of standardized testing procedures, the quality of movements and the sensorimotor components that are missing or impaired in abnormally performed motor activities. Treatment based solely on an inventory of motor milestones easily deteriorates into the training of splinter skills that do not effectively serve long-term motor development. Furthermore, assessment as we described it is an ongoing process that continues throughout treatment. Not only should the effects of intervention be actively monitored in therapy sessions, but also carryover to other activities and more natural environments must be probed. The types of assessment tasks described here are well suited to this ongoing diagnostic treatment process.

Standardized tests do, however, serve a number of purposes. They help clinicians to organize their assessment. For those clinicians not familiar with a pediatric population, tests direct attention to those behaviors and skills that are important at specific ages. Norm-referenced tests provide valuable normative information that may, for example, be useful in decisions regarding school placement. Finally, tests can yield useful baseline information against which to measure progress.[91] Informal assessment procedures can also be made relatively objective by using serial videotaping of target behaviors. These videos can then be used for feedback or motivational purposes with patients or their families.

With these caveats in mind, we present in Table 37–3 brief descriptions of selected standardized motor assessments. None of these tests has been developed for or validated on a population of head injured children. Indeed, several of the tests presuppose

levels of attentional, language, and memory ability that make the tests unrealistic for many head injured children.

REHABILITATIVE MEDICAL ASSESSMENT

The importance of thorough medical assessment during the rehabilitation phase of

Table 37–3. SELECTED TESTS OF MOTOR DEVELOPMENT

Brigance Diagnostic Inventory of Early Development[92]
Age range: birth to 6 years
Content areas: preambulatory motor skills; gross motor skills; fine motor skills; prespeech, speech, and language skills; general knowledge, reading, writing, math
Comments: not standardized, but field-tested and norm-referenced; provides performance records expressed in developmental ages; provides guides to writing objectives; does not address quality of movement in test items, but does break components of skills into testable units

Developmental Programming for Infants and Young Children[93]
Age range: birth to 6 years
Content areas: cognitive skills, motor skills, sensorimotor skills, language skills, social growth
Comments: not standardized; concurrent validity established with other assessment tools; scores can be converted to developmental levels; separate volumes for infants and young children; includes stimulation activities useful for head injured children; describes the quality of responses and how to modify the items for use with motorically impaired children

Erhardt Developmental Prehension Assessments[94]
Age range: birth to 6 years
Content areas: fine motor skills, including involuntary arm and hand patterns and cognitively directed prewriting skills
Comments: not standardized; provides developmental norms; can be used to sequence developmental skills; provides guidance on moving from assessment to treatment

Vulpe Assessment Battery[95]
Age range: birth to 6 years
Content areas: Basic senses and functions, gross motor skills, fine motor skills, language skills, cognitive skills, organizational skills, assessment of environment
Comments: not standardized, yields developmental levels in the form of a narrative report rather than a score; provides guidance in analyzing the interaction among developmental skills; some description of the quality of responses; the "organization behaviors" and "basic senses and functions" sections are particularly applicable to head injured children

Purdue Perceptual-Motor Survey[96]
Age range: 6 to 10 years
Content areas: balance and postural flexibility; gross motor skills; perceptual-motor match; ocular control; form perception
Comments: standardized; primarily useful with mildly to moderately involved patients; designed to detect perceptual-motor impairments

Bruininks-Oseretsky Test of Motor Proficiency[97]
Age range: 4½–14½ years
Content areas: gross and fine motor skills; running speed and agility; balance; bilateral coordination; strength; upper limb coordination; response speed; upper limb speed and dexterity; visual-motor control
Comments: standardized; primarily useful with mildly to moderately involved children in the assessment of higher-level coordination and balance (although said to be useful for children with severe motor impairments as well); gives information as to residual deficits post-trauma

Jebsen Hand Function Test[98, 99]
Age range: 6 to 19 years
Content areas: fine motor skills; hand function for use in activities of daily living
Comments: standardized, relates speed of performance to age-level group norms

a patient's recovery following severe head injury is underscored by the finding of Kalisky and coworkers[100] that 16 percent of the medical problems found on admission in a series of 180 consecutive admissions of patients with severe head injury to a rehabilitation center (aged 6 to 71 years) were present but not identified in the acute-care setting. An additional 18 percent of the medical difficulties occurred for the first time after admission to the rehabilitation center. Rehabilitative medical assessment of head injured patients—children and adults alike—begins with a comprehensive and detailed history and physical examination that emphasizes the neurologic and neuromuscular systems. There are many respects, however, in which the assessment of children is different from that of adults. In this section we briefly highlight some of these differences.

Somatic Growth

Clearly, somatic growth is a significant factor that affects children and adults differently. Assessment of growth is based on serial measurements of height and weight that are compared to standards for age-appropriate peers.[101, 102] Growth *rate* based on serial assessment is essential because it is an important indicator of a child's overall health status. Previous records of a child's growth are of particular value in assessing endocrine function as well as nutritional status.

Nutritional and Gastrointestinal Problems

A comprehensive nutritional assessment of head injured children involves investigation of the metabolic and physical changes caused by the trauma as well as of nutritional requirements for growth and development.[103–105]

Nutritional assessment of children in a rehabilitation setting should follow specific guidelines for comprehensive metabolic and feeding needs, and includes the following components:

1. **Clinical Findings:** Age; sex; usual weight prior to injury; present level of physical and cognitive activity and emotional status; anthropometric measurements (including height, weight, triceps skin fold, mid-arm circumference, and mid-arm muscle circumference); multiple trauma or other medical conditions (e.g., fractures, decubiti, stress ulcers, gastritis); feeding in acute-care setting (method of delivery, food consistency, amount consumed in 24 hours); present medications; and vitamin and mineral supplements

2. **Laboratory Aides:** Blood count; urinalysis; chemistries for electrolytes, glucose, calcium, creatine, blood urea nitrogen, serum protein (specifically, albumin), occasionally amylase and lipids, and 24-hour urine for nitrogen balance[104, 106]

3. **Physical Problems Related to Fluids and Food:** Ability to suck, swallow, and chew; oral reflexes (e.g., gag, root, suck); fever (including fever of central origin and/or infection); diaphoresis; constipation or diarrhea; spasticity; and gastrointestinal reflux

4. **Food Habits:** Typical day's intake prior to injury; appetite prior to injury and currently; favorite and strongly disliked foods; time of day when most hungry; food allergies; and behavior and attitudes toward eating

Children have larger surface areas than do adults and can become rapidly dehydrated if adequate fluid requirements are not met. Depending on the child's age and size, the metabolic rates are greater than for adults, and children therefore require more calories per kilogram of weight. This is especially true of infants. Children's resting oxygen consumption per unit of body weight is approximately twice that of adults. The child's growth and nutritional status should be monitored closely during and after discharge from rehabilitation. Once a stable anabolic state is achieved, care should be given to provide sufficient calories for adequate growth without causing obesity.[107] Additionally, children presenting with anemia, especially infants, should have serum iron, total iron binding capacity, and ferritin levels obtained in addition to the standard blood count and reticulocyte count, as well as blood testing of stool to look for gastrointestinal bleeding prior to institution of therapy. If vomiting is present, the emesis should also be tested for blood.

A barium esophagram, esophageal manometry, esophageal Ph probe monitoring, gastroesophageal scintiscan, and fiberoptic endoscopic evaluation may be necessary in the assessment of children with gastrointestinal bleeding if prophylactic therapy with histamine H2-receptor antagonist and antacids is not effective.[108–113]

Hypertension

To assess hypertension a blood pressure cuff of the appropriate size must be used, as a cuff that is too narrow can produce falsely elevated readings and one that is too wide may produce readings that are falsely low. Spasticity may also affect the accuracy of the reading by increasing vascular tone. Blood pressure readings in children should be compared with age-appropriate norms before treatment is considered.[114]

In the assessment of patients with multiple trauma, especially to the abdomen and flank area, and of patients who manifest signs of hypercalcemia (because of long-term consequences of kidney stones), care should be taken to rule out kidney injury as a possible cause of hypertension. In such cases, an intravenous pyelogram (IVP) and an indepth urologic workup are indicated.

Genitourinary Problems

Normal developmental factors must be taken into account in assessing and managing bowel and bladder function in very young children with head injury. This necessitates obtaining a thorough history of toilet training and/or enuresis. Urinary incontinence may be a developmental phenomenon, the result of an uninhibited bladder, or detrusor outlet dyssynergia.[115]

Because urinary tract infections are common complications of indwelling catheters, all head injured children admitted to rehabilitation from an acute care setting should have a urinalysis and urine culture performed. Cultures should also be obtained when the child runs a fever without obvious focus or cause for infection. Ideally, all children should be observed for adequacy of stream and for voiding problems, especially males who have had prolonged indwelling catheters. For such children, as well as for those who have frequent urinary tract infections or a history of multiple trauma (especially to the spinal cord or abdomen), an indepth urologic assessment including an IVP, a voiding cystourethrogram (VCUG), and urodynamic studies,[115] should be considered.

Fever and Infection

Assessment of fever in children and in adults is essentially the same process—i.e., to look for the cause of the fever. All children with fever should undergo a complete physical re-examination. Appropriate cultures should be obtained from the throat, urine, blood, spinal fluid, stool, skin, ear, and sinus. Findings can be related to laboratory studies (e.g., blood counts, sedimentation rate, chest and bone radiographs, and computer tomography scans) in order to confirm clinical impressions.

A high index of suspicion can direct the clinician to the most revealing studies with least delay. Middle ear infections, so frequent during early childhood, are easily diagnosed through direct visualization and pneumatic otoscopy. With a basilar or compound fracture or penetrating brain injury, cultures of cerebrospinal fluid (CSF) are mandatory.[116] Computerized tomography (CT) of the cranium can help localize an abscess or exclude hydrocephalus before a lumbar puncture is performed.

Severely head injured children with no physical findings of infection and with multiple negative cultures may have fever of central origin. Since the mechanisms involved in fever due to infection differ from those in fever of central origin, aspirin treatment can assist in differential diagnosis.[117, 118] Fever from an infection process usually responds to aspirin, whereas central fever does not.

Respiratory Problems

Since obstruction of the airway is life threatening, accurate assessment of respiratory functioning and problems is critical. Assessment procedures and techniques vary, depending on the nature and acuteness of the problem. Careful clinical observation of the child, including vital signs, is basic.

Since aspiration and choking are a consideration in head injured children, especially when changes in the feeding regimen are instituted (e.g., the transition from tube to oral feeding), assessment of the adequacy of the swallow, protective cough, and gag reflexes is basic to the therapeutic feeding evaluation. A videofluorographic swallowing study (modified barium swallow), using both thin and thick fluids, should be obtained if aspiration or posterior swallowing disorders are suspected.[119] A chest radiograph, when positive for aspiration pneumonia, can aid in diagnosis. However if it is minimal and absorbed, aspiration can be missed on routine radiography.

Head injured children with tracheostomies present additional problems and require special assessment. Because of their short necks, infants may obstruct their tracheostomy tube simply by flexing their head. Tracheostomy dependency can be assessed at bedside by occluding the tube with the child's own hand or the examiner's finger and observing respiratory effort.[107] In order to prepare for possible complications, such assessment is mandatory before changing the tracheostomy. Studies such as anterior/posterior and lateral radiograms of the neck and chest, pulmonary function studies, and direct bronchoscopy and laryngoscopy aid in the diagnosis of complications of tracheostomy. Children should undergo endoscopic evaluation of the entire airway immediately prior to decanulation, and blood gases should be monitored with the tracheostomy tube plugged. Feeble cry, hoarseness, stridor, brassy cough, and aphonia are all signs of phonatory dysfunction that also merit endoscopy. Children should be reassessed by an ear-nose-throat (ENT) specialist 3 months postdecanulation.

Endocrine Problems

Dysfunction of the posterior pituitary may be expressed as a syndrome of inappropriate secretion of antidiuretic hormone (SIADH) or central diabetes insipidus (DI). Both SIADH and DI may be detected through the routine monitoring of fluid intake, urinary output, body weight, serum sodium concentration, and urine specific gravity or osmolarity. Partial or complete DI may be especially difficult to diagnose. Water deprivation testing with vasopressin supplementation may be needed to evaluate mild abnormalities of antidiuretic hormone.

Anterior pituitary dysfunction is assessed by specific assay of its hormones. Specific age norms must be used in the interpretation of the results when evaluating children. Diurnal variations in hormone release must also be kept in mind especially for growth hormone and ACTH. In addition to basal measurement of anterior pituitary hormone levels, the combined assessment of target-gland status and the investigation of responses of pituitary hormones to the administration of hypothalamic releasing factors as well as other stimulatory tests may be necessary for an indepth assessment of endocrine function. Consultation with a pediatric endocrinology specialist is very often needed.

Assessment of sexual development is an essential component of the physical evaluation. Accurate Tanner staging of children should be done for future reference.[120–122]

Visual Problems

A comprehensive ophthalmologic evaluation of all head injured children should be performed as soon as possible after the injury, with follow-up evaluations scheduled at intervals commensurate with the injury. These evaluations establish baseline visual acuity and document early eye findings so that progress during recovery can be measured. The nature of the evaluation depends on the child's age and level of responsiveness. In infants and very young children, visual acuity is assessed by the fixation response and optikokinetic drum testing. Otherwise, the assessment is similar to that used for adults. Occasionally, the more objective electrophysiologic tests, such as visual evoked potentials (VEP) and electroretinography, may be needed to confirm clinical findings of visual pathway dysfunction.[123] Early assessment and immediate treatment are necessary for globe injuries, hyphema, iris prolapse, subconjunctival blood, blow out fractures, and lacerated extraocular muscles. In these cases, early ophthalmologic consultation is imperative.

Auditory and Vestibular Dysfunction

Children with suspected problems are referred for complete ENT examination, audiologic evaluation, electronystagmography, and brainstem evoked responses as clinically indicated. Brainstem evoked potential measurements have the advantage of being completely objective and not affected by the patient's psychologic state, level of consciousness, or medications. However, in infants (under 2 years of age) the patterns of electrophysiologic response differ from older children and adults and must be interpreted properly.[124, 125] These assessment procedures are described elsewhere in this volume and are similar in adults and children.

Heterotopic Ossification

Serum alkaline phosphatase determinations usually parallel the activity of heterotopic ossification. However, since alkaline phosphatase levels vary according to the phase of normal bone growth, this test may be less useful in children than in adults. Technetium bone scanning is positive earlier than radiography, which may be negative until calcification occurs.[126]

Immobilization Hypercalcemia

Laboratory investigation should include determination of serum calcium and protein levels, phosphate and alkaline phosphate levels (which are age related), and the urinary calcium-to-creatinine ratio. If this ratio is equal to or greater than 0.4:1, then hypercalcemia is likely. Parathormone levels are helpful adjuncts in distinguishing primary hyperparathyroidism from other causes of hypercalcemia.[127]

Seizures

Assessment of seizures in children is essentially the same as in adults—that is, observation of clinical manifestation followed by electroencephalographic (EEG) confirmation. However, the interpretation of the EEG must be done by an experienced pediatric encephalographer, since the unique rhythms of infants and young children may be misinterpreted if adult standards are used.[128] If seizures are suspected but cannot be distinguished from nonconvulsive behavior, then more sophisticated assessment techniques may be indicated, including a 24-hour ambulatory EEG recording and closed circuit prolonged video monitoring with simultaneous EEG recording.[107, 128] Since anticonvulsant medications are known to affect behavior and cognition, children receiving such medication should be closely monitored for side effects.

SUMMARY

Our focus in this chapter has been on issues in pediatric assessment that relate directly to practical management decisions. We have stressed the importance of a developmental perspective and of assessments that highlight functional needs of the child. Finally, we have promoted an interdisciplinary approach to assessment so that fragmentation is avoided and so that the total child stands in sharp relief as the focus of the rehabilitative enterprise.

REFERENCES

1. Cohen, SB et al: Educational programming for head injured students. In Ylvisaker, M (ed): Head Injury Rehabilitation: Children and Adolescents. College-Hill Press, San Diego, 1985, p 383.
2. Miner, ME, Fletcher, JM and Ewing-Cobbs, L: Recovery versus outcome after head injury in children. In Miner, ME and Wagner, KA (eds): Neurotrauma: Treatment, Rehabilitation, and Related Issues. Butterworths, Boston, 1986, p 233.
3. Rutter, M: Psychological sequelae of brain damage in children. Am J Psychiatry 138:1533, 1981.
4. Taylor, HG, Fletcher, JM and Satz, P: Neuropsychological assessment of children. In Goldstein, G and Hersen, M (eds): Handbook of Psychological Assessment. Pergamon Press, New York, 1984.
5. Reitan, RM: Psychological effects of cerebral lesions in children of early school age. In Reitan, RM, and Davison, LA (eds): Clinical Neuropsychology: Current Status and Applications. VH Winston and Sons, Washington, 1974.
6. Sweet, J et al: Relations between the Luria-Nebraska Battery–Children's Revision and the WISC-R: Further examination using Kaufman's factors. Int J Clin Neuropsychol 8:177, 1986.
7. Chadwick, O et al: A prospective study of children with head injuries, IV: Specific cognitive deficits. J Clin Neuropsychol 3:101, 1981.
8. Klonoff, H, Low, MD and Clark, C: Head injuries in children: A prospective five year follow-up. J Neurosurg 40:1211, 1977.

9. Ylvisaker, M: Cognitive and behavioral outcomes in head injured children. Paper presented at the International Symposium on the Traumatic Brain Injured Adult and Child, Boston, 1981.

10. Boll, TJ and Barth, JT: Neuropsychology of brain damage in children. In Filskov, F and Boll, TJ (eds): Handbook of Clinical Neuropsychology. John Wiley & Sons, New York, 1981.

11. Rourke, BP et al: Child Neuropsychology: An Introduction to Theory, Research, and Clinical Practices. Guilford Press, New York, 1983.

12. Kaufman, AS and Kaufman, NL: Kaufman Assessment Battery for Children: Administration and Scoring Manual. American Guidance Service, Circle Pines, MN, 1983.

13. Neglieri, JA: Assessment of mentally retarded children with the Kaufman Assessment Battery for Children. Am J Ment Def 89:367, 1985.

14. Neglieri, J and Haddad, F: Learning disabled children's performance on the Kaufman Assessment Battery for Children: A concurrent validity study. J Psychoeduc Assess 2:49, 1984.

15. Golden, CJ: The Luria-Nebraska Children's Battery: Theory and formulation. In Hynd, GW and Orbzut, JE (eds): Neuropsychological Assessment and the School-Age Child: Issues and Procedures. Grune & Stratton, New York, 1981.

16. Plaistad, JR et al: The Luria-Nebraska Neuropsychological Battery—Children's Revision: Theory and current research findings. J Clin Child Psychol 12:13, 1983.

17. Adams, KM: In search of Luria's battery: A false start. J Consult Clin Psychol 48:511, 1980.

18. Spiers, PA: Have they come to praise Luria or bury him? The Luria-Nebraska controversy. J Consult Clin Psychol 49:331, 1981.

19. Stambrook, M: The Luria-Nebraska Neuropsychological Battery: A promise that may be partly fulfilled. J Clin Neuropsychol 5:247, 1983.

20. Reitan, RM: Methodological problems in clinical neuropsychology. In Reitan, RM and Davison, LA (eds): Clinical Neuropsychology: Current Status and Applications. VH Winston and Sons, Washington, 1974.

21. Reitan, RM and Davison, LA (eds): Clinical Neuropsychology: Current Status and Applications. VH Winston and Sons, Washington, 1974.

22. Fay, G and Janesheski, MS: Neuropsychological assessment of head injured children. J Head Trauma Rehabil 1:16, 1986.

23. Boll, TJ: Behavioral correlates of cerebral damage in children aged 9 through 14. In Reitan, RM and Davison, L (eds): Clinical Neuropsychology: Current Status and Applications. VH Winston and Sons, 1974.

24. Klonoff, H and Low, M: Disordered brain function in young children and early adolescents: Neuropsychological and electroencephalographic correlates. In Reitan, R and Davison, L (eds): Clinical Neuropsychology: Current Status and Applications. Wiley & Sons, New York, 1974.

25. Reed, H, Reitan, R and Klove, H: The influence of cerebral lesions on psychological test performance of older children. J Consult Psychol 29:247, 1965.

26. Hart, T and Hayden, M: The ecological validity of neuropsychological assessment and remediation. In Uzzell, B and Gross, Y (eds): Clinical Neuro-

psychology of Intervention. Martinus Nijhoff, Boston, 1986.

27. Leton, D: Reitan-Indiana Neuropsychological Test Battery for Children. In Keyer, DJ and Sweetland, RC (eds): Test Critiques. Westport Publishers, Kansas City, 1984.

28. McCarthy, D: Manual for the McCarthy Scales of Children's Abilities. Psychological Corp, New York, 1972.

29. Kaufman, AS and Kaufman, NL: Clinical Evaluation of Young Children with the McCarthy Scales. Grune & Stratton, New York, 1977.

30. Uzgiris, IC and Hunt, JM: Assessment in Infancy. University of Illinois Press, Urbana, IL, 1975.

31. Foster, R, Giddan, JJ and Stark, J: Assessment of Children's Language and Comprehension (rev). Consulting Psychologists Press, Palo Alto, CA, 1973.

32. Semel, EM and Wiig, EH: Clinical Evaluation of Language Functions. Charles E Merrill Publishing, Columbus, OH, 1980.

33. Kirk, S, McCarthy, J and Kirk, W: Illinois Test of Psycholinguistic Abilities (rev ed). University of Illinois Press, Urbana, IL, 1968.

34. Jorgenson, C et al: The Word Test. Lingui Systems, Moline, IL, 1981.

35. Spreen, O and Benton, AL: Neurosensory Center Comprehensive Examination for Aphasia: Manual of Directions. Neuropsychology Laboratory, University of Victoria, Victoria, BC, 1969.

36. Gaddes, WH and Crocket, DJ: The Spreen-Benton Aphasia Tests: Normative data as a measure of normal language development. Brain Lang 2:257, 1975.

37. Levin, HS and Eisenberg, HM: Neuropsychological impairment after closed head injury in children and adolescents. J Pediatr Psychol 4:389, 1979.

38. Ewing-Cobbs, L, Fletcher, JM and Levin, HS: Neuropsychological sequelae following pediatric head injury. In Ylvisaker, M (ed): Head Injury Rehabilitation: Children and Adolescents. College-Hill Press, San Diego, 1985.

39. Gardner, MF: Test of Visual Perceptual Skills (non-motor). Special Child Publications, Seattle, WA, 1982.

40. Colarusso, RP and Hammill, DD: Motor Free Visual Perception Test. Academic Therapy Publications, Novato, CA, 1972.

41. Beery, KE: Revised Administration, Scoring, and Teaching Manual for the Developmental Test of Visual-Motor Integration. Modern Curriculum Press, Cleveland, 1982.

42. Gardner, MF: Test of Visual-Motor Skills. Children's Hospital Publication Department, San Francisco, 1986.

43. LeMay, DW, Griffin, PM and Sanford, AP: Learning Accomplishment Profile—Diagnostic Edition. Kaplan School Supply Corp, Winston-Salem, NC, 1977.

44. Sanford, AR: Learning Accomplishment Profile. Kaplan Press, Winston-Salem, NC, 1974.

45. Glover, ME, Preminger, JL and Sanford, AR: Early Learning Accomplishment Profile. Kaplan School Supply Corporation, Winston-Salem, NC, 1978.

46. Cohen, MA and Gross, PJ: The Developmental Resource: Vol I. Behavioral Sequences for Assessment and Program Planning. Grune & Stratton, New York, 1979.

47. Slingerland, BH: Revised Pre-reading Screening Procedures. Educators Publishing Service, Cambridge, MA, 1977.
48. Slingerland, BH: Slingerland Screening Tests for Identifying Children with Specific Language Disability—Forms A, B, and C. Educators Publishing Service, Cambridge, MA, 1970.
49. Slingerland, BH: Slingerland Screening Tests for Identifying Children with Specific Language Disability—Form D. Educators Publishing Service, Cambridge, MA, 1974.
50. Malcomesius, N: Specific Language Disability Test. Educators Publishing Service, Cambridge, MA, 1967.
51. Dunn, LM and Markwardt, F Jr: Peabody Individual Achievement Test. American Guidance Service, Circle Pines, MN, 1970.
52. Woodcock, RW: Woodcock Reading Mastery Tests. American Guidance Service, Circle Pines, MN, 1973.
53. Spache, GD: Diagnostic Reading Scales. CTB/McGraw-Hill, Monterey, CA, 1981.
54. Monroe, M and Sherman, EE: Group Diagnostic Reading Aptitude and Achievement Tests. CH Nevins Printing Company, Bradenton, FL, 1966.
55. Woodcock, RW and Johnson, MB: The Woodcock-Johnson Psychoeducational Battery. DLM Teaching Resources, Allen, TX, 1977.
56. Hammill, DD: Detroit Tests of Learning Aptitude (DTLA-2). Pro-Ed, Austin, TX, 1985.
57. Connally, AJ, Nachtman, W and Pritchett, EM: Key Math Diagnostic Arithmetic Test. American Guidance Service, Circle Pines, MN, 1976.
58. Gates, AI and McKillop, AS: Gates-McKillop Reading Diagnostic Tests. Teachers College Press, Columbia University, New York, 1962.
59. Brigance, AH: Inventory of Basic Skills. Curriculum Associates, Woburn, MA, 1977.
60. Brigance, AH: Comprehensive Inventory of Basic Skills. Curriculum Associates, Woburn, MA, 1983.
61. Brigance, AH: Inventory of Essential Skills. Curriculum Associates, Woburn, MA, 1981.
62. Baxter, R, Cohen, SB and Ylvisaker, M: Comprehensive cognitive assessment. In Ylvisaker, M (ed): Head Injury Rehabilitation: Children and Adolescents. College-Hill Press, San Diego, 1985, p 247.
63. Szekeres, S, Ylvisaker, M and Cohen, SB: A framework for cognitive rehabilitation. In Ylvisaker, M (ed): Community Re-entry for Head Injured Adults. College-Hill Press, San Diego, 1987.
64. Thorndike, R, Hagen, E and Sattler, J: The Stanford-Binet Intelligence Scale: Fourth Edition—Technical Manual. Riverside Publishing, Chicago, 1986.
65. Siegler, RS: Children's Thinking. Prentice-Hall, Englewood Cliffs, NJ, 1986.
66. Flavell, JH: Cognitive Development. Prentice-Hall, Englewood Cliffs, NJ, 1977.
67. Kail, R: The Development of Memory in Children, ed 2. Freeman, New York, 1984.
68. Dunn, L and Dunn, L: Peabody Picture Vocabulary Test—Revised. American Guidance Service, Circle Pines, MN, 1981.
69. Cohen, SB: Educational reintegration and programming for children with head injuries. J Head Trauma Rehabil 1:22, 1986.
70. Ylvisaker, M: Language and communication disorders following pediatric head injury. J Head Trauma Rehabil 1:48, 1986.
71. Gilfoyle, EM, Grady, AP and Moore, JC: Children Adapt. Charles B Slack, Thorofare, NJ, 1981.
72. Weeks, ZR: Sensorimotor integration theory and the multisensory approach. In Farber, SD (ed): Neurorehabilitation: A Multisensory Approach. WB Saunders, Philadelphia, 1982, p 186.
73. Bly, L: The Components of Normal Movement During the First Year of Life and Abnormal Motor Development. Pittengerand Associates Pathway, Birmingham, England, 1983.
74. Curry, JD and Butler, G: The mechanical properties of bone tissue in children. J Bone Joint Surg 57-A:810, 1975.
75. Palmer, CE: Studies on the center of gravity in the human body. Child Dev 15:134, 1944.
76. Bray, L et al: Physical rehabilitation. In Ylvisaker, M (ed): Community Re-entry for Head Injured Adults. College-Hill Press, San Diego, 1987.
77. Jaffe, M, et al: Intervention for motor disorders. In Ylvisaker, M (ed): Head Injury Rehabilitation: Children and Adolescents. College-Hill Press, San Diego, 1985.
78. Hensinger, RN and Jones, ET: Developmental orthopedics. I. The lower limb. Dev Med Child Neurol 24:95, 1982.
79. Farber, SD: Neurorehabilitation: A Multisensory Approach. WB Saunders, Philadelphia, 1982.
80. Bobath, B: Abnormal Postural Reflex Activity Caused by Brain Lesions, ed 3. Aspen Systems, Rockville, MD, 1985.
81. Kendall, FP and McCreary, EK: Muscles: Testing and Function. Williams & Wilkins, Baltimore, 1983.
82. O'Sullivan, SB, Cullen, K and Schmitz, TJ: Physical Rehabilitation: Evaluation and Treatment Procedures. FA Davis, Philadelphia, 1981.
83. Ayres, AJ: Southern California Postrotary Nystagmus Test. Western Psychological Services, Los Angeles, 1977.
84. Lowry, GH: Growth and Development of Children. Year Book Medical Publishers, Chicago, 1978.
85. Omamoto, T and Kunamoto, M: Electromyographic study of learning process of walking in infants. Electromyography 12:149, 1972.
86. Burnett, CN and Johnson, EW: Development of gait in children: Part III. Dev Med Child Neurol 13:207, 1971.
87. Bobath, B: Adult Hemiplegia: Evaluation and Treatment, ed 2. Wm Heinemann, London, 1978.
88. Ayres, AJ: Sensory Integration and Learning Disorders. Western Psychological Services, Los Angeles, 1972.
89. Ayres, AJ: Southern California Sensory Integration Tests. Western Psychological Services, Los Angeles, 1980.
90. Coley, IL: Pediatric Assessment of Self-Care Activities. CV Mosby, St Louis, 1978.
91. Bagnato, SJ and Mayes, SD: Patterns of developmental and behavioral progress for young brain-injured children during interdisciplinary intervention. Devel Neuropsychol 2:213, 1986.
92. Brigance, AH: Inventory of Early Development. Curriculum Associates, Woburn, MA, 1978.

93. Schafer, DS and Moersch, MS: Developmental Programming for Infants and Young Children. University of Michigan Press, Ann Arbor, 1981.

94. Erhardt, RP: Developmental Hand Dysfunction: Theory, Assessment and Treatment. RAMSCO Publishing, Laurel, MD, 1982.

95. Vulpe, SG: Vulpe Assessment Battery. National Institute on Mental Retardation, Toronto, 1979.

96. Roach, EG and Kephart, NC: The Purdue Perceptual Motor Survey. Charles E Merrill Publishing, Columbus, OH, 1966.

97. Bruininks, RH: Bruininks-Osteretsky Test of Motor Proficiency. American Guidance Service, Circle Pines, MN, 1978.

98. Jebsen, R et al: An objective and standardized test of hand function. Arch Phys Med Rehabil 50:311, 1969.

99. Taylor, N, Sand, PL and Jebsen, RH: Evaluation of hand function in children. Arch Phys Med Rehabil 54:129, 1973.

100. Kalisky, Z et al: Medical problems encountered during rehabilitation of patients with head injury. Arch Phys Med Rehabil 66:25, 1985.

101. Smith, DW: Growth and its disorders: Basics and standards, approach and classification, growth deficiency disorders, growth excess disorders, obesity. Maj Probl Pediatr 15:1, 1977.

102. Vaughan, VC: Developmental pediatrics: Growth and development. In Behrman, R and Vaughan, VC (eds): Nelson Textbook of Pediatrics, ed 12. WB Saunders, Philadelphia, 1983.

103. Hargrave, M: Nutritional care of the physically disabled. Sister Kenny Institute, Minneapolis, 1979.

104. Krick, J: Nutritional status during the rehabilitation process. Diet Phys Med Rehabil 5:3, 1986.

105. Barness, LA: Nutrition and nutritional disorders. In Behrman, R and Vaughan, VC (eds): Nelson Textbook of Pediatrics, ed 12. WB Saunders, Philadelphia, 1983.

106. Young, B et al: Metabolic and nutritional sequelae in the non-steroid treated head injury patient. Neurosurgery 17:784, 1985.

107. Chamovitz, I et al: Rehabilitative medical management. In Ylvisaker, M (ed): Head Injury Rehabilitation: Children and Adolescents. College-Hill Press, San Diego, 1985.

108. Lloyd, CW et al: Pharmacokinetics and pharmacodynamics of cimetidine and metabolics in critically ill children. J Pediatr 107:295, 1985.

109. Arasu, et al: Gastroesophageal reflux in infants and children—comparative accuracy of diagnostic methods. J Pediatr 96:798, 1980.

110. Christie, DL: The acid reflux test for gastroesophageal reflux. J Pediatr 94:78, 1979.

111. Ramenofsky, ML, Powell, RW and Curreri, PW: Gastroesophageal reflux: pH probe-directed therapy. Ann Surg 203:531, 1986.

112. Sondheimer, JM: Continuous monitoring of distal esophageal pH: A diagnostic test for gastroesophageal reflux in infants. J Pediatr 96:804, 1980.

113. Wilkinson, JD, Dudgeon, DL and Sondheimer, JM: A comparison of medical and surgical treatment of gastroesophageal reflux in severely retarded children. J Pediatr 99:202, 1981.

114. Report on Task Force on Blood Pressure Control in Children. Pediatrics (Suppl) 59:797, 1977.

115. Hald, T and Bradley, WE: The Urinary Bladder: Neurology and Dynamics. Williams & Wilkins, Baltimore, 1982, p 230.

116. Hirschmann, JV: Bacterial meningitis following closed cranial trauma. In Sande, MA, Smith, AL and Root, RK (eds): Bacterial Meningitis. Churchill-Livingstone, New York, 1985, p 95.

117. Wright, PF et al: Patterns of illness in the highly febrile young child: Epidemiologic, clinical and laboratory correlates. Pediatrics 67:694, 1981.

118. Kluger, MJ: Fever. Pediatrics 66:720, 1980.

119. Ylvisaker, M and Longemann, J: Therapy for feeding and swallowing disorders following head injury. In Ylvisaker, M (ed): Head Injury Rehabilitation: Children and Adolescents. College-Hill Press, San Diego, 1985, p 195.

120. Brown, DR and McMillin, JM: Posttraumatic anterior hypopituitarism-revisited: The role of TRH provocative release prolactin in the confirmation of anterior pituitary damage. Pediatrics 59:948, 1977.

121. Copeland, KC, Brookman, RR and Rauh, JL: Assessment of pubertal development. Pediatr Rev 8:47, 1986.

122. Tanner, JM: Growth at Adolescence, ed 2. Blackwell Scientific, Oxford, 1962.

123. Matsuzaki, H, Kunita, M and Kawai, K: Optic nerve damage in head trauma: Clinical and experimental studies. J Ophthalmol 26:447, 1982.

124. Mochizuki, Y et al: Developmental changes of brain stem auditory evoked potentials (BAEPs) in normal human subjects from infants to young adults. Brain Dev 4:127, 1982.

125. Lutschag, J et al: Brain-stem auditory evoked potentials and early somatosensory evoked potentials in neurointensively treated comatose children. Am J Dis Child 137:421, 1983.

126. Freed, JH et al: The use of the three-phase bone scan in the early diagnosis of heterotopic ossification (HO) and in the evaluation of didronel therapy. Paraplegia 20:208, 1982.

127. Cristofaro, RL and Brink, JD: Hypercalcemia of immobilization in neurologically injured children: A prospective study. Orthopedics 2:485, 1979.

128. Dreifuss, FE: Pediatric Epileptology: Classification and Management of Seizures in the Child. J Wright, PSG, Inc, Boston, 1983.

129. Buschke, H and Fuld, PA: Evaluating storage, retention, and retrieval in disordered memory and learning. Neurology 24:1019, 1974.

APPENDIX: A CONCEPTUAL FRAMEWORK AND SELECTED PROBES FOR EXPLORING COGNITIVE FUNCTIONING IN HEAD INJURED CHILDREN

I. COMPONENT PROCESSES

A. ATTENTIONAL PROCESSES

1. Is the child adequately *alert/aroused?*
   a. Observe level of arousal in relation to time of day, people in the environment, and levels and modalities of sensory stimulation (e.g., varying interactive styles; novel versus familiar objects, music, games) (E, M, A).*

2. Can the child *maintain attention* long enough to accomplish age-appropriate tasks? If not, what factors appear to improve attention span?
   a. Time continuous attention during formal assessment tasks; compare with attention during group therapy or classroom tasks and with caregivers' reports of attention to favorite activities (e.g., play, TV watching) in natural settings (E, M, A).
   b. Does attention span increase: when distractions are reduced? when the task is more interesting/enjoyable for the child? when the task is a familiar practical activity? when there is a reward for task completion? when the task instructions/expectations are made clearer, or when the child is instructed to pay attention? when the task is made easy to accomplish? during specific times of day following medication? (E, M, A)

3. Can the child attend to *selected* stimuli and disregard stimuli not relevant to the task? If the ability to selectively attend is not age-appropriate, what are the effects on selective attention of the variables listed in 1a and 2b?
   a. Observe responses to distractions in a variety of tasks and settings; e.g., abrupt topic shifts in conversation? deterioration in performance with distractions (e.g., reduced comprehension with background noise)? (M, A)

4. Can the child *shift* attentional focus adequately for effective classroom or social functioning?
   a. Can the child: flexibly change activity in a classroom or nursing unit? interrupt TV watching for a short conversation and return to the show? play video games that require rapid shifting of attention from stimulus to stimulus? shift from topic to topic during conversation? (E, M, A)

---

*E = early childhood (roughly 2–5 yr)
 M = middle childhood (roughly 6–11 yr)
 A = adolescence (roughly 12–18 yr)

*See also planning tasks under Executive System.

584

b. Is perseveration observed during formal assessment (e.g., during rapid naming tasks or set-shifting tasks)? (M, A)
5. Can the child *divide* attention adequately for effective academic and social functioning?
   a. Can the child maintain conversation and/or comprehend instructions while engaged in a motor activity (like walking or eating)? pick up objects with one hand while holding the container in the other? (E, M, A)

B. PERCEPTUAL PROCESSES

Care must be taken to distinguish visual-perceptual problems from visual acuity problems, limited ocular range of motion, and cognitive problems such as impaired attention, organization, or executive functions.

1. Does the child *focus* on selected objects?
   a. Observe eye movements and duration of visual fixation with familiar people and highly meaningful objects/pictures in his or her visual field. (E, M, A)
2. Does the child visually *track* objects/people?
   a. Observe sustained fixation on moving objects or light source. Does the child track across midline? Does tracking systematically end/begin at certain points in the visual field? (E, M, A)
   b. Observe visual regard while attempting to have the child rapidly alternate visual fixation from one object to another (saccades). Gradually move the objects into different quadrants of the visual field (E, M, A).
3. Can the child *identify* and *discriminate* among objects and features of objects?
   a. Have the child find familiar photos in a photo album; complete large piece inset puzzles; place shapes into sorting boxes; stack stacking boxes by size; complete pegboard designs; color selected shapes on a page (E, M, A).
   b. Have the child match increasingly complex pictures; identify which of four increasingly complex shapes is different; complete math problems on increasingly complex (visually) worksheets; decode words/sentences on increasingly full pages; select correct coins from a group (E, M, A).
   c. Figure-ground mechanisms: Observe the child's search for a specified item in a toy box, in a clothing drawer, or in a complex picture (E, M, A).

C. MEMORY/LEARNING PROCESSES

1. Is there a "memory problem" to be explored?
   a. Interview teachers, family members, and nursing staff about the child's functional ability to remain oriented (person/place/time), retain information from day to day about personally experienced events, and learn new information/skills at an age-appropriate rate.
   b. Observe (1) recall of events from day to day, (2) recognition of the examiner, examiner's name, and route to the office from day to day, (3) prospective recall of interesting events that have been planned for the next day. Observe the effects of cues (E, M, A).
   c. Assess performance on a sensitive test of memory/learning.[55, 129]
2. Since *encoding, storage,* and *retrieval* are all tested by testing for retrieval of information, it is not possible to obtain a clear and quantified picture of the relative contributions of each of these aspects of memory to memory problems. However, significant disparities

among free, cued, and recognition memory do give insight into this issue. If performance on recognition memory tasks is substantially better than performance on free recall tasks, then it is likely that the problem may be largely at the retrieval stage. If performance is poor even on recognition memory tasks, then it is likely that encoding or storage is weak. If immediate recognition memory is good, but delayed recognition memory is poor, then *perhaps* storage is weak. Only if differences are extreme can inferences be drawn. *Qualitative* analysis of what the child recalls (e.g., significant versus insignificant details? main idea? sequences?) is often more revealing than quantity of information remembered.

  a. Immediate versus delayed recognition memory (visual): Have the child look at and name a small number of objects or pictures; then have the child identify those objects or pictures in a larger set; repeat after 30 minutes (M, A). Preschoolers: same task, but in the context of familiar activities.

  b. Immediate versus delayed recognition memory (auditory): Read a story that the child can easily understand; ask yes/no or multiple choice questions immediately and again 30 minutes later —compare results (M, A).

  c. Free versus cued recall: read a story that the child can easily understand. Ask the child to retell as much as he can remember. Then read another story (same level and length) and ask wh-questions about the information — compare results (could add a yes/no condition to compare recognition memory) (M, A). Preschoolers: act out the story with props; ask questions.

  d. Show a picture of a room with furniture and accessories; take the picture away and ask the child to recreate the room with flannel board props; does performance improve substantially with spatial cues? (E, M, A)

  e. Use tests of naming and word retrieval (e.g., controlled word fluency) to measure the ability to access stored lexical items (E, M, A).

3. *Attention versus memory:* Is the observed memory problem specific to memory processes or is it a result of weak attention?

  a. Using the same task (e.g., story recall or nonverbal task) with materials at the same level, compare results in a nondistracting environment (one-on-one, with attempts to guarantee attention) with results in a more distracting setting or group context with no special attempts to prompt the child to manipulate, name, or focus on salient aspects of the objects (E, M, A).

4. *Comprehension versus memory processes:* Is the observed memory problem specific to memory or is it a result of weak comprehension?

  a. Compare recall of stories that are challenging in terms of academic/language level with recall of stories that are below the upper limits of the child's academic/language level. Alternatively, use two stories at the same academic/language level, but allow the child to act out or draw aspects of the story in one case but not the other; compare results (M, A).

5. *Executive system versus memory processes:* Is the observed memory problem specific to memory processes or is it (in part) a failure of the executive system (e.g., to deliberately pay special attention to material that has to be remembered or to initiate and maintain an organized search of memory)?

  a. Compare story recall results when the child is simply read a story and then asked to recall vs. when he is encouraged to pay attention and remember. Compare results when the child is simply asked to retell the story versus when he or she is given repeated encouragement to search his or her memory and to ask self questions that might help the search (M, A).

b. Using a word retrieval task (e.g., listing words in categories or starting with a specific letter), compare results of uncoached performance versus performance with some encouragement, rewards, and suggestions to approach the task systematically (M, A; E = words in concrete categories).

6. *Characteristics of the information to be remembered:* Is it substantially easier for the child to remember one type of information than another?

a. Compare the child's ability to remember (1) *recent episodes in own life* with (2) *factual information that has nothing to do with own life* with (3) *procedures to accomplish a task or rules of a game* with (4) *routes and locations in the building* with (5) *new faces* with (6) *new names* (E, M, A).

b. Compare the child's ability to remember information that is emotionally *significant* versus information that is interesting but not at an emotional level versus information that is neither (bearing in mind that personally meaningful information is normally easier to remember (E, M, A).

7. *Aspects of presentation of the information:* Does the child's ability to remember vary with the way the information is presented?

a. *Input and output channels:* Compare recall of a story that is read to the child versus a story of the same level and length that the child reads (M, A). (All combinations of input and output channels can be systematically varied to detect relative strengths and weaknesses.)

b. *Processing time:* Compare recall of a story that is read with normal pauses after clauses with recall of a story of the same level and length that is read with extended pauses after clauses (E, M, A).

c. *Task orientation* (incidental versus deliberate learning): Compare results in word list learning tasks: when the child is told (1) to remember as many words as possible from the list; versus (2a) to listen to the words and indicate each time a word of a certain sort is heard; or (2b) to get a set of items to accomplish some activity; or (2c) to join in an activity with the items and in the context of the activity name each item once; the child is later asked to recall what things were used in the activity (E, M, A).

d. *Incentive to remember:* Compare recall when the child is simply asked to remember something versus when child is promised a reward for remembering (E, M, A).

e. *Repetition and spacing:* Compare recall of a story that is read just once with recall of a story of the same level and length that is read twice (or more) and at planned intervals (E, M, A).

f. *Feedback:* Does the child profit from informational feedback in a learning task? (M, A)

8. Does the child *spontaneously use strategies* to learn/remember?

a. During memory/learning tests or functional activities, does the child show evidence of repetition/rehearsal or grouping/organizing information? ask for repetition/clarification? ask to take notes? (M, A)

b. Ask the child what he or she did to insure a better performance on the test (M, A) or what he or she would do to remember last year's Christmas present (E, M, A) or what he or she would do to remember to go to a friend's birthday party (E, M, A).

   c. Go through a list of common strategies and ask the child if he or she used any of them to help self remember (M, A).

9. *Effects of memory strategies:* Does performance improve when the child is instructed to use specific strategies? Which strategies are most effective?

   a. Use a paragraph recall task (using paragraphs matched for length and level; reading or listening) with and without the following strategy instructions — compare results (M, A):

      "Repeat important information in your head as you listen," "re-read or ask for repetitions," "draw a vivid picture in your head of the story as you listen," "draw little pictures on paper to represent important events," "find something in your own experience to relate the information to," "take notes," "ask yourself questions during pauses."

   b. *Elaboration:* Use two paragraphs of the same level and length. Read one to the child twice, then test recall 24 hours later. Read the other once and then discuss the information, including relevant elaboration of the key points, then test recall 24 hours later. Compare results (M, A). With preschoolers, analogous probes can be constructed using play materials; elaboration is accomplished by relating the objects in play.

   c. *Organization:* Compare recall of paragraphs without versus with a proposed system for *organizing* the information (e.g., who, what happened, where, when, why). Compare results (M, A).

   d. *Mnemonics:* Compare memory for names or word lists with and without instruction to use "tricks" such as unusual associations (M, A).

   e. *Retrieval strategies:* Compare recall without versus with suggestions on how to search memory. Base suggestions on the strategies that were suggested at the time of encoding (M, A).

D. ORGANIZING PROCESSES

It is necessary to eliminate the confounding effects of other cognitive processes/systems; e.g., in probing organizing processes, avoid straining attentional, perceptual, comprehension, memory, and "executive" skills.

1. Can the child *analyze* objects into their component parts? concepts into their component features? tasks into their component steps?

   a. Ask the child to describe a familiar object or explain a familiar activity or game to a person who has no idea about the activity or object. Have the child explain what he or she is doing throughout a block design task (M, A).

   b. Present a novel task; have the child select the materials/tools needed to complete the task (E, M, A).

2. Can the child *compare* features, *identify* similarities/differences, and *classify/categorize/associate?*

   a. Use concept formation/analysis or semantic association tests (M, A).

   b. Have the child sort/group objects or pictures (E, M, A).

   c. Give the child a set of pictures that could be sorted *categorically* or *sequentially/thematically;* which way does he or she sort? Have the child organize furniture in a room for a snack, for watching a movie, and so on (E, M, A).

   d. Ask the child how he or she would pack grocery bags at a super-

market. Give a list of items and a set of conditions (e.g., it is hot outside; the customer is small; the customer has to put things away in a hurry) (M, A).
3. Can the child *sequentially* organize events?
    a. Use a test of sequencing (e.g., Picture Arrangement from WISC-R); how many sequence cards (and at what level) can the child sequence? (M, A)
    b. Propose a script for play (e.g., let's go to the store; let's make a sandwich). Observe how effectively the child directs the events (E, M, A).
    c. Does the child progress through routine daily events in correct sequence without cues (e.g., get up, get dressed, eat breakfast, brush teeth)? describe his or her daily schedule in correct sequence? (M, A)
    d. Can the child follow the sequence of steps in a structured activity like cooking? with (or without) a guide? (M, A)
4. Can the child *integrate/synthesize* events into *main ideas/themes/scripts??*
    a. Preschoolers: Present an increasing number of toys that relate to one another thematically. How many can the child organize into a play theme? (E)
    b. Ask the child to make something out of construction toys. How many of the objects are used? Is the construct an organized whole? (E, M, A)
    c. Have the child answer main idea questions from paragraphs (M, A).
    d. Have the child select the best words to express a complex idea in a short telegram; explain a favorite game: does the child start with a general orienting statement about the overall nature of the game? (M, A)

E. REASONING/PROBLEM-SOLVING PROCESSES

Again, it is necessary to rule out the confounding effects of attentional problems, perceptual problems, comprehension problems, memory problems, and executive control problems.
1. *Inductive reasoning:* Can the child make appropriate generalizations, given a set of instances? see single principles in a set of instances? see the rule that guides a progression or a grouping of things?
    a. Use concept formation/categories types of tests/tasks (M, A).
    b. With objects that could be sorted in a variety of ways (e.g., to animals), begin sorting into two bins according to a rule (e.g., two-legged in one, four-legged in the other); can the child continue the sorting? (E)
2. *Causal reasoning:* Can the child infer causes from effects? predict effects from causes?
    a. Using picture cards or descriptions of hypothetical events, have the child (1) predict what would happen if a certain event occurred or (2) explain why a certain event occurred (M, A). Preschoolers: Place a desired object in a precarious position, in which an undesired event is likely (e.g., a favorite doll falls); cause the event to occur; repeat; does the child do anything to prevent the event from occurring? (E)
3. *Deductive reasoning:* Can the child draw logical conclusions on the basis of formal logical relations signaled by terms such as "all," "some," "if-then," "and," "or," "not"?
    a. Use a test of reasoning skills (e.g., Ross Test of Higher Cognitive

Functions [Deductive Reasoning; Missing Premises]).[130] Reasoning tests are often best used informally; have the child explain why each answer is selected. If child cannot do the task, teach the task with one or two items, then probe again (A).

  b. Use graded reading comprehension materials, especially "Drawing Conclusions" components (M, A).

4. *Analogic reasoning:* Can the child detect indirect relationships among words, ideas, and events?

  a. Use word analogy tests. Used informally, the largest amount of information is obtained by (1) having the child complete some items in the standard way; (2) having the child describe the relationship as he sees it; (3) then, if necessary, teaching the type of thinking involved and trying additional items (M, A). Preschoolers: Analogical relationships may be best tested with objects; e.g., the clinician shows the child a foot and a sock, then gives the child a hand and asks what should go with it, given a choice of objects.

  b. Have the child explain proverbs. Again, use the progression: (1) child attempts to explain proverb; (2) examiner teaches the process involved in explaining proverbs; (3) child tries again (A).

5. *Divergent thinking:* Can the child suggest varied solutions to problems? varied interpretations of events or actions?

  a. Present a number of concrete problem situations (e.g., candy in a jar with a tight lid); how many possible solutions does the child explore to solve the problems? (E, M).

  b. Present hypothetical problems and ask for as many possible solutions as the child can imagine (M, A).

  c. Give the child a selection of animal or person figures; ask him or her to make the figure do as many things as the child can think of (E).

6. *Problem solving/decision making*

  a. Using tasks 5a and 5b, have the child select and justify the best solution (M, A).

  b. Look for patterns in the child's problem solving (e.g., trial and error? ask for help? give up? random ineffective? or impulsive behavior?) (E, M, A).

  c. Give math word problems; look for recognition of the problem, selection of appropriate operations, and calculation (M, A).

  d. Ask family members if the child spontaneously engages in organized problem-solving behavior in natural settings (M, A).

II. **COMPONENT SYSTEMS**
  A. WORKING MEMORY
    1. What is the child's immediate memory span for *unrelated* items (e.g., digits, unrelated words, visual symbols)? Compare with memory span for *related* items (e.g., semantically related words, sentences). Does the child frequently need directions repeated? (E, M, A)
  B. KNOWLEDGE BASE
    1. What is the child's level of language knowledge and organization?
      a. Use a receptive picture vocabulary test. Start testing well below anticipated basal and look for gaps in the knowledge base (E, M, A).
      b. Use tests of word definitions, multiple definitions, antonyms, synonyms (M, A). (See also organization probes.)
    2. What is the child's level of general knowledge?

  a. Specifically probe knowledge in the child's areas of pretraumatic interest, activity, and/or education (E, M, A).
 3. What is the child's level of academic achievement?
  a. Compare current with pretraumatic academic achievement (M, A).
 4. What is the child's level of knowledge of pretraumatically acquired social and nonsocial skills, rules, and procedures (e.g., how to ride a bike, use a calculator, play a game, interact with adults)?
  a. Specifically probe skills and knowledge of rules and procedures in areas of pretraumatic interest, activity, and education (E, M, A).
C. EXECUTIVE SYSTEM
 1. *Awareness of strengths and weaknesses:* Is the child's awareness of own strengths and weaknesses age-appropriate?
  a. Use a self-report questionnaire (A) or ask the child open-ended questions about why he or she is in a rehabilitation center; what sorts of activities he or she now has trouble with; if he or she is ready to return to school (M, A).
  b. Ask more specific questions about the ability to remember; to understand what others say; to understand what he or she reads; to concentrate (M, A).
   Assess the child's comprehension of cognitive terms. Can he or she meaningfully discuss cognitive strengths and weaknesses? (M, A).
  c. Before giving a test, ask the child to predict how well he or she will do? After the test, ask child how well he or she thinks performance was (M, A).
 2. *Goals:* Does the child understand and engage in goal-directed activity?
  a. Does the child accept and work toward short-term goals (e.g., attempt to achieve a set goal within a therapy activity) and intermediate goals (e.g., attempt to achieve a set goal within a few days or weeks)? (E, M, A) Compare goal-directedness with and without incentives.
  b. Ask about long-term goals (e.g., What do you plan to do when you are done with school?) and mid-term goals (e.g., What courses do you plan to take next term at school?); compare with abilities (A). Ask family members the same questions about the child's goals (A).
  c. Does the child set goals for self and pursue them in play (E, M, A) and in therapy or school? (M, A)
 3. *Planning:* Does the child give evidence that he or she actively creates plans to achieve own goals?
  a. Ask specific questions about what the child plans to do to achieve long-term/mid-term goals (M, A).
  b. Give the child a complex task that requires some planning (e.g., making a model; baking a cake); observe for evidence of spontaneous planning; if the child begins without a plan, ask him or her to stop and create a plan; evaluate the plan for organization and completeness (M, A).
 4. *Self-Initiating:* Does the child evidence age-appropriate initiation of activities and of cognitive processes?
  a. Ask family members about the child's initiation of activity at home or in other natural settings (e.g., "Does he think up things to do as much as before?"). Ask the same question of nursing

staff. Observe the child's initiation of social interaction, play, and daily living activities (E, M, A).

  b. In testing sessions, does child initiate conversation? spontaneously offer information? begin tasks without a direct command? (E, M, A)

  c. In therapy tasks, does the child require cueing to use the cognitive abilities that he has, e.g., to search memory, to organize a task, to use a log book or other compensatory device/strategies, to ask questions when information is needed? (E, M, A)

5. *Self-Inhibiting:* Does the child demonstrate age-appropriate ability to inhibit behavior, thoughts, and emotions that are inappropriate or nonfunctional?

  a. Is there evidence of perseveration? Observe performance during tests that can elicit perseveration (e.g., confrontation naming or rapid automatized naming tasks)? (E, M, A)

  b. Are there perseverative motor behaviors? (E, M, A)

  c. Does the child's conversation remain fixed on a given topic? Does the child wander from topic to topic with no orientation for the listener? (E, M, A)

  d. Does the child do things that are considered socially inappropriate? Does he or she recognize that they are inappropriate but continue anyway? (E, M, A)

6. *Self-Monitoring:* Does the child demonstrate age-appropriate ability to monitor (attend to) own behavior? monitor own orientation to the tasks? monitor the adequacy of own knowledge to accomplish a task? monitor own remembering?

  a. Is there evidence during testing or other structured activities that the child notices and tries to correct mistakes? (M, A)

  b. Does the child request information, repetition, or slowing of rate when needed? (M, A) Given incomplete instructions for task completion (written or oral), does the child recognize the need for more information? (E, M, A)

7. *Self-Evaluating:* Does the child show age-appropriate ability to evaluate own performance?

  a. Ask the child "How do you think you did?" following a test or other structured activity. Are the answers accurate? (M, A)

8. *Ability to change set:* Does the child demonstrate age-appropriate ability to consider alternative hypotheses/courses of action?

  a. Observe for flexibility in natural problem-solving situations (E, M, A).

9. *Strategic Behavior:* Does the child demonstrate age-appropriate ability to use strategies?

  a. Spontaneous use of strategies: Look for use of pretraumatically rehearsed strategies in informal activities like card or board games? Look for spontaneous use of strategies during testing (e.g., does child ask for help? rehearse or organize information in obvious ways during memory testing? use sentence completion to help with word finding?) (M, A).

  b. Ability to describe strategies: After a test in which strategic behavior was observed or was at least relevant, ask the child what he or she did to help self accomplish the task (M, A).

  c. Ability to recognize strategies: After a test for which strategies are useful (e.g., a memory or learning test), give the child a list of possible strategies and ask if he or she used any of them (M, A).

  d. Ability to profit from strategy suggestions: See strategy probes under Memory/Learning Processes.

Chapter 38

Rehabilitation Management Approaches

BRUCE M. GANS, M.D.
NANCY R. MANN, M.D.
MARK YLVISAKER, Ph.D.

The overwhelming majority of pediatric head injuries are minor and without visible effects. Yet head injury is the most common diagnosis among seriously injured children.[1] The occurrence of a severe traumatic brain injury (TBI) in childhood represents a major catastrophe in not only the life of the child but also the lives of the parents, siblings, and extended family. While in general those children who survive have a better functional prognosis than similarly affected adults,[2-4] they nevertheless have major functional impairments that require sophisticated evaluation and management for an extended period of time.[5]

DIFFERENCES BETWEEN CHILDREN AND ADULTS

The child with a TBI is substantially different from an adult with the same injury in many physiologic, social, and functional aspects. A child is not merely a small adult. Children vary from adults in a variety of obvious and subtle ways. The two most important aspects of difference are that a child is a growing organism, and that functional development is incomplete.

Physical and Neurologic Development

In the physical sense, children grow along generally predictable patterns. The most rapid phase of growth occurs in the first year of life. A second and important period of rapid growth occurs during puberty (11 to 14 years of age, depending upon sex and individual differences).[6] Attention to patterns of growth is a guiding principle in managing the child with brain injury. Persisting dynamic deformities (e.g., flexible scoliosis) influence the pattern of bone growth and convert a positional deformity to a structural one. This is most noticeable during periods of rapid growth. Hence, the closest and most frequent attention to spinal alignment should be paid during adolescence.[7]

Neurologic patterns of maturation are more important to observe in the first 2 years of life. The normal presence of primitive reflex postures such as the asymmetric tonic neck reflex, the symmetric tonic neck reflex, and others, should be distinguished from the pathologic persistence and dominance of these patterns in older brain injured children.[8] Hyperactive phasic stretch reflexes, clonus, and Babinski's sign all may be normal phenomena in infants as well, needing distinction from the pathologic finding of the upper motor neuron syndrome in brain injured children.

The immaturity of the nervous system seems to allow the child to be more responsive to external manipulations of reflex behaviors. For example, inhibitive casts seem more effective for spasticity management and the use of dynamic vestibular stimulation appears more helpful in developing protective extension reflexes with children than with adults.

The physical size of children makes them easier to handle by therapists as well. Control of extension posturing by holding a child in the lap, for instance, is much easier than in a full grown adult patient.

Cognitive Development

Normal patterns of cognitive development similarly guide the assessment and treatment of children following brain injury. Attention to the following dimensions of development is important:

☐ **Centration to Decentration:** Ranging from an exclusive concern with self and the immediate surroundings to an ability to take other people's perspectives and to consider events that are distant in time and space

☐ **Concrete to Abstract:** Ranging from considering only concrete things and people and solving problems only by trial and error to considering abstract attributes, relationships, and principles, thinking about possibilities, and solving problems in a hypothetical manner

☐ **Surface to Depth:** Ranging from attention to superficial (usually perceptual) characteristics of things and people to a focus on underlying causes and inferred meanings

☐ **Growth of the Knowledge Base:** Including the addition of factual information as well as principles and associational ties that promote increasingly efficient learning of new information

☐ **Increased Capacity and Efficiency:** Including increased speed of processing, capacity of working memory, and flexibility of the retrieval system

☐ **Improved Situational Discrimination:** Ranging from indiscriminant behavior to an appreciation of the situational appropriateness of specific types of behavior

☐ **Improved "Metacognitive" Functioning:** Including increasingly deliberate and goal-directed behavior, improved ability to plan and monitor activity (including cognitive activity), and behavior that is increasingly strategic

General outlines of cognitive development are presented by Flavell[9] and Siegler;[10]

Ylvisaker and coworkers[11] discuss the treatment implications of cognitive development.

An understanding of cognitive development plays several significant roles in rehabilitation. First, it enables professionals to make accurate judgments about the effects of the injury. A preschooler who is egocentric, impulsive, and nonstrategic and who lacks situational discrimination may simply be a normal preschooler. The type of frontal lobe damage that is associated with these cognitive deficits in older people may not have identifiable effects on the functioning of a preschooler until that child reaches an age at which maturation of these functions is expected. For this reason, long-term follow-up of children injured early in life is essential.

Second, normal development places certain limits on approaches to cognitive rehabilitation with young children. For example, whereas adults may be encouraged to compensate in a deliberate way for residual cognitive deficits, this is not a reasonable goal for preschoolers and young school-age children. The metacognitive maturity that is presupposed when teaching compensatory cognitive strategies is normally not present in very young children.

Finally, these areas of cognitive development suggest general goals for a rehabilitation program. By creating tasks that encourage movement along these dimensions, clinicians can promote more mature cognitive functioning, recognizing at the same time that all of us on occasion revert to thinking that is concrete, superficial, and egocentric.

Psychosocial Development

In addition to physical, neurologic, and cognitive differences from adults, children are very different social and functional creatures. Most importantly, they are not considered to be competent, in either the operational or legal sense. Parents or other caretakers are explicitly responsible for all medical decisions made about a child's care. This means that rehabilitation providers should regularly consult with the parents when any significant therapeutic decision is to be made.

A combination of factors following severe

brain injury interfere with psychosocial development. Under normal circumstances, children are dependent on their parents, and parents nurture and protect their children. Severely injured children are unusually dependent, and parents understandably feel an intense need to nurture and protect them. These factors combine with a set of common psychosocial deficits—disinhibition, impaired social judgment, and egocentrism—to block normal social experiences and maturation. It requires extraordinary skill and understanding both to encourage parents to be active members of the rehabilitation team, and to promote the development of autonomy and independence in the child which are essential to psychosocial maturation.

Parents or others who are willing to assume the role of caretaker for even the most severely involved child frequently seek early discharge to the home setting. The desire to see a child return to the home needs to be balanced by consideration of the therapeutic needs of the child, resources in the community to meet those needs, and the capacity of the family to care for the child over a long period of time. For the severely physically disabled child (such as the child in the persistent vegetative state), constant unrelieved physical care can destroy even the most enduring of families. Supplemental home nursing care services are critical to ensure long-term viability of this type of placement.

Similarly, for the higher functioning but behaviorally impaired child, home placement frequently necessitates monitoring and supplemental caretaker assistance. The constant supervision needed by this type of child has the potential to trap a parent or family in an unending demand for care. The availability of respite care and supplemental home-based child care is essential for long-term success.

Siblings are frequently ignored or experience limited attention in households of children with TBI. Families must be able to attend to the care and emotional needs of other children in the home, or serious emotional disorders may develop that lead to further home chaos. Professionals caring for children with TBI and their families should remain cognizant of this fact and "give permission" to families to seek out respite and other supplemental care options to attend to the needs of siblings.

DEVELOPMENTAL ASPECTS OF SPECIFIC REHABILITATION PROBLEMS

Mobility for a child is not simply ambulation or wheelchair propulsion. Small children normally first acquire floor mobility (creeping and crawling) and this may be an early gross motor goal for restoration of function. Similarly, wheelchair mobility at the floor level is frequently more appropriate than mobility with a standard wheelchair. Furthermore, when a child does require a wheelchair, the ability to descend to the floor (either by transfer or through descent of the seat electrically) may deserve particular consideration (Fig. 38-1).[12]

Older children who are marginal walkers because of weakness and spasticity may "outgrow their ability to walk" as further physical growth occurs. This change does not necessarily represent a deterioration in neurologic function, but rather a decline in biomechanical efficiency. Alternative mobility systems should be available in these cases.

Dressing skills are greatly influenced by developmental state. Parents and rehabilitation providers must have realistic expectations of levels of function. For example, a normally developing 3-year-old child should not be expected to show proficiency at tying shoelaces, let alone a 3-year-old impaired by a TBI.

Similarly, self-feeding skills are age dependent, and food choices and eating behaviors are also influenced by normal development. Finger feeding and limited food choices are typical of young children, and should be distinguished from pathologic states associated with the brain injury.

Bathing needs for the child should be addressed in relationship to the home setting. Bathrooms may be difficult access areas, and tub-bathing may prove awkward or dangerous without the use of a bath seat or other modification. For more functional children, careful supervision of bathing will frequently be necessary for hygiene effectiveness and safety. Parental counseling is usually necessary.

Communication skills need to be developmentally assessed. In many cases, the use of augmentative communication strategies such as pointing boards, manual signing, or other methods will be necessary. Children tend to adapt well to the use of supplemen-

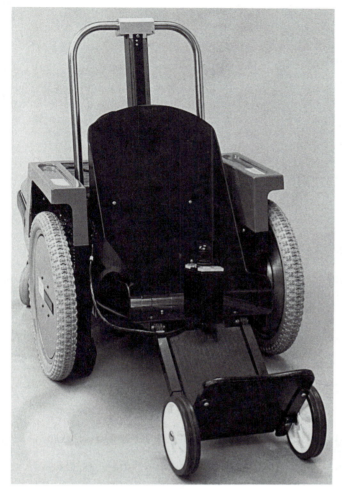

Figure 38–1. Pediatric powered wheelchair that allows vertical rise and descent to floor level, in addition to horizontal travel. (Courtesy of Everaids Turbo, Invacare Corporation.)

tal communication aids and these can have a facilitative effect on the development of language. Furthermore, the presence of a communication board or other device on a lap tray, even if not actively used, often serves as an invitation to others to initiate interaction with the child. This situation is particularly advantageous if the child does not appear to be capable of functional communication.

There are, however, important cautions surrounding the introduction of communication aids. Sensitive counseling is required to keep family members from interpreting the presence of an aid as a tacit statement that the child will never speak. Staff and family members must also recognize that some children who are physically capable of using a communication system may not use it functionally, because of initiation problems or because the system places too great a demand on their capacity for new learning.

Cognitive function is a critical developmental area for long-term attention. Children ordinarily participate in educational programs; therefore, much of what would otherwise be called cognitive rehabilitation is accomplished in the traditional educational environment. Issues in school re-entry are discussed later in this chapter.

Since children commonly show behavioral changes following brain injury, support for the parents is necessary. Frequently, parents may be found to have had limited parenting skills before the injury occurred. Counseling about techniques of parenting, establishing expectations of the child's performance, and dealing with impulsive activity levels should be offered.

Rehabilitation of the child with a traumatic brain injury occurs throughout the natural history of the injury. Specific highlights of the rehabilitation approach during the various stages of this injury are described further on.

ACUTE MANAGEMENT

It is essential that rehabilitation management of the child with traumatic brain injury begin in the intensive care unit. The rehabilitation team should be consulted on the day of admission and actively participate in the patient's care in the intensive care setting. Early intervention in this way may prevent complications that could take months to resolve if left unmanaged during the acute care period.

SKIN INTEGRITY

Infants are at relatively low risk for skin breakdown because of their light body weight. The one common site of exception is the posterior aspect of the head. A T-foam pillow with a cut out for weight relief of the occipital tuberosity is helpful if frequent repositioning is not possible because of airway management or intravenous access needs.

The most frequent sites of skin breakdown in older children are the heels, malleoli, and sacrum. Placement of pillows between the calves and thighs while side lying helps to relieve pressure over the bony prominences at the knees and ankles. Placement of pillows between the knees and ankles should be avoided since this increases the pressure over sensitive bony prominences. A water or air mattress may be helpful if frequent repositioning is contraindicated because of difficulty in controlling increased intracranial pressure.

Decubitus ulcers that develop during the acute period can interfere with rehabilitation during the rapid recovery phase, prolong hospital stays, and greatly increase the cost of rehabilitation. Sacral ulcers may limit sitting and transfers severely, restricting mobility. This limitation may also impact on cognitive improvement as attentional function and sensory stimulation are diminished in the sidelying and prone positions. Skin breakdown in the extremities can interfere with casting and splinting needed to maintain range of motion, and bracing necessary to enhance functional skills such as transfers and ambulation.

SPASTICITY

Management of spasticity in the pediatric patient is similar in many aspects to adult management but there are several notable exceptions. Children are more sensitive than adults to the side effects of medications to control spasticity. Antispasticity medications should be avoided whenever possible. For children with severe spasticity not adequately managed with other therapeutic modalities, medication will be necessary. The team should observe the child for possible effects on arousal, attention, and cognitive functioning.

Diazepam, baclofen, and dantrolene sodium are the most commonly used antispasticity drugs.[13, 14] Diazepam has significant sedative side effects. Brain injured children often accommodate poorly to these side effects and tend to remain underaroused even at low dosages. The effects on attention and arousal may not be apparent during the early phases of recovery until the medication is withdrawn.[15]

Baclofen has been most effective in treating spinal cord mediated spasticity associated with spinal cord injuries and multiple sclerosis. It has also been effective in some head injured patients. Baclofen is less sedating than diazepam but can have deleterious effects on attentional function and memory.[16] The drug is associated with a low incidence of hallucinations, both on therapeutic doses and upon sudden withdrawal.[17, 18] No parenteral form of baclofen is available. This may be a problem in the child with erratic oral intake due to medical complications or behavioral problems.

Dantrolene sodium appears to be the least sedating of the antispasticity agents. Its mechanism of action is at the muscle level and thus dosage may require careful titration to prevent generalized weakness. It is essential that liver function tests be monitored closely, especially with changes in dosage.[13] Dantrolene sodium is the drug of choice in head injured children with normal liver function studies because of its limited deleterious effects on cognitive function.[19]

Physical modalities can be useful in the treatment of spasticity. Children often respond very well to sustained static stretch of tight muscles. The biarticular muscles, including the gastrocnemius, hamstrings, and long flexors of the feet and hands are particularly susceptible to tightness. Heat can be effective in reducing generalized tone. In young children, a Hubbard tank or therapeutic pool has many advantages. Generalized superficial sedative heat, buoyancy, and an excellent environment for early active assisted exercises against resistance are all provided by this modality. Other modalities such as cold, neutral warmth, and vibration are occasionally helpful.

The use of casting, especially inhibitive casting, can be remarkably effective for the reduction of spasticity in the pediatric patient. In the early stages of motor recovery, casting can provide decreases in spasticity. Proposed mechanisms of action include inhibition of mass reflexes by maintaining neutral joint positioning and decreasing hypertonia by virtue of total skin contact. A patient's reaction to foot positioning can be assessed at the bedside by manipulation of the foot into a position of neutral dorsiflexion with toe extension and abduction. If this is a relaxing manipulation, inhibitive casts can be fabricated to incorporate this posture.[20]

In the later stages of motor recovery, bivalved inhibitive casts are a useful therapeutic tool. These inhibitive casts should only be used as an adjunct to an intensive physical therapy program with a neurodevelopmental approach. They provide stability of the foot and ankle and can directly enhance knee stability. The stabilization of these joints allows the child and therapist more freedom to concentrate on improving proximal stability, trunk, and head control. Foot positioning can be incorporated into custom molded plastic orthotics for persisting problems. The use of orthotics must be closely monitored in a pediatric population. Modifications may be necessary as often as every 3 months during periods of rapid growth.

As with adults, chemical neurolysis can be greatly beneficial in the management of spasticity. Phenol nerve and motor point blocks have been used successfully in children. They should be employed in the following situations: when spasticity is not generalized but limited to a few localized problem areas; when use of medications is contraindicated secondary to liver function abnormalities, sedation, or other deleterious effects on cognitive function; or when other therapeutic modalities have not been adequate to control spasticity.[21, 22]

Chemical neurolysis of individual muscle groups may have more widespread effects by decreasing the stimulus for flexor or extensor synergy patterns. For example, an obturator nerve block to decrease adductor spasticity may allow the hips to be abducted to a neutral position, thereby decreasing the stimulus for extensor posturing during wheelchair positioning.

A decrease in spasticity in an agonist muscle group may unmask active voluntary control in a weaker antagonist muscle group. For example, a tibial nerve block resulting in decreased gastrocnemius-soleus spasticity may unmask voluntary movement in the anterior tibialis. Strengthening of the anterior tibialis during the effective period of the block may help to decrease spasticity over the long term by increasing reciprocal inhibition of the plantarflexors.

Diagnostic Marcaine blocks can be extremely useful in assessing the potential effect of spasticity reduction prior to performing a longer duration phenol block. Performance of the preliminary block is especially warranted when significant spasticity is present in both agonist and antagonist muscle groups. Reduction of tone in one muscle group may allow for an increase in tone in the opposing group, creating a new positioning or functional problem. Intramuscular neurolysis may be more effective in these situations as the effect of the block can be titrated more easily. The assessment of motor patterns is particularly critical when there is a dominance of primitive reflex patterns or a superimposed movement disorder.

Chemical neurolysis may be useful in the treatment of spasticity at any stage of recovery. In the acute period, it can help to prevent progressive loss of range of motion that cannot be maintained with positioning, therapy, and modalities. In later stages, it can be a beneficial adjunct to serial casting in the treatment of contractures. Spasticity reduction in the lower extremities can aid in achieving adequate wheelchair positioning and sitting tolerance. Chemical neurolysis has also been helpful in reducing clonus which interferes with transfers and ambulation training. Reduction of tone in the upper extremities can prevent disabling contractures, aid in splinting and positioning, and facilitate active movement.

Phenol blocks should be performed using 6.5 to 7 percent aqueous phenol. The peripheral nerve or motor point is located using percutaneous electrical stimulation. A teflon-coated needle attached to flexible tubing and a syringe is used to inject the phenol. This apparatus is shown in Figure 38-2.

Phenol blocks of peripheral nerves have a duration of action of approximately 6 to 12 months.[23] Phenol blocks at the intramuscular level generally have a shorter duration of action.[24] Duration may vary, depending on the number of motor points that are blocked. Phenol blocks of peripheral nerves may be preferable in children because of the relative ease of performance, compared with blocking multiple intramuscular sites, and the longer duration of effect. In our experience with children, the incidence of persistent pain problems following phenol blocks of peripheral nerves, including mixed motor and sensory nerves, is extremely low.

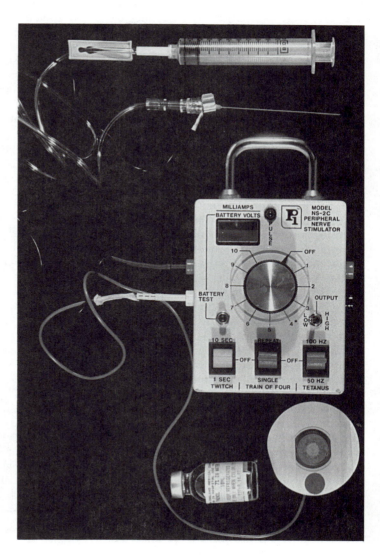

Figure 38-2. Apparatus for performing phenol nerve and motor point blocks with constant current stimulator (Courtesy of Life Tech Incorporated), extention tubing, and teflon-coated, 22-gauge open lumen needle (Courtesy of TECA Corporation).

In cases when rapid improvement is occurring but short-term control of spasticity is essential, alcohol muscle washes, with a duration of effect of 4 to 6 weeks, may be useful.[25]

POSITIONING

Careful attention should be paid to bed positioning to maintain skin integrity and to decrease spasticity and posturing.

In the acute stage, children often exhibit rigidity and posturing in response to minimal stimulation. The posturing is usually in a decorticate or decerebrate position. With decorticate posturing, the upper extremities are rigidly flexed and the lower extremities are extended. The trunk may be fully extended. With decerebrate posturing, both the upper and lower extremities are extended. Passive range of motion is extremely difficult during this stage, and the stimulation may exacerbate rigid posturing. Careful static positioning with the trunk and lower extremities in flexion can be helpful. A side-lying positioner can be used if this position cannot be maintained with pillows and towel rolls.

Mobilization should begin as soon as the child is medically stable. The upright position has many benefits, including providing increased awareness of the environment. Mobilization should begin with short sitting periods in a reclining wheelchair at 30 degrees with careful monitoring for orthostatic hypotension. The angle should be increased gradually until the child can tolerate a more vertical position. The time spent out of bed should be slowly increased as sitting tolerance improves. The child should be carefully observed for signs of discomfort or fatigue. These are most commonly demonstrated with an increase in agitation. Once reasonable sitting tolerance has been achieved, changes in environmental stimuli can be tried. Short periods of time out of the room can be spent at the nurses' station in the beginning.

Proper upright positioning in a well designed seating system can significantly reduce spasticity. Any seating system should begin with a solid seat of appropriate depth and a solid back. A high-back chair is helpful when head and trunk control are poor. The back should be slightly reclined to improve head and trunk control. The seat should be wedged anteriorly to maintain a 90-degree flexed position at the hips and knees. A low-slung pelvic belt on the chair is essential to keep the pelvis firmly stabilized in the chair. Cushions should be firm to provide a stable base. Two or three inches of a dense closed-cell foam is usually adequate. Pelvic obliquities should be carefully evaluated and asymmetric cushions made to accommodate them. If the pelvic obliquity is rigid, the foam cushion should be built up under the higher ischial tuberosity to provide more evenly distributed weight bearing. If the deformity is flexible, height should be added to the cushion beneath the lower ischial tuberosity to shift the pelvis into a more symmetric position. Pelvic blocks will help to control external hip rotation. An abduction wedge can be used if hip adduction is a problem. The wedge should never be used to push the child back into the chair. Lateral trunk supports can improve trunk stability. Proper positioning of the trunk decreases the risk of scoliosis in the growing child with neurologic impairment (Fig. 38–3).[26, 27]

An additional chest strap can be used if

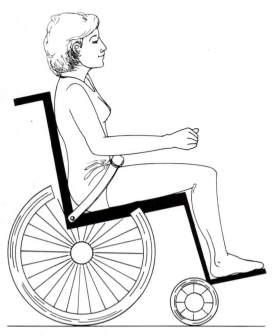

Figure 38–3. Idealized seating system demonstrating solid seat and back with wedged seat maintaining 90-degree hip and knee position.

trunk flexion posturing is a problem. This may also be improved by adding lumbar support to decrease posterior pelvic tilt. Appropriate head support and a lap tray for upper extremity positioning are also important.

A commercially available seating system which is flexible enough to adapt to a child's rapidly changing neurologic and functional status can be very useful during the rapid recovery phase and can facilitate early mobilization. The Mulholland wheelchair system can provide maximal control of trunk and head positioning with a variety of interchangeable positioning components. This seating system can be adapted to gradually decrease the amount of control it furnishes as the child improves. A power base can be added to provide early powered mobility. A new Mulholland positioning system will soon be available that has the option of active manual propulsion.

The Safety Travel Chair is another system that can provide good proximal control for the smaller child. It also permits changes of position in space while maintaining a 90-degree hip and knee angle to decrease spasticity. The chair can greatly contribute toward achieving the goals of increasing sitting tolerance and improving ability to tolerate a more vertical position. Frequent changes in position throughout the day may be necessary to allow for rest periods. Many head injured children make rapid progress during an inpatient rehabilitation phase and do not require wheelchair mobility at the time of discharge. Appropriate positioning during the early recovery period facilitates their functional rehabilitation and helps avoid potentially disabling complications.

CONTRACTURES

Contractures can severely limit functional abilities following traumatic brain injury. Passive range-of-motion exercises should be performed at least once and preferably twice a day in the intensive care unit (ICU) setting after intracranial pressure has been adequately controlled. This program requires the participation of the ICU nursing staff and also of families, if possible. Special attention should be paid to the shoulder, as external rotation range is often compromised very early.

Static positioning is critical in the maintenance of functional range of motion. Splinting of the wrist in extension and the fingers in a neutral position is optimal. The use of a small roll in the palm of the hand is often helpful in maintaining hand positioning. In infants, orthoplast splints are useful for positioning the thumb in abduction and maintaining the palmar web space. Serial casting of the upper extremity is rarely feasible in the ICU setting because of the urgent need for intravenous (IV) access.

Plantarflexion contractures at the ankle are common sequelae of traumatic brain injury. A combination of static positioning and frequent range-of-motion exercises is necessary for prevention. Passive range of motion should be performed with the knee in extension as well as flexion to prevent shortening of the gastrocnemius. Ranging the ankle with the knee in flexion will only adequately stretch the soleus since the gastrocnemius crosses the knee as well as the ankle joint. High-top sneakers worn in bed are useful positioning aids for the child without significantly increased tone. In the presence of increased extensor tone, well-padded fiberglass casts are the best positioning aids. They may be fabricated at the bedside and may be quickly bivalved for access to the lower extremities if needed for intravenous access. Frequent checks for skin tolerance to the casts, with modification of casts if needed, are integral management responsibilities.

When the child is medically stable, fixed contractures of the extremities are best treated with serial casting. These casts should be well padded and changed at weekly intervals until no further gains in range can be obtained. Drop-out casts can be very useful for the treatment of contractures at the elbow and knee. The use of therapeutic modalities such as ultrasound and electrical stimulation can be combined with drop-out casting. Bivalve casts can be fabricated to maintain a range when no further gains are being made with serial casting.

Contractures of the long finger flexors can be a difficult problem in the pediatric population. Casting is sometimes poorly tolerated because of the forces being applied over a small surface area. Initially casting may need to be done with the wrist in flexion to gain some extension of the fingers. Alternating splinting of the wrist in flexion with fingers in extension, and the wrist in extension with fingers in flexion may help to maintain range of motion.

Surgical intervention during the first year postinjury should be discouraged because of the potential for neurologic improvement. Patterns of spasticity and the resulting musculoskeletal deformities may show significant change over the first 1 to 2 years after injury. An aggressive physical therapy program supplemented by casting is the best initial management strategy. Adequate spasticity management is of paramount importance in preventing major deformities.

One major exception to the general rule of timing of surgical intervention is in the case of hip deformities. Children with hip flexor and adductor spasticity are at high risk for hip dislocation. This risk is particularly great in young children who do not have a fully developed acetabulum. Early intervention with positioning of the hips in abduction, neutral rotation, and slight flexion when in bed is necessary. Obturator nerve blocks may be helpful if severe adductor spasticity is present. Early surgical intervention may be needed if there is progressive loss of abductor range of motion and evidence of hip subluxation. Soft tissue releases, muscle releases, obturator neurectomy, or varus derotational osteotomy of the femur may be indicated.[28]

Scoliosis is often a late sequela of traumatic brain injury in children with persistent neurologic deficits. This is especially true in children with asymmetric spasticity. Scoliosis can be exacerbated by pelvic obliquity and hip dislocation. Seating systems designed to keep the pelvis level and to provide trunk control will improve postural alignment, but a seating system alone will not prevent the progression of spastic scoliosis. Properly fitted, custom molded, total contact orthoses may slow progression of the curve, but are not a definitive solution to the problem. Orthoses may assist in controlling scoliosis to delay surgical fusion in order to allow for growth and an attainment of an acceptable adult height. Long spinal fusions, often including the sacrum, are necessary when significant scoliosis develops. Fusions performed early, prior to the development of severe fixed deformities and large pelvis obliquities, are technically easier and result in better functional outcomes. Clinical follow-up for scoliosis should be done routinely, as the risk for development of neurogenic scoliosis continues beyond the end of the growth spurt in adolescence.[28]

MOTOR FUNCTION

Once the child is medically stable and out of the intensive care unit, a more intensive rehabilitation program can begin. In the early stages of the rapid recovery phase, the general approach should be toward as much hands-on therapy as possible. Family and nursing staff should be intensively involved in range-of-motion, positioning, and sensory stimulation programs.

Physical therapy should be directed toward preserving or recovering full range of motion and maximizing returning motor function. Therapy must be developmentally mediated, taking into account the child's present and premorbid developmental status. A neurodevelopmental treatment approach works well with children.[29] The neurodevelopmental postural support sequence should be worked through with emphasis on facilitation of protective reflexes and balance activities. Most therapists also use a variety of therapeutic modalities from several of the established schools of therapy as a basis for treatment as the child's needs change.[30] A skillful pediatric therapist can use play to engage a child in therapeutic activities directed toward the acquisition of new skills.

It is fundamental that the setting in which the therapy is performed be developmentally suitable. Therapeutic equipment should not be too large for small children. Toys should be used to aid in the development of gross and fine motor skills. In the young child, floor play is developmentally appropriate and should be encouraged. Alternate forms of mobility such as scooter boards and adapted tricycles can be explored prior to the achievement of independent ambulation.

Additional therapeutic settings such as swimming or riding programs can be most effective. The child's motivation is often significantly improved in these settings. Therapeutic horseback riding programs can improve lower extremity strength and positioning. Positioning of the hips in abduction combined with the rhythmic movement of the horse may aid in reducing spasticity. Exercises can target equilibrium and righting reactions. A well-conceived program can also focus on goals in many other areas, including: self-image, peer relations, social and pragmatic skills; orientation and spatial relations; following directions; motor planning and sequencing; gross and fine motor skills; and symbol discrimination.[31]

Peer group activities are quintessential for children. A small group setting with appropriate peers can be a forceful motivator. Socialization skills are readily incorporated into therapy sessions directed at improvement of motor skills.

In normal children, play activities are a major form of developing new motor skills. With the head injured child, play activities should be used to improve newly established gross and fine motor skills. Toys consonant with the child's cognitive level should be selected to enhance developing motor skills. For example, large pop beads can be used to encourage mid-line activities for the child who is beginning to be able to perform bimanual tasks.

Opportunities for play should be structured to allow for a successful play experience. Structured play activities can be helpful in refining motor skills, but one should ensure that these are not stressful or frustrating experiences for the child.[32]

A therapy program should not be all-consuming for child and family. There must be a balance between time spent on therapeutic activities for specific benefit and time focused on family life. Families must be able to spend time enjoying what the child can do and not solely concentrate on the child's disabilities. Families often need help in adapting play activities to take advantage of their child's abilities. Guides such as "Recipes for Fun" can be a good starting point.[33]

AMBULATION

Orthotics can be assistive in gait training if the child is unable to control motion in all joints. For example, stabilizing the foot and ankle in ankle-foot orthoses (AFOs) or plaster casts can allow the child to concentrate on trunk, hip, and knee control. Young children may achieve ambulatory status even if extensive bracing is required for joint control. Their short stature and low center of gravity enhance mechanical efficiency. A regression of these skills during the adolescent growth spurt is not unusual. The change in mechanical relationships with growth may tremendously increase the energy consumption necessary for ambulation. Other factors including emotional turmoil and increasing emphasis on social, intellectual, and vocational goals may play a role in the decrease in ambulatory function.

SENSORY STIMULATION

The rationale for carefully modulating the child's sensory environment in the early acute stage of recovery is based largely on the need to prevent secondary complications resulting from prolonged sensory deprivation, or overstimulation of a nervous system that is dramatically reduced in its capacity to filter and process stimuli and that may react pathologically (e.g., increased muscle tone) to inappropriate stimulation. In general, nursing care, therapists' interventions, and family interaction with the child are a natural context for sensory stimulation. *Specific* types of stimulation—for example, perioral stimulation designed to normalize oral responsiveness in preparation for feeding—should be provided by staff trained in the relevant techniques.[34]

Family and staff are encouraged to eliminate background noise and activity when interacting with the child, to alert and prepare the child for the care or treatment to come, and to monitor the child's responsiveness so that the sensory environment can be adjusted to promote the most adaptive responses. Families are invited to make audio tapes of the child's favorite music or familiar voices which can be played, in 10- to 15-minute segments, when no treatment is occurring. Families are also requested to bring in favorite toys and pictures of family, friends, and home so that the environment in which the child finally becomes alert has some degree of familiarity. These pictures and objects also help the nursing staff to associate a normal personality with the child who, at this stage of recovery, is minimally responsive.

ATTENTION AND AROUSAL

During the rapid recovery stage, children often have major problems with arousal and attention. At this stage, they are readily overwhelmed by the increased stimuli of the busy hospital environment. Children respond to overstimulation by either increased agitation or decreased arousal. Trials of therapy should be limited to short periods with close attention to agitation and level of arousal. In the rapid recovery phase, therapy is most effective when performed one-on-one in a quiet environment with a minimum of external distractions. As the child's attention and arousal improve, periods of time spent outside of the room can be increased.

Sedative drugs should be avoided whenever possible. When it is necessary to use medications, careful attention should be paid to their potential deleterious effects on cognitive and attentional function.[35]

Attention deficits may persist in milder forms during later stages of recovery. Stimulant medications are commonly used in the treatment of children with attention deficit disorders (ADD).[36, 37] They have been shown to diminish hyperactivity, decrease distractibility, and improve sustained attention. Methylphenidate hydrochloride (Ritalin) and dextroamphetamine are used most often.

The literature on the use of stimulants in head injured children is extremely limited. A trial of stimulant medication may be warranted when problems of attention and arousal are interfering with a child's progress in a rehabilitation program. Specific target behaviors should be identified prior to the trial of medication and monitored closely during the trial to assess effectiveness of treatment.

Trials of oral stimulants require close monitoring of pulse, blood pressure, and seizure-free status. Possible side effects of stimulants include anorexia, tachycardia, arrhythmias, hypertension, insomnia, headaches, and abdominal pain.

Although stimulants should be used with caution in patients with seizure disorders, they are not likely to provoke seizure activity. Stimulants can increase undesirable behaviors including unprovoked tearfulness, oversensitivity to reproach, irritability, lethargy, increased aggression, choreiform movements, and tics. Higher doses of stimulants can cause an increase in perseveration and stereotyping.[38]

Frequent reassessment is needed to determine their effectiveness in controlling the problem behavior. A double-blind trial of stimulants versus placebo may be needed to assess the true effect of stimulants on arousal and attentional functioning. Drug holidays should be planned as part of the long-term management strategy.[39]

Recent research has indicated some response to therapy with tricyclic antidepressants in children with attention deficit disorder with hyperactivity.[40, 41] A trial of antidepressants may be warranted in the child who does not respond to stimulant therapy, especially if there appears to be a depressive component to the attentional problems. Antidepressants can lower the seizure threshold; therefore, risk for seizure activity must be carefully considered.[38]

BEHAVIOR

Behavior problems frequently occur during all stages of recovery following traumatic brain injury. Aggressive behavior usually provokes the most anxiety among staff and family, but all forms of behavioral difficulties can adversely affect a person's functional reintegration into the community.

It is common for children to regress behaviorally during the early period after head injury. They often show clinging and overdependency on family members. It is important to discuss behavioral issues early with families. Regressive behavior must be explained in the context of the recent head injury. Behavior management strategies with positive reinforcement should begin early. During this period, children often behave in a way that is inappropriate, impulsive, and even bizarre. A salient goal of behavior management is to prevent these behaviors from becoming learned behavior patterns. This requires consistent responses from family and staff as well as control of the environment so that factors that elicit inappropriate behavior can be reduced. Effective responses to the undesirable behavior include a skillful mix of ignoring the behavior and redirecting the child's attention. If the behavior is perseverative or purely impulsive rather than attention seeking, then ignoring the behavior may be insufficient. In this case, the child should be redirected to another task, but not in a way that unintentionally rewards the inappropriate behavior. Consultation with a behavioral psychologist is often advisable.

The most common behavioral patterns in

children less than 8 years old involve hyperactivity, short attention span, poor sustained attention, temper tantrums, impulsiveness, aggressive and destructive behavior, and enuresis. Older children tend to show poor initiation with motivational problems, apathy, and lethargy. Other frequently observed problems include depression, denial, euphoria, acting-out behavior, emotional regression, poor judgment, and overdependency.

These children often display inappropriate social behavior with general disinhibition. They are often unaware of social boundaries and may initiate physical contact with casual acquaintances. Because of these personality changes many severely injured children lose the friends they had before the injury, compounding the psychosocial adjustment difficulties that they face.

The lack of inhibition may result in increased vulnerability to the actions of others. Parents must be exceptionally cautious to control the younger child's willingness to approach strangers, with the potential risk of abduction being increased. For older children and adolescents, particularly females, organically based disinhibition can result in sexual vulnerability or promiscuity. Provision of a suitably structured and protective environment is necessary to avoid these additional problems.

Affect is often inappropriate. Parents will often describe their child as "silly," with frequent giggling. It is instructive to help families and teachers understand that these behavioral patterns are related to the child's brain injury and must be managed with that perspective.

The most effective behavioral management strategy at this stage involves clear and consistent limit setting, combined with attempts to guarantee as much social and academic success for the child as possible. Parents need to understand that consistently applied limits within the child's physical capabilities and cognitive abilities are fitting and necessary. This is often a difficult management plan of action for families of children who have so recently been critically ill. The emotional burden of family members who are in a phase of active grief for their child's losses frequently limits their ability to engage in consistent limit setting and behavioral management strategies.

Children with behavior problems must be carefully assessed in all settings to identify situations provoking specific problematic behaviors. Specific baseline data including frequency, duration, intensity, and environmental factors should be collected. Reactions of other people to the behavior and its consequences should be evaluated. In the inpatient setting, the entire rehabilitation team must be involved in behavior management planning. Emphasis of the plan should be on the reinforcement of appropriate behavior rather than the consequences and punishment of unsuitable behavior. For the child living in the community, behavioral planning must include significant people from both home and school. Behavior management must be consistent throughout the child's day to be effective.[42-44]

Careful assessment of attentional function and arousal is an important first step in the study of aggressive behavior. Withdrawal of sedating medications such as benzodiazepines can be helpful. Brain injured children seem to be especially sensitive to the cognitive side effects of medications. Many children are placed on phenobarbital or Dilantin for seizure prophylaxis. Tapering of these sedating anticonvulsants and initiation of carbamazepine may improve a child's attention and arousal, leading to a significant decrease in aggressive and inappropriate behavior. If attention and arousal problems persist, a trial of stimulants may be indicated.[45]

The use of pharmacologic therapy for behavioral management in head injured children and adolescents has been extrapolated from the literature on the use of medications in psychiatric and mentally retarded populations. Very few data are available on the use of medications in head injured children. One must be cautious in the comparison of these populations, as the etiology of their behavior problems may be quite different.

We do not recommend the use of neuroleptic agents such as haloperidol and chlorpromazine in head injured children. Studies in the mental retardation literature indicate that neuroleptics may impair learning and performance.[46] There are also significant risks of problematic side effects, especially tardive dyskinesia.

With many children, behavioral functioning improves over time, particularly with return to a normal routine. However, it is not uncommon for behavioral disturbances to worsen over the course of 2 to 3 years following the injury.[47] This is emphatically the case with children who return to families poorly equipped to understand and manage behavior problems. The problems that persist usually involve disinhibited and inappropriate social behavior, poor judgment, and attentional deficits.

COGNITIVE RETRAINING

Cognitive retraining begins with early informal neuropsychological testing and speech and language therapy during inpatient rehabilitation. Detailed formal cognitive assessment does not yield results that are meaningful for rehabilitation planning until the child's recovery has slowed and he or she is sufficiently attentive and oriented to respond appropriately to test items. Therefore, informal but careful tracking of cognitive functioning is indicated during the recovery phase, characterized by rapid change and some degree of confusion. Cognitive assessment is discussed at length in Chapter 37.

Cognitive rehabilitation is best understood as a variety of interventions designed to promote adaptive and successful behavior that otherwise is blocked by cognitive deficits. Understood in these broad terms, cognitive rehabilitation includes much of the treatment provided by speech pathologists, occupational therapists, teachers, recreation therapists, psychologists, and others. Furthermore, it includes the following:

☐ Environmental modifications (e.g., posting orientation reminders in the child's environment, reducing expectations for the child's performance)

☐ Remedial exercises (e.g., practicing systematic left-right perceptual scanning, practicing clear and concise expression of thoughts; practicing organized problem solving)

☐ Content instruction (e.g., teaching the child academic content, teaching the child about head injury and his or her deficits)

☐ Training in compensatory strategies (e.g., requesting speakers to repeat their message, recording information in a memory book)

One of the dominant themes of the rapid recovery phase is confusion, resulting from general disruption of the cognitive system.

Despite their increasing alertness, children at this stage lack adequate orientation to their condition and surroundings, process information slowly and incompletely, have shallow recall of the recent past, and have poor access to their stored knowledge. Small increases in cognitive stress (the amount or complexity of information to be processed, the rate of its presentation, or interference in the environment) may result in substantial functional breakdowns. The general goals of rehabilitation at this stage are to (1) reduce the child's confusion; (2) increase adaptive, purposeful behavior; (3) systematically increase the efficiency of information processing; and (4) re-establish basic organized thinking (relative to age expectations).

A major component of cognitive intervention at this stage is environmental support. Places, schedules, staff, and routines should be as consistent as possible to promote orientation. Throughout the day, children should be given meaningful orienting information (e.g., where they are and why; what therapy they are going to, with whom, and why) in the context of easy-to-understand conversational exchanges. Personal items should be stored in consistent places. The child's room should include age-appropriate orientation cues such as a calendar and printed schedule. Events of the day should be recorded in a log book that is reviewed several times a day by family members or nursing staff. Routine daily living activities should be analyzed into component parts so that, with cueing, the child can successfully perform some part of the task (e.g., taking the lid off the toothpaste). As processing abilities improve, the child can be given more of the task and be expected to complete the task with systematically decreasing cues. In this way, activities that occur naturally over the course of the day can be used by family and nursing staff to systematically encourage improved information processing and organized functional behavior. Staff and family members should be trained to respond to inappropriate language and bizarre behavior in a way that promotes learning and communicates understanding, but without reinforcing undesirable behavior.[48]

At this stage, specific cognitive treatment activities are also designed to promote more efficient and organized processing of information, without expecting children to understand their deficits or compensate for them in a deliberate way. Structured activities in occupational or recreation therapy sessions (puzzles, games, projects) can be designed so that the focus is on one or two cognitive dimensions of the task (e.g., attending selectively, organizing the parts, remembering the instructions), with improvement measured by systematic increases in performance in those dimensions.

Language therapy sessions during this phase of recovery should include activities designed to improve the efficiency of language processing (both receptive and expressive) and to promote more organized thinking and retrieval of information. Since conceptual organization of preschoolers is largely idiosyncratic, based on their concrete experiences, it is useful to rehearse "real-event scripts" in play and in descriptive language tasks. If, for example, the child had attended a preschool before the accident, a therapy session could include the creation of a "school script" with toys, followed by the child's dictating the story to the therapist. Children then may carry the written story—an organized description of an event that was an important part of their lives—with them so that it can be read to the children by family and staff or repeated by the children several times a day. In this way the children recreate meaningful organizational schemas and practice the organized expression of ideas. Progress is measured by the number of toys that the child can meaningfully organize in play and by the amount of information that can be clearly expressed in language.

Older children can be given language organizational tasks that represent more mature thinking. For example, the child may be asked to (1) consider some familiar person, object, or event; (2) analyze it: what type of thing is it? what does it do? what is it used for? where is it found? what attributes/parts does it have? what does it make you think of?; (3) consider ways in which it is similar to and different from a related object or event; and then (4) write a short descriptive paragraph about the object or event. Activities of this sort help children to re-establish access to their stored knowledge, to retrieve information in an organized manner, to classify and organize effectively, and to express themselves clearly. Haarbauer-Krupa and colleagues present a number of therapy activities appropriate for children at this stage of recovery.[49]

It is important to modify expectations for language and articulation by recognizing what is developmentally germane to each child. As with adults, the use of computer software has been facilitative in providing structure, repetition and feedback in cognitive retraining. There is a great deal of commercially available software, but each program must be assessed individually to determine if it is compatible with the goals of the therapeutic program. Anecdotally, video games have been ascribed as a motivating force in children, especially useful in focusing on attentional problems and fine motor skill deficits.

Many severely injured children evidence residual cognitive deficits that cannot be remediated through practice, however intensive and well conceived the exercises may be. General aspects of cognitive functioning such as memory should not be conceptualized as "mental muscles" that are strengthened by exercise. Long-term cognitive deficits are frequently observed in these areas:

☐ Concentration and attentional flexibility
☐ Efficiency (especially speed) of information processing
☐ Memory/new learning
☐ Organization of behavior and of language expression
☐ Abstract thinking
☐ Organized problem solving
☐ Executive functions, including self-awareness of strengths and weaknesses, goal setting, planning, self-initiating, self-inhibiting, self-monitoring, self-evaluating

Faced with cognitive deficits that do not resolve spontaneously or with targeted remedial exercises, clinicians must consider either adaptations in environment that can promote efficient learning and successful performance of meaningful tasks, or strategies that children can use to compensate for their cognitive weaknesses. Environmental compensations, including the classroom adaptations listed later in this chapter, may indefinitely continue to be necessary for traumatically brain injured children.

Compensatory strategies are procedures that children deliberately use to achieve a goal that is difficult to attain because of impaired functioning. Strategies may include external aids, such as a memory book or tape recorder to compensate for impaired memory, or a task guide to compensate for organizational problems. Alternatively, strategies may include overt behavior (e.g., asking a teacher for written directions or for additional time to complete a task) or covert behavior (e.g., mentally organizing, elaborating, or rehearsing information so that it is easier to remember.)[49]

Successful strategy intervention begins with the selection of appropriate candidates. Although it may be possible to train preschoolers or older children with severe cognitive impairments to use alternative behaviors (e.g., to use gestures when they cannot retrieve the appropriate word), it is unreasonable to expect them to engage in *deliberate* compensatory behavior. As a rough guide, children should have the cognitive maturity of average students in the early to middle grades before they can be expected to master compensatory behavior and use it effectively in the appropriate situations. Good candidates for this intervention should have meaningful goals to which strategies apply, should recognize that they have deficits, and should have adequate attentional functioning so that they can attend to strategies and also the task at hand. Furthermore, they should be capable of learning to recognize situations in which use of the strategy is suitable, and not be so impulsive that they would inevitably act before considering the use of a strategic procedure. Successful intervention also presupposes that significant individuals in the child's environment, especially teachers and parents, support and encourage the use of strategies.

Effective strategy instruction includes active engagement of the child in identifying the problem and experimenting with different procedures that might be useful. It is much more likely that a compensatory strategy will be used if the child has selected it and appreciates its value in relation to real-world goals than if it is simply presented by the teacher or therapist as another task to master. Instruction should also be intensive and systematic so that the strategic procedure becomes automatic. To promote generalization, strategies must be practiced in a variety of settings and tasks and with functional materials. For example, if an adolescent needs to take notes when reading a text and to organize the notes in a specific way to ensure comprehension of the material, this activity should be practiced in a real or simulated classroom setting with actual texts. Generalization of strategic procedures from a training situation to functional application in the child's academic or social setting rarely occurs without deliberate efforts to ensure generalization. Issues in cognitive strategy intervention are discussed in several recent texts.[50–52]

FAMILY ADJUSTMENT

A major role of the rehabilitation team in the acute stage is to help families cope with the stressful environment of the ICU. It is of critical importance to interpret the early signs of recovery for families and to distinguish between involuntary posturing and evolving voluntary movement. Although families often over-react to the early signs of recovery, it is necessary to take all reports seriously. Early volitional responses to stimuli are frequently inconsistent, and often first occur with familiar family members. The rehabilitation team should work closely with the family to objectively assess any observed change in status.

It is beneficial for families to be actively involved in the care of their child in the acute care environment. This activity can aid in reducing their fears and anxiety while instilling a sense of constructive caring. Parents can be taught exercises and positioning techniques by the physical therapist and can be encouraged to participate in nursing care (e.g., feeding and bathing) if such activities are considered safe.

Families can also be encouraged to participate in sensory stimulation. Parents should be advised to talk to the child since it is unclear at what point he or she becomes responsive to familiar auditory stimulation.

Early introduction of the families to other parents of brain injured children, possibly through contact with a local chapter of the National Head Injury Foundation, may be therapeutic for all involved persons. Sharing of experiences with peers offers a level of support not easily obtained in other ways.

The entire family unit must be considered during discharge planning for the child with traumatic brain injury. Home may not always be the optimal environment, especially for the severely disabled child. The team must assess the magnitude of the child's daily physical, emotional, and behavioral needs and the family's ability to provide this level of care. When a home discharge is planned, arranging for adequate home services, including respite care, is essential to maintain the family unit. The stress of caring for a disabled child at home can be overwhelming if adequate support services, including family counseling, are not available. These problems can lead to a more unstable environment for the disabled child and siblings, or even to breakup of the family unit.

SIBLINGS

The entire family unit is affected when a child suffers a severe traumatic brain injury. Siblings should be given accurate information at a level they can understand throughout the hospital admission. They should be prepared for the changes in their sibling prior to visiting. It is sometimes advisable to engage older siblings in volunteer roles in the hospital to help them gain perspective. Group discussions, particularly for adolescent siblings, may promote an understanding of head injury and provide a forum for the expression of concerns. For example, the group can discuss appropriate responses to peers who ridicule the injured family member and effective ways to deal with parents who do not openly discuss the problems posed by the injured sibling's behavior. Many siblings express feelings of vulnerability, anxiety, guilt, fear, and jealousy during the grieving period. Families must allow siblings to express their fears and emotions. Professional counseling may be necessary.

Particular attention should be paid to the siblings and their reactions during the discharge planning process. Family life has been significantly disrupted during the inpatient phase of recovery. Siblings will often react to the attention the "special" child has received during the acute phase. If possible, parents should include siblings in the planning process for the return home of the "special" child. Siblings may demonstrate behavior problems themselves, either as a reaction to their relative loss of parental attention, or due to feelings of guilt over the cause of injury (whether justified or not). Helping the family to find ways of preserv-

ing attention to the sibling's emotional needs may facilitate a more successful long-term home placement for the injured child.

Case 1. R.P. is a 5-year-old boy whose 9-year-old sister suffered a traumatic brain injury when hit by a school bus while crossing the street. He visited her several times during her 2-month hospitalization, the first time while she was still in a coma. At discharge, his sister could walk independently but was still mildly ataxic. She had mild cognitive deficits, emotional lability, and poor endurance. R.P. was extremely overprotective of his sister, assuming the role of an older brother. He hovered over her, offering constant supervision which was not necessary. As her functional skills improved, he was unable to accept her increasing independence, leading to frequent conflicts. Family therapy was helpful in resolving these issues.

As this case example illustrates, sibling roles may be significantly altered following discharge. Parents must be sensitive to changes in sibling relationships. Professional family counseling may be needed if there are behavioral changes that interfere with the function of the family unit.

Finally, injured children and their families should receive long-term follow-up by the rehabilitation team. This is particularly important for young children, since the brain injury may manifest itself in new and unpredictable ways as the child enters new developmental phases. For instance, children injured as preschoolers may experience greater than expected difficulty when they begin their formal education: children injured in the early grades may have unusual difficulty during the normally problematic early adolescent years. Scheduled re-evaluations during these important transitional periods may be needed to ensure continuity of services. Family follow-up is equally important, since stresses on the family system may grow following reintroduction of the injured family member into the home.

RETURN TO SCHOOL

Early close collaboration with the educational system is necessary to successfully reintegrate the child into the school system. A teacher should be included as a member of the rehabilitation team. Education should begin with tutoring in the hospital when the child's cognitive and attentional functions are adequate for participation.

For school-age children, community schools are often the setting in which long-term rehabilitative care is delivered. This is particularly true in an era of reduced lengths of stay in hospitals and rehabilitation facilities alike. However, very few school systems have specialized programs for traumatically brain injured children; indeed, few teachers, supervisors, or school administrators have been exposed to this disability group in their preservice or inservice training.[53] Consequently, rehabilitation professionals must pay special attention to the transition from hospital to school to ensure that the child's program of rehabilitation is maintained and continues to be adjusted as the child recovers neurologically and responds, positively or negatively, to the demands of school.

In the absence of a planned transition, the most likely consequence is academic failure and behavioral maladjustment. Since the common cognitive and psychosocial deficits that underlie this failure are often difficult to detect, school personnel who are poorly oriented to traumatic brain injury may respond punitively to the child's substandard work or behavioral inappropriateness. This easily sets in motion a downward spiral of failure, misinterpretation of that failure, and negative behavioral response that is an all-too-common natural history following traumatic brain injury in children.

There are three general approaches to school re-entry for severely head injured children: (1) to use established criteria for classroom placement and provision of special services; (2) to place these children in special TBI classrooms, either transitional or permanent; (3) to create a customized package of services, without regard to established criteria, that supports the child's academic and social growth in a setting that is as close to normal as possible.

Traditional Placement. There is a natural resistance on the part of school officials to considering traumatic brain injury a separate special education category, analogous to categories such as hearing impairment, visual impairment, learning disability, mental retardation, physical handicap, and emotional disturbance. Traumatic brain injury

appears to be strictly an etiologic, rather than a disability category; depending on many factors, these children may have no special education needs or they may fall into one of the existing categories. Thus, it is common for school authorities to offer special services only if the head injured child meets established criteria for classification in one of the traditional special education categories.

This approach has many shortcomings. Unlike the other special education categories, traumatic brain injury is a dynamic neurologic condition for a period of from several months to several years following a severe injury. Classification of a child as mentally handicapped or learning disabled at the time of hospital discharge may be completely inappropriate within weeks of school re-entry. Furthermore, even at the time of re-entry, such classification rarely represents a good fit with the injured child and his or her educational needs.

For example, TBI students with substantial brain damage and severe learning impairment may resemble, in global intellectual functioning, mentally retarded students. However, unlike most students with mental retardation, head injured students generally evidence a sharply varied profile of skills and knowledge, and continue to reacquire skills for years following the injury. Furthermore, placement in a setting for mentally retarded students is socially inappropriate and educationally counterproductive for most head injured students and can be emotionally explosive for the students and their families.

Like learning disabled students, many TBI students score within normal limits on tests of intelligence despite substantial difficulty learning new information, weak attentional and organizational skills, slow processing of information, impulsive and disinhibited behavior, and reduced tolerance for stress. However, in important ways these TBI students are also different from their learning disabled peers. For example, they frequently reacquire basic academic content (reading—at least at the level of word recognition and phonics—as well as spelling and arithmetic calculation) that children who have been learning disabled from birth have great difficulty acquiring. Hence, much of the curriculum in a learning disabilities classroom may be irrelevant to the needs of the TBI student. These students also have an academic and cognitive profile that is not only varied (like many learning disabled students) but also "gappy"; for example, a student injured in ninth grade may remember much of the algebra that was learned in ninth grade, but be weak at third grade–level calculation. To approach the education of this child in a "bottom-up" hierarchical fashion characteristic of learning disabilities curricula may be inefficient, in that it fails to capitalize on the surprising strengths at higher levels of skill acquisition and on the child's motivation to do ninth grade work.

These examples illustrate some of the problems in placing a TBI child within the special education system. An entirely different set of problems is illustrated by those children who have legitimate special education needs, but whose test results fail to qualify them for those services. For example, TBI students with significant learning deficits but good recovery of pretraumatically acquired information may not evidence a significant disparity between their actual academic achievement scores and the scores predicted by their IQ. Therefore, they may not technically qualify for learning disabilities or any other services.

TBI Classrooms. A small number of school districts, university laboratory schools, and private rehabilitation facilities have classrooms specifically for students following head injury. In most cases, they are transitional settings, designed for students who are discharged from the hospital or rehabilitation facility while they are still confused, disoriented, and changing rapidly. These classrooms provide a useful service in expertly managing the children during a pivotal stage of recovery and in systematically investigating the variables (environmental, instructional, motivational) that influence academic and social success, thereby enabling the community school to educate the child in the most efficient manner possible.

Creative and Unique Packages of Services. For most traumatically brain injured children, the most reasonable approach to school re-entry is to abandon traditional criteria for services (which, in any case, have not been validated with this population) and to customize a set of services that includes as much regular classroom learning

as possible along with whatever support is needed to allow the child to progress academically and socially. These supports may include

1. Special education resource room intervention
2. Tutorial or itinerant specialist services
3. Remedial programs
4. Ancillary services/therapies
5. Consulting services (e.g., behavioral psychology)
6. Classroom adaptations, including
    a. Individualized instruction
    b. Ability grouping
    c. A shortened day (gradually increasing to a full day)
    d. Rest periods
    e. Seating/environmental modification
    f. Materials modification (e.g., enlarged print books, fewer mathematics problems on a page)
    g. Compensatory equipment (e.g., tape recorder, calculator)
    h. Additional processing or work time
    i. Reduced assignments
    j. Testing modifications (e.g., oral, open-book, or take-home tests)
    k. Posted/written assignments, schedules, and task guides
    l. An assignment and accomplishment notebook
    m. A buddy system
    n. Peer tutoring

Cohen and colleagues[54] discuss in some detail classroom strategies suitable for many traumatically brain injured children.

Essential to the success of this approach is a designated program coordinator who serves as a consultant to the staff teachers and therapists, ensures the integration of services, and monitors the adequacy of the service mix over time. Without such a person, good educational programs readily disintegrate into poor programs because the services fail to keep pace with the student or because deterioration in the services over time is not recognized. The program coordinator may or may not be an employee of the school district but must have expertise in traumatic brain injury in children, must be familiar with resources in the school system and in the hospital system, and must be a skilled negotiator and an effective teacher of professionals and family members.

Rehabilitation professionals must work with school personnel to create an individualized academic program for each traumatically brain injured child. This cooperative effort requires flexibility and a departure from eligibility criteria that were created for quite different groups of children. Often the most general special education classification ("Other Health Impaired") is useful for purposes of enabling the child to receive special education services without thereby dictating the nature of those services or imposing a stigmatizing label. If the child's community school cannot create an educational program that is suitable, then the family, together with the local education authority and the hospital staff, should consider transitional placement in a residential school/rehabilitation facility for traumatically brain injured children.

The foundation for a smooth and ultimately successful school re-entry is created by active and open communication between hospital and school personnel. Shortly after the child's admission to the hospital or rehabilitation center, the school (in most cases the principal) should be contacted. The goals of this communication are to give the school an update on the child's status, to establish a working relationship with school personnel, and to raise the possibility that the child may require a special set of services when he or she returns to school.

Several weeks before discharge to home and community school, the family, together with the rehabilitation staff, should initiate development of an individual education program (IEP) with the local school district. Although specific regulations and practices vary from state to state, it is always the right of parents to approve or reject the proposed educational program. Recommendations for the content of the IEP should be made by the rehabilitation team, including specific goals and frequencies of treatment as well as classroom placement and adaptations. The school system may require an evaluation by its own staff before completing the IEP. If there is a discrepancy between the program recommended by the rehabilitation staff and that proposed by the school district, a period of negotiation should ensue that includes providing the school staff with educational materials on traumatic brain injury and, if necessary, inservice training.

It is also advisable to bring brain injured adolescents to the attention of the appropriate vocational rehabilitation agencies. Even if specific vocational services will not be needed in the immediate future, the office of vocational rehabilitation is in a position to track the adolescent's progress and have services available when they are indicated. States have the responsibility to provide transitional services to vocational training for special-needs students who are outgrowing their eligibility for publicly sponsored special education services.

Shortly before discharge, teachers and therapists from the school should be invited to the rehabilitation facility to observe the child's program and discuss plans for continuation of the rehabilitation program in the school setting. Often, however, it is logistically easier for hospital staff to visit the school than for school staff to visit the hospital. The school visit is designed to evaluate the school from a physical perspective (accessibility, distance from class to class, and so on) as well as from a cognitive and behavioral perspective (e.g., level of activity in the halls and in the classrooms, suitability of the educational materials and curriculum in the proposed classroom). The visit also creates an opportunity to assess the school staff members' understanding of traumatic brain injury and of interventions that are indicated for this group. It is useful to give the school relevant educational materials such as the National Head Injury Foundation's *Educator's Manual*[55] and to offer inservice training for the school staff.

A treatment videotape, made shortly before discharge from the rehabilitation facility, is an effective medium for communicating important treatment ideas. For example, physical therapists can demonstrate techniques of physical management (positioning, therapeutic handling, transferring) and educators in the rehabilitation setting can demonstrate instructional strategies and environmental modifications of known value to the child.

It is often constructive to prepare peers before the child's return to school. In terms that they can easily understand, fellow students should learn that the child may be different from before the accident and that these differences can include cognitive and emotional changes as well as physical changes. Concrete suggestions on how classmates can interact with the child may prevent some of the awkwardness and apparent rejection of the injured child that frequently occurs following a severe injury.

The re-establishment of peer relationships may proceed slowly. Initially, children are most comfortable interacting with one peer in a noncompetitive environment. Pragmatic skills are often significantly impaired. Impaired nonverbal communication skills can contribute to problems with peer relationships. Once the child is able to interact with several different peers in a one-to-one situation, an introduction to group dynamics can begin. Structured noncompetitive group settings such as Boy Scouts or Girl Scouts can be a good starting point.

School planning for head injured adolescents is especially difficult. As the following case illustrates, returning to a large high school can be problematic for an adolescent with even minor cognitive, attentional, perceptual, or motor deficit.

Case 2. T.S. is a 16-year-old boy who suffered a severe traumatic brain injury in a motor vehicle accident 6 months ago. He has made excellent progress but still has minor attentional, perceptual, and fine motor deficits. He has had individual tutoring at home and his academic skills are now at grade level. He is returning to a large high school where each of his classes is in a separate classroom. He arrives at school and has difficulty locating his locker. Once he finds it, he tries the combination several times but is unable to open the lock. He checks the combination in his pocket and realizes that he has reversed the numbers. He succeeds in opening his locker but the bell has rung and he is now late for class. He is unsure of what books he should take with him and whether he will be able to return to his locker before lunch. Arriving at a history class already in session, he finds his seat, dropping his books as he attempts to sit down. Finally he gets settled into the seat but has difficulty in paying attention to the teacher. He has reviewed this material recently with his tutor but finds his attention wandering to the charts on the wall, the noises from the street outside, and the turning notebook pages of his classmates. The bell rings and his teacher gives the assignment for tomorrow. T.S. is distracted by sounds from the hallway and does not note the assignment. After class he stops to ask the teacher to repeat the assignment, but the teacher is talking with another student and becomes impatient when T.S. interrupts. He realizes he's late for the next class and leaves without his homework assignment. In the crowded hallway, he must concentrate on keeping his balance, becomes disoriented, and is unable to locate his next class.... He returns home from school and his mother asks how his day went. "Fine," he responds.

Head injured adolescents are at high risk for developing social problems. If they are returning to their premorbid school setting, their friends may initially be supportive. Over time, these peer relationships tend to fade. The head injured adolescent often does not fit well into his previous peer group because of diminished social, pragmatic, and athletic skills. These adolescents are extremely vulnerable and are at risk for developing drug and alcohol problems in their attempts to be accepted socially.

Adolescent girls often become involved in inappropriate sexual relationships. Promiscuity may not be consistent with their premorbid personality but is often related to their low self-esteem, disinhibition, and need for acceptance in peer relationships. Parents of head injured adolescents need to be aware of these potential problems. It is essential that both parents and teenagers receive adequate education about contraceptives if these problems exist.

At the age of 16 or 17, driving becomes a common issue. Head injured people need careful evaluation prior to receiving a driver's license. It is mandatory to assess multiple factors including reaction time, distractibility, and neglect, as well as motor and cognitive performance. Driver training should be done with instructors who are familiar with the deficits that can result from traumatic brain injury. Training should occur in a dual-controlled car over a period of time adequate to provide experience in all situations including variations in time of day, weather conditions, and traffic patterns.

Long-term neuropsychologic follow-up is essential. These children may demonstrate progressive cognitive improvements several years after their initial injury. Children will also continue to gain skills on the basis of normal growth and development. These changes must be serially analyzed and documented so that appropriate modifications of educational programs can be planned.

SUMMARY

The rehabilitation management of head injured children is complex and requires a coordinated team approach. In addition to appreciating that children are not small adults, professionals must maintain an awareness of the processes of growth and maturation. Rehabilitation programs should be designed to take advantage of this poten-tial for further progress. The impact of the child's injury on the entire family must be considered. The family can be a valuable resource and should receive the education necessary to become an active member of the rehabilitation team. Careful follow-up of the child and family is obligatory. Attention should be paid to family dynamics and the social functioning of the child in home and school environments. Serial neuropsychologic testing should be done to assess for learning disabilities and attentional problems in all head injured children including those with good recovery. Cautious optimism is usually warranted in predicting the outcome of children with significant brain injuries.

REFERENCES

1. Gans, BM: Pediatric Trauma Registry, unpublished data, 1987.
2. Bruce, DA: Outcome following severe head injuries in children. J Neurosurg 48:679, 1978.
3. Brink, JD et al: Recovery of motor and intellectual function in children sustaining severe head injuries. Dev Med Child Neurol 12:565, 1970.
4. Brink, JD et al: Physical recovery after severe closed head trauma in children and adolescents. Pediatrics 97:721, 1980.
5. Levin, HS et al: Neuropsychological outcome of closed head trauma in children and adolescents. Child Brain 5:281, 1979.
6. Behrman, R et al: Nelson Textbook of Pediatrics. WB Saunders, Philadelphia, 1987.
7. Cailliet, R: Scoliosis Diagnosis and Management. FA Davis, Philadelphia, 1975.
8. Bobath, B: Abnormal Postural Reflex Activity Caused by Brain Lesions, ed 2. Wm Heinemann, London, 1971.
9. Flavell, JH: Cognitive Development. Prentice-Hall, Englewood Cliffs, NJ, 1977.
10. Siegler, RS: Children's Thinking. Prentice-Hall, Englewood Cliffs, NJ, 1986.
11. Ylvisaker, M, Szekeres, S and Cohen, SB: A framework for cognitive rehabilitation therapy. In Ylvisaker, M (ed): Community Re-entry for Head Injured Adults. College-Hill Press, San Diego, 1987, p 87.
12. Gans, BM and Hallenborg, SC: Advances in wheelchair design. In Redford, JB: Physical Medicine and Rehabilitation: State of the Art Reviews. Vol 1. 1987, p 95.
13. Young, R and Delwaide, P: Spasticity, Part I. N Engl J Med 304:28, 1981.
14. Young, R and Delwaide, P: Spasticity, Part II. N Engl J Med 304:96, 1981.
15. Romney, DM and Angus, WR: A brief review of the effects of diazepam on memory. Psychopharmacol Bull 20:313, 1984.
16. Sandy, KR and Gillman, MH: Baclofen-induced memory impairment. Clin Neuropharm 8:294, 1985.
17. Mann, NR and Gans, BM: Hallucinations associated with acute baclofen withdrawal: Report of two pediatric cases. Arch Phys Med Rehabil 66:564, 1985.
18. Terrence, CF and Fromm, GH: Complications of baclofen withdrawal. Arch Neurol 38:588, 1981.
19. Glenn, MB and Wroblewski, B: Antispasticity medications in the patient with traumatic brain injury. J Head Trauma Rehabil 1(2):71, 1986.
20. Watt, J et al: A prospective study of inhibitive casting as an adjunct to physiotherapy for cerebral-palsied children. Dev Med Child Neurol 28:480, 1986.
21. Glenn, MB: Nerve blocks in the treatment of spasticity. J Head Trauma Rehabil 1(3):72, 1986.
22. Easton, JKM, Ozel, T and Halpern, D: Intramuscular neurolysis for spasticity in children. Arch Phys Med Rehabil 53:179, 1972.
23. Khalili, AA and Betts, HB: Peripheral nerve block with phenol in the management of spasticity. JAMA 200:103, 1967.
24. Halpern, D and Meelhuysen, FE: Duration of relaxation after neuromuscular neurolysis with phenol. JAMA 200:100, 1967.
25. Carpenter, EB and Seitz, DG: Intramuscular alcohol as an aid in the management of spastic cerebral palsy. Dev Med Child Neurol 22:497, 1980.
26. Wilson, AB: Wheelchairs: A Prescriptive Guide. Rehabilitation Press, Charlottesville, VA, 1986.
27. Trefler, E: Seating for Children with Cerebral Palsy: A Resource Manual. University of Tennessee, Knoxville, 1984.
28. Lovell, WW and Winter, RA: Pediatric Orthopedics. JB Lippincott, Philadelphia, 1986.
29. Bobath, K: A Neurophysiological Basis for the Treatment of Cerebral Palsy. JB Lippincott, Philadelphia, 1980.
30. Scherzer, AL and Tscharnuter, I: Early Diagnosis and Therapy in Cerebral Palsy. Marcel Dekker, New York, 1982.

31. Joswick, et al: Aspects and Answers: A Manual for Therapeutic Horseback Riding Programs. WK Kellogg Foundation, Battle Creek, MI, 1986.
32. Tizard, B and Harvey, D: Biology of Play. JB Lippincott, Philadelphia, 1977.
33. Rappaport, L: Recipes for Fun. Let's Play to Grow. New York, 1986.
34. Ylvisaker, M and Logemann, J: Therapy for feeding and swallowing disorders following head injury. In Ylvisaker, M (ed): Head Injury Rehabilitation: Children and Adolescents. College-Hill Press, San Diego, 1985, p 195.
35. Evans, RW, Gualtieri, CT and Patterson, D: Treatment of chronic closed head injury with psychostimulant drugs: A controlled case study and an appropriate evaluation procedure. J Nerv Ment Dis 175(2):106, 1987.
36. Gittleman, R: Experimental and clinical studies of stimulant use in hyperactive children and children with other behavioral disorders. In Creese, I (ed): Stimulants: Neurochemical, Behavioral and Clinical Perspectives. Raven Press, New York, 1986.
37. Campbell, M and Spencer, EK: Psychopharmacology in child and adolescent psychiatry: A review of the past five years. J Am Acad Child Adolesc Psychiatry 27(3):269, 1988.
38. Glenn, MB: CNS stimulants: Applications for traumatic brain injury. J Head Trauma Rehabil 1(4):74, 1986.
39. Creese, I: Stimulants: Neurochemical, Behavior and Clinical Perspectives. Raven Press, New York, 1983.
40. Biederman, J, Gastfriend, DR and Jellinek, MS: Desipramine in the treatment of children with attention deficit disorder. J Clin Psychopharmacol 6(6):359, 1986.
41. Pliszka, SR: Tricyclic antidepressants in the treatment of children with attention deficit disorder. J Am Acad Child Adolesc Psychiatry 26:127, 1987.
42. Glenn, MB: A pharmacologic approach to aggressive and disruptive behaviors after traumatic brain injury (Part 1). J Head Trauma Rehabil 2(1):71, 1987.
43. Glenn, MB: A pharmacologic approach to aggressive and disruptive behaviors after traumatic brain injury (Part 2). J Head Trauma Rehabil 2(2):80, 1987.
44. Glenn, MB: A pharmacologic approach to aggressive and disruptive behaviors after traumatic brain injury (Part 3). J Head Trauma Rehabil 2(3):85, 1987.
45. DeLisa, JA: Rehabilitation Medicine: Principles and Practice. JB Lippincott, Philadelphia, 1988.
46. Ferguson, DG: Effects of neuroleptic drugs on the intellectual and habilitative behaviors of mentally retarded persons. Psychopharmacol Bull 18(1):54, 1982.
47. Brown, G et al: A prospective study of children with head injuries: III. Psychiatric sequelae. Psychol Med 11:63, 1981.
48. Haarbauer-Krupa, J et al: Cognitive rehabilitation therapy: Middle stages of recovery. In Ylvisaker, M (ed): Head Injury Rehabilitation: Children and Adolescents. College-Hill Press, San Diego, 1985, p 287.
49. Haarbauer-Krupa, J et al: Cognitive rehabilitation therapy: Late stages of recovery. In Ylvisaker, M (ed): Head Injury Rehabilitation: Children and Adolescents. College-Hill Press, San Diego, 1985, p 311.
50. Pressley, M and Brainerd, C (eds): Cognitive Learning and Memory in Children. Springer-Verlag, New York, 1985.
51. Pressley, M and Levin, JR (eds): Cognitive Strategy Research: Educational Implications. Springer-Verlag, New York, 1983.
52. Forrest-Pressley, DL, MacKinnon, GE and Waller, TG (eds): Metacognition, Cognition and Human Performance, Vol 2: Instructional Practices. Academic Press, Orlando, 1985.
53. Savage, RC: Educational issues for the head-injured adolescent and young adult. J Head Trauma Rehabil 2:1, 1987.
54. Cohen, SB et al: Educational programming for head injured students. In Ylvisaker, M (ed): Head injury Rehabilitation: Children and Adolescents. College-Hill Press, San Diego, 1985, p 383.
55. National Head Injury Foundation, Special Education Task Force: An Educator's Manual: What Educators Need to Know About Students With Traumatic Brain Injury, Revised Edition. National Head Injury Foundation, Framingham, MA, 1988.

Section VI
Conclusion

ERNEST R. GRIFFITH, M.D.

Just as the child is not a miniature adult, the brain injured child is not a replica of the brain injured adult. The four chapters of this section allude to many distinctions between adults and children as well as those within segments of the pediatric population.

Bruce points out demographic variations within age groups. In infancy the home rather than the highway is the most dangerous place. The high incidence of falls and child abuse in toddlers suggests entirely different preventive approaches than do the pedestrian and bicycle-related injuries of older children. Bruce differentiates mechanisms of injury, primary and secondary responses of brain to injury, and emergent priorities of management that in certain respects contrast with those same aspects covered in Miller's chapter on adults.

Jaffe, Brink, Hays, and Chorazy review specific problems of pediatric injuries, noting similarities and differences from those associated with adult injuries. For example, young children have a lesser frequency of heterotopic bone formation, more often are ataxic, and rarely incur thrombophlebitis. Hypercalcemia is most often encountered in adolescents with rapid bone growth.

This chapter identifies a spectrum of psychosocial, medical, and communicative sequelae as the background for the ensuing discussion of assessment by Ylvisaker and his associates. We are afforded a survey of a multitude of evaluative instruments and techniques of specific areas of function: their indications, scope, and limitations for various ages and degrees of severity of disability. The accompanying tables and appendix provide considerable detail in the clinical utilization of these tools.

Gans, Mann, and Ylvisaker present a review of rehabilitation management strategies and tactics that reflect the peculiar needs of children and their families. As with adults, the hospital program is generally the first phase of a protracted, constantly modified design of interdisciplinary management. Inevitably, pediatric management strategies must incorporate the effects of growth and development of the child, the integration of the child into community educational systems, and the re-establishment of parental and sibling relationships.

Each of the four chapters is, in many respects, an extension of the information presented in a corresponding section of the book relating to adults. Therefore, it is especially useful for the reader to preface his or her reading of this section by studying the pertinent preceding adult material.

From the offerings of this section, one must conclude that pediatric brain trauma is a major health issue, an epidemic as dire, and as menacing, as that of the brain injured adult. Our previously optimistic view of relatively good outcomes for children must be tempered by fresh disturbing evidence that certain subsets of children may fare as poorly as, or worse than, adults. Despite heightened attention to the issues of brain injury, the particular problems of children are only now being more fully addressed. Resources such as treatment facilities, knowledgeable professionals, sources of funding, and community liaisons are still woefully inadequate to serve the needs of these children and their families. Current enthusiasm for deinstitutionalization and mainstreaming of disabled children places a mounting burden upon schools whose teachers, other personnel, and students are often unprepared for the child with sequelae of brain injury. Family stresses may burgeon as its members attempt to assimilate the disabled child into the home. Yet the alternatives of institutional care are too often unacceptable. Many of these younger children may be arbitrarily clustered under the rubric of cerebral palsy. Although this categorization may bring such benefits as financial support, there may be disadvantages to being considered and managed as children with cerebral palsy. The various systems of neuromuscular facilitation and inhibition that have been used for cerebral palsy are being applied to brain injured children, at times with the same quasireligious fervor and lack of assurance of their efficacy. The determination of effectiveness of any rehabilitation treatment hinges upon specific outcome measurements, a formidable task in the growing, developing child.

In our litigious society, the settlement of liability for brain injury poses some vexing problems. What is the lifetime expense of having a brain injury? How does one project 60 to 70 years of optimal "quality of life" with the assignment of a monetary value? How does a prospective payoff affect the potential of the child? Does the strategic downgrading of the child's functions for purposes of obtaining a maximal settlement become the subsequent functional reality?

These are a smattering of the many issues that confront us. Fortunately, the issues are being articulated in the forums of publications, seminars, classrooms, clinical settings, and institutions that provide all manner of services for children. At last these pediatric concerns are "on the table," under scrutiny and debate by an increasingly sophisticated, discerning audience of consumers and professionals. The enigma unravels; answers become revealed; light emerges.

INDEX

(A page number followed by an "F" indicates a figure; a "T" following a page number indicates a table.)

pediatric, 542–543
Extended care, period of, behavior dysfunction treatment during, 427–430
Extensor responses, 54
Extinction, behavior management method of, 422
Extradural hematoma, CT scanning of, 241–242, 242T
Extraoculomotor (EOM) paresis, 96
Extremity injuries, 120–122. *See also specific type, e.g.,*
    Fracture(s)
Eye(s). *See also* Vision; Visual *entries*
    complications involving, 109–110
    pupillary light response and, 55–56
    raccoon's, 37, 552
Eye exercises, vestibular, 349
Eye movements, 56–57
    outcome and, 48
    saccadic, decrease in, 352T
Eye opening
    consciousness level and, 36T, 37, 53–54
    recovery of, 46
Eye position, resting, 56

Facial injuries
    intensive care unit management of, 43
    sexual dysfunction and, 213
Facial nerve (cranial nerve VII)
    early sequelae involving, 96
    lesions of, 57
Facial palsy, 57, 96
Facial recognition, 167
Facilitation
    aphasia treatment with, 378
    movement, 333
    neuromuscular, proprioceptive, 338
Falls, 11
    pediatric, 522
False localizing signs, 22
Family
    adjustment of, pediatric head injury and, 608–609
    behavior dysfunction and, 181, 182
    behavioral training of, 442, 444–445
    burden of, 228T, 228–229
        pediatric patient and, 541–542
    community re-entry and, 466
    education of head injured student and, 491
    familiar items contributed by, reality orientation
        therapy and, 368–369
    head injury effects on, 433–434
        case studies of, 232
        pediatric patient and, 541–542
        social impact, 230–231
    homemaking skills and, 200–201
    information provision to, 76. *See also* Family education
    interpersonal skills and, 201, 202
    pediatric injury and
        motor function of child and, 603
        sensory stimulation of child and, 603
    physiatrist interaction with, 257–258
    problems described by, 225–228, 226T, 227T
    psychologic distress in, 229–230, 230T
        crisis resolution and, 256–257
    reactions of, sexual dysfunction and, 210–211
    recovery and, 7
    rehabilitation of, 231–235, 438
    respite care for, 442–443, 474
    roles in, 434–435

sensory stimulation by, 336
sex education and, 215–216
social roles and, 201, 202
support groups for, 233, 443, 444
symptoms reported by, 226T, 226–227, 227T
therapeutic recreation and, 450
time management problems and, 202
transfers and, 199
vocational potential and, 495–496
vocational training and, 501
Family Assessment Device, 445
Family conferences, 439
Family counseling, 440–441
    behavior dysfunctions and, 424
    NYU Head Trauma Program and, 403
    sexual dysfunction and, 216
Family education. *See also* Patient education; Patient-
        family education
    behavior dysfunction and, 418, 424
    reality orientation therapy and, 370
Family environment, physiatric assessment of, 260
Family groups, NYU Head Trauma Program and, 403
Family interventions, 446
    case studies of, 435–436, 438, 441, 442
    family as personal system and, 434–436
    mourning and, 436–437
    need for, assessment of, 437–439
    types of
        behavioral family training, 442
        evaluation of, 443–445
        family counseling, 440–441. *See also* Family counseling
        family therapy, 441–442
        patient-family education, 439–440. *See also* Family education
        respite care, 442–443, 474
        support groups, 443
Family therapy, 441–442
Fat embolism, 44
Fat/carbohydrate ratio, 114
FCP (Functional Communication Profile), 156
Federal education legislation, 477–478
Feeding
    dysphagia and, 388. *See also* Dysphagia
    enteral, 113–114
        discontinuation of, medicolegal issues of, 509
    nasogastric tube, 43, 113
Feeding behavior, control of, 114
Feeding disorders, pediatric, 547, 577–578, 595
Feeding program, 196
Feeding skills, 193
    behavioral, cognitive, and perceptual problems with, 195–196
    cerebellar ataxia and, 141
    oral-motor skills and, 194
    physical skills and, 194–195
    treatment model for, 196
    unilateral hemiparesis and, 139
Feigned death state, children and, 540–541
Femur fractures, 119
FES (functional electrical stimulation) treatment, 342
Fever, 44–45
    pediatric, 548, 578
Fifth cranial nerve (trigeminal nerve), early sequelae
        involving, 96
Figure-ground perception deficits, 356T, 357–358
Financial costs, family interventions and, 444
Financial management skills, 202–203